Nora and Fraser

Medical Genetics: Principles and Practice

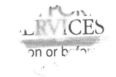

Nora and Fraser

Medical Genetics: Principles and Practice

JAMES J. NORA, M.D., M.P.H.
University of Colorado School of Medicine
Denver, Colorado

F. CLARKE FRASER, Ph.D., M.D.C.M., F.R.S.C., F.R.C.P.(C), D.Sc. (Acadia)
McGill University
Montreal, Quebec

JOHN BEAR, Ph.D.
Memorial University of Newfoundland
St. John's, Newfoundland

CHERYL R. GREENBERG, M.D.C.M.
University of Manitoba Faculty of Medicine
Winnipeg, Manitoba

DAVID PATTERSON, Ph.D.
Eleanor Roosevelt Institute for Cancer Research
University of Colorado School of Medicine
Denver, Colorado

DOROTHY WARBURTON, Ph.D.
College of Physicians and Surgeons
Columbia University
New York, New York

FOURTH EDITION

Lea & Febiger
PHILADELPHIA·BALTIMORE·HONG KONG
LONDON·MUNICH·SYDNEY·TOKYO
A WAVERLY COMPANY
1994

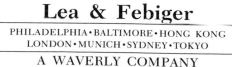

Lea & Febiger
Box 3024
200 Chester Field Parkway
Malvern, Pennsylvania 19355-9725
U.S.A.
(215) 251-2230

Executive Editor—J. Matthew Harris
Development Editor—Lisa Stead
Project/Manuscript Editor—Jessica Howie Martin
Production Manager—Michael DeNardo

Library of Congress Cataloging-in-Publication Data

Medical genetics : principles and practice/James J. Nora . . . [et
al.]. -- 4th ed.
        p.   cm.
    Includes bibliographical references and index.
    ISBN 0-8121-1663-1
    1. Medical genetics.   I. Nora, James J., 1928–
RB155.N67   1993
616′.042—dc20

93-19984
CIP

First Edition, 1974
Reprinted, 1976
Second Edition, 1981
Third Edition, 1989
Fourth Edition, 1993

Translated Editions
Spanish: La Prensa Medica Mexicana, Mexico D.F.
Italian: Idelson, Napoli
Portuguese: Guanabara Koogan, Rio de Janeiro

NOTE: Although the author(s) and the publisher have taken reasonable steps to ensure the accuracy of the drug
information included in this text before publication, drug information may change without notice and readers are
advised to consult the manufacturer's packaging inserts before prescribing medications.

Reprints of chapters may be purchased from Lea & Febiger in quantities of 100 or more. Contact Sally Grande in
the Sales Department.

PRINTED IN THE UNITED STATES OF AMERICA

Print number: 5   4   3   2   1

To
Audrey Hart Nora, M.D. and Joseph J. Nora, M.D.,
and the late
Frank Fraser and Nan Fraser

Preface

This is the sixth edition of our collaboration, beginning in 1974, in which we have alternated the publication of *Medical Genetics* with *Genetics of Man*. For this edition, we are forced to acknowledge that it is difficult for two authors to cover adequately the many rapid changes in human genetics. However, we are pleased to bring on board four excellent coauthors whose expertise greatly enhances the value and content of this edition.

Our objective continues to be to provide, in sufficient detail and depth, what we believe the student of human genetics wants and needs to know in an introductory course. The chapters fit well with the topics in the human genetics courses at our own universities and medical schools and, we believe, at many others. *Medical Genetics* is intended not only for medical, dental, and other students in the health sciences, but for graduate and undergraduate students taking courses in human

genetics. And in *Medical Genetics* we provide physicians, nurses, and other health workers who see patients with a reference source that covers common clinical conditions and counseling situations.

By judicious pruning and condensing, we have tried to accommodate new information without substantially increasing the text. As in the previous editions, the references are not intended to be comprehensive, but rather to offer supplementary information. For detailed information on genetic theory, diagnosis, and treatment, the reader is referred to more extensive and specialized texts in genetics, pediatrics, and medicine.

We hope that this book will continue to find its place in the classroom, the clinic, and the counseling center.

Denver, Colorado   James J. Nora
Montreal, Quebec   F. Clarke Fraser

Acknowledgments

Many people have helped us in many ways over the several editions, and should we fail to acknowledge assistance we have received, it is not because of lack of appreciation, but through unintentional oversight.

Our gratitude is expressed to: Audrey Hart Nora, Marilyn Preus, Victor A. McKusick, Harold P. Klinger, Arthur Robinson, Anil Sinha, Joy Ingram, Brian Ward, Elizabeth Nora, Wayne Persutte, Stephen Goodman, Ronald Gotlin, Herbert Lubs, James J. Nora, Jr., David W. Smith, Eva Sujansky, Janet Stewart, and Chris Heughan.

Studies and projects that accounted for much of the material in this book have been funded during the past two decades by the U.S. National Institutes of Health; the Medical Research Council, Canada; the Department of National Health and Welfare, Canada; the March of Dimes—National Foundation; the American Heart Association; the Helen K. and Arthur E. Johnson Foundation; and the Junior League of Denver.

J.J.N.
F.C.F.

Contents

Section I

Heredity and Disease

Chapter *1*
Heritability of Diseases and Traits

From the beginning of Western medicine, the heritability of physical traits and diseases has been recognized. Hippocrates not only observed that blue eyes and baldness ran in families, but that diseases such as epilepsy (the sacred disease) followed a similar pattern. Before the early twentieth century, inheritance was considered to be a blending, a continuous variation, and this is probably what Hippocrates had in mind. However, the emphasis shifted away from blended inheritance following the rediscovery of Mendel[6] and unit inheritance, and the locating of the hereditary particles, the genes, in chromosomes. Indeed, among the earliest published examples of mendelian inheritance was the disease alkaptonuria, described by Sir Archibald Garrod in 1902.[4] A large number of diseases attributed to single mutant genes followed this remarkable observation. The current catalog of disorders considered to have a firm mendelian basis lists 3307 conditions.[5] The terms "dominant" and "recessive" entered the medical vocabulary, and many diseases which have later been demonstrated to have no true basis in mendelian inheritance still carry such labels. If a disease was presumed to have a genetic basis, an effort at mendelian interpretation was made.

A further shift in emphasis began in 1959, when the first disorders were described that could be traced to abnormalities of chromosome number. During the next few years, several more syndromes associated with a chromosomal aberration were discovered. Then, in the minds of many students (and physicians), the erroneous idea took root that if a disease has a genetic basis, a chromosome karyotype must be ordered to establish the diagnosis. However, the consultant in genetics appreciates that a large percentage of the patients he is asked to see have disorders that can be attributed to neither a single mutant gene nor a chromosomal anomaly. If there is a genetic basis for these diseases, then we must return through the full circle to Hippocrates and discuss the hereditary aspect of disease in its earliest sense, that is, predisposition or diathesis.

In the past, the major causes of disease and death were infection and malnutrition, and the genetic causes did not attract much attention. As social conditions have improved and medicine has begun to control infections, the genetic causes of ill health have become much more important.

About 1 in 20 North Americans have a disorder with a major genetic component,[2] as do over 40% of patients admitted to a pediatric hospital and 12% of patients admitted to a general hospital.[7] These figures can only increase unless there is a major deterioration in our environment.

Most recently the phenomena of mitochondial inheritance, genomic imprinting, germline mosaicism, and uniparental disomy have attracted investigative interest. These processes may temporarily be pooled together under the sobriquet: nontraditional inheritance.

A useful classification of diseases having a genetic background would thus be:
1. Single mutant gene (mendelian) disorders.
2. Chromosomal aberration syndromes.
3. Diseases determined by multifactorial inheritance—genetic predisposition with environmental interaction.
4. Nontraditional inheritance.
5. Somatic cell genetic diseases (neoplasia, aging, autoimmune disease).

One may ask, how does an investigator determine whether or not genetic factors are important in a disease whose cause is unknown? Several tools are available, and these are discussed in their appropriate chapters.

First, if a disease has a genetic basis, it will occur in **familial aggregates**. This does not mean that all diseases found in more than one member of a family are necessarily genetic: take, for example, an epidemic of chickenpox or a bout of food poisoning. How then can one distinguish between familial environmental causes and genetic causes? One may begin by testing the data to see whether they fit the expectation for mendelian or multifactorial in-

heritance. If they do, a nongenetic cause is unlikely, although one must carefully rule out environmental causes.

Second, **twin studies** measuring the differences in concordance between monozygotic and dizygotic twins with respect to a given disease offer a means to determine whether the familial distribution results from genetic factors and to assess the contribution of these genetic factors to the disorder.

Finally, **animal homologies** are used to aid in the understanding of etiologic mechanisms in the human subject.

RECURRING THEMES

It is useful to state at the outset certain themes, concepts, and definitions that are so central that they must be repeated frequently in any treatment of genetics. It is likely that a reader with modest sophistication will find this discussion too elementary. We apologize, but submit that the most elementary material is not familiar to everyone and must be stated somewhere in an introductory text.

Mendel, Genes, and Chromosomes. Although this is a textbook of human genetics, and our examples will generally be confined to the human subject, it is entirely appropriate that mendelian inheritance be given its first exposure in the light of original materials and methods. Laws of heredity became apparent when certain highly distinctive traits in garden peas were selected and studied by the Austrian monk, Gregor Mendel.[6] These traits are defined by what we now know to be segments of deoxyribonucleic acid (DNA), called **genes**. Genes are linked together within a larger structure, the **chromosome**. In higher organisms, chromosomes come in pairs. Alternative forms of a gene exist, which are called **alleles**. Alleles occupy the same **locus** or position on homologous chromosomes. Each pair of homologous chromosomes is identical with respect to its loci (unless there is a structural anomaly). When Mendel was looking at round peas and wrinkled peas, he was looking at the alleles at the same locus on one pair of homologous chromosomes of the seven pairs in

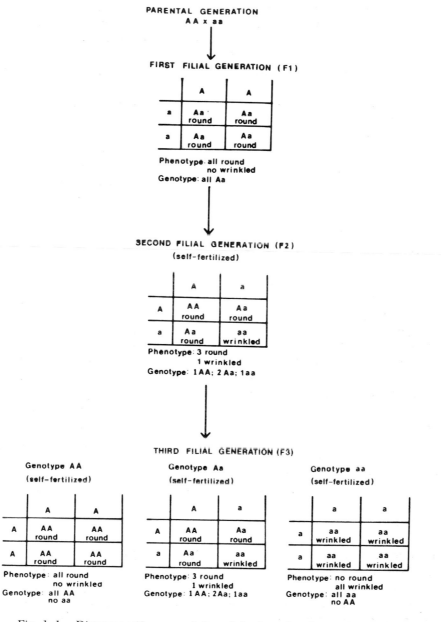

Fig. 1–1. Diagrammatic representation of the law of random segregation.

garden peas—the locus which defines a surface characteristic of the pea. In discussing one set of different chromosomes (7 in the garden pea and 23 in the human), the term **haploid** number is used. Actually there are 14 chromosomes in the pea and 46 in the human. These are the **diploid** numbers of chromosomes—the chromosomes that one can count and photograph under a microscope. The

chromosomes may then be displayed in homologous pairs in what is called a **karyotype**.

Referring to Figure 1–1 may help the reader through the next several paragraphs. When Mendel crossed two true-breeding strains, round peas × wrinkled peas, the progeny that the F_1 (first filial) generation yielded would not have been expected within the prevailing dogma of blended inheritance. Instead of finding peas with surface characteristics halfway between round and wrinkled, he found all of the peas to be round. Then he allowed the F_1 generation to fertilize itself. Something occurred that completely violated intuition: three fourths of the peas were round and one fourth of the peas were wrinkled. Further self-fertilizing of wrinkled peas yielded *only* wrinkled peas in subsequent generations. The separation of the genetic determinants of the traits round and wrinkled is termed **segregation**. These observations are the basis of Mendel's first law, the **law of random segregation**. They showed that, contrary to previous belief, hereditary differences did not blend in the next generation, but were based on hereditary factors (genes) that maintain their individuality unchanged from generation to generation.

Mendel called the trait of roundness, which was fully expressed in the F_1 generation and expressed in a 3:1 ratio in the F_2 generation, the **dominant** form. A dominant trait, by a convention that goes back to Mendel, is given a capital letter, for example, "A." The wrinkled surface of the pea, which did not even appear in the F_1 generation and was only found in a 1:3 ratio in F_2, he called a **recessive** trait. A recessive trait at the same locus is designated by a lowercase letter, "a." The 3:1 (or 1:3) ratio is called a **segregation ratio**.

A continuation of the experiment revealed that one third of the round peas in the F_2 generation, when self-fertilized, produced only round peas in subsequent generations. Two thirds of the peas produced round:wrinkled progeny in a 3:1 ratio. It was then apparent that there had been three types of offspring in the original F_2 generation. In one fourth of the peas, both alleles carried the genetic trait, round (AA). **Homozygous** is the term used when both alleles are identical. In one half (two fourths) of the progeny, a dominant "round" allele was paired with a recessive "wrinkled" allele (Aa), but the **phenotype** of the seed surface, the observable property of the pea, was round. When the two alleles are not identical, the individual is **heterozygous**. In the final one fourth with a wrinkled phenotype, the genetic constitution (*genotype*) consisted of two "wrinkled" alleles. The seg-

regation ratio of the genotype in the F_2 generation was then: 1AA:2Aa:1aa. The segregation ratio of the phenotype was 3 round: 1 wrinkled.

Thus, in this first experiment, the important genetic segregation ratios, with one exception, were disclosed. The phenotypic ratios are 3:1, 1:3, 0:4, or 4:0. The final genetic ratio would be disclosed by a backcross from the heterozygous individual or **heterozygote** (Aa) to the recessive **homozygote** (aa). The term **backcross** is usually confined to infrahuman subjects and in the broadest sense implies a mating between a heterozygous and a homozygous (usually recessive) parental genotype. This produces offspring with the phenotypic feature of interest in a 1:1 ratio.

Figure 1–1 helps us to visualize how the alleles for round and wrinkled seed surface segregate through several generations. Such diagrams must be relied on in our following of genotypes and phenotypes. Remember, in this illustration of the law of segregation, we are dealing with alleles at the same locus on homologous chromosomes. The capital letter, A, represents the dominant allele. The lowercase letter, a, stands for a recessive allele at the same locus.

In these two-by-two tables, a single letter appears at the head of each of the columns and rows. This letter is for the single allele which is transmitted in the **gamete**, the mature reproductive cell of either parent. When the male reproductive cell fertilizes the female reproductive cell, a **zygote** is formed. In the normal human somatic cell there are 46 chromosomes, and in the garden pea, 14. After fertilization, an organism grows by cell division, and the genetic information of each cell is passed to two new cells by a process called **mitosis**. Chapter 2 offers a more detailed discussion of this subject. To avoid providing duplicate illustrations, the reader is asked to scan Figure 2–9. In mitosis in the human, each of the 46 chromosomes (23 pairs) divides to form new ones, and each new cell also has 46 chromosomes. But **meiosis**, which is the process by which reproductive or germ cells divide to form gametes, is different from mitosis, reducing two sets of 23 (46) chromosomes to a single set of 23.

In meiosis (see Chap. 2), the homologous chromosomes join together and, having joined, may exchange genetic material before each of the 23 paired chromosomes separates from its homologue and is incorporated into a daughter cell, having not 46 chromosomes, but 23. The 23 chromosomes are not random but one from each of the 23 pairs. A second meiotic division then takes place which is similar to mitosis in that each of the 23 individual chromosomes divides, and this process ends with the formation of a mature gamete with 23 chromosomes. The gametes then unite at fertilization, and the original 46 chromosomes are reconstituted in the zygote.

If Mendel had selected traits that were all on the same chromosome, the second law, the **law of independent assortment,** would not have been readily apparent (because the traits would have tended to segregate together as **linked** alleles on the same chromosome). He was fortunate in his selection of subsequent characteristics. The gene for color of seed, yellow or green, is located on another chromosome. This permitted Mendel to recognize that peas could be yellow and wrinkled, green and round, green and wrinkled, or yellow and round. The genes for yellow and green are allelic on one pair of chromosomes and the genes for round and wrinkled are alleles on a different chromosome.

In his original paper published in 1865, Mendel looked at seven differentiating characters in garden peas and described experiments with hybrids of other species of plants. Unfortunately, Mendel's work was about 35 years ahead of the *Zeitgeist*. The enormous importance of the studies was simply not recognized until 1900, when not one, but three investigators independently confirmed Mendel's experiments. And what happened to Mendel after the landmark discoveries that laid the foundation of the science of genetics? He did what many good researchers do. He left investigative work for administration.

BEYOND MENDEL

Almost as soon as Mendel was rediscovered, applications of his laws of inheritance to the human subject were found. Mendel's laws remain one of the most valued stocks in trade for the geneticist dealing with humans. But, of course, the clinical geneticist is asked to see patients for several different reasons.

Often an infant or child is born with a common malformation, and the parents are concerned about the risk of recurrence. Is the malformation inherited? Is there something that the parents did to cause this problem? What is the chance that this may recur and what can be done to prevent it?

In another category of patients referred to the clinical genetics consultant is an individual with a pattern of anomalies in search of a diagnostic label. The hope here is that naming a disease will help to explain it. In some cases this is true. Determining that a patient has the Marfan syndrome provides a reasonable basis for medical management, prognosis, and counseling. Often, however, suggesting a label for a group of anomalies implies a greater understanding of the disease than actually exists. The cause of the condition is uppermost in the minds of the anxious parents. Invoking a difficult-to-pronounce eponym makes the geneticist appear to be a scholar, but he is deceiving both himself and his patients unless he acknowledges the limits of his diagnostic label. Does naming this disease answer the question of etiology? Does it provide a reasonably firm basis for discussing prognosis in the patient and risk of recurrence in the family? And how precise is the diagnosis of the Balderdash syndrome, anyway? Could this be another condition entirely?

If the patient has a common malformation, the familial aspects of which have been well investigated (e.g., atrial septal defect), then meaningful genetic counseling may be offered. If the patient clearly has a specific syndrome about which there is usable etiologic and prognostic information (e.g., Hurler syndrome or 21 trisomy), it is possible for the geneticist to answer many urgent questions.

As our data base increases, so does its complexity. Heterogeneity and polymorphisms are becoming more widely recognized. In **genetic heterogeneity,** the same or similar physical characteristics may be produced by different genes (loci) or different mechanisms. **Genetic polymorphism** means that there are at least two alleles at a given locus that are not uncommon (i.e., the less common one has a frequency of greater than 1%). The ABO blood type is a typical example of a genetic polymorphism. It has been estimated that, in man, one third of the loci are polymorphic. An additional concept is that of **pleiotropy,** in which a single gene or gene pair may produce multiple different effects (e.g., anomalies of the heart, the eye, and the skeleton in Marfan syndrome).

A few years ago, it was possible to talk about Ehlers-Danlos syndrome as if it represented one disease with one mode of inheritance. Now we must distinguish at least 17 types of the disease with three modes of inheritance. The more we know about a disease, the more we appreciate that the disease in question may be several diseases with several separate etiologies.

DIAGNOSIS OF GENETIC DISORDERS

Advances in genetic diagnosis are discussed throughout this book. The opportunity to detect genetic disorders and high-risk individuals is increasing so rapidly that one wonders how far we can afford to go. "Triple testing" of maternal serum for alpha-fetoprotein (AFP) and various other markers is done routinely in more and more prenatal care programs. Prenatal diagnosis using fetal cells from maternal serum is becoming feasible. This noninvasive procedure makes prenatal screening simpler and cheaper, resulting in more widespread application and an increased load on genetic-counseling services.

Population screening in high-risk populations has brought about major decreases in specific disorders, such as the hemoglobinopathies. Cystic fibrosis is likely to be the next candidate for population screening, again with increasing pressure on laboratories and counseling services. Progressive refinement of DNA technology and fluorescent in situ hybridization (FISH) increases the number of specific disorders that can be tested for in a popula-

tion or within families, particularly when testing for susceptibility genes for common disorders (e.g., coronary disease, hypertension, diabetes) is considered.

It may be possible to justify the necessary expansion of diagnostic and support services in terms of cost-effectiveness, even when measured only in dollars. But how much can we afford to invest?

TREATMENT OF GENETIC DISORDERS

Rather than sequester genetic treatment to a chapter of its own, we have distributed this topic throughout the book in the appropriate contexts, such as in the chapters on molecular and biochemical genetics. As in the case of genetic diagnosis, the issue of what we can afford in genetic treatment must be addressed. To select dramatic examples, the treatment of hemophilia may cost as high as $200,000 a year, and enzyme replacement for Gaucher disease may reach $300,000 a year. It is clear that unrestrained demand for genetic services can divert funds from the urgent needs of those suffering from environmental causes of ill health, such as infections, malnutrition, and poverty. Earlier, we noted that improved control over environmental causes of disease had made genetic causes more important. Is the pendulum beginning to swing back? We can only hope that those who allocate resources will reach an optimal compromise.

OBJECTIVE OF THIS BOOK

Knowledge in fundamental genetics has expanded explosively during the past decade to the point where it may be considered the central and unifying biologic science. The aim of this book is to explore medical genetics following the map provided by investigation into the fundamental areas of genetics.

COMMUNICATING BREAKTHROUGHS IN GENETICS

Writing a textbook on genetics is a daunting task. Electronic media are better suited to the transmission of important advances in the field, which may occur weekly if not daily. At the stage of final page proofs of this book, two developments have occurred that must be mentioned. To avoid costly alterations, we have added some recent information in this available space and cross-referenced it in the appropriate chapters.

Colon Cancer

This disease is the second leading cause of cancer deaths (55,000 annually) in the USA. Two major forms of predisposition to colorectal cancer (CRC) are recognized: familial adenomatous polyposis (FAP), discussed in Chapters 8 and 21, which accounts for about 1% of CRC; and hereditary nonpolyposis colorectal cancer (HNPCC), which is also called familial colon cancer (FCC), and which is much more common (about 15% of CRC). The breakthrough is in this second form of CRC, the discovery of a dominantly inherited susceptibility gene for FCC by the de la Chapelle and Vogelstein groups.[1] The gene is estimated to be carried by one person in every 200—10 times more common than the gene for cystic fibrosis—and is projected by Vogelstein to lead to colon cancer (or one of the other forms of cancer that have clustered in large FCC families) in 90 to 100% of those who carry the gene. The associated cancers involve the breast, ovary, endometrium, stomach, duodenum, pancreas, and kidney.

The FCC gene has been defined by anonymous microsatellite (short repetitive DNA sequences) markers on chromosome 2 and represents a new class of cancer gene in addition to tumor suppressors and proto-oncogenes. This gene acts by causing DNA triplets to repeat themselves many times over, which produces microsatellite instability and may contribute to some other gene changes found in colon cancer.

Repetitive DNA triplets have previously been found in four hereditary diseases: myotonic dystrophy, fragile-X syndrome, Huntington disease, and spinal and muscular bulbar atrophy. (See Chapters 7 and 8.) Instead of one copy of a triplet, 10 or 100 copies may be made. In many cases, the more the triplets are repeated, the more severe the disease. Some investigators have been led to speculate that expanding DNA triplets represent a bridge concept between certain hereditary diseases, hereditary cancers, and other cancers.

Familial Breast Cancer

The April 1993 issue of *The American Journal of Human Genetics* contained a series of 17 articles produced by the members of the Breast Cancer Linkage Consortium and other authors, investigating linkage between a dominantly inherited breast cancer susceptibility gene (BRCA1) and various markers on chromosome 17q21 (first reported by Hall et al. in 1990). Easton and colleagues summarized the findings of the 13 collaborating groups.[3] A gene (or genes) on the long arm of chromosome 17 (17q12-q21) accounts for most of the families with both early-onset breast cancer and ovarian cancer. They noted that other genes also predispose to breast cancer. The estimation of the cumulative risk associated with the susceptibility gene(s) on 17q was 59% by age 50 and 82% by age 70.

REFERENCES

1. Aaltonen, L.A., et al: Clues to the pathogenesis of familial colorectal cancer. Science 260:812, 1993.
2. Baird, P.A., et al.: Genetic disorders in children and young adults: A prospective study. Am. J. Hum. Genet. 42:677, 1988.
3. Easton, D.F., et al: Genetic linkage analysis in familial breast and ovarian cancer: Results from 214 families. Am. J. Hum. Genet. 52:678, 1993.
4. Garrod, A.E.: The incidence of alkaptonuria: A study in chemical individuality. Lancet 2:1616, 1902.
5. McKusick, V.A.: Mendelian Inheritance in Man, 10th ed., Baltimore, Johns Hopkins Press, 1992.
6. Mendel, G.: Experiments in Plant-Hybridization. *In* Classic Papers in Genetics, edited by J.A. Peters, New York, Prentice-Hall, Inc., 1959.
7. Science Council of Canada: Genetics in Canadian Health Care Report 42. Ottawa, 1991.

Chapter 2

Chromosomal Basis of Heredity

THE GENERAL CONCEPTIONS HERE ADVANCED WERE EVOLVED PURELY FROM CYTOLOGICAL DATA, BE-
FORE THE AUTHOR HAD KNOWLEDGE OF THE MENDELIAN PRINCIPLES . . . AS WILL APPEAR HEREAFTER
THEY COMPLETELY SATISFY THE CONDITIONS IN TYPICAL MENDELIAN CASES, AND IT SEEMS THAT MANY
OF THE KNOWN DEVIATIONS FROM THE MENDELIAN TYPE MAY BE EXPLAINED BY EASILY CONCEIVABLE
VARIATIONS FROM THE NORMAL CHROMOSOMIC PROCESSES.
WALTER S. SUTTON: THE CHROMOSOMES IN HEREDITY. BIOLOGICAL BULLETIN, 4:231, 1903.

The chromosomes are thread-like bodies, visible under the microscope in dividing cells. Each species has its characteristic chromosome number, and the chromosomes vary in size and other properties that make them unique. Chromosomes consist chiefly of DNA and proteins. The DNA specifies, in its nucleotide sequence, the genetic code. The proteins are involved in maintaining chromosome structure, replication and repair of the DNA, and the movements of the chromosomes at cell division. In most species, the chromosomes occur in pairs, the members of each pair specifying the same genetic information.

HISTORY

Even before the rediscovery of Mendel's laws, it was recognized that the chromosomes, visible under the microscope, could be the vehicles for hereditary factors. In both Europe and America, cytologists such as Roux, Boveri, Wilson, and Sutton were working out the details of mitosis and meiosis. Immediately after the rediscovery of mendelian prin-

ciples, Sutton and Boveri realized that the behavior of chromosomes was exactly what was expected of the units of inheritance, and independently proposed the chromosomal theory of heredity.

Over the next decades, the major contributions to chromosomal research were, of necessity, derived from studies in plants and lower animals, particularly the genus Drosophila. As early as 1910, T.H. Morgan was able to locate a specific gene locus on a specific chromosome in *Drosophila melanogaster*. The human, however, was in many ways an unsatisfactory subject for genetics research, so that the correct human chromosome number (46) was not determined until 1956.[8] Technical advances in tissue culture and methods of chromosome preparation were necessary to allow good visualization of mammalian chromosomes in mitosis. Human diseases (Down syndrome, Turner syndrome, Klinefelter syndrome) were first attributed to abnormal human chromosome numbers in 1959. Originally, human chromosome preparations had to be made from either fibroblast cultures after

10

tissue biopsy, or bone marrow samples. A major advance that made study of human chromosomes a widely applied diagnostic procedure was the discovery, in 1960, that a plant lectin, phytohemagglutinin, would induce cell division in cultured lymphocytes from the blood. Chromosome analysis within 72 hours was then possible from a peripheral blood sample, and the major contribution of cytogenetic abnormalities to the causes of congenital abnormalities and miscarriages was quickly established. In 1970, the discovery of methods of chromosome banding (which will be discussed subsequently) greatly improved the resolution of chromosome analysis, and initiated the second log-phase of growth in the study of human chromosomes. In the 1990s the application of molecular genetic methods to cytogenetics ushered in another major phase of rapidly advancing knowledge.

Recognizing that the hereditary material was carried by the chromosomes did not, of course, define the nature of the unit of inheritance, which the Danish botanist Johannsen labeled the gene. This side of the story will be taken up in Chapter 5.

CHROMOSOME STRUCTURE

A chromosome consists of the basic hereditary material deoxyribonucleic acid (DNA) organized into a complex structure along with histone and nonhistone proteins; isolated chromosomal material is known as **chromatin.** Proteins account for about 58% of the weight of chromatin, DNA 39%, and RNA 3%.

The human genome (one copy of each chromosome, or the **haploid** number) has been estimated to contain approximately 3 billion nucleotide base pairs [note: 3×10^9 base pairs (bp) $= 3 \times 10^6$ kilobases (kb) $= 3 \times 10^3$ megabases (mb)]. The largest human chromosome is estimated to contain about 300 mb of DNA, and the smallest contains about 50 mb. Although there is sufficient DNA to code for several million genes of average length, only about 5% actually consists of active genes, of which it is estimated that there are between 10,000 and 100,000 in the human genome. The rest of the DNA consists of noncoding se-

quences, many of which are repetitive units of various kinds. Some of these are known to be components of important chromosomal structures such as the centromere and the telomere (see subsequent text), whereas others may cluster in particular areas and then are known as **heterochromatin** because they have different staining properties than the surrounding **euchromatin.** Other repetitive sequences, such as those known as Alu (after an enzyme that cuts in this sequence) and LINES, are widely dispersed in the genome, have some of the properties of viral elements and may occasionally jump about in the genome. The function, if any, of most of these repetitive and non-coding sequences, is unknown.

A normal **diploid** human cell (with two copies of each chromosome) contains about 6 billion base pairs (bp) of DNA, which would stretch about 6 feet in length if simply extended. This must be packaged into a very small nuclear volume: in interphase the "packing ratio" is estimated at 1 to 80, while in a chromosome which has contracted and entered mitotic metaphase, the ratio is as high as 1 to 8000. The precise way in which this packing is accomplished is still the subject of research,[5] but it is principally through an increasing hierarchy of supercoils of the basic DNA chromatin fibre.

There is good evidence that an entire chromosome contains one single continuous DNA molecule, in the form of a Watson-Crick double helix roughly 3 nm in diameter (Chap. 5). The first unit of chromosome structure consists of a chain of a repeating subunit, the **nucleosome** (Fig. 2–1). This is composed of 166 DNA bp wrapped in two full turns around a core of eight small histone proteins (H2a, H2b, H3, H4), with a connecting stretch of DNA bound to another histone (H1). Nucleosomes are connected by spacer DNA which may vary from 0–80 bp. Under certain conditions the basic repeating subunit can be seen under the electron microscope as a chain of beads, with a width of about 10 nm. This 10 nm filament is in turn coiled into a 30 nm solenoid. Every 50th or so turn of this helix is anchored to a scaffold or matrix protein, so that the fiber is

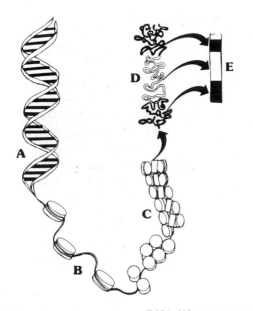

Fig. 2–1. Chromatin structure. DNA (A) wraps around a disc-shaped core of histones (B), which constitutes a nucleosome, separated by spacer DNA, which in turn coil around each other to form a solenoid structure (C). The further coiling of these chromatin threads (D) leads to the chromatin fiber of interphase and (E) to the metaphase chromosome.

thrown into a series of loops projecting laterally from a central protein. Nonhistone proteins consist largely of enzymes involved in the DNA functions of repair, replication and transcription (e.g., DNA and RNA polymerases and ligases), as well as some, such as the scaffold proteins, which are thought to contribute to the structure of the chromosome. There is evidence that histone binding differs in transcriptionally active and inactive chromatin, and that unwinding of the chromatin fibre is associated with transcription. Histones may be modified in various ways, such as acetylation and phosphorylation, and this may be associated with changes in DNA binding and functions such as replication and transcription. The histones are coded for by clustered repetitious genes, and for some, such as H1 and H2, there may be variation in the sequence among different copies. For others, such as histone 4, there is almost no variation in the amino acid sequence from copy to copy. These sequences have also been highly conserved throughout evolution, having the lowest mutation rate yet observed.

HUMAN CHROMOSOMES: MORPHOLOGY AND BANDING PATTERNS

As noted in Chapter 1, the chromosomal constitution of each individual is derived equally from mother and father; in the human, 23 chromosomes are contributed by each gamete (egg or sperm). Thus at fertilization, the fusion of two haploid gametes results in a diploid zygote with 23 pairs of **homologous chromosomes** (chromosomes containing the same gene loci). There are 22 pairs of **autosomes** in which the male and female chromosomes are identical, and one pair of **sex chromosomes** which vary between the sexes, the female having a pair of identical **X** chromosomes, and the male having one **X** chromosome and a much smaller **Y** chromosome.

Chromosomes are individually distinguishable only during cell division, at which time they appear under the microscope as rod-like bodies which stain with various dyes (chromos = color; soma = body). During the first stage of mitosis, prophase, the chromosomes begin to condense. During the next stage, metaphase, the chromosomes become maximally contracted and the two replicated chromatids are distinguishable. The **centromere,** the site of attachment to the mitotic spindle fibers by means of a protein structure known as the **kinetochore,** is visible as a constriction where the chromatids remain together. Another chromosomal landmark is the **telomere** which is the structure maintaining the integrity of the ends of the chromosome. Chromosomes can be described as **metacentric,** with the centromere near the middle, **submetacentric,** with the centromere closer to one end than the other, and **acrocentric,** with the centromere very near one end. The centromere divides the chromosome into two arms, a short arm and a long arm. In the case of metacentric chromosomes, one arm is arbitrarily designated the short arm.

Preparations of metaphase chromosomes are used to analyze a chromosome complement. In humans, these are usually obtained from 72 hour cultures of peripheral lymphocytes stimulated with phytohemagglutinin. Bone marrow cells need no stimulation to divide,

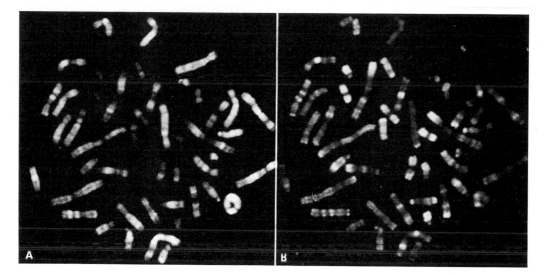

Fig. 2–2. The same chromosome preparation sequentially stained by (A) quinacrine mustard (Q-banding) and (B) acridine orange (R-banding). That the fluorescence in R-banding is the reverse of Q-banding (and G-banding) may be observed most readily in the chromosomes located at 11 o'clock. Courtesy H.E. Wyandt and H. Lebowitz.

and can be examined either directly after sampling, or after a short culture period. This tissue is commonly sampled in studies of leukemia, or can be used when a very quick turnaround time is needed (as with a seriously ill newborn). Chromosome preparations can also be made from any other dividing cells in culture, for example from fibroblast cultures from skin or muscle, from placental tissues in the case of miscarriage or chorionic villus sampling, or from amniotic fluid cells (see Chap. 15). For analysis, well-spread metaphase chromosomes are usually photographed, and the chromosomes cut out and matched in pairs to form a **karyotype.** Computerized image-processing can also be used to assist in this procedure.

Since 1960, human cytogeneticists or a representative committee have met regularly to standardize the system of nomenclature. The resulting International System of Human Chromosome Nomenclature (ISCN) is published at regular intervals, and provides the rules for writing karyotype designations.[2] Early on, it was decided to use the letter "p" (for petit) to designate the short arm, and "q" to designate the long arm. Autosomes are numbered approximately in order of decreasing size. Before chromosome banding, length and

centromere position were all that could be used to classify the chromosomes into pairs. The original classification scheme used the letters A–G to refer to the groups of chromosomes that could be easily distinguished from one another.

The Swedish cytologists Caspersson and Zech[1] discovered in 1970 that some fluorescent dyes such as quinacrine mustard produced alternating bands of bright and dull fluorescence along human chromosomes. It was possible to distinguish all chromosome pairs on the basis of these banding patterns, known as **Q-bands,** which were reproducible from cell to cell, tissue to tissue, and person to person. (Fig. 2–2A). Soon afterwards, it was shown that the same banding patterns could be produced by pretreating slides containing metaphase preparations with salt solutions or proteolytic enzymes, and then staining with standard blood stains such as Giemsa (**G-banding**). With a few exceptions, those regions which fluoresce brightly when Q-banded stain darkly when G-banded. G-banding methods, usually involving pretreatment of slides with a weak trypsin solution, have become standard in most American laboratories. A G-banded metaphase and karyotype are shown in Figure 2–3. Other methods of producing banding

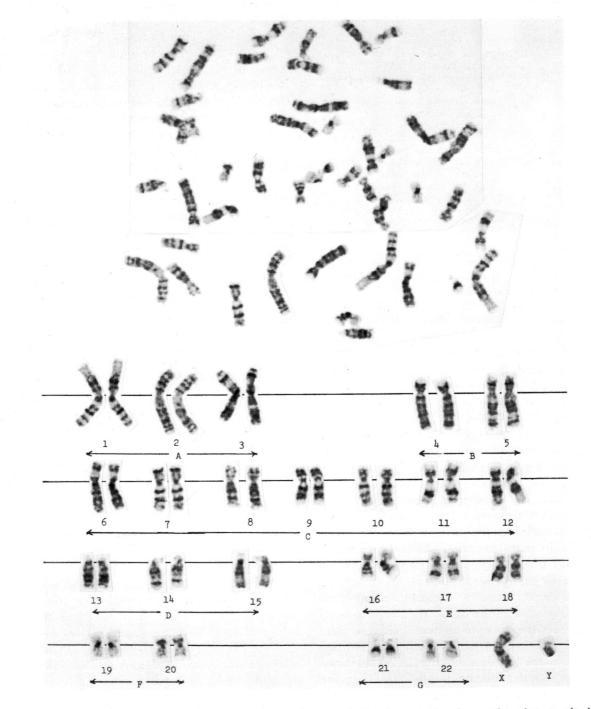

Fig. 2–3. Chromosomes from a normal human male are shown as they appear in metaphase and as they are displayed in a karyotype for study. The chromosomes have been individually cut out of the photomicrograph and arranged on the basis of size, position of centromere and banding pattern.

Table 2–1. Karyotype Nomenclature for Numerical Abnormalities

Karyotype	Description
46,XX	normal female
46,XY	normal male
45,X	female with only one X chromosome (Turner syndrome)
47,XXY	male with two X chromosomes (Klinefelter syndrome)
49,XXXXY	male with four X chromosomes
47,XX,+21	female with additional chromosome 21 (Down syndrome)
47,XY,+18	male with additional chromosome 18 (trisomy 18 syndrome)
46,XY,−21	male with missing chromosome 21
45,X/46,XX	mosaic, some cells with 45,X, some with 46,XX

patterns can give what is called a reverse or R-banding pattern: in this type of banding the same patterns are seen, but the bands have an opposite intensity to that seen in Q- or G-banding (Fig. 2–2B).

After chromosome banding was discovered, each chromosome pair was assigned a number, roughly in order of length. The number of chromosomes is put first in designating the karyotype, followed by the sex chromosome complement, and then any abnormalities of number or rearrangements are defined. Table 2–1 shows the karyotype formulas for some commonly found numerically abnormal chromosome complements. The clinical correlates of these karyotypes are described in Chapters 3 and 4. The nomenclature for structural rearrangements of chromosomes will be described later. The use of chromosome banding greatly increased the precision and scope of cytogenetic analysis because aberrations involving different chromosomes in the same group could be told apart, and many more structural rearrangements could be recognized and precisely identified. It also allowed the precise mapping of human genes to particular chromosomes and chromosome bands. The location of a gene is commonly given as the chromosome band in which it is known to reside.

In an early stage of metaphase (prometaphase), the chromosomes are more extended, and many more and finer bands can be observed than in chromosomes that are more contracted. The resolution of the banding pattern can be expressed as the total number of visible bands in the haploid chromosome complement. This is about 400 for the more or less standard chromosome preparations shown in Figure 2–3, and can be 1000 or more in very extended ("high resolution") chromosomes. Various technical tricks can be used to catch the chromosomes at an earlier stage, or to reduce their contraction. The higher the resolution of the chromosome preparations, the greater the potential for detection of very small chromosome changes, especially if one knows where to look. Figure 2–4 shows several human chromosomes from an early metaphase cell, in which many more bands can be seen than in the same chromosome in Figure 2–3. It should be realized that even at a 1000 band resolution a single chromosome band will consist of about 3 mb of DNA. This is sufficient to harbor hundreds of genes.

The International System of Human Chromosome Nomenclature provides a standardized numbering system for all chromosome bands, which is illustrated in Figure 2–5. The arms, designated as p and q, are first divided into regions, then into subregions or bands, according to a sort of decimal system. As the chromosome is observed at higher resolution, single bands can be seen to break up into multiple finer bands. The regions and bands

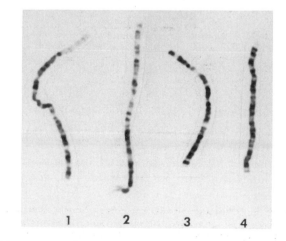

Fig. 2–4. G-banded chromosomes 1 through 4 in early metaphase division, at a resolution of approximately 850 bands per haploid complement.

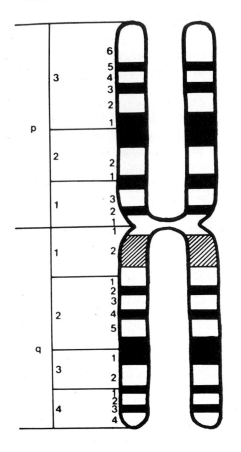

Negative or pale staining Q and G bands
Positive R bands

Positive Q and G bands
Negative R bands

 Variable bands

Fig. 2–5. Diagrammatic representation of chromosome bands in chromosome No. 1 as observed with Q-, G-, and R-staining methods.

By using these band numbers and a standard system of abbreviations for various kinds of chromosomal structures and rearrangements (given in Table 2–2), it is possible to describe each abnormal karyotype unambiguously, so that cytogeneticists all over the world will understand what is meant. The system is somewhat complicated, and a detailed treatment is beyond the scope of this book, but some examples of how the system is used to describe structural chromosome aberrations will be discussed later.

Chromosomal Heteromorphisms

Certain chromosome regions show differences among individuals in size and staining intensity, which are transmitted in regular Mendelian fashion from parent to child. These are called **heteromorphisms** and can be used as genetic markers in the same way as other polymorphic genetic traits. These heteromorphisms involve noncoding, repetitive DNA sequences that are associated with hetero-

Table 2–2.   Selected Symbol Nomenclature for Karyotypes

ace	acentric
cen	centromere
del	deletion
der	derivative chromosome
dup	duplication
end	endoreduplication
h	secondary constriction
i	isochromosome
ins	insertion
inv	inversion
inv ins	inverted insertion
mar	marker chromosome
mat	maternal origin
pat	paternal origin
r	ring chromosome
rcp	reciprocal translocation
rec	recombinant chromosome
rob	Robertsonian translocation (centric fusion)
s	satellite
t	translocation
tan	tandem translocation
ter	terminal or end (pter = end of short arm qter = end of long arm)
tri	tricentric
:	break (no reunion, as in a terminal deletion)
::	break and join
→	from-to

are numbered, proceeding from the proximal arm (near the centromere) to the distal arm (near the telomere). Note that band 1q32 is not the 32nd band on the long arm of chromosome 2: it is the 2nd band in region 3 of the long arm (and in fact should be read as "q three two" not "q thirty-two." In Appendix A, the banding diagrams for all the human chromosomes are given at three different resolutions: these diagrams are taken from the International System of Human Chromosome Nomenclature.[2]

chromatin. They are most clearly revealed through special banding techniques such as C-banding, where most of the chromosome is palely staining, and only the heterochromatin is darkly staining. Such regions are found at the centromere of all chromosomes, in large blocks close to the centromere on chromosomes 1, 9 and 16, in the short arms of the acrocentric chromosomes, and in the distal end of the Y chromosome. These may vary greatly in size without phenotypic effects (Fig. 2–6A). Some of these regions may also vary in the intensity with which they fluoresce when Q-banded (Fig. 2–6B); such variation often does not show up with G-banding, so that Q-banding is the method of choice when searching for such variants. It is important to recognize that such normal variants exist, so as not to mistake them for significant abnormalities. Sometimes these variations may be in the position of the heterochromatic blocks as well as their size; a common variant, particularly in African-Americans, is an inversion of the heterochromatic region of chromosome 9 so that it is in the short arm of the chromosome rather than the long arm (Fig. 2–6C).

The Biochemical Basis of Visible Chromosome Structures

The chromosome banding patterns revealed by special staining techniques are correlated with a number of properties of the DNA within the bands. In general, G-dark and Q-bright regions ("positive" bands) are richer in AT base pairs than the G-light and Q-dull regions ("negative" bands). The basis for the difference in staining reactions is probably related to a mean difference in base composition between negative and positive bands. Although this is reasonably easy to understand for fluorescein dyes that bind directly to the DNA, it is not well understood how this is mediated by a pretreatment such as the trypsin digestion used in G-banding. G-positive bands replicate later in the cell cycle than G-negative bands. Some of the standard methods of chromosome banding rely on this fact; DNA base-analogues such as 5-bromodeoxyuridine (BrdU), which change staining properties, are introduced into the culture medium so that the observed metaphase chromosomes will have incorporated BrdU only in late replicating regions. G-negative bands also are richer in the common Alu repetitive sequence than G-positive bands, and appear to contain more transcribed genes.

The centromere of each chromosome consists largely of a class of repetitive DNA known as alpha-satellite: although built of essentially the same repetitive 161 bp units, the centromere of each chromosome has a slightly different sequence and arrangement of these repeats, allowing it to be distinguished by specially designed DNA probes. This is the basis of the chromosome specific centromere staining that can now be achieved with in situ hybridization, as will be discussed in the following section.

A specific short repetitive sequence, (TTAG)n, occurs at the telomere and forms a hairpin structure, which defines the end of the

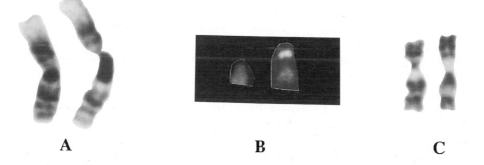

A   **B**   **C**

Fig. 2–6. A. C-band heteromorphism at the centromere of chromosome 1. B. Q-band heteromorphism in the short arm of chromosome 22. C. Heteromorphic variant of chromosome 9, inv(9qh).

chromosome. Unlike the centromere sequences, in which homology to the human can be demonstrated only in other primates, the telomeric sequences are similar in all eukaryotes. At each cell division, some of the telomeric sequences are lost and must be replaced, through the action of a specific telomerase. This repair must be imperfect because in aging cells, both in culture and in vivo, the length of the telomeric repeat is reduced over that in younger cells.

Another variety of heterochromatin deserving special mention belongs to the moderately repetitive class of DNA sequences (occurring several hundred but less than a 1000 times per genome). This is the DNA coding for the 18 and 28S ribosomal RNA, which are structural components of ribosomes (the **rDNA**). These sequences are transcribed, though not translated, and are found in the short arms of all the human acrocentric chromosomes 13, 14, 15, 21, and 22. These rDNA containing regions are also known as "nucleolar organizing regions" or **NORs** because of the association of this region with the nucleolus in prophase. Each acrocentric short arm contains a virtually nonstaining region known as the "stalk" at the end of which may be more darkly staining dot-like regions known as "satellites" because of their apparent separation from the rest of the chromosome (see Fig. 2–3). The rDNA is found in the stalks, with a total of about 400 copies per diploid genome. This redundancy means that chromosomal abnormalities involving the short arms of the acrocentrics are usually benign. These are also very heteromorphic chromosome regions with large differences in the size of the stalks (and number of copies of the rDNA) and in the size and staining properties of the satellites.

CHROMOSOMAL IN SITU HYBRIDIZATION

Beginning in the 1970s, it was recognized that DNA and RNA hybridization procedures would work on intact chromosomes spread on glass slides. This made it possible to take known fragments of DNA (**probes**) and find out where the complementary sequence was on a chromosome. Both the slide containing the chromosomes and the probe are subjected to a procedure that denatures DNA into single strands, and then allowed to hybridize. By labelling the probe with a radioactive nucleotide, and then detecting the radioactive sites with photographic film, the chromosomal position of particular kinds of DNA can be examined. This was first done for repetitive DNA regions such as the rDNA genes and the centromeric repeats; later, as recombinant DNA technology became more advanced and "hotter" probes could be produced, single copy sequences could be detected in the same way. However, the use of radioactive probes for single copy sequences stretched the technique to its limits, because even after a week's developing time, only one or two significant silver grains would be expected on the film. This meant that the level of tolerable background had to be extremely low, and that statistical analysis of many cells had to be carried out to determine the most likely site of the probe. Nevertheless, many genes and DNA sequences were localized in this manner.

A significant advance came with the demonstration that nonradioactive labelling with DNA binding substances such as biotin, coupled with detection by fluorochrome dyes visible under ultraviolet light, could significantly increase the sensitivity of the technique. Again, the first applications used repetitive signals such as centromeric repeats: later, single copy probes as small as 1 kb were successfully localized on metaphase chromosomes by this or similar methods (see Plate 1). An advantage of using fluorochrome dyes is that multiple colors can be used to distinguish between different signals; by labelling two probes with different DNA binding agents, and detecting them after hybridization with antibodies labelled with red and green fluorochromes dyes such as FITC and Texas Red, one could order probes with respect to one another on the same metaphase chromosome preparation (Figure 2–7). The reliability of the signal with these procedures is such that only a few metaphase spreads need to be examined, and the signal can be finely localized without the spread typical of radioactive detection.

Fluorescent in situ hybridization (FISH) has already been used for various research prob-

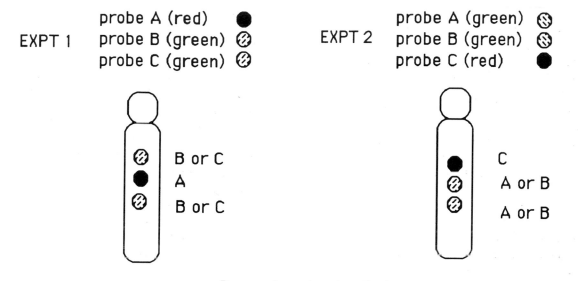

Fig. 2–7. Use of two different colored fluorochromes to order three probes on a chromosome segment by fluorescent in situ hybridization. Two labelling experiments are necessary using only two colors.

lems, particularly for genome mapping, and its potential is just beginning to be realized in clinical cytogenetics.[1,3,6] Chromosome-specific centromere probes are now available for most chromosomes, making possible the identification of the origin of small chromosomes with unidentifiable banding patterns. "Chromosome paints" consisting of a mixture of chromosome-specific sequences have been developed that light up only one homologous chromosome pair (see Plate 2): the use of multiple colors can allow recognition of many different chromosomes at once. This has application in the identification of complex rearrangements such as those seen in tumor cells, and of subtle rearrangements involving chromosome segments too short to identify by banding pattern. Probes that recognize single copy sequences are also available for many chromosome regions, and are the method of choice for recognition of small deletions and subtle translocations. It is interesting to realize that DNA analysis cannot distinguish between a normal karyotype and one in which a balanced rearrangement has occurred. This can be achieved only by karyotype analysis for gross rearrangements, and in situ hybridization for rearrangements that cannot be recognized under the light microscope.

Cytogenetic analysis has long implied examination of chromosomal spreads. However, with in situ hybridization, DNA organization can now also be examined in interphase nuclei. The DNA condensation in such nuclei is an order of magnitude less than that in mitotic chromosomes. Although two probes less than 1 mb apart cannot be distinguished on metaphase chromosomes, two distinct spots can readily be seen in interphase nuclei for loci as close as 100 kb. This resolution is extremely useful in ordering closely placed DNA sequences along the chromosome, and is necessary in mapping the human genome.

Another advantage of interphase nucleus cytogenetics is that it makes it unnecessary to have a rapidly dividing cell population for analysis. By using chromosome-specific probes on interphase nuclei, one can determine the presence of numerical abnormalities for any chromosome: e.g., trisomy 21 would give three signals, rather than the normal two (see Plate 3). This makes it possible to perform prenatal chromosome analysis, at least for the common trisomies and sex chromosome abnormalities, without the need to wait for the fetal cells to grow in culture. Interphase analysis is also useful in cancer cytogenetics, in which the malignant cells may be difficult to establish in

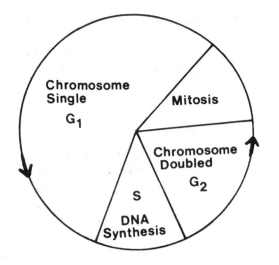

Fig. 2–8.   Periods of the cell cycle: G_1, after division the chromosomes are single and do not synthesize DNA; S, the period of DNA synthesis; G_2, the chromosomes are now doubled; mitosis occupies a relatively small portion of the cell cycle.

culture. Developments in this area are being made rapidly, and clinical validation studies are in progress to compare these techniques with standard cytogenetics.[2] Although interphase analysis has the advantage of being both faster and cheaper than standard cytogenetic analysis, it has the disadvantage of being limited at the present time to detection of the common numerical chromosome abnormalities.

MITOSIS

Dividing cells pass through the cell cycle diagrammed in Fig. 2–8. Mitosis is the relatively brief period during which somatic cells are observed to be in the process of replicating themselves. Interphase occupies the majority of the cycle, and is the period during which the cells are engaged in their normal metabolic activities. Chromosomes are not individually visible during this time. During the S period, the DNA replicates in preparation for cell division; G2 is the period after S before cell division takes place, and G1 the period after mitosis before DNA replication begins again.

In mitosis, four stages are recognized: prophase, metaphase, anaphase and telophase.

During this process, the nucleus undergoes a series of changes resulting in two daughter cells with the exact chromosome complement of the parental cell.

Prophase. During this stage, the chromosomes condense and become visible under light microscopy. The DNA content has already doubled, and each chromosome is visualized as two parallel strands, the **chromatids,** joined together at the centromere. The nuclear membrane disappears, and two small bodies, the **centrioles,** start to migrate to opposite poles from a position immediately external to the nuclear membrane (Fig. 2–9A).

Metaphase. This is the stage at which the individual chromosomes are most clearly seen. The nuclear membrane has disappeared and the chromosomes come to lie in a single plane at the equator of the cell, between the two poles. By their kinetochores they are connected to protein spindle fibres which radiate from the centriolar regions at the poles (Fig. 2–9B).

Anaphase. At anaphase, the two chromatids separate from each other at the centromeres, and are propelled by the spindle fibers toward the poles. Each pole of the dividing cell

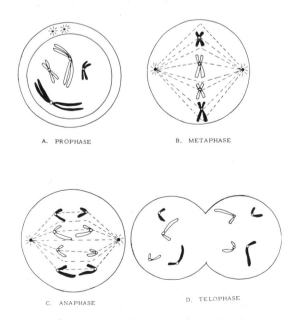

Fig. 2–9.   Mitosis. Two of 23 pairs of chromosomes are shown passing through the four stages. Observe that double-stranded chromosomes separate at anaphase. See text.

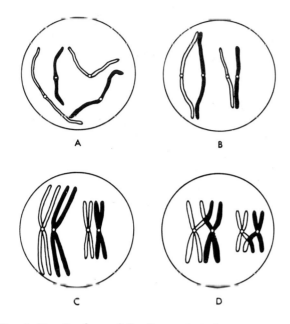

Fig. 2–10.   Prophase of the first meiotic division. Two of 23 pairs of chromosomes are shown in the stages of prophase: A. Leptotene; B. Zygotene; C. Pachytene; D. Diplotene. Diakinesis is not illustrated. Note that there is pairing of homologous chromosomes and crossing over. See text.

thus receives one copy of each chromosome (Fig. 2–9C).

Telophase. The daughter chromosomes arrive at the poles as the cytoplasm begins to divide in the area of the equatorial plane (Fig. 2–9D). The chromosomes become less condensed and gradually become indistinguishable once again.

MEIOSIS

Meiosis is a form of cell division that occurs only in the cell lineage which gives rise to the gametes, i.e., the germ cell line. Three critical events occur in meiosis that do not occur in mitosis: (1) pairing of homologous chromosomes, (2) exchanges between the homologous chromosomes in one or more places, (3) two successive divisions that reduce the number of chromosomes to the haploid number, so that only one member of each pair is present in each nucleus. The **segregation** of homologous chromosomes from one another provides the first source of variability in the gametes, since there are 2^{23} possible combinations with 23 chromosome pairs. A second

source of variability results from **recombination,** the exchanges between homologous chromosomes that produce new combinations of variable regions along the chromosome.

First Meiotic Division

Prophase. Before the first visible signs of meiotic division, each chromosome has duplicated, as in mitotic division. Prophase is arbitrarily divided into five stages, in which the important events of chromosome pairing and recombination occur:
1. Leptotene. The chromosomes first become visible and appear as single threads even though DNA replication has already occurred. (Fig. 2–10A).
2. Zygotene. Each chromosome pairs with its homologue in a very precise way so that identical, or nearly identical, DNA sequences are associated. If there have been chromosome rearrangements, chromosomes still form associations that permit this precise pairing to occur (see Fig. 2–24). A protein structure called the synaptonemal complex appears between the paired homologues, and can be demonstrated by electron microscopy. These synapsed chromosomes, or **bivalents,** do not form in mitosis (Fig. 2–10B).
3. Pachytene. Each chromosome now becomes visible as a double strand, and areas of exchange (**chiasmata,** singular **chiasma**) can be seen between single strands of the chromosome pairs. (Fig. 2–10C). Each chiasma results in a genetic **crossover,** or recombination event.
4. Diplotene. The two members of the pair begin to repel each other, and are held together only where the chiasmata have occurred (Fig. 2–10D).
5. Diakinesis. In this final stage of prophase, the chromosomes become very condensed and darkly staining.

Metaphase. This stage is the same in meiosis as in mitosis except that the homologues are paired as bivalents. The bivalents line up at the equatorial plane, connected to the spindle fibres radiating from the centrioles (Fig. 2–11E).

Anaphase. Each chromosome, still consisting of two chromatids joined at the centromere, separates from its homologue, so that 23 double-stranded chromosomes go into each of two daughter cells (Fig. 2–11F). In first meiotic anaphase we find the chromosomal basis of two of Mendel's laws of inheritance: **segregation** and **independent assortment**. The separation of the homologous chromosomes is the basis of segregation. Notice that, because of crossing over, there have been exchanges between these homologues in some places. The decision as to whether the maternally inherited copy or the paternally inherited copy goes to each pole is independent for each pair. This is the basis of independent assortment.

Telophase. At meiotic telophase, the cytoplasm divides into two, as in mitotic telo-

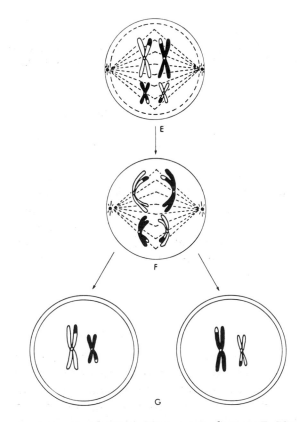

Fig. 2–11.   Continuation of first meiotic division: E. Metaphase; F. Anaphase; G. Telophase. Note that *double-stranded* chromosomes go into the daughter cells (23 randomly assorted double-stranded chromosomes instead of 46 single-stranded chromosomes as in mitosis). See text.

phase, but the double-stranded chromosomes do not decondense until after meiosis II (Fig. 2–11G).

Second Meiotic Division

This is essentially the same as a mitotic division in which the 23 double-stranded chromosomes separate into daughter cells, each of which contains 23 single-stranded chromosomes, i.e., a complete haploid set (Fig. 2–12). In the male, the cytoplasm divides evenly in cells destined to become sperm, so that four sperm result from one meiotic division. In the female, however, the cytoplasm is unevenly divided, and only one functional ovum is produced from each meiotic division (see subsequent text).

GAMETOGENESIS AND FERTILIZATION

The products of meiosis are the gametes. Fusion of the maternal and paternal gametes produces the first cell of the new individual, the **zygote**. Within this single cell resides all the genetic information required for growth and differentiation into a complex, multicellular organism.

Spermatogenesis. This is the process through which the early male germ cells (**spermatogonia**) undergo a series of changes terminating in the differentiation of mature sperm. Spermatogenesis occurs in the seminiferous tubules of the testis, and begins at puberty. The entire process takes about 64 days. During the first meiotic division, the spermatogonia become the primary spermatocytes; during the second meiotic division they are called secondary spermatocytes. The first stage of differentiation is known as the spermatid, which undergoes major changes in nuclear proteins and chromatin condensation during differentiation into the sperm. About 200 million sperm are normally present in one ejaculate; only one will fertilize the egg.

Oogenesis. In the human, the process in which the primary female germ cells, the oogonia, differentiate into ova, may take from 12 to 45 years, depending upon the age at which the egg is released. The oogonia begin to dif-

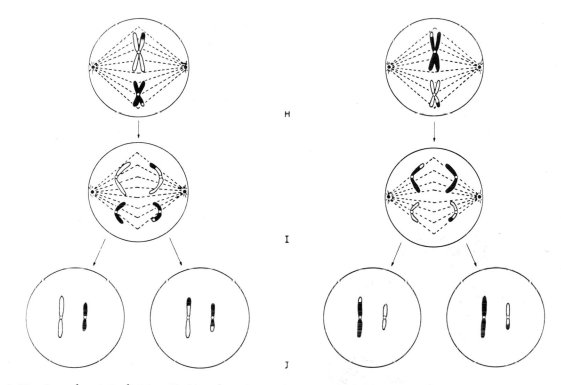

Fig. 2–12.   Second meiotic division: H. Metaphase; I. Anaphase; J. Telophase. The 23 double-stranded chromosomes now separate into 23 single-stranded chromosomes. Note that the 8 strands in J derive from the two bivalents shown in Figure 2–10.

ferentiate into primary oocytes at about three months of intrauterine development in the female fetus. After pairing and formation of chiasmata, they remain arrested in meiotic prophase, in a stage known as **dictyotene**. It is believed that, at birth, a female infant has all the primary oocytes she will ever possess. Even before puberty, a large number of oocytes have begun the process of differentiation into mature ova, but eventually die because the pituitary hormones necessary for completion of the maturation process are not present. After puberty, a wave of oocytes enters the differentiation process every month, but usually only one becomes a mature ovum, which is extruded from the ovarian follicle during ovulation. Only at ovulation is the first division of meiosis completed, with the daughter cells consisting of the large secondary oocyte or ovum and a small **first polar body** which is not functional.

Fertilization usually occurs in the lateral portion of the fallopian tube, when one of the many sperm that surround the ovum penetrates it. The second meiotic division of the ovum is completed only at this time, with the formation of a **second polar body.**

The sperm head decondenses inside the ovum, and becomes the male pronucleus. After DNA replication in the male and female pronuclei, both enter mitosis, forming a single metaphase plate with 46 chromosomes. Continued mitotic division then gives rise to the embryo.

NUMERICAL CHROMOSOME ABERRATIONS

An abnormal chromosome number in an individual can be produced by errors in meiosis, errors in the mitosis of embryonic cells, or errors in fertilization. In general, any change from the normal diploid number of 46 chromosomes is associated with severe developmental abnormalities, which are often lethal in the early stages of gestation. The clinical

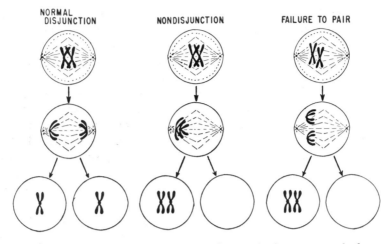

NORMAL DISJUNCTION   NONDISJUNCTION   FAILURE TO PAIR

Fig. 2–13.   Mistakes in first meiotic division leading to aneuploidy.

consequences of these changes are detailed in the next chapter.

Any exact multiple of the haploid chromosome number (n = 23) is called **euploid.** In humans both **triploidy** (n = 69) and **tetraploidy** (n = 92) are observed chiefly in spontaneous abortions, and tetraploidy and higher degrees of **polyploidy** are seen in a few differentiated tissues and tumors. In about 80% of cases, triploidy results from the fertilization of one ovum by two sperm (**dispermy**). In the rest an unreduced diploid gamete, either egg or sperm, is the problem. Tetraploidy, on the other hand, results from a failure of the first mitotic cell division of the zygote, with a resulting doubling of the chromosome number.

Sometimes the chromosome complement is aberrant in having two copies of each chromosome derived from the same parent, although the normal diploid chromosome number is present. If two male complements and no female complement are present, the resulting conception is said to have **diandry**; such conceptions develop a large cystic placenta without visible embryonic structures—the so-called hydatidiform mole—which may develop into a placental tumor, choriocarcinoma. Two female complements, **digyny,** has been observed in parthenogenetic embryos observed in vitro, and in ovarian tumors. Occasionally only one chromosome pair may have an aberrant origin. Such **uniparental disomy** is discussed in Chapter 14.

Aneuploidy occurs when the chromosome number is not an exact replica of the haploid. **Trisomy** is present when there are three copies of one chromosome, and **monosomy** when there is only one copy. Monosomy for an autosome is usually an early embryonic lethal. So are most autosomal trisomies, although trisomies for a few chromosome pairs are compatible with survival, leading to the clinical syndromes described in the next chapter. The sex chromosomes, to be discussed in Chapter 4, are exceptions to the rule that numerical chromosome abnormalities are associated with severe developmental defects.

Aneuploidy can result from errors in meiosis or in mitosis. These errors are often collectively referred to as **chromosomal nondisjunction,** although this term can imply a number of different sorts of errors, some of which do not really involve failure to disjoin.

When chromosome pairs fail to separate properly during the first division of meiosis, both copies of the chromosome from one parent are present in the zygote. This can be caused by (1) failure of pairs to separate, resulting in one daughter cell with both copies of a chromosome, and one daughter cell with no copies; or (2) failure of chromosomes to pair or to stay paired, resulting in random distribution of the two members of a pair to daughter cells (Fig. 2–13). Although the causes of these two kinds of error may be different, their consequences are similar. One difference is that imperfect pairing might lead to fewer exchanges than usual between homologues (reduced recombination), whereas failure of pairs to separate might be associated with more exchanges than usual.

Chromosomes may also fail to separate properly during the second meiotic division, leading to two copies of the same parental chromosome in the zygote (Fig. 2–14). Again, this can be caused by failure of chromatids to separate, or by random distribution of unpaired chromatids. Sometimes a chromatid may move too slowly in anaphase to be incorporated into a new daughter cell, and simply be lost. This is called **anaphase lag**, and leads to monosomy. It is believed to be one of the chief causes of monosomy X, which is viable, unlike autosomal monosomies, and associated with Turner syndrome.

In spite of an enormous amount of research, which has looked for associations between the frequency of aneuploidy and almost everything else, the only clear-cut association remains that which was documented more than 50 years ago by the distinguished English geneticist, Lionel Penrose—the increase in frequency of trisomy 21 with increasing maternal age. We now know that this increase extends to trisomies for most other chromosomes as well, most of which lead to spontaneous abor-

tion. Although maternal and paternal ages are correlated, sophisticated statistical analyses have shown that it is the maternal age that matters and not the paternal age.

It has long been postulated that the effect of maternal age is related to the long period of "suspended animation" in female meiosis, which may last as long as 40 years before completion of meiosis I at the time of ovulation. This would predict that most trisomies will result from a maternal meiotic error, and that this would most often be in the first meiotic division.

A large number of studies have examined the source and timing of the meiotic error in cases of Down syndrome, because this is the most easily ascertained trisomy. At first, chromosome heteromorphisms on the short arm of chromosome 21 were used to assign the parent of origin and stage of meiosis. Fig. 2–15 shows an example of how this can be done. These early studies indicated that about 75% of cases were caused by a maternal error, but a surprisingly high 25% were caused by a paternal error. Informative cytogenetic polymorphisms are not always present, and they are somewhat subjective to score.

When large numbers of polymorphic DNA markers became available, they were used to re-examine the question of the origin of tri-

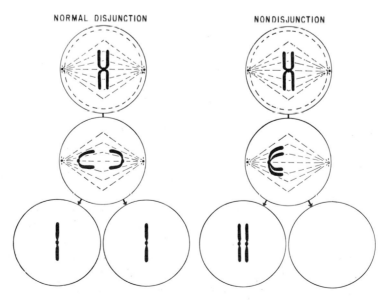

Fig. 2–14.   Mistake in second meiotic division leading to aneuploidy.

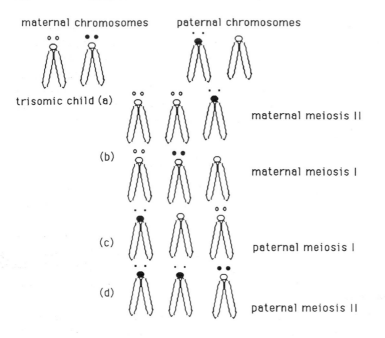

maternal chromosomes   paternal chromosomes

trisomic child (a)   maternal meiosis II

(b)   maternal meiosis I

(c)   paternal meiosis I

(d)   paternal meiosis II

Fig. 2–15. Diagram showing how short-arm and centromere heteromorphisms were used to assign parental origin and meiotic stage of nondisjunction in trisomy 21. It is assumed that there is no crossing over in the short arm, which may not be correct.

somy, as well as to examine the degree of crossing-over which had occurred. Fig. 2–16 illustrates the method. Parental origin can almost always be readily assigned. However, the distinction between meiosis I and meiosis II error is not so easy. In the absence of crossing over, a maternal meiosis I error always results in the trisomic child having both copies of the maternal 21 (which may carry different gene variants), whereas a meiosis II error results in the trisomic child having two identical maternal chromosomes. However, crossing over *does* occur, and confuses the picture. Heterozygous markers, so close to the centromere that crossing over is unlikely, are required to assign the stage of meiosis accurately.

Studies using the less subjective and more informative DNA markers demonstrated that

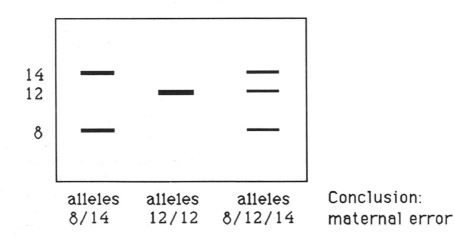

mother   father   DS child

14
12

8

alleles   alleles   alleles   Conclusion:
8/14   12/12   8/12/14   maternal error

Fig. 2–16. Determining parental origin of extra chromosome 21 in a Down syndrome patient, using DNA analysis of dinucleotide repeat polymorphism on chromosome 21. Gel analysis of PCR products reveals differences in repeat size. The child with Down syndrome inherits two alleles from the mother and one from the father.

only about 5% of cases of trisomy 21 have a paternal origin, and that about 2/3 arise at meiosis I.[7] Because crossing over can be demonstrated to have taken place between the homologous chromosomes which segregated together, complete failure of pairing cannot have occurred. However, some evidence suggests there is a reduction in crossing-over as compared to normally segregating chromosomes.

What happens at the second meiotic division can also occur during cell division in the zygote. This **mitotic nondisjunction** may result in two cell lines, one with an aneuploid number and one with a normal number (Fig. 2–17). The resulting mixture of cell lines with different genetic make-up is known as **mosaicism.** Cell lines with a missing autosome are not commonly observed, indicating that loss of a chromosome usually results in poor cell growth or death. In the early development of the fertilized egg, the first cellular differentiation leads to a large number of cells, which will develop into the placental villi, and a smaller number of cells, which will develop into the actual embryo. As a result, an abnormal mitotic division may result in aneuploid cells in the placenta but not in the embryo, or vice versa. This "confined" mosaicism may complicate prenatal diagnosis based on sampling of chorionic villi from the placenta. When mosaicism is present in an embryo, there may also be differing proportions of the two cell lines in different tissues.

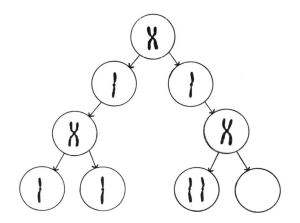

Fig. 2–17.   Nondisjunction at second cell division producing two viable cell lines, one euploid and one aneuploid (mosaicism).

When only part of a chromosome is present in triplicate, this is sometimes described as **partial trisomy**; deletion of one copy of a chromosome segment is similarly called **partial monosomy.** These imbalances usually occur as a result of structural chromosome changes, as discussed in the next section.

STRUCTURAL ABERRATIONS

Structural rearrangements may occur as a result of chromosome breakage and rejoining either in interphase or during meiotic or mitotic cell division. Many physical and chemical agents are known to increase chromosome breakage, but there is an underlying background frequency of breakage due to unknown causes. In the laboratory, lymphocyte cultures from normal human subjects show as many as 1 in 50 cells with a detectable structural abnormality. Common tests for genotoxicity involve assessment of the frequency of chromosome aberrations after exposure to potential chromosome-damaging agents. Most chromosome breaks are repaired by part of a complex DNA repair system involving multiple enzymes. In a few genetic diseases (e.g., Bloom syndrome, Fanconi anemia, xeroderma pigmentosum), a defect in part of this DNA repair system leads to an increase in the observed frequency of "spontaneous" chromosome rearrangements. Challenge of cultured cells with specific DNA-damaging agents can serve as a diagnostic test for these diseases.

With standard banding techniques, the frequency with which structural abnormalities can be observed is a function of the banding resolution of the chromosome preparation. In situ hybridization with specific locus probes or specific chromosome "paint" can reveal aberrations not visible with nonmolecular techniques, either because they involve too small a chromosome segment, or because the rearrangement has not changed the visible chromosome banding patterns (e.g., exchange of one G-negative band with another).

Chromosome rearrangements can involve only one chromosome or more than one. They may also be classified according to whether they are **balanced**, resulting in no net change

Table 2–3. Karyotypic Formulas for Chromosome Rearrangements

Karyotype	Description
46,XX,del(5)(p15)	terminal deletion of the short arm of chromosome 5, in band p15
46,XY,del(13)(q22q32)	interstitial deletion of the long arm of chromosome 13, with breaks in bands q22 and q32
46,XX,dup(8)(q21)	female with duplication of band q21 in chromosome 8
46,XY,inv(7)(p15q32)	pericentric inversion of chromosome 7, with breaks in bands p15 and q32
46,XX,inv(14)(q11.2q24)	paracentric inversion of chromosome 14, with breaks in bands q11.2 and q24
46,X,r(X)(p22q26)	female with ring X chromosome, with breaks in bands p22 and q26
46,X,i(Yq)	female with a normal X and an isochromosome for the long arm of the Y
45,XY,t(14q21q)	male with balanced Robertsonian translocation between chromosomes 14 and 21
46,XX,t(5;14)(p13;q32)	female with balanced translocation between the chromosome 5 short arm at p13 and the chromosome 14 long arm at q32
46,XX,−5,+der(5)t(5;14)(p13;q32) mat	female with unbalanced translocation as the result of adjacent segregation of maternal translocation between 5p and 14q
46,XY,−14,+t(14q21q)	male with unbalanced Robertsonian translocation (2 copies of 14q, 3 copies of 21q)

in chromosome material, or **unbalanced**, resulting in net gain (**duplication**) or loss (**deletion**) of chromosome material. The nomenclature for chromosomal rearrangements is complex, but is described briefly in the following sections. Table 2–3 gives examples of karyotypic formulas for more common types of rearrangements.

Rearrangements within Chromosomes

An **inversion** results from two breaks, with the intervening segment being reversed before healing (Fig. 2–18). If the breaks are on

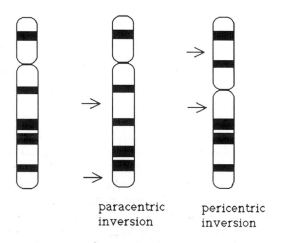

paracentric   pericentric
inversion   inversion

Fig. 2–18. Types of inversions. In a paracentric inversion, both breaks occur in the same chromosome arm; in a pericentric inversion, the breaks are on different chromosome arms.

opposite sides of the centromere, the inversion is **pericentric**; if the breaks are on the same chromosome arm, the inversion is **paracentric**. Pericentric inversions often cause a change in the relative length of the two arms; paracentric inversions do not, and can be observed only by changes in banding patterns. Individuals carrying one inverted chromosome are usually normal because this is a balanced rearrangement. However, at meiosis the two homologues can only pair along their length by forming an "inversion loop" (Fig. 2–19). If crossing over occurs within this loop, unbalanced gametes may result, so that offspring may have congenital defects caused by partial trisomy and monosomy. The various unbalanced gametes resulting from a paracentric and pericentric inversion are shown in Figure 2–22. The unbalanced gametes always have a duplication of the part of the chromosome on one side of the inversion breakpoint, and a deletion of the part of the chromosome on the other side of the breakpoint. Those resulting from a paracentric inversion are usually not compatible with embryonic development because they involve unstable configurations—either a **dicentric** chromosome with two centromeres or an **acentric** chromosome with no centromere. Pericentric inversions can result in viable offspring with chromosome imbalance. In both cases, half the balanced offspring will inherit the inverted chromosome. An example is shown in Fig. 2–

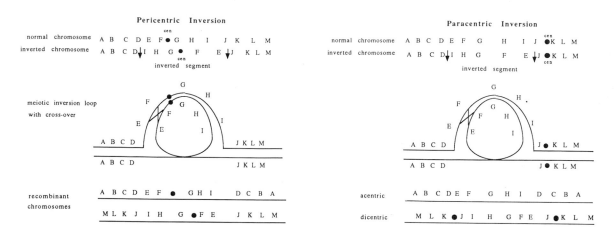

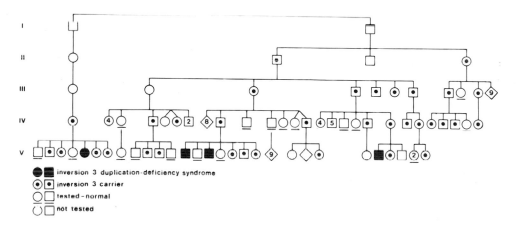

Fig. 2–19. Meiotic pairing and segregation in inversions. If a crossover occurs in the inverted segment, recombinant chromosomes have duplications and deficiencies. If the inversion is paracentric, these recombinant chromosomes will be dicentric or acentric.

Fig. 2–20. A Newfoundland pedigree illustrating segregation of an inversion of chromosome 3. Carriers are indicated by a single dot, chromosomally normal individuals by a horizontal line. Unbalanced offspring with a duplication-deletion syndrome are fully shaded. Note how the unbalanced children show up in several branches of the family. Courtesy of Dr. P. Allderdice.

20 of a family in Newfoundland in which a pericentric inversion of chromosome 3 was inherited over several generations and caused multiple cases of a duplication-deletion syndrome.

A **deletion** occurs when there is loss of material from one chromosome arm because of either one break (a **terminal** deletion) or two breaks (an **interstitial** deletion) (Fig. 2–21). A terminal deletion must heal by addition of telomeric sequences to the broken end. A **ring** chromosome is produced when a break occurs in each arm, with rejoining of the broken ends. Breaks very near the telomeres result in minimal imbalance; more proximally placed breaks lead to deletion in both the short and long arms. Ring chromosomes are commonly lost during mitosis because of complications in mi-

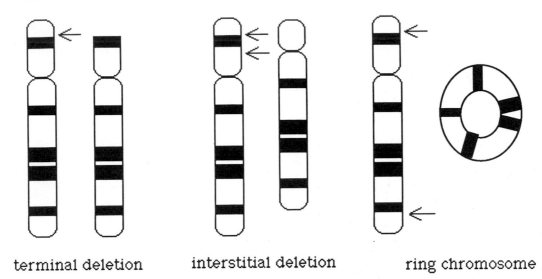

terminal deletion   interstitial deletion   ring chromosome

Fig. 2–21.   Types of deletions. A terminal deletion results from one break, with repair of telomere; an interstitial deletion results from two breaks in the same arm, and a ring chromosome results from two breaks in different arms.

totic disjunction of duplicated chromatids. This leads to mosaicism involving a monosomic line and a line with a ring chromosome.

A **duplication** occurs when there is a duplication of a chromosome segment, usually due to exchange between homologous chromosomes or sister chromatids. A duplication which involves a change in orientation of the duplicated segment is known as an **inverted duplication**, as opposed to a **direct duplication**, which does not change the orientation.

An **isochromosome** is a chromosome in which there are two copies of one arm and none of the other. It may result from exchange between homologues at meiosis, or from breakage and rejoining of sister chromatids near the centromere (Fig. 2–22). Although it used to be said that isochromosomes resulted from "misdivision of the centromere" in the horizontal rather than the longitudinal plane of the chromosome, it is uncertain that this mechanism ever actually occurs.

The nomenclature system for single chromosome rearrangements involves using an abbreviation to define the type of rearrangement, and, in brackets, the bands where breaks are assumed to have occurred. For example, a terminal deletion of the long arm of chromosome 1 can be written: del(1)(q31), whereas

an interstitial deletion would be written: del(1)(q31q34). In the first case, all of chromosome 1 distal to q31 is missing; in the second case, bands q32 and q33 are missing. Notice that the band(s) in the brackets are not the missing bands, but the breakpoints. Similarly a pericentric inversion of chromosome 3 would be written inv(3)(p12q32), and a paracentric inversion in the long arm would be written inv(3)(q21q28).

Rearrangements between Chromosomes

A **translocation** is a rearragement in which a piece of one chromosome is transferred to another chromosome. In a **balanced reciprocal** translocation, two chromosomes exchange broken pieces (Fig. 2–23). A **Robertsonian** translocation is a special case in which two acrocentric chromosomes join near their centromeres to form a single new chromosome. The chromosome number, as counted by the number of centromeres, is reduced by one, with loss of chromosome material on the short arms (Fig. 2–23). Because in the human acrocentric chromosomes the short arms contain only copies of the ribosomal DNA, which is redundant in the genome, this loss results in no

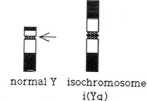

normal Y   isochromosome
i(Yq)

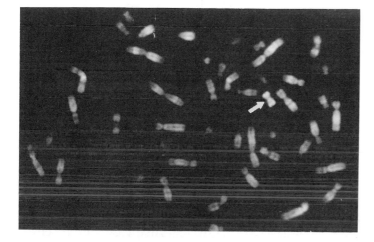

Fig. 2–22. Q-banded meta-phase showing isochromosome for Yq.

change in phenotype, and the rearrangement is said to be balanced.

The nomenclature system for translocations uses one bracket to describe the chromosomes involved (in numerical order), and another to describe the breakpoints. Thus, a female with a balanced reciprocal translocation between the long arm of 2 and the short arm of 5 would be described: 46, XX, t(2;5)(q23;p14). Robertsonian translocations are described by the arms which they contain, e.g., a balanced Robertsonian translocation between 14 and 21 would be written: 45, XX, t(14q21q). Notice that, in the reciprocal translocation, a semicolon is used between the chromosomes because *two* abnormal **derived** chromosomes are being described; for Robertsonian translocations, only one abnormal chromosome is present, and no semicolon is used.

More than 1 in 1000 normal newborns carries a balanced translocation; some are inherited from a parent, and some are **de novo**; that is, they have arisen anew during gametogenesis. Carriers of balanced rearrangements are usually normal. However, occasionally a break may interrupt a gene, leading to clinical abnormalities. Sometimes these abnormalities fit those of a known single-gene disorder, pinpointing the exact chromosomal location of the gene. Cell lines from such patients have provided important material that has led to the isolation, for example, of the genes for neurofibromatosis and muscular dystrophy. Chromosome rearrangements may also occasionally cause abnormalities as a result of a change in gene activation. The latter is well documented in the chromosomal rearrangements that are associated with cancer (see Chap. 21).

Normal balanced translocation carriers are at risk to produce chromosomally unbalanced gametes at meiosis. This is because, to achieve pairing of homologous segments, more than one pair of chromosomes must participate in meiotic pairing. The resulting configuration of three chromosomes (in the case of a Robertsonian translocation) or four chromosomes (in the case of a reciprocal translocation) may separate in a number of different ways, some of which result in chromosomally balanced gametes, and some which do not. Fig. 2–24 illustrates the ways in which this may occur.

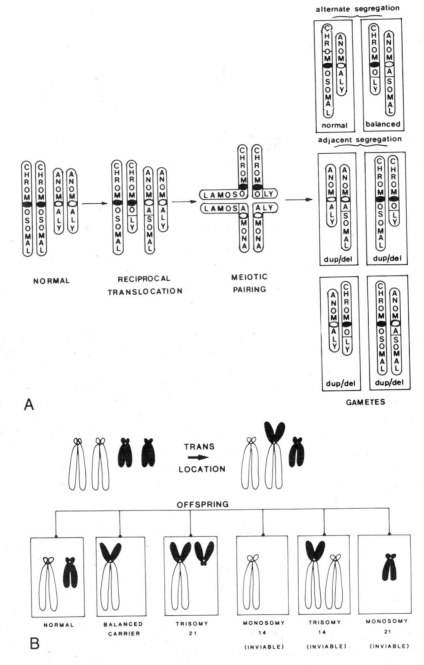

Fig. 2–23.   A. Reciprocal translocation involves a mutual exchange of segments between two nonhomologous chromosomes. In this case, the two chromosomes are designated "chromosomal" and "anomaly." Reciprocal exchange results in two "new" chromosomes, "chromoly" and "anomasomal." If a gamete carrying these chromosomes combines with a normal gamete, the resulting zygote is a balanced translocation carrier and will be phemotypically normal, because all the chromosomal material is there. However, at meiosis, a balanced carrier may form various types of gametes, as illustrated. The chromosomes form a cross-shaped bivalent. If the two centromeres on opposite corners of the cross go to the same pole (alternate segregation), the gametes will be normal or will carry a balanced translocation. Otherwise (adjacent segregation), the gamete will be unbalanced—for instance, carrying "chromosomal" and "chromoly," which has "chromo" in duplicate and "anoma" missing. The resulting zygote will be abnormal. The proportions of the various types of gametes depend on the length and position of the translocation; they are not necessarily equal. Courtesy Dr. Margaret Corey. B. Robertsonian ("centric fusion") translocations involve end-to-end fusion of acrocentric chromosomes, with loss of the short arms. The balanced carrier has 45 chromosomes and is phenotypically normal (the short arms do not seem to carry any significant gene loci). Again, the carrier may form unbalanced gametes, in nonrandom proportions.

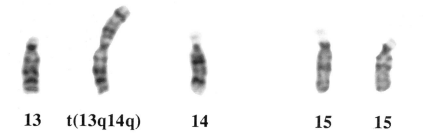

13   t(13q14q)   14   15   15

Fig. 2–24.   D-group chromosomes from a patient with a balanced Robertsonian translocation, 45, XY, t(13q14q).

The nomenclature for an unbalanced translocation is complex, and involves describing which normal chromosome is missing, and which derived chromosome is present (see Table 2–3).

The relative frequencies of the various kinds of segregation depend on factors such as the position of the breakpoints and the centromeres of the chromosomes, and cannot be exactly predicted. Many of the unbalanced conceptions may be nonviable beyond the early embryonic stage, and in general, the larger the unbalanced segment, the greater the chances for nonviability. As a result of all these complexities, there is no theoretical prediction for the rate of unbalanced offspring to be expected for any translocation. However, empirically derived estimates may be available, as discussed in the next chapter.

SUMMARY

Chromosomes consist of the basic hereditary material, deoxyribonucleic acid (DNA), organized into a complex structure along with histone and nonhistone proteins. The human genome (one copy of each chromosome) contains about 3 billion nucleotide base pairs. Only about 5% consist of active genes, of which it is estimated there are between 10,000 and 100,000. The rest of the DNA consists of noncoding sequences, many of which are repetitive units of various kinds. The 6 feet of DNA in the diploid cell must be compacted into a very small nuclear volume. The first step in this process involves a subunit of DNA wound around a histone core (the nucleosome): further hierarchical coiling eventually produces the interphase chromatin fiber, and the even more contracted metaphase chromosome.

The 23 pairs of human chromosomes consist of 22 pairs of autosomes in which the male and female chromosomes are identical, and one pair of sex chromosomes, which vary between the sexes. Analysis of the human karyotype is usually made from slides of metaphase chromosomes prepared from 72-hour cultures of peripheral lymphocytes. Special staining techniques, such as G-banding, produce banding patterns that, together with length and centromere position, define each chromosome pair. Bands are numbered and karyotypes described by an international system of nomenclature. A larger number of bands can be resolved in the less contracted chromosomes of early metaphase than in standard preparations.

Some chromosome regions are variable in size and staining proportions, without affecting the phenotype. These heteromorphisms involve noncoding, repetitive DNA sequences which are associated with heterochromatin, usually at or near the centromere. Staining properties of chromosomes reflect underlying differences in DNA base composition.

DNA hybridization may be performed on slide preparations of chromosomes in metaphase or interphase to define the number and position of cloned DNA segments. In situ hybridization is usually carried out with fluorescently labelled probes (FISH). This technique can identify chromosomal changes too small to see in banded preparations, identify complex rearrangements, and determine aneuploidy in interphase nuclei as well as metaphase plates. Multicolored fluorescent labels can be used to analyze several sequences at once.

Mitosis, or somatic cell division, is the process by which cells duplicate themselves. The DNA replicates during the interphase between cell divisions. During prophase, the chromosomes condense and become visible under light microscopy. At metaphase, the duplicated chromosomes are seen as discrete bodies, with their two chromatids held together at the centromere, which is also attached to the spindle. At anaphase, the 46 single-stranded chromatids migrate to opposite poles. Cytoplasmic division takes place at telophase.

Meiosis, or reduction division, takes place during the formation of gametes, and differs from mitosis in that (1) there is pairing of homologous chromosomes and exchange (crossing over) between them, and (2) there are two successive divisions of nuclear material, resulting in gametes containing 23 chromosomes. Fusion of two haploid gametes then produces a diploid zygote.

Excesses or deficiencies of chromosomal material generally result in abnormal development, often resulting in embryonic or fetal loss, but sometimes to liveborn offspring with developmental defects. Errors in meiosis and mitosis can lead to aneuploidy, the gain or loss of individual chromosomes. Trisomy, the presence of three copies of one chromosome, is usually caused by an error in maternal meiosis (nondisjunction), and increases in frequency with maternal age. Gain of additional complete chromosome sets (triploidy and tetraploidy) is generally not compatible with survival beyond early gestation.

Structural abnormalities are produced as a result of chromosome breakage and rearrangement. This may lead to inversion of chromosome segments, loss or duplication of chromosomal material, or exchange of material between chromosomes (translocation). Individuals with balanced rearrangements (no loss or gain of chromosome material) are at risk to produce offspring with unbalanced complements as a result of segregation of chromosomes from the complex pairing arrangements that occur in meiosis.

REFERENCES

1. Breuning, M.H., et al.: Rubinstein-Taubi syndrome caused by submicroscopic deletions within 16p13.3. Am. J. Hum. Genet. 52:249, 1993.
1a. Caspersson, N., and Zech, L. (eds.): Chromosome Identification. Nobel Symposia on Medicine and Natural Sciences. New York, Academic Press, 1973.
2. ISCN (1985): An International System for Human Cytogenetic Nomenclature. Harnden, D.G. and Klinger, H.P. (eds). Published in collaboration with Cytogenet. Cell Genet., Basel, Karger, 1985.
3. Klinger, K., et al.: Rapid detection of chromosome aneuploidies in uncultured amniocytes by using fluorescence in situ hybridization (FISH). Am. J. Hum. Genet. 51:55, 1992.
4. Lichter, P., et al.: High resolution mapping of human chromosome 11 by in situ hybridization with cosmid clones. Science 247:64, 1990.
5. Manuelidis, L., and Chen, T.L.: A unified model of eukaryotic chromosomes. Cytometry 11:8, 1990.
6. Pinkel, D., et al.: Fluorescence in situ hybridization with human chromosome-specific libraries: Detection of trisomy 21 and translocations of chromosome 4. Proc. Nat. Acad. Sci USA 85:9138, 1988.
7. Sherman, S.L., et al.: Trisomy 21: association between reduced recombination and nondisjunction. Am. J. Hum. Genet. 49:608, 1991.
8. Tjio, J.H., and Levan, A.: The chromosome number in man. Hereditas 42:1, 1956.

Chapter 3

Clinical Consequences of Autosomal Chromosome Abnormalities

". . . IT MAY BE POSSIBLE THAT WE ARE DEALING WITH A HUMAN EXAMPLE OF A CERTAIN CHROMOSOME
ABERRATION. WHY SHOULD IT NOT OCCUR OCCASIONALLY IN HUMANS, AND WHY WOULD IT NOT BE
POSSIBLE THAT—UNLESS IT IS LETHAL—IT WOULD CAUSE A RADICAL ANOMALY OF CONSTITUTION?"
WAARDENBURG, P.J. BIBLIOGR. GENET. 7, 1932

Before abnormalities of human chromosomes could be recognized, satisfactory preparations and knowledge of normal human chromosomes were required. Tjio and Levan set the stage in 1956 when they demonstrated the correct human chromosome number as 46, and described techniques for making good chromosome spreads. In 1958, a young French pediatrician, Jerome Lejeune, reported his finding of a chromosomal abnormality in Down syndrome at a seminar at McGill University during the Tenth International Congress of Genetics. The report of this discovery was published in 1959,[15] the same year that Jacobs described the chromosome abnormality in Klinefelter syndrome and in Turner syndrome. Since then, chromosome anomalies visible under the microscope have been shown to be among the major causes of human mortality and morbidity, and a very large number of specific clinical syndromes attributable to specific chromosome abnormalities have been

described. In a textbook of this size and intent, it is not possible to provide clinical details of this ever-enlarging body of information. In the next two chapters, we present only an arbitrary selection of the more common and illustrative examples.

FREQUENCY OF HUMAN CHROMOSOMAL ABNORMALITIES

In the 1960s and 70s, several groups determined the frequency of chromosome anomalies at birth by karyotyping over 60,000 consecutive newborn infants. From these studies[11] we derive the estimates of the frequencies of particular numerical chromosome abnormalities at birth, as shown in Table 3–1. Although these early studies are fairly accurate for numerical abnormalities, they underestimate structural abnormalities because no chromosome banding was carried out in most of them. It has been estimated that about 50% of struc-

Table 3–1. Approximate Incidence of Chromosome Abnormalities at Birth

Category	Frequency	
Sex chromosome aneuploidy*		
all	1/500 live births	
47,XXY	1/1000 male births	
47,XYY	1/1000 male births	
47,XXX	1/1000 female births	
45,X	1/10,000 female births	
Autosomal aneuploidy*		
trisomy 21	1/800 live births	
trisomy 18	1/8000	
trisomy 13	1/20,000	
triploidy	1/60,000	
Structural abnormalities†	de novo	inherited
balanced Robertsonian	1/3000	1/2000
balanced reciprocal	1/2000	1/1000
balanced inversions	1/5000	1/1000
all balanced	1/1000	1/400
all unbalanced	1/1000	1/2000

*Data from Hook, E.B., and Hamerton, J. L.[11]
†Data from Hook, E.B., and Cross, P.K.[8]

tural abnormalities would not have been visible without banding. The estimates for structural abnormalities in Table 3–1 are derived from studies by Hook and Cross[8] on prenatal samples.

Approximately 1 in 200 live births has a visible chromosome abnormality: this includes sex chromosome abnormalities and balanced rearrangements that are not usually associated with any phenotypic abnormalities. The number of chromosome abnormalities observed at birth is only a small proportion of those that occur

Table 3–2. Incidence of Chromosome Abnormalities in Embryonic and Fetal Deaths, by Gestational Age*

Weeks of Gestation	Percentage of Chromosome Abnormalities
<8	27.1
8–11	53.5
12–15	47.9
16–19	23.8
20–23	11.9
24–27	13.2
Stillbirths†	6.0
Neonatal deaths†	5.5

†Data from Angell, R.R., Sandison, A., Bain, D.A.[2]

at conception. Current estimates are that about 9% of sperm and 15% of ova in normal individuals have a visible chromosome abnormality. Most of the anomalies in sperm are structural, whereas most of those in ova are numerical. During gestation, most chromosomally abnormal conceptions are lost as spontaneous abortions. (miscarriages)[21] Table 3–2 shows the proportion of chromosome anomalies in embryonic and fetal deaths at

Table 3–3. Frequency of Types of Chromosome Abnormalities among Spontaneous Abortions*

Karyotype	Percentage of All Karyotyped Spontaneous Abortions
Normal	60.2
Autosomal trisomy	19.5
Sex chromosome trisomy	0.2
Mosaic trisomy (with normal line)	1.8
Double Trisomy	1.1
45,X	6.1
45,X mosaic	0.5
Triploidy	6.0
Tetraploidy	2.4
Structural rearrangements	1.5
Others (double anomalies, etc.)	0.6

*Data from 3300 karyotyped spontaneous abortions from Warburton, Byrne and Canki; Chromosome Anomalies and Prenatal Development. An Atlas. New York, Oxford University Press, 1991.

Table 3–4. Incidence of Chromosome Abnormalities in Various Populations (Not Including fragile-X)*

Population Studied	Percentage with Abnormal Karyotypes
Live births	0.5
Induced abortions, <12 weeks	5
Stillbirths and perinatal deaths	6
Infants with congenital anomalies	4–8
Mental retardation (moderate and severe)	12–35
Congenital anomaly + mental retardation	6–21
Infants with congenital heart disease	10–13
Pseudo or true hermaphroditism	20–25
Females with delayed puberty	27
Males with infertility	2
Couples with two or more spontaneous abortions	4

*Data from Hook, E.B.[10]

Table 3–5.   Risks of Unbalanced Offspring for Rearrangement Carriers*

Type of Rearrangement	Percentage of Unbalanced Offspring
Robertsonian translocations	
D/21, female	10–15
D/21, male	2–5
13/14, both sexes	1–2
21/22, female	10–15
Reciprocal translocations	
pooled, both sexes	6–12
identified by unbalanced child	20
identified by unbalanced child with small unbalanced segment	50
identified other than by abnormal child	2–5
t(11;22)(q23;q11)	5–7
Pericentric inversions	
identified by unbalanced child	5–10
identified otherwise	2

*Data from Daniel, A., Hook, E.B., and Wulf, G.[5] Also from Bouć, A., and Gallano, P.[3]

various gestational ages; about 50% of first trimester losses are the result of visible chromosome aberrations, the rate gradually decreasing in later gestations to about 10% at 28 weeks. Pregnancies resulting in a stillbirth or neonatal death have a 6% rate of chromosome anomalies, making karyotype analysis of such pregnancies an important diagnostic procedure.[2] The types and frequencies of the common chromosome anomalies found in spontaneous abortions are given in Table 3–3. The commonest anomaly is trisomy, which may occur for any chromosome (although trisomy 1 has only been observed in an in vitro fertilized embryo). Trisomy 16 accounts for about a third of all trisomies seen in spontaneous abortions, although this karyotype is never seen in a live birth. The trisomies that often survive to birth, trisomies 21, 13 and 18, do not occur at conception more often than many other kinds of trisomy. They are exceptional only in their potential for viability. Even for trisomy 21, 70% of all known conceptions with this chromosome complement do not survive to term, and for trisomy 13 and 18, the proportion is greater than 90%.

Examples of the frequency of chromosome anomalies in patients presenting in various ways are shown in Table 3–4. Karyotype analysis is indicated in any child with unexplained mental retardation or congenital anomalies. In one survey, 13% of all infants with congenital heart

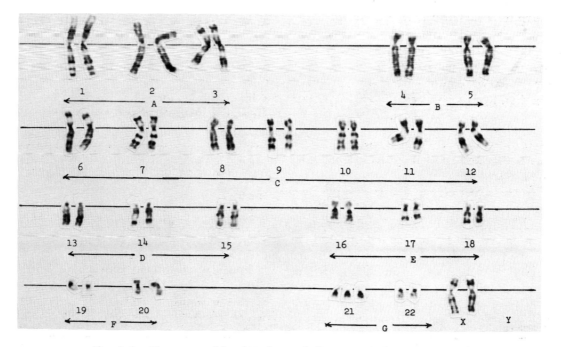

Fig. 3–1.   Karyotype of female infant with Down syndrome, trisomy 21.

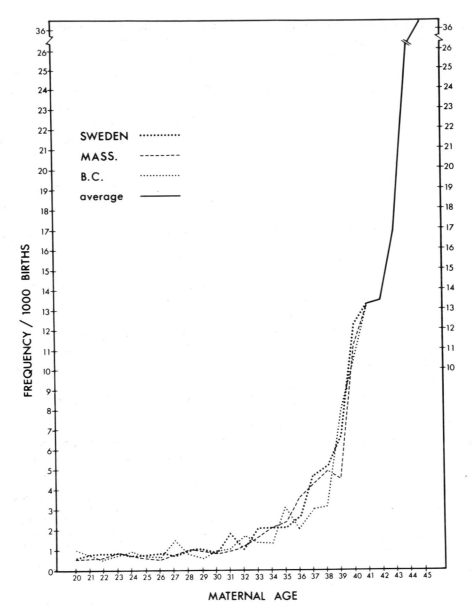

Fig. 3–2.   Frequency of Down syndrome at birth related to maternal age in three population surveys: Sweden, Massachusetts, and British Columbia.[11,28]

disease had a chromosome abnormality.[10] Chromosome studies are also indicated in couples who have had either two or more spontaneous abortions or an unexplained neonatal death. In about 4% of such couples (about 10 times the expected frequency), one parent is found to have a balanced translocation, in which unbalanced segregation has led to abnormal pregnancies.

RECURRENCE RISKS FOR CHROMOSOMAL ABNORMALITIES

Parents who have one child with a chromosome anomaly want to know the chances of this happening again. The only situation in which there is a relatively high probability of recurrence involves parents who are carriers of a balanced rearrangement such as an in-

Table 3-6. Risks of Down Syndrome at Birth and Amniocentesis, by Maternal Age*

Maternal Age	Live Births	Rate per 1000 Amniocentesis
<20	0.7	
20–24	0.7	
25–29	0.9	
30–34	1.3	
33	1.6	2.4
35	2.9	3.7 (1/270)
37	4.4	6.1
40	10.0	13.1 (1/76)
42	15.4	21.8
45	40.0	46.8 (1/21)

*Data from Hook and Lindsjo[9] and Hook.[12]

version or translocation. It is therefore important to perform chromosome analysis on patients with autosomal trisomy syndromes to rule out the small proportion of cases that result from a translocation rather than simple trisomy. Parental chromosome analysis should also be performed whenever there is a child with an unbalanced rearrangement such as a deletion or duplication. About half of such cases occur de novo, and half have a parent who is a balanced translocation carrier.

As discussed in the previous chapter, the chance of an unbalanced offspring differs with each rearrangement, and may vary with the sex of the carrier parent. Empirically derived estimates are available for some commonly occurring translocations, such as the Robertsonian 14/21, 21/22 and 13/14 translocations.[3,5] For many others, all that is available is an estimate based on pooling all translocation or inversion carriers who have had prenatal diagnosis. To make things even more complicated, risks are sometimes different for male and female carriers of the same rearrangement. Table 3–5 gives empirically derived risks for some common situations. The risk is substantially higher for couples in whom the parental rearrangement was found because of a liveborn child with an unbalanced rearrangement, because this identifies unbalanced chromosome complements that are compatible with survival to term.

In the case of a de novo rearrangement in a child, few data exist concerning recurrence risk, but theoretical considerations suggest that there should be little, if any, increased risk of recurrence.

In the case of numerical anomalies, significant data on recurrence are available only for trisomy 21. One study in women with multiple karyotyped spontaneous abortions[20] suggests that there are no "trisomyprone" couples with an increased chance for all kinds of aneuploid conceptions. Trisomy for any chromosome tended to recur with about the frequency expected for the appropriate maternal age. However, this study was not large enough to examine recurrence for individual trisomies. Such data are available for prenatal diagnoses following a trisomy 21 pregnancy. The recurrence risk in parents with normal chromosomes is about 1%, regardless of maternal age. This indicates that, for younger women, the risk is increased above that expected for their age, whereas in older women, the risk remains that associated with their age. The increased recurrence risk could be explained by a small proportion of parents who

Table 3–7. Features of Trisomy 21

Area	Findings
General	Male sex preponderance (M, 3:F, 2); variable lengths of survival
Neurologic	Hypotonic; psychomotor retardation
Head	Characteristic facies, flat occiput
Eyes	"Mongoloid slant;" epicanthic folds; Brushfield spots
Ears	Small, frequently low-set
Nose	Low nasal bridge
Mouth and chin	Protruding fissured tongue secondary to maxillary hypoplasia and narrow palate
Neck	Broad, frequently webbed
Heart	Congenital heart lesions in 50%, VSD and AV canal most common
Abdomen	Diastasis recti; umbilical hernia; duodenal atresia
Hands	Short hands and fingers; clinodactyly fifth finger
Feet	Gap between first and second toes with plantar furrow
Urogenital	Occasional cryptorchism
X-ray	Pelvic x-rays iliac index <60°; hypoplasia midphalanx fifth finger
Dermatoglyphics	Simian line; distal axial-triradius; ten ulnar loops or radial loops on fourth and fifth fingers
Incidence	1 in 700

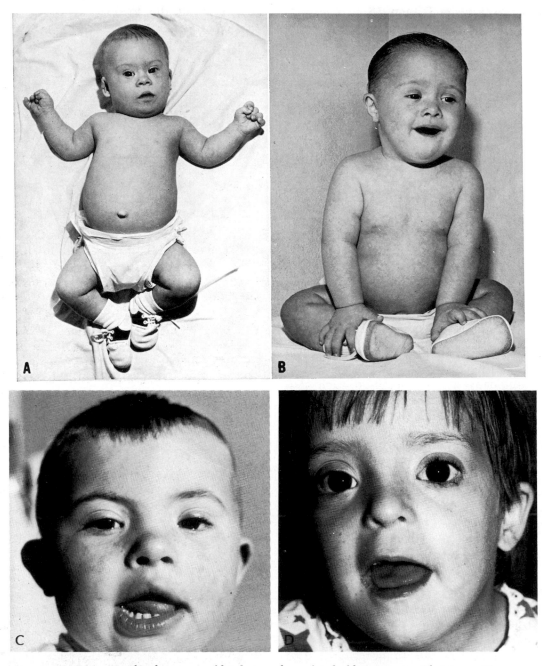

Fig. 3–3.   Unrelated one-year-old infants and unrelated older patients with trisomy 21.

are themselves mosaic for trisomy 21 in their germ cell precursors. For other trisomies such as trisomy 18 and 13, there are fewer data. However, it is reasonable to think that the same situation may apply. A previous trisomy 21, 13, or 18 is therefore an indication for prenatal diagnosis.

TRISOMY 21 (DOWN SYNDROME)

Cytogenetic Findings

This clinical disorder was first recognized by J. Langdon Down in 1866.[13] Although he coined the term "mongolism" for this syn-

Table 3–8.   Features of Trisomy 18

Area	Findings
General	Female sex preponderance (M,1:F,4); low birth weight for gestational age; failure to thrive; early death
Neurological	Mental and growth retardation; hypertonic
Head	Prominent occiput
Eyes	Epicanthic folds; small palpebral fissures
Ears	Low-set; malformed
Mouth and chin	Micrognathia, narrow palatal arch, microstomia; infrequently, cleft lip and/or palate
Thorax	Short sternum; eventration of diaphragm
Heart	Congenital heart anomalies in 99%, most often VSD or PDA
Abdomen	Meckel's diverticulum; inguinal hernia
Hands	Third and fourth fingers clenched against palm with second and fifth fingers overlapping them
Feet	Rocker-bottom shape; great toe dorsiflexed
Pelvis	Small pelvis; limited hip abduction
Urogenital	Renal anomalies; cryptorchism
X-ray	Hypoplastic sternum; thin tapered ribs; hypoplastic mandible; "antimongoloid" pelvis
Dermatoglyphics	Characteristic digital pattern of 6 to 10 low arches; high axial triradius; single flexion crease on digits
incidence	1 in 3500 to 1 in 8000

drome, based on the apparently mongoloid facial features, it is now known as Down syndrome. The association with older mothers was recognized in the 1930s, and at that time it was also suggested that a chromosome anomaly could be responsible for the syndrome. However, this could not be demonstrated until 1959, after human cytogenetic analysis had become reliable. Because chromosomes 21 and 22 could not be distinguished in the early unbanded chromosome studies, Down syndrome was first described as due to G trisomy. The majority of babies born with Down syndrome have 47 chromosomes with complete trisomy 21 (Fig. 3–1); a small proportion (5%) have trisomy for all or part of chromosome 21 as a result of a chromosome rearrangement. About 2% have mosaicism, with both a normal cell line and a cell line with trisomy 21.

Patients who have Down syndrome as a result of a translocation involving the whole long arm have all the features of those having a "free" extra 21. Studies of patients with translocations involving only part of chromosome 21 have shown that many of the characteristic features of the syndrome are associated only with trisomy for the distal region of the long arm, and are attempting to find precise genetic loci leading to particular features. Patients who have trisomy only for the proximal region also have mental retardation and multiple anomalies, but would not be classified clinically as having Down syndrome.

When a child is suspected to have Down syndrome, cytogenetic analysis is necessary even if the diagnosis is not in doubt clinically. This is because it is important to distinguish between straight trisomy 21 and cases involving a translocation. Almost all translocations involved in Down syndrome are Robertsonian, usually involving either a 14/21 translocation or a 21/22 translocation. In about half these cases, one parent carries a balanced translocation, and may have a greatly increased risk of another child having Down syndrome. Other family members may also need to be studied to determine if they too are carriers. Prenatal diagnosis can be offered to couples carrying such a translocation.

Occasionally a child with Down syndrome is found to have the karyotype 46,t(21q21q). This is almost always a sporadic event, but in rare cases a parent is found to have a balanced 21q/21q translocation. This is one of the few examples in genetics of a 100% re-

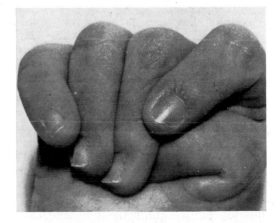

Fig. 3–4.   Typical conformation of hand in trisomy 18.

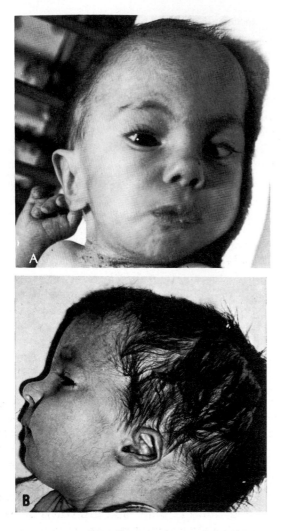

Fig. 3–5. Two infants illustrating craniofacial characteristics of trisomy 18 (prominent occiput, low-set malformed ears and small chin).

icism for trisomy 21 appears usually to arise after anaphase lag in a conception that was originally trisomic, rather than as a result of nondisjunction in a chromosomally normal conception. As a result, there is an increased maternal age in mosaic patients, and the recurrence risk for their parents should be the same as if they had a fully trisomic child. Of interest is the fact that there may be gradual loss over time of the trisomic line in peripheral blood cultures of mosaic patients.

Incidence

Trisomy 21 is the most common autosomal abnormality, with a frequency of approximately 1 in 700 births in North America. For many decades, physicians have recognized that there is a relationship between maternal age and the risk of having an offspring with Down syndrome. The risk increases from approximately 1 in 1500 in a woman under 25 to 1 in 350 in a woman of 35, and 1 in 100 in a woman of 40. Plotting the risk by single year of maternal age gives an exponentially rising curve, which is reasonably flat until a sudden upturn at about age 32 (Fig. 3–2 and Table 3–6).[9] At the usual time of amniocentesis for prenatal diagnosis (16 weeks of gestation), the incidence for each age is somewhat higher than these figures (Table 3–6), because there is about a 30% chance that a Down syndrome pregnancy diagnosed at 16 weeks will end in a fetal death before term.[11]

currence risk. Because both chromosomes 21 are united, gametes from this parent can have only two or no copies. No normal children can be born. In the days before chromosomal studies were routinely performed, we saw two tragic families in which five successive children were born with Down syndrome as the result of such a translocation in a parent.

Patients with trisomy 21 mosaicism may have the classic appearance of Down syndrome, or may look essentially normal, depending, presumably, on the tissue distribution and preponderance of the abnormal cell line. Mosa-

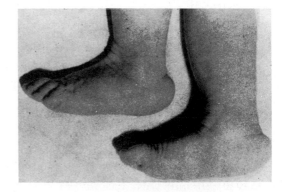

Fig. 3–6. Rocker-bottom foot of infant with trisomy 18.

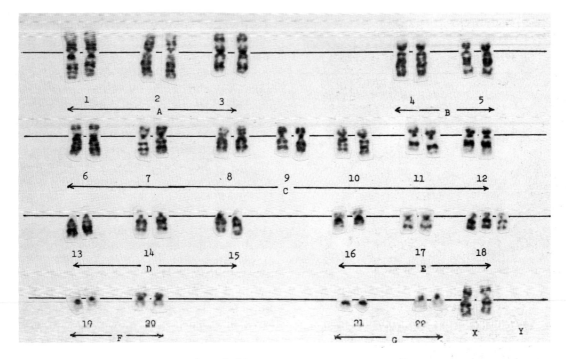

Fig. 3–7. Banded karyotype of female with trisomy 18.

The maternal age association in Down syndrome and other trisomies is the rationale behind the screening by prenatal diagnosis of pregnancies in women over 35. The proportion of all cases of Down syndrome born to women over 35 is a function of the distribution of ages of child-bearing in the population. At the present time in North America, only about 25% of cases of Down syndrome are born to women over 35, so that other ways of detecting high-risk situations are needed. One such screening tool became available when it was recognized in 1984 that low maternal serum alpha-fetoprotein is associated with a small but significant increase in the risk of trisomy.[16] Other biochemical markers that indicate increased risk are now also known. This subject is discussed in more detail in Chapter 15.

Clinical Features

These are summarized in Table 3–7. For Down syndrome, as for all chromosomal syndromes, one can list the characteristic features, but any particular feature may or may not be present in an individual patient. Also, some features, such as poor muscle tone, poor growth, and psychomotor retardation, are common to most syndromes and do not provide a differential diagnosis.

In infancy, patients with Down syndrome have poor muscle tone, and growth is slower than normal. Psychomotor development is the major area of concern, and there is a fairly broad spectrum of achievement. Although most patients are in the IQ range of 25 to 50, an occasional patient may learn to read and write, and the stimulus of early training programs and parental involvement may improve the outcome. Adult stature is usually below normal.

The facial appearance of Down syndrome is often diagnostic (Fig. 3–3). The tendency of the palpebral fissures to slant upward at the lateral borders, and the presence of an epicanthic fold, give a "mongoloid" appearance. The iris may be speckled with round, grayish Brushfield spots. The back of the head is somewhat flat, and the nasal root is also flat-

Table 3–9. Features of Trisomy 13

Area	Findings
General	Slightly more common in females; failure to thrive; apneic spells; early death
Neurological	Mental and motor retardation; hypertonic or hypotonic; defects of the forebrain (holoprosencephaly, arhinencephaly)
Head	Sloping forehead; scalp defects; microcephaly
Eyes	Colobomata; microphthalmia; anophthalmia
Ears	Low-set, malformed
Mouth and chin	Usually cleft lip and/or palate; micrognathia
Heart	Congenital heart lesions in 88%, most often VSD, PDA, and rotational anomalies
Abdomen	Rotational anomalies; hernias, absent spleen; accessory spleens
Hands	Polydactyly; frequently third and fourth fingers clenched against palm with second and fifth fingers overlapping; hyperconvex nails
Feet	Polydactyly, frequently rocker-bottom shape
Urogenital	Polycystic kidneys; hydronephrosis; cryptorchism; bicornuate uterus
Dermatoglyphics	Ridge hypoplasia; radial loops and arches; high triradius; single palmar flexion crease; hallucal arch fibular or fibular-S pattern
Incidence	1 in 4000 to 1 in 15,000

tened. Because the maxilla is small and the palate narrow, the tongue frequently protrudes, and may be fissured in appearance. In the newborn, there may be a third fontanelle.

Common to many syndromes are webbing of the neck, umbilical hernias, and cryptorchidism in the male. About half of the patients with Down syndrome have congenital cardiac malformations, with endocardial cushion defects being the most common. Many other heart lesions may occur, including ventricular septal defect, atrial septal defect, and patent ductus arteriosius.

The hand is broad, the fingers short, and the fifth finger incurved as a result of hypoplasia and asymmetry of the middle phalanx. There may be a gap between the first and second toes, with a furrow extending down the plantar surface from this gap. Characteristic features of the dermal ridge patterns (**dermatoglyphics**) will be described in Chapter 17. Two of the most useful and easily observed

are the presence of a bilateral simian crease, and of a single flexion crease on the fifth finger.

The presence of congenital heart disease, duodenal atresia, and other life-threatening conditions leads to the death of 50% of patients before the age of 5 years, but if this period is passed, life expectation may extend to 50 years or more. Accelerated aging and the brain changes typical of Alzheimer's disease are often found in patients over 30, a fact of interest because two genes that may be mutated in familial Alzheimer's disease are found on chromosome 21. A child with Down syndrome has about a 20-fold increase of risk of leukemia.

Adult males with Down syndrome do not have normal spermatogenesis and are sterile. Females are apparently normally fertile, and the few existing reports indicate about a 50% risk of producing a child with Down syndrome because of maternal trisomy 21.

TRISOMY 18 (EDWARDS SYNDROME)

Trisomy 18 was the first chromosomal syndrome to be described which was unknown as a clinical entity before cytogenetic analysis; in 1960, Edwards and colleagues described the findings in a child with an extra chromosome in the E group, and Patau, Smith, and co-workers described two other patients.[6,17] Trisomy 18 is the second most common of the autosomal trisomy syndromes, with an estimated incidence between 1 in 4000 and 1 in 8000 births. The clinical features are summarized in Table 3–8. A preponderance of patients are female, perhaps reflecting differential survival. In contrast to patients with Down syndrome, intrauterine growth retardation is common. Postnatal growth retardation ("failure to thrive") and severe developmental retardation with early death before 6 months are typical. However, some patients may survive for years, and in such cases there is profound psychomotor retardation, often with inability to sit alone or walk.

At birth, the affected individual is usually hypertonic, and holds her hands in the peculiar manner illustrated in Figure 3–4, with

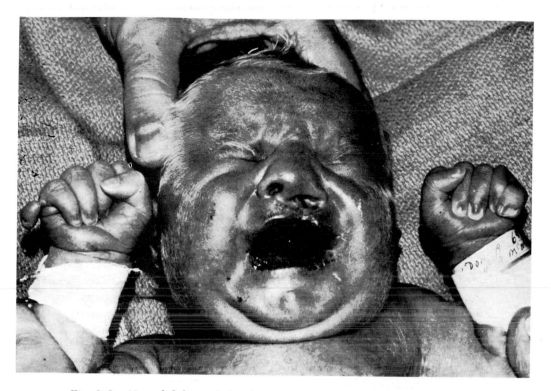

Fig. 3–8. Note cleft lip, polydactyly, and microphthalmia typical of trisomy 13.

the third and fourth finger clenched tightly against the palm and the second and fifth fingers overlapping them. When the fingers are straightened out, the most distal flexion crease is missing. There is microcephaly, a prominent occiput, low-set malformed ears, and a small chin (Fig. 3–5). A short sternum, small pelvis with limited hip abduction, and rocker-bottom feet (Fig. 3–6) are common. Almost all patients have congenital heart lesions, most often ventricular septal defect and patent ductus arteriosus. Dermatoglyphics provide useful diagnostic evidence, such as a preponderance of arch patterns on the fingers (see Chap. 17).

Almost all patients have a full trisomy 18 (Fig. 3–7). As with patients with Down syndrome, a small proportion of cases of trisomy 18 may have mosaicism with a normal cell line. Full trisomy 18 is not possible as a result of a translocation, but partial trisomy for the long arm produces many of the same features. Although the data are sparse, it appears that the risk of another trisomy after a child with tri-

somy 18 is approximately the same 1 or 2% as after a child with Down syndrome.

TRISOMY 13 (PATAU SYNDROME)

Although the pattern of anomalies found in trisomy 13 has been traced back through 300 years, the first report that they were associated with a chromosomal anomaly was presented by Patau and colleagues in 1960.[17] Trisomy 13 is the least common of the major autosomal trisomies, with an estimated incidence of 1 in 5000 to 1 in 20,000 births. This reflects its higher intrauterine mortality.

A patient with trisomy 13 often has more obvious severe malformations than patients with the other trisomies. (Table 3–9 and Figs. 3–8 through 3–10). Most patients have cleft lip and palate and eye abnormalities that range from coloboma of the iris through microphthalmia to complete absence of the eye. Polydactyly is common. Seventy-five percent of patients have defects of the midface and forebrain, including arrhinencephaly and hol-

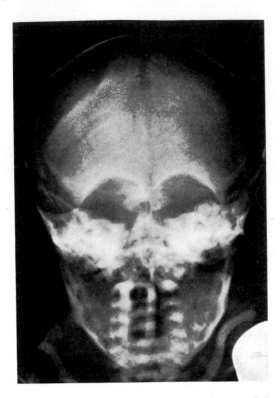

Fig. 3–9. Radiographic appearance of arhinencephaly in trisomy 13.

location involving chromosome 13. A balanced Robertsonian translocation, t(13q14q), is the most common translocation in the population, occurring in about 1 in 1000 normal individuals. Carriers of such a translocation have only about a 2% chance of having a liveborn child with trisomy 13, probably because of the high rate of intrauterine loss of unbalanced conceptions. Partial trisomy for the 13 long arm as the result of a reciprocal rearrangement may give many of the features of the complete trisomy. Mosaicism of trisomy 13 with a normal cell line also occurs, and may be associated with a less severe phenotype. As with Down syndrome, even if the phenotypic picture appears diagnostic of trisomy 13, karyotype analysis should be done for purposes of genetic counselling.

OTHER AUTOSOMAL TRISOMIES

Although trisomies for all chromosomes except chromosome 1 have been found in spon-

oprosencephaly. The head is small, the forehead slopes, and there is often a scalp defect. As in trisomy 18, the ears are low-set and malformed, the chin is small, and the hands may be held in a clenched position. Many patients have seizures and apneic spells. Survival beyond a few months is rare, and in cases with longer survival, there is severe psychomotor retardation, and often deafness.

The most frequently encountered cardiovascular lesions are ventricular septal defect and patent ductus arteriosus, but rotational cardiovascular lesions are highly characteristic (e.g., dextroposition of the heart without abdominal situs inversus). The spleen may be absent or there may be accessory spleens. Urogenital anomalies are common. Dermatoglyphic anomalies are also present (see Chapter 17).

Most patients with trisomy 13 have a complete trisomy with 47 chromosomes (Fig. 3–11). However, complete duplication of 13q may occur as the result of a Robertsonian trans-

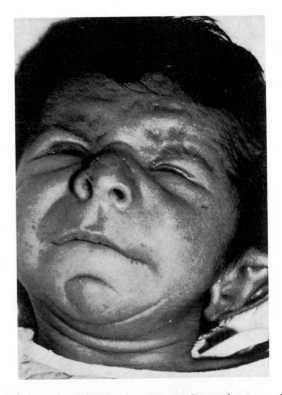

Fig. 3–10. Midfacial appearance of infant with trisomy 13 but without cleft lip and palate.

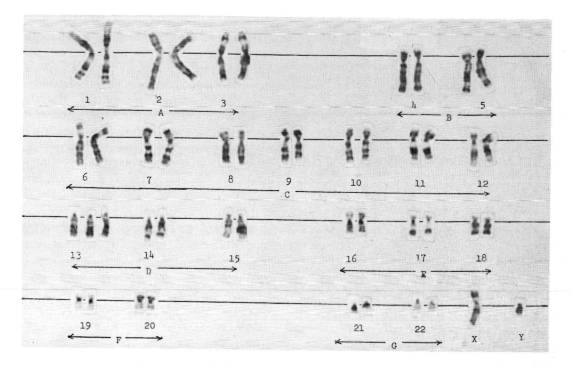

Fig. 3–11. Giemsa-banded karyotype of male patient with trisomy 13.

taneous abortions, most are either never found in live births or occur only occasionally as mosaics together with a normal cell line. Such mosaics are now sometimes identified because mosaicism found in prenatal diagnosis leads to chromosome studies after birth. A maternal age relationship has been found for all trisomies except for those of the largest chromosomes: this is the major cause of the increasing rate of spontaneous abortion with maternal age. By the time a woman reaches 40, there is a 60% probability that any miscarriage she has will be trisomic.[21]

Trisomy 8 has been described relatively frequently in a nonmosaic state, and is associated with specific clinical findings. (Table 3–10, Figs. 3–12 and 3–13). The mental retardation in trisomy 8 may be relatively mild.[4]

PARTIAL MONOSOMIES AND TRISOMIES (DELETIONS AND DUPLICATIONS)

These abnormalities can occur as de novo deletions or duplications, or as the result of

Table 3–10. Features of Trisomy 8

Area	Findings
General	Male preponderance (M,3:F,1)
Neurological	Mild to moderate retardation
Facies	Prominent lower lip; micrognathia; occasional strabismus; often similar to Williams' syndrome
Ears	Large, low-set, sometimes simple
Thorax	Kyphoscoliosis; vertebral anomalies; extra ribs; occasional spina bifida
Heart	<50% prevalence; discrete lesions (e.g., VSD, ASD, PDA)
Limbs	Ankylosed joints; clubfoot; camptodactyly; clinodactyly; arachnodactyly; brachydactyly; absent patella
Urogenital	Hypogonadism
Dermatoglyphics	Deep grooves (plis capitonnés) on palms and soles

unbalanced segregation in a parent carrying a balanced rearrangement such as a translocation or inversion. The breakpoints are unlikely to be exactly the same in any two non-related cases, even when the same cytogenetic band seems to be involved, and the situation is further complicated by the common presence of both monosomy for one segment and

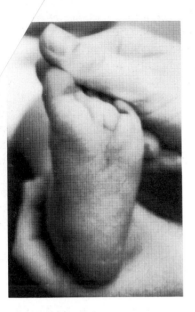

Fig. 3–12. Prominent grooves in the foot are characteristic of patients with trisomy 8.

trisomy for another segment in cases involving translocation. The phenotypes of most such cases are therefore highly variable, and not easy to fit into distinct syndromes. Several useful compendiums of the phenotypic features of specific partial trisomies and monosomies exist (e.g., Schinzel, 1984[18]) and a detailed discussion will not be presented here. However, a few clear-cut syndromes are associated with particular chromosome regions. In many cases, detailed cytogenetic and molecular analysis have shown that the main clinical features are associated with deletion or duplication of a very small chromosome region. Most cases are sporadic, but the transmission of a deletion or duplication from parent to child may mimic dominant inheritance, or segregation in cases with a parental balanced rearrangement may mimic recessive inheritance. In the following paragraphs we describe a few of the more common or illustrative duplication or deletion syndromes.

The concept of a **contiguous gene syndrome** has been developed to describe a situation in which deletion or duplication of several different closely spaced genes may be responsible for various individual features of a syndrome. However, in most cases evidence is insufficient to distinguish this idea from the competing one that all the features are caused by an abnormality in a single gene with wide-ranging effects on development.

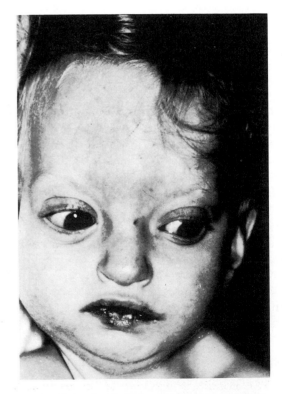

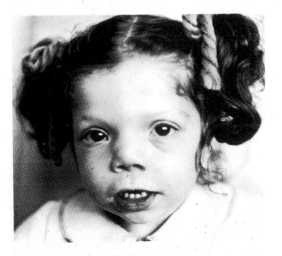

Fig. 3–13. The facies reminiscent of Williams syndrome is common in patients with trisomy 8. This patient has an 8 duplication resulting from an inversion.

Fig. 3–14. Craniofacial appearance of patient with 4p–syndrome. Note prominent glabella and widely spaced eyes with inner cathic folds—the "Greek warrior helmet" facies.

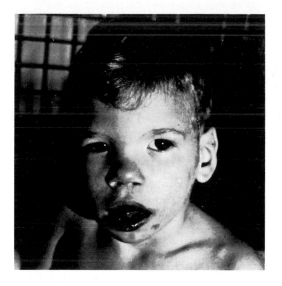

Fig. 3–15.   Patient with the cri-du-chat syndrome. The eyes are widely spaced with an inner canthic fold, but there is nothing pathognomonic about the facial features of this syndrome.

Monosomy 4p (4p- Syndrome or Wolff-Hirschhorn Syndrome)

The syndrome is produced by deletion of part of the most terminal band, 4p16 on the short arm of chromosome 4. There is severe mental retardation and a midline facial defect consisting of marked hypertelorism, a broad nasal root and bridge, and a prominent glabella. The facial appearance has been likened to that of a "Greek warrior helmet." (Fig. 3–14). Coloboma, large, low-set ears with preauricular tags, carp-mouth, cleft lip or palate, and midline scalp defects are present. Heart defects are common, but survival into adulthood can occur. Mental retardation is severe. A minute deletion has been demonstrated molecularly by in-situ hybridization in several patients with typical features but no cytogenetically detectable deletion.[1] If the clinical picture is suggestive, such studies should be pursued to rule out an inherited rearrangement as the source of the problem.

Monosomy 5p (Cri-du-Chat Syndrome)

This condition was one of the earliest deletion syndromes to be described,[14] but is rare, with an incidence of about 1 in 50,000 births.

The most striking feature of this syndrome, which gave it its original name of the "cri-du-chat" syndrome, is the peculiar mewing cry, like that of a kitten in distress, which is found in infants. The rest of the physical features are less diagnostic. The head is small, the eyes slant downwards (an "antimongoloid" slant), and the jaw is small (Fig. 3–15). Heart anomalies occur in about 20%. Mental and growth retardation are severe, but survival into adulthood is common. Although diagnosed cases commonly have a substantial deletion of chromosome 5p (Fig. 3–16), the syndrome may be seen in patients who have only a small very distal deletion of p15, and patients with deletions detectable only at the molecular level have been observed.

Monosomy 11 p13 (WAGR Syndrome)

This syndrome is discussed in more detail in Chapter 21. The initials WAGR stand for Wilms tumor (nephroblastoma), aniridia, genital abnormalities, and retardation of growth and development. (Table 3–11). The association of this syndrome with a specific small deletion made it possible to clone a gene for Wilms tumor in this region. This is one contiguous gene syndrome in which the involvement of several different genes has been demonstrated, because cases with different deletions at the molecular level may have some of the features of the syndrome but not others.

Duplication 11p15 (Beckwith-Wiedemann Syndrome; Exomphalos-Macroglassia-Gigantism)

Children with this syndrome are often large at birth and grow rapidly. There is macro-

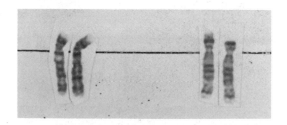

Fig. 3–16.   Banded preparation showing 5p–deletion.

Table 3–11.   Features of Monosomy 11p13

Area	Findings
General	Growth retardation
Neurologic	Mental retardation
Eyes	Aniridia (bilateral), glaucoma, cataracts, nystagmus
Heart	Cardiomyopathy
Urogenital	Wilms tumor, ambiguous genitalia, gonadoblastoma, gonadal dysgenesis
Enzymes	Catalase deficiency

glossia in 80% (Fig. 3–17), and often omphalocele or umbilical hernia. There is cytomegaly of the adrenal cortex, and visceromegaly involving kidneys, liver, spleen, pancreas, adrenal cortex, gonads, and pituitary. The kidneys show medullary dysplasia. Mild mental retardation may be present, and 8% have tumors which are often Wilms tumors.

This syndrome has been shown to be the result of duplication of a small region in chromosome 11p15 (distal to the region involved in the WAGR syndrome). The region involved appears to be imprinted (see Chapter 14), and inheritance of two paternal copies of 11p15 or inactivation of the maternal copy are apparently required to cause the syndrome.

Trisomy 11q32-qter (with Partial Monosomy 22q)

This syndrome was once thought to be caused by trisomy 22, because a 47th chromosome resembling 22 was present. However, the extra chromosome turned out to be a derived chromosome from a parental translocation between chromosomes 11 and 22 (Fig. 3–18). This translocation occurs nonrandomly, and is the most common reciprocal translocation in the population, so that many families with similarly chromosomally unbalanced offspring have been described.[7] The child receives 47 chromosomes as a result of 3:1 seg-

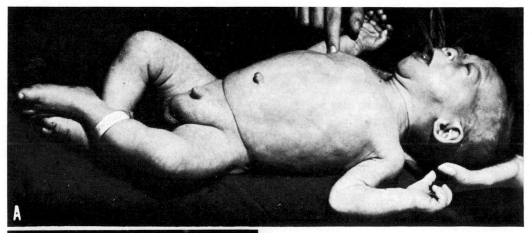

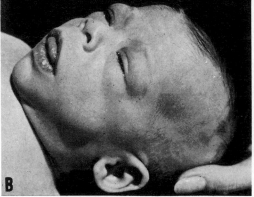

Fig. 3–17. Beckwith-Wiedemann syndrome. Full length view and view of head of patient (to better illustrate macroglossia).

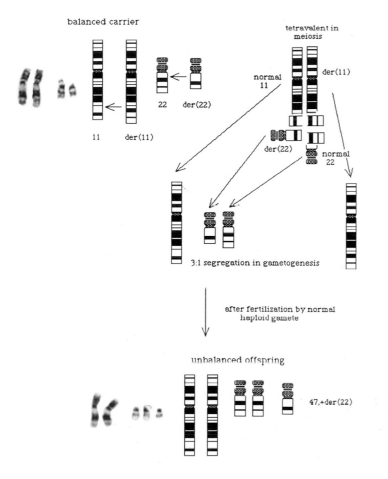

Fig. 3–18. 3:1 segregation at meiosis in reciprocal translocation t(11;22).

regation of the four chromosomes in the tetravalent formation at meiosis: the child inherits a normal 11, a normal 22, and a derived 22 from one parent. Although other forms of unbalanced gametes have been demonstrated to occur in sperm, these do not appear to result in liveborn offspring.

The features of the syndrome are anteverted nares, epicanthic folds, low-set malformed ears, preauricular tags, microcephaly, micrognathia and sometimes cleft palate and cardiac anomalies. Redundant skin folds of the neck, abnormal thumbs, and congenitally dislocated hips also occur. Severe growth and mental retardation are present.

Monosomy 13q

Many patients have been described with deletions of the long arm of chromosome 13. The phenotypic features depend on the position of the deleted segment.[19] Those with deletions including band 13q14.3 usually have retinoblastoma; it was the existence of patients with such deletions that led to the localization and cloning of the retinoblastoma gene (see Chap. 21). Growth retardation, mild to moderate mental retardation, and minor

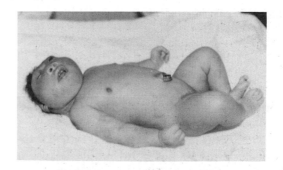

Fig. 3–19. Infant with del(13)(q32q34). Visible are severe microcephaly with nearly missing frontal lobes, and absent thumbs and great toes.

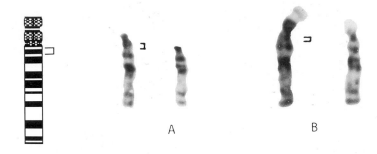

A   B

Fig. 3–20.   Deletion in Prader-Willi syndrome. Two cases showing deletion including bands q11 and q12. Deleted chromosome is on the right.

dysmorphic features are also usually present when the deletion includes only the more proximal bands of 13q. Major malformations including severe microcephaly, absent or hypoplastic thumbs, congenital heart defects, and abnormalities of the kidney and intestinal tract occur when the distal part of the chromosome is deleted (Fig. 3–19).

Prader-Willi Syndrome and Angelman Syndrome (Monosomy 15q11)

Both of these syndromes are associated with deletions of band 15q11 (Fig. 3–20). This is a region in which imprinting occurs; a paternal deletion in this region leads to Prader-Willi syndrome and a maternal deletion to Angelman syndrome. For a further discussion of the role of imprinting and uniparental disomy in these conditions, see Chapter 14.

Patients with Prader-Willi syndrome are characterized by hypotonia and poor feeding in early infancy, followed by obesity and an enormous appetite beginning in the second year. Mental retardation, small hands and feet, short stature, and hypogonadism are present. The progressively increasing obesity is illustrated in Figure 3–21. About 50% of patients have a cytogenetically detectable deletion, and another 20% a molecularly detectable deletion. The rest are the result of uniparental disomy or mutation.

Angelman syndrome is characterized by severe motor and mental retardation, ataxia with jerky movements, hypotonia, unusual facies with large mandible, and bouts of inappropriate laughter. It was also known as the "happy puppet syndrome." It is rarer than Prader-Willi syndrome, and a smaller propor-

tion of patients have a cytogenetically demonstrable deletion in 15q11.

Other Contiguous Gene Syndromes

Table 3–12 lists several other syndromes that have been associated with deletions or duplications of particular chromosome regions. These include Miller-Dieker syndrome, Langer Giedion syndrome, diGeorge syndrome, the "cat-eye" syndrome, and Smith-Magenis syndrome. Cytogenetic analysis may confirm the diagnosis in some cases, when a visible deletion, duplication, or translocation is present. However, cytogenetically undetectable deletions may be present, and the use of specific probes for either DNA analysis or in-situ hybridization is the method of choice for diagnostic purposes.

SUMMARY

About 1 in 200 live births has a visible chromosome abnormality. However, the number observed at birth is only a small proportion of those that occur at conception because most chromosomally abnormal conceptions end in spontaneous abortion. About 50% of first-trimester losses are the result of visible chromosome aberrations, with the most frequent being triploidy, monosomy X, and trisomy for many different chromosomes. Many anomalies, including most trisomies, are seen only in miscarriages. Karyotype analysis is indicated in any child with unexplained mental retardation or congenital anomalies, and in couples with multiple reproductive losses.

The recurrence risk for trisomy 21 is about 1% at all maternal ages, representing a sig-

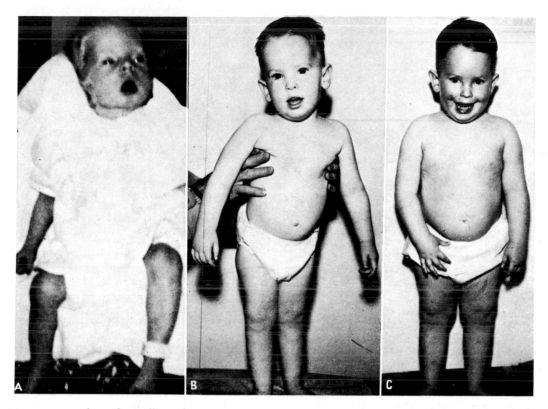

Fig. 3–21.   Patient with Prader-Willi syndrome as neonate and at 20 and 30 months. (Courtesy D.W. Smith. From Hall, B.D., and Smith, D.W.: Prader-Willi syndrome. J. Pediatr. 81:286, 1972.)

nificant increase in risk for younger mothers, though not for older mothers. Parental chromosome analysis should be performed when a child has an unbalanced rearrangement because about half of cases involve a parent with a balanced rearrangement who is at increased risk for miscarriages and other unbalanced offspring. Empirically derived risks are available for particular kinds of rearrangements. Prenatal diagnosis is recommended in couples with a previous trisomic birth or a known chromosomal rearrangement, as well as for women at increased risk for trisomy because of age.

The most common autosomal trisomy syndromes at birth are trisomy 21 (Down syndrome), trisomy 18, and trisomy 13. Most cases are the result of a free trisomy, but a few cases are the result of translocation. Chromosomal syndromes, caused by either whole trisomies or segmental aneuploidy, involve a wide variety of abnormalities, and often overlap in clinical features. In a subset of cases, the characteristic phenotypic features of the syndrome have been associated with duplication or deletion of a relatively small chromosomal region. In such cases, cytogenetically undetectable chromosome changes may be present. These may be recognizable with in-situ hybridization or DNA analysis.

Table 3–12.   Microdeletion or Contiguous Gene Syndromes

Syndrome	Region
Deletions	
Miller–Dieker	17p13
Di George	22q11
Langer–Giedion	8q24.1
WAGR	11p13
Prader–Willi, Angelman	15q11–12
Alagille	20p11.2–12
Smith–Magenis	17p11.2
Duplications	
Cat–eye	22q11
Beckwith–Wiedeman	17p15

REFERENCES

1. Alther, M.R., et al.: Molecular confirmation of Wolf-Hirschhorn syndrome with a subtle translocation of chromosome 4. Am. J. Hum. Genet. 49:1235, 1991.
2. Angell, R.R., Sandison, A., and Bain, D.A.: Chromosome variation in perinatal mortality: A survey of 500 cases. J. Med. Genet. 21:39, 1984.
3. Boué, A., and Gallano, P.: A collaborative study of the segregation of inherited chromosome structural rearrangements in 1356 prenatal diagnoses. Prenat. Diag. 4:45, 1984.
4. Cassidy, S.B., et al.: Trisomy 8 syndrome. Pediatrics 56:826, 1975.
5. Daniel, A., Hook, E.B., and Wulf, G.: Risks of unbalanced progeny at amniocentesis to carriers of chromosome rearrangements: Data from United States and Canadian laboratories. Am. J. Med. Genet. 31:14, 1989.
6. Edwards, J.H., et al.: A new trisomic syndrome. Lancet 1:787, 1960.
7. Fraccaro M., et al.: The 11q;22q translocation: A European collaborative study of 43 cases. Hum. Genet. 56:21, 1980.
8. Hook, E.B., and Cross, P.K.: Rates of mutant and inhertied structural cytogenetic abnormalities detected at amniocentesis. Results on about 63,000 fetuses. Ann. Hum. Genet. 51:27, 1987.
9. Hook, E.B. and Lindsjo, A.: Down syndrome in live births by single year maternal age interval in a Swedish study. Am. J. Hum. Genet. 30:19, 1978.
10. Hook, E.B.: The impact of aneuploidy upon public health. In Aneuploidy: Etiology and Mechanisms. Edited by Dellarco, V.L., Voytek, P.E., and Hollaender, A. New York, Plenum Press, 1986, p. 7.
11. Hook, E.B., and Hamerton, J.L.: The frequency of chromosome abnormalities detected in consecutive newborn studies, difference between studies, results by sex and by severity of phenotypic involvement. In Population Cytogenetics. Edited by Hook, E.B., and Porter I.H. New York, Academic Press, 1977, p. 63.
12. Hook, E.B.: Chromosome abnormalities and spontaneous fetal death following amniocentesis; further data and associations with maternal age. Am. J. Hum. Genet. 35:110, 1983.
13. Langdon-Down, J.: Observations on the ethnic classification of idiots. Lond. Hosp. Clin. Lec. Rep. 3:259, 1866.
14. Lejeune, J., et al.: Trois cas de délétion partielle de bras court d'un chromosome 5. C. R. Acad. Sci. (Paris) 257:3098, 1963.
15. Lejeune, J., Gautier, M., and Turpin, R.: Etude des chromosomes somatique de neuf enfants mongoliens. C. R. Acad. Sci. (Paris) 248:1721, 1959.
16. Merkatz, I.R. et al.: An association between low maternal serum alphafetoprotein and fetal chromosomal abnormalities. Am. J. Obstet. Gynec. 148:886, 1984.
17. Patau, K., et al.: Multiple congenital anomalies caused by an extra autosome. Lancet 1:790, 1960.
18. Schinzel, A.: Catalogue of Unbalanced Chromosome Aberrations in Man. New York, Walter de Gruyter, 1984.
19. Tranebjaerg, L., et al.: Interstitial deletion 13q: Further delineation of the syndrome by clinical and high resolution chromosome analysis of five patients. Am. J. Med. Genet. 29:739, 1988.
20. Warburton, D., et al.: Does the karyotype of a spontaneous abortion predict the karyotype of a subsequent abortion? Evidence from 273 women with two karyotyped spontaneous abortions. Am. J. Hum. Genet. 41:465, 1987.
21. Warburton, D.: Chromosomal Causes of Fetal Death. Clin. Obstet. Gynec. 30:268, 1987.

Chapter *4*

Sex Chromosomes and Their Abnormalities

EARLY STUDIES OF SEX CHROMOSOMES

The first two sex chromosome anomalies were reported in 1959, the same year the first autosomal chromosome anomaly was described. Jacobs and Strong[8] described a patient who had the clinical features of Klinefelter syndrome and a 47, XXY chromosome constitution. In the same year, Ford and coworkers[6] demonstrated monosomy for a C-group chromosome in a patient with Turner syndrome, and deduced that only one X chromosome was present. These findings first demonstrated the sex-determining nature of the Y chromosome, a fact that came as a surprise because of the very different and well-understood situation in the geneticists' favorite experimental animal, Drosophila, in which sex is determined by the ratio of autosomes to X chromosomes.

Earlier work on interphase nuclei had led to the discovery by Barr and Bertram,[1] in 1949, that female nuclei contained a dense mass of chromatin that was not present in male nuclei. First made in cats, the observation was extended to other mammals and humans. Although the exact percentage depends on

staining techniques and other factors, a normal female with an XX chromosome constitution will have a sex chromatin (or Barr) body in 20 to 60% of cells from a scraping of buccal mucosa (Fig. 4–1). A normal XY male has no cells with a true Barr body. In individuals with abnormal sex chromatin complements, the number of Barr bodies is equal to one less than the number of X chromosomes. Thus, an XXX female has two Barr bodies, whereas an XYY male has none. Females with Turner syndrome, who have only one X, have no Barr body, whereas males with Klinefelter syndrome, who have an XXY complement, have one Barr body. At one time, this sex chromatin test was commonly performed as a diagnostic tool for sex chromosome abnormalities. Today it is not generally used because karyotypic analysis is easily available, and is a much more reliable and informative procedure.

In the 1960s, studies of chromosome replication patterns using incorporation of tritiated thymidine showed that one of the human X chromosomes in females consistently replicated very late in the S period, and that this

55

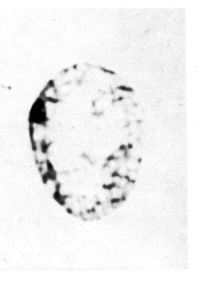

Fig. 4–1. Barr body. Note that this densely staining mass lies against the nuclear membrane.

late-replicating X chromosome remained highly condensed in interphase, to form the Barr body. In males, there is only one X chromosome, and thus no late-replicating X. In individuals with more than two X chromosomes, all but one of the X chromosomes becomes late-replicating.

THE LYON HYPOTHESIS

In 1961, Mary Lyon and others[11] put forward a concept to explain many of the puzzling facts about X chromosome behavior in mammals. This has come to be known as the Lyon hypothesis, and can be summarized as follows:

1. The late-replicating, condensed X chromosome in females is inactive, i.e., does not undergo transcription.
2. The inactivation may occur in either the paternally or maternally inherited X chromosome.
3. During an early stage of embryonic life, inactivation occurs in each cell, at random with respect to the paternal or maternal X. The same X remains inactive in all the descendants of each cell.
4. Each female is a mosaic, with some cells having an active paternal X and some an active maternal X.

The hypothesis was based on observations in the mouse. Female mice heterozygous for X-linked coat color mutations had patchy coats of two different colors, whereas male mice with only one X chromosome had single color coats. The same effect on coat pattern is seen in the female tortoise-shell cat, which has inherited one X chromosome with a gene giving orange coat color, whereas the other X chromosome has an allele giving black color. The color of each skin patch depends upon which X is active.

The Lyon hypothesis explains the phenomena of the sex chromatin body and the late replicating X by equating them with the inactive X chromosome. The single-active-X hypothesis also resolves the problem of why a female with two X chromosomes does not make twice as much of an X-linked gene product as does a male with only one X chromosome. "Dosage compensation" occurs because in any one cell only one X is functional. Inactivation occurs at an early stage when there are about 64 total cells in the embryo. Random X inactivation leads to about half the cells having an active paternal X and half an active maternal X; however, chance, or selection against one cell type, may sometimes lead to a preponderance of cells with one particular active X.

Many observations have confirmed the Lyon hypothesis.[12] Human females heterozygous for X-linked mutations can be demonstrated to be mosaic. For example, in a female heterozygous for an abnormal variant of the enzyme glucose-6-phosphate dehydrogenase (G6PD), about half of the red blood cells have the abnormal variant and half have the normal variant. Cells in tissue culture can be shown to express only one X-linked allele, and active and inactive X chromosomes have been separated in rodent-human somatic cell hybrid cells.

The sex-determining nature of the human Y chromosome, and the presence of a single active X in female cells, can explain most of the observations concerning the phenotype of individuals with sex chromosome anomalies. However, certain exceptions to these rules have been important in furthering our understanding of the structure and function of the sex chromosomes.

THE Y CHROMOSOME

The human Y chromosome is a small acrocentric chromosome, in which about half of the long arm consists of heterochromatin, which fluoresces brilliantly with Q-banding and is C-band positive. This part of the chromosome is heteromorphic in size, and may even be completely missing without affecting the phenotype. Because there are no traits which clearly show Y-linked inheritance, it is believed that few genes reside only on the Y chromosome except those that influence sexual differentiation. A subset of genes on the Y chromosome are homologous to genes on the X chromosome. These are known as **pseudoautosomal** genes because their pattern of inheritance will be indistinguishable as a rule from autosomal loci.[3]

The pseudoautosomal region is at the distal end of the Y short arm, and forms the pairing segment with the X chromosome at meiosis. Just proximal to the pseudoautosomal region is the region containing the gene or genes (SRY and perhaps others) that control the development of the embryonic gonad into a testis. (Fig. 4-2). This embryonic switch is necessary (but not sufficient) to ensure male differentiation of the internal and external organs (see Chapter 11). There is also some evidence for the presence of a gene controlling spermatogenesis and a gene controlling stature on the proximal long arm of the Y.

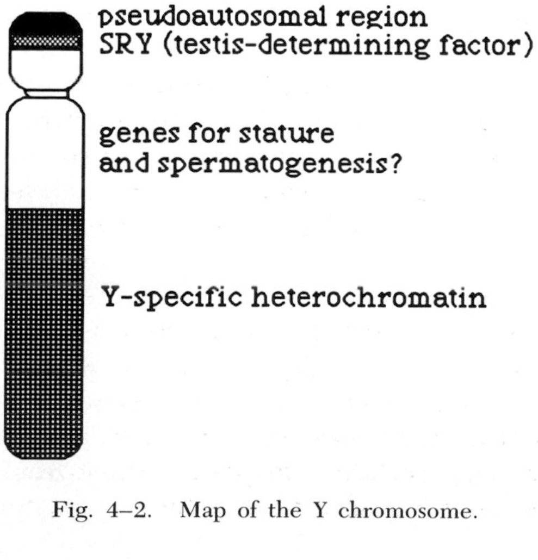

In the pseudoautosomal region, there is an obligatory cross-over between the X and Y chromosomes, necessary for proper segregation of the X and Y chromosomes. Occasionally crossovers occur in the more proximal region of the Y, transferring the segment containing the sex determining genes to the terminal short arm of the X, and leaving a Y chromosome lacking these genes. Offspring receiving the chromosomes resulting from such exchange may be **XX males** or **XY females**: their sex chromosomes usually look entirely normal cytogenetically. The study of individuals with such unusual chromosomes was of critical importance in pinpointing the exact location of candidate genes for the testis-determining factors.[15]

Most of the Y chromosome appears to consist of many different families of repeat DNA sequences. These have been cloned from the centromere, the long arm and the short arm of the Y chromosome, and can be used as probes for in situ hybridization to identify the Y chromosome or Y chromosome rearrangements. This is illustrated in Plate 4.

THE X CHROMOSOME

The X chromosome is a large submetacentric chromosome that appears to be as gene-dense as any autosome. More genes have been assigned to the X chromosome than to any other, because the pattern of inheritance makes it comparatively easy to make this assignment. The genes on the X do not have any special relationship to sexual differentiation, but may affect any tissue.

One specialized region of the X of great interest is the **X-inactivation center.** When there is an interchange between an X chromosome and an autosome, inactivation of the autosome may occur. Studies of such cases and of abnormal X chromosomes have indicated that X-inactivation starts at a particular region of the chromosome and spreads outward in both directions. The inactivation center can be localized to band Xq13 in the proximal long arm.

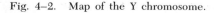

pseudoautosomal region
SRY (testis-determining factor)

genes for stature
and spermatogenesis?

Y-specific heterochromatin

Fig. 4-2. Map of the Y chromosome.

Investigation of rodent-human hybrid cell lines containing only an inactive X chromosome led to the isolation of a gene product produced only by the inactive X, which was coded for by a gene in Xq13.[2] Studies of the function of this gene, known as XIST, may shed light on the mechanism of X inactivation. Although changes in DNA methylation have been found to be associated with X inactivation, it is not known whether this is a primary or secondary event.

As will be described in the next section, individuals with abnormal numbers of X chromosomes often do not have normal gonads, and may have other abnormalities as well. This would not be expected if the inactivated X chromosomes had no functional activity. Although most genes on the inactive X chromosome are not transcribed, there are exceptions. Genes that escape inactivation occur in the pseudoautosomal region at the distal end of the X short arm, and there are also genes just proximal to this region, such as those determining the Xg blood group and steroid sulfatase, that are not inactivated. Other genes escaping inactivation are known in the more proximal short arm and in the long arm near the inactivation center (Fig. 4–3).

THE 45, X TURNER SYNDROME (GONADAL DYSGENESIS, BONNEVIE-ULLRICH)

Most of the phenotypic features of what is now called the Turner syndrome were de-scribed in 1930 by Ullrich, who reported a combination of anomalies in an 8-year-old girl, including webbing of the neck, cubitus valgus, congenital lymphangiectatic edema, prominent ears, ptosis, small mandible, dystrophy of the nails, and hypoplastic nipples.[17] In 1938, Turner[16] observed webbing of the neck and cubitus valgus together with sexual infantilism in young women. Ullrich did not describe sexual infantilism in his first or subsequent reports because his patients were children, whereas Turner's patients were young adults. After the discovery of sex chromatin, it was recognized that patients with what had come to be called Turner syndrome were sex chromatin negative. In 1959, Ford and colleagues[6] could relate this to the presence of a 45,X karyotype (Fig. 4–4).

The incidence of Turner syndrome is approximately 1 in 5000 female births. About half the cases have a 45,X chromosome constitution.[7] (Although this is sometimes written in the literature as 45,XO, this designation is incorrect because there is no "O" chromosome). About 7% of spontaneous abortions also have the 45,X karyotype, so that the incidence of this abnormality at conception must be at least 1%. This means that about 99% of all conceptions with a 45,X chromosome complement die in utero; the usual phenotype is an embryonic lethal. This is somewhat surprising in view of the usually benign features of Turner syndrome at birth. One explanation that has been put forward is that all surviving cases may be mosaics with a normal cell line, or were so in embryonic life. It appears that pseudoautosomal genes must be present in duplicate for normal development to proceed. One must postulate such loci to explain why having a single X chromosome leads to embryonic lethality or Turner syndrome, whereas the presence of either an additional inactive X or a Y leads to fairly normal development.[15]

Studies on the parental origin of the X chromosome in Turner syndrome have found that the single X chromosome is of maternal origin in about two thirds of cases. One can conclude that most cases do not arise from maternal nondisjunction, but either from pa-

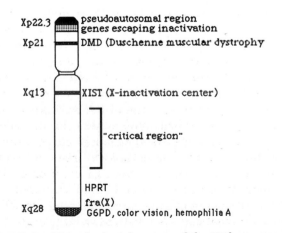

Fig. 4–3.   Map of selected regions of the X chromosome.

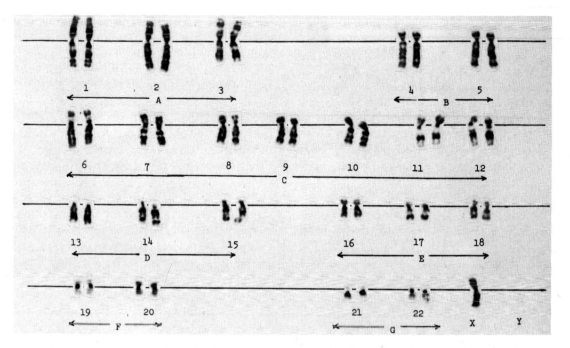

Fig. 4-4.   Giemsa-banded karyotype of patient with 45,X Turner syndrome.

ternal nondisjunction or anaphase lag during an early cell division. No difference in phenotype has been found between cases with a maternally derived X and those with a paternally derived X. There is no relationship to advanced maternal age; among spontaneous abortions the 45,X karyotype has been found to be especially common in young mothers.

Table 4-1 summarizes the features of Turner syndrome. The most constant feature of Turner syndrome is shortness of stature, which begins before puberty but is especially pronounced in adulthood; adult height rarely exceeds 60 inches. The mean verbal IQ is normal, but the mean performance IQ is about 10 points below average because of specific space-form perception and visual-motor deficits. Patients may have difficulty in map-reading, figure drawing, and mathematics. The appearance of the face is distinctive, with a narrow maxilla, small chin, low-set ears, epicanthic folds and ptosis (Fig. 4-5). Only about 50% of patients have the webbing of the neck that is often considered the characteristic anomaly of the syndrome (Fig. 4-6). Spontaneously aborted fetuses with the 45,X karyo-

type, and 45,X fetuses observed with ultrasound during the second trimester often have large cystic hygromata of the neck (Fig. 4-7); this may be the forerunner of the loose neck skin or webbing seen at birth. A low posterior hairline and pigmented nevi are frequently found. A useful diagnostic sign in infants and children is the lymphedema of the hands and feet (Fig. 4-8). Short fourth and fifth metacarpals are another characteristic sign. (Fig. 4-9).

A shield-shaped chest with widely spaced and hypoplastic nipples are common features. Approximately 50% of patients have cardiovascular disease. Many of the somatic stigmata of Turner syndrome (though not the gonadal dysgenesis) are also found in patients with Noonan syndrome, which is inherited as an autosomal dominant, and may occur in males as well as females (see Chapter 8). A useful dichotomy in cardiac pathology exists between Turner syndrome and Noonan syndrome. In Turner syndrome, coarctation of the aorta is the most common lesion, accounting for 70% of malformations. No patient with confirmed Turner syndrome has been reported to have

Table 4–1. Features of Turner Syndrome*

Area	Findings
General	**Female**. Normal life expectancy may be altered by cardiovascular or renal disease. **Invariably small stature** for age with eventual height attainment rarely exceeding 60 inches; chromatin-negative
Neurological	Intellectual development is generally good but is usually below the attainment of siblings; perceptive hearing loss is common
Skin	Frequent pigmented nevi
Head	Characteristic facies; narrow maxilla; small mandible
Eyes	Frequent epicanthic folds; occasional ptosis; infrequent hypertelorism
Ears	**Usually normal**, sometimes prominent
Mouth	Sharklike—curved upper lip, straight lower lip
Neck	Low posterior hairline; webbed in about 50% of patients
Chest	Shield shaped; widely spaced hypoplastic nipples; underdevelopment of the breasts
Cardiovascular	Anomalies in approximately 35%; **coarctation of the aorta** is most common; pulmonic stenosis rarely if ever occurs; occasional idiopathic hypertension
Extremities	Cubitus valgus; lymphedema of dorsum of hands and feet in infancy; dystrophic nails; short fourth and fifth metacarpals; short fifth finger with clinodactyly; medial tibial exostosis
Urogenital	**Ovarian dysgenesis with infertility** (only 6 reported instances of fertility)
Roentgenogram	Hypoplasia of lateral ends of clavicles and sacral wings; platyspondylia; metaphyseal dysplasia of long bones; "positive metacarpal sign" (short fourth and fifth metacarpals)
Dermatoglyphics	Distal axial triradius in 20 to 30% higher than average ridge count
Incidence	1:5000 (1:2500 females)

*Many findings are similar to or identical with those observed in the Noonan syndrome. (See Table 8–3.) Features that help to distinguish between the syndromes are in **bold face**.

pulmonic stenosis. The opposite is true of the Noonan syndrome, in which the characteristic cardiac lesion is pulmonic stenosis, and coarctation of the aorta is rare.

Patients with Turner syndrome have a uterus and normal female external genitalia, but as a rule do not undergo the changes of puberty,

do not menstruate, and are infertile. In the adult, the ovaries are replaced by connective tissue—so-called "streak gonads"—and ovulation does not occur. Although the ovaries in Turner syndrome differentiate normally and

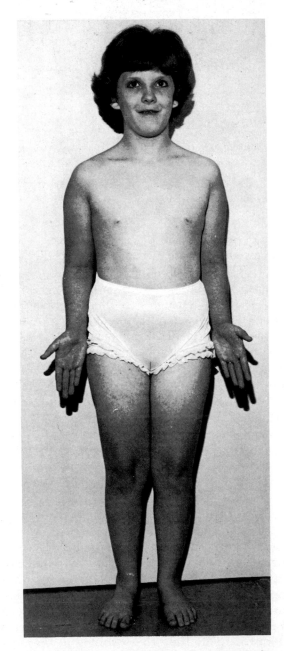

Fig. 4–5.   Fourteen-year-old girl with Turner syndrome. Note that she has the facies and somatic features of the disorder, but like 50% of patients with Turner syndrome, she does not have webbing of the neck. Her height at this age is 55 inches.

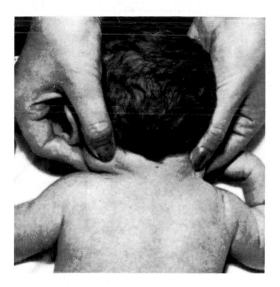

Fig. 4–6. Prominent webbing of the neck and low posterior hairline in newborn with Turner syndrome.

nal testicular material there is a risk of gonadoblastoma or other gonadal tumors, so that removal of the gonads is recommended.

Nonmosaic structural anomalies of the X chromosome are also sometimes associated with gonadal dysgenesis. Patients with an isochromosome for the X long arm, karyotype 46,X, i(Xq), are missing one copy of the X short arm, and have most of the features of Turner syndrome (Fig. 4–10). Such patients are sex chromatin positive because the i(Xq) is inactivated. Patients with large short arm deletions may also have gonadal dysgenesis, although some patients with only small terminal deletions have only short stature.

Patients with deletions of the X long arm, or occasional patients with i(Xp), have gonadal dysgenesis, but not short stature or the other somatic features of Turner syndrome. There is

oocytes are present in fetal life, the primary oocytes degenerate and are usually absent at birth. The rate of attrition of germ cells is somewhat variable, so that a few individuals with Turner syndrome have been reported to menstruate, and a very few have reproduced.

Patients with Turner syndrome can be treated with hormonal therapy, which must be carefully timed and administered to achieve significant improvement in growth. With hormonal therapy, breast development, pubarche, and menarche can occur. Women with Turner syndrome have borne children through appropriate hormone treatment to maintain pregnancy, and implantation of a donor egg fertilized in vitro.

OTHER CHROMOSOME CONSTITUTIONS IN GONADAL DYSGENESIS

Almost 50% of patients with Turner syndrome are mosaic, with one of the cell lines being 45,X.[7] The other cell line may be XX, XXX, XY, or contain a structural anomaly of the X or Y chromosome. The phenotype may be modified by the presence of the other cell line: for example, some patients with an XY line may have some masculinization of the external genitalia, and the gonads may contain testicular tissue. In all patients with abdomi-

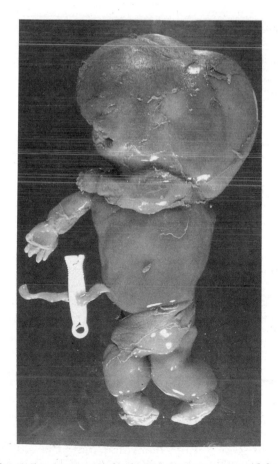

Fig. 4–7. Spontaneously aborted 20-week macerated fetus with huge cystic hygromata, edema, and karyotype 45,X.

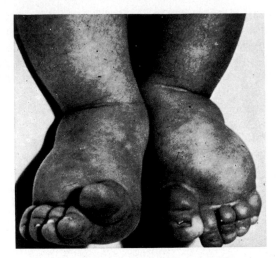

Fig. 4–8.   Pedal lymphedema and nail dysplasia of Turner syndrome.

also a group of patients with gonadal dysgenesis who have an apparently balanced translocation involving an autosome and the long arm of the X chromosome. For unknown reasons, if the breakpoint in the X long arm is in the so-called "critical region," between Xq13 and Xq27, gonadal dysgenesis often occurs.

In X chromosome structural abnormalities, one generally finds that the abnormal X chromosome is inactive in all or most cells. This has been ascribed to "preferential inactivation." However, it is more likely to be caused by a selective disadvantage of cells that have inactivated the normal X, since they will lack expression of that part of the X chromosome which is absent from the abnormal chromosome. This principle is illustrated by what is observed in X/autosome translocations. Here, the normal X is usually found to be inactivated in balanced translocation carriers because inactivation of the other X can spread to the autosomal material and lead to functional partial monosomy. However, in unbalanced X/autosome translocations the opposite occurs because inactivation of the X bearing the translocation eliminates the functional trisomy for the autosomal material (Fig. 4–11).

Some female patients with short stature and features of Turner syndrome may also have a structurally abnormal Y chromosome, in which the male determining factor has been lost. For example, the karyotype 46,X, i(Yq) is also associated with full-blown Turner syndrome. Other variant Y chromosomes (ring Y, Yp-) may also be found.

Gonadal dysgenesis may also occur in patients who have apparently normal sex chromosome complements, either XX or XY. These cases may result from either cytogenetically invisible sex chromosome rearrangements or mutation of genes involved in sex determination.

47,XXY (KLINEFELTER SYNDROME)

In 1942, Klinefelter and coworkers[10] recognized a pattern of anomalies in males that did not become evident until adolescence. These include small testes, absent spermatogenesis, high urinary gonadotropins, and frequently eunuchoid habitus and gynecomastia (Fig. 4–12). Jacobs and Strong observed an XXY karyotype in such a patient in 1959, and that same year the simultaneous anomalies of Klinefelter and Down syndrome were re-

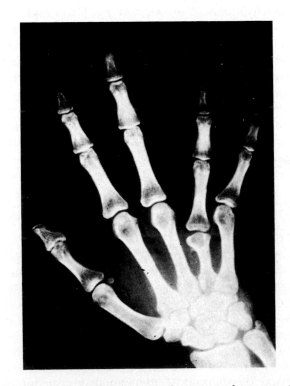

Fig. 4–9.   Unusually short fourth metacarpal common in Turner syndrome.

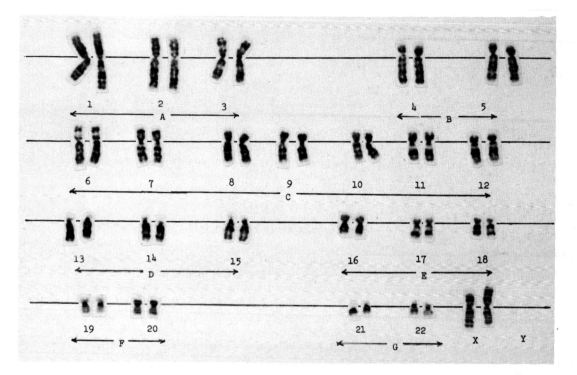

Fig. 4-10.   Isochrome X made up of two long arams [X,i(Xg)].

ported in the same patient by Ford and co-workers.[5] Patients with the 47,XXY karyotype are sex chromatin positive because one X is inactivated. Recent studies using X-linked markers have demonstrated that about half the cases result from nondisjunction in spermatogenesis, and half from nondisjunction in oogenesis. The 47,XXY karyotype is associated with advancing maternal age just like the autosomal trisomies.

Klinefelter syndrome occurs in approximately 1 in 1000 male births, but is not usually diagnosed in infancy or childhood. Studies have found, however, that the 47,XXY karyotype is not as benign as previously thought because there is a higher than normal rate of loss in intrauterine life, and life expectancy is significantly reduced. Because most children with the 47,XXY karyotype do not look abnormal, it is rarely diagnosed in children usually because of behavioral problems or mild mental retardation. Most cases are found after adolescence because of inadequate sexual development, gynecomastia, or infertility (Table 4-2). Body hair may be sparse,

and the patient may not have to shave. The most consistent features are the small testes, which usually do not exceed 2 cm in length, and the lack of spermatogenesis. Biopsy re-

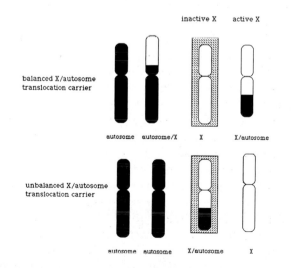

Fig. 4-11.   In the case of an X/autosome translocation, X chromosome inactivation is not random: cells preferentially survive that preserve normal diploid function of the autosomal segment.

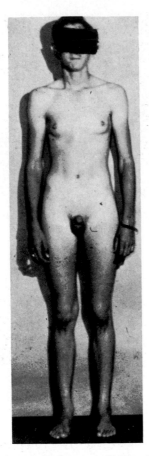

Fig. 4–12. Phenotypic features of Klinefelter syndrome (although gynecomastia is found in only 25% of patients with the XXY anomaly).

veals hyalinized or small immature seminiferous tubules and Leydig cell hyperplasia. Dermatoglyphic patterns may also be unusual (see Chapter 17). Intellectual achievement is often below that of siblings, but is highly variable. In patients who have been diagnosed prenatally or at birth in screening programs, problems in both learning and behavior at school have been seen more often than in controls.[13]

OTHER ABNORMAL KARYOTYPES IN KLINEFELTER SYNDROME VARIANTS

Mosaicism with an XY karyotype is not uncommon in Klinefelter syndrome. Less common are patients who have a Y chromosome plus more than two X chromosomes, e.g.,

karyotypes 48,XXXY and 49,XXXXY. The degree of intellectual impairment increases with the number of X chromosomes, even though all but one are inactivated. The 49,XXXXY karyotype is associated with characteristic congenital malformations, which may even be confused with Down syndrome. Retardation is significant, and there is a low nasal bridge, inner epicanthic folds, mongoloid slant, and occasional Brushfield spots. (Table 4–3 and Fig. 4–13). X-rays often reveal radioulnar synostosis, and occasional heart lesions have been described. The buccal smear shows three sex chromatin bodies (Fig. 4–14).

Rarely, males with features of Klinefelter syndrome turn out to have an XX karyotype. These **XX males** can almost always be found to have material from the sex-determining region of the Y chromosome, which has been transferred from the Y to the X during meiosis by crossing over. Their hypogonadism is similar to that in Klinefelter syndrome, but they are not usually as tall, and have normal intelligence.

47,XYY MALES

The first report of a male with two Y chromosomes was published by Sandberg and co-workers in 1961.[14] The frequency of the 47,XYY karyotype is about 1 in 1000 male births. All cases of 47,XYY must result from nondisjunction at meiosis II in the father, and as expected, there is no association with advanced maternal age.

Table 4–2. Features of Klinefelter Syndrome

Area	Findings
General	Phenotypic males with chromatin-positive buccal smear; no detectable somatic abnormality in childhood; diagnosis usually made in adolescence or adult life; tall eunuchoid habitus common
Neurological	Intellectual development fair to good but usually less than that of sibs
Chest	Frequent gynecomastia
Urogenital	Small testes in adolescence and adult (<2 cm in length); infertile
Dermatoglyphics	Average ridge count is low
Incidence	Approximately 1:850 live male births

Table 4–3. Features of XXXXY Syndrome

Area	Findings
General	Phenotypic males may have some genital ambiguity; small stature
Neurological	Retarded: IQ between 25 and 50; moderate hypotonia and joint laxity
Head	Characteristics facies (often confused with mongoloid); low nasal bridge; protruding mandible; occasional flat occiput
Eyes	Epicanthic folds, mongoloid slant; occasional Brushfield spots; strabismus
Ears	Malformed; low-set
Neck	Short; occasionally webbed
Cardiovascular	Occasional congenital heart lesions (e.g., PDA)
Extremities	Limited elbow pronation; genu valgum; clinodactyly of fifth finger
Urogenital	Small penis and testes; frequent cryptorchism
Roentgenogram	Radioulnar synostosis
Dermatoglyphics	Average ridge count is low (<60); frequent low arches; occasional simian line
Incidence	Undetermined; relatively uncommon

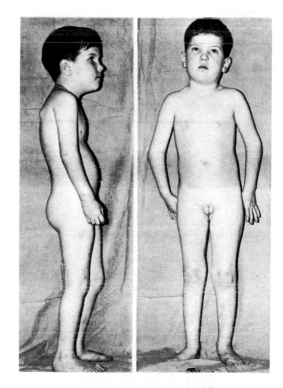

Fig. 4–13. Five-year-old boy with XXXXY syndrome. His IQ was 50. Note arm deformity of severe radioulnar synostosis.

Public attention was first directed to these patients in 1965, when Jacobs and coworkers[9] discovered that men in maximum security hospitals had a higher frequency of the 47,XYY karyotype than could be ascribed to chance. This and other studies suggested that males with two Y chromosomes were taller, tended to have severe acne, and were more aggressive than XY males. Other surveys have borne out the increased incidence of the XYY sex chromosome constitution in prison populations, although they also found an increased frequency of the 47,XXY karyotype. Physical anomalies such as hypogonadism, seizures, early acne, and radioulnar synostosis have also been associated with the 47,XYY karyotype. However, many men with the 47,XYY karyotype are normal.

The possible relationship of the XYY chromosome constitution to criminal behavior became an area of intense controversy and public interest in the 1960s and 70s. Investigators in several countries set out to do prospective studies by screening newborn males at birth to detect those with the XYY chromosome constitution. Although these studies were eventually stopped because of opposition from those who felt they were unethical, they did provide a group of XYY males who have continued to be followed, and have provided important information on the phenotype. Another group of patients has been provided by

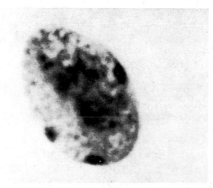

Fig. 4–14. Three Barr bodies in patient with XXXXY syndrome.

cases that are now diagnosed prenatally during routine screening because of advanced maternal age.

The follow-up studies[13] indicate that, on the average, patients with XYY have normal IQ and no serious medical problems. They may be unusually tall, and often have significant behavioral and learning problems as children and young adults. However, the stereotypic picture of excessively aggressive behavior does not seem to be borne out by these studies. XYY males are generally fertile, but do not produce male offspring with additional sex chromosomes, for reasons not yet understood.

47,XXX FEMALES (TRIPLE-X; TRISOMY X)

This karyotype occurs in about 1 in 1000 female births, and is associated with advanced maternal age. Most patients have no distinguishing physical features, although menstrual disorders and early menopause may occur. Early studies that found these patients in homes for the mentally retarded presented a biased picture of outcome. However, follow-up studies of cases diagnosed at birth or prenatally have confirmed a significant reduction in average IQ, and found learning disabilities in many of the children.[13] Like XYY males, XXX females are generally fertile, but do not have offspring with additional sex chromosomes.

Patients with four and five X chromosomes are also found rarely, and like the males with multiple X chromosomes, are more severely retarded than the 47,XXX females. The **penta-X female** is similar in phenotype to the XXXXY male. Four sex chromatin bodies are present.

SUMMARY

The phenotypic sex of an individual is determined with few exceptions by the presence (male) or absence (female) of a Y chromosome. Most of the X chromosome is subject to inactivation, and a single active X is usually present in any cell. In females, one of the two Xs is randomly inactivated in each cell during early embryonic development. The inactive X is visible as a sex chromatin or Barr body on the nuclear membrane. The Y chromosome contains sequences on the distal short arm that have homologues on the X chromosome, the pseudoautosomal segment. Proximal to this is the region containing the sex-determining gene or genes. Most of the Y long arm consists of inactive heterochromatin.

The X chromosome contains some genes that are not inactivated, mainly in the distal short arm. These may be responsible for the phenotypic abnormalities found in individuals with missing or extra X chromosomes. However, much less developmental abnormality results from sex chromosome aneuploidy than from autosomal aneuploidy. Females with the 45,X karyotype and males with the XXY karyotype are generally sterile, with absence of germ cells in the gonads. The 45,X karyotype also results in the somatic features of Turner syndrome, including short stature and frequent heart defects. The same phenotype is often associated with mosaicism for the presence of a second normal or structurally abnormal sex chromosome. Most other sex chromosome aneuploidies are associated with few development defects, although mild to moderate mental retardation and behavioral problems may be present.

REFERENCES

1. Barr, M.L., and Bertram, E.G.: A morphological distinction between neurones of the male and female, and the behaviour of the nucleolar satellite during accelerated nucleoprotein synethesis. Nature 163:676, 1949.
2. Brown, C.J., et al.: A gene from the region of the human X inactivation center is expressed exclusively from the inactive X chromosome. Nature 349:38, 1991.
3. Ellis, N., and Goodfellow, P.N.: The mammalian pseudoautosomal region. Trends Genet. 5:406, 1989.
4. Fisher, E.M.C., et al.: Homologous ribosomal protein genes on the human X and Y chromosomes: Escape from X inactivation and implications for Turner syndrome. Cell 61:1205, 1990.
5. Ford, C.E., et al.: The chromosomes in a patient showing both mongolism and the Klinefelter syndrome. Lancet 1:711, 1959.
6. Ford, C.E., et al.: A sex-chromosome anomaly in a case of gonadal dysgenesis (Turner's syndrome). Lancet 1:711, 1959.
7. Hook, E.B., and Warburton, D.: The distribution of chromosomal genotypes associated with Turner syndrome: Livebirth prevalence rates and evidence for diminished fetal mortality and severity in genotypes associated with structural X abnormalities or mosaicism. Ann. Hum. Genet. 64:24, 1983.

8. Jacobs, P., and Strong, J.A.: A case of human intersexuality having a possible XXY sex-determining mechanism. Nature 183:302, 1959.

9. Jacobs, P.A., et al.: Aggressive behaviour, mental subnormality and the XYY male. Nature 208:302, 1959.

10. Klinefelter, H.F., Reifenstein, E.C., and Albright, F.: Syndrome characterized by gynecomastia, aspermatogenesis without A-Leydigism and increased excretion of follicle stimulation hormone. J. Clin. Endocrinol. 2:615, 1942.

11. Lyon, M.F.: Sex chromatin and gene action in the mammalian X-chromosome. Am. J. Hum. Genet. 14:135, 1962.

12. Lyon, M.F.: X-chromosome inactivation and the location and expression of X-linked genes. Am. J. Hum. Genet. 42:8, 1988.

13. Ratcliffe, S.G., and Paul, N. (eds.): Prospective studies on children with sex chromosome aneuploidy. March of Dimes Birth Defects Foundation, Birth Defects Original Article Series 22(3). Alan R. Liss, New York, 1986.

14. Sandberg, A.A., Koepf, C.F., Ishihara, T., and Hauschka, T.A.: An XYY human male. Lancet 1:488, 1961.

15. Sinclair A.H., et al.: A gene from the human sex-determining motif. Nature 346:240, 1990.

16. Turner, H.H.: A syndrome of infantilism, congenital webbed neck and cubitus valgus. Endocrinology 23:566, 1938.

17. Ullrich, P.: Turner's syndrome and status Bonnevie-Ullrich: A synthesis of animal phenogenetics and clinical observations on a typical complex of developmental anomalies. Am. J. Hum. Genet. 1:179, 1949.

Chapter 5

Genetic Basis of Heredity

ELEMENTARY, MY DEAR WATSON.

DR. A. CONAN DOYLE

One of the most exciting discoveries in biology and, indeed, in all science of the last two decades has been the biochemical nature of the gene and its mechanism of action, in precise biochemical terms. Further details can be found in Chapter 7. A summary of the current view of the gene's biochemical structure and functions will be presented here.

THE STRUCTURE AND FUNCTION OF THE GENE

In bacteria, the genetic material is a strand of deoxyribonucleic acid, or DNA. The brilliant work of Watson and Crick showed this material to consist of a double-stranded helix, like a rope ladder, in which the ropes are made up of alternating deoxyribose (a sugar) and phosphate molecules, and the rungs consist of purine and pyrimidine bases, held together by hydrogen bonds, the ladder being twisted into a double helix (Fig. 5–1).

The purine bases are adenine (A) and guanine (G), and the pyrimidine bases are cytosine (C) and thymine (T); the stereochemical restrictions are such that G on one strand can pair only with C on the other, and A with T. Thus the sequence of bases on one strand is **complementary** to that on the other (Fig. 5–2).

A deoxyribose, a phosphate group, and a base constitute a **nucleotide**, so a DNA strand is a nucleotide polymer, or polynucleotide. Because the deoxyribose is linked to one phosphate group at the 3′ position, and to the other at the 5′ position, the strand has polarity and the complementary strands run in opposite directions.

When the DNA replicates, the two strands separate and each, with the aid of an enzyme, DNA polymerase, lays down a new complementary strand to form two new helices, identical in base sequence with the original (Fig. 5–1). In higher organisms, the DNA is associated with proteins, particularly histones, to form the microscopically visible chromosomes depicted in Chapter 2.

It is now well established that genes act by determining the amino acid sequences of polypeptides and, thereby, the structures and properties of proteins. For each polypeptide being synthesized there is a corresponding region of a chromosome in which the sequence of base pairs in the DNA determines the amino acid sequence of the polypeptide, and that particular sequence of the DNA is said to be

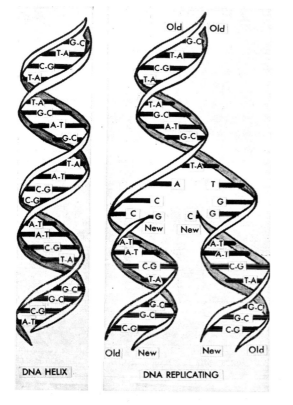

DNA HELIX

DNA REPLICATING

Fig. 5–1. Diagrams of the DNA double helix, and of DNA replicating.

the gene for the polypeptide. A mutant gene results in an altered amino acid sequence, which may alter the structure of the polypeptide, and hence its properties, thus leading to a genetically determined defect in the corresponding protein, be it an enzyme as in the inborn errors of metabolism, or other protein as in the abnormal hemoglobins.

This concept was first suggested by the observation that in sickle cell anemia the mutant gene causing the disease resulted in an abnormal hemoglobin. Sickle cell hemoglobin differed from normal hemoglobin only in that the sixth amino acid from the N-terminal was a valine instead of a glutamic acid. Thus a single gene difference was associated with a single amino acid substitution in a particular polypeptide. Evidence from microbial genetics confirmed that *a gene is that portion of the DNA responsible for the primary structure (amino acid sequence) of a particular polypeptide.*

The means by which the gene determines the amino acid sequence of its polypeptide is, briefly, as follows (Fig. 5–2). The sequence of bases in the DNA constitutes a code for the amino acid sequence of the polypeptide, a triplet of three bases (or codon) corresponding to one amino acid. For instance, the triplet CTT at a particular place on the DNA codes for a glutamic acid at the corresponding place on the polypeptide. Evidence from study of the amino acid substitutions in mutant hemoglobins suggests that the genetic code in man is the same as in bacteria (Chap. 6).

The **translation** of the DNA code into protein is done by means of a special type of ribonucleic acid, or RNA, called messenger RNA, or mRNA. RNA differs from DNA in being single-stranded, with ribose instead of deoxyribose and the pyrimidine uracil (U) instead of thymine. The mRNA is synthesized on the DNA strand (by the action of the enzyme RNA polymerase) with the same kind of complementary pairing as the two DNA strands; for instance, a CTT triplet in the DNA would correspond to a GAA triplet in the RNA. Thus *the mRNA has a sequence of bases determined by that of the corresponding DNA strand.* The mRNA migrates from the nucleus to the cytoplasm and becomes associated with a ribosome (which contains another kind of RNA, the ribosomal RNA, or rRNA); there it acts as a mold, or template, on which the amino acids are assembled into polypeptides in the following way.

A third type of RNA, the transfer RNA, or tRNA, exists in the cytoplasm in many varieties, one or more for each amino acid. It serves to bring the amino acids to the messenger, for incorporation into the polypeptide. To do this, the transfer RNA must be able to recognize a specific amino acid, on the one hand, and a specific place on the mRNA, on the other. Thus each species of tRNA has a site—the recognition site—that combines specifically with a particular amino acid, and another site with a particular triplet—an "anticodon"—that can attach to the appropriate codon in the messenger. The structures of the various tRNAs (known as "adaptors" because they adapt the amino acids for incorporation

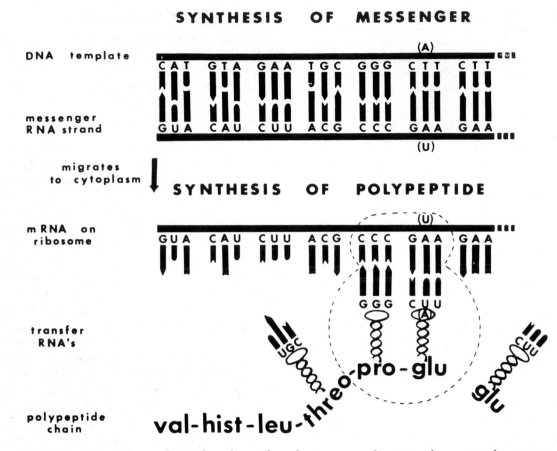

Fig. 5–2.   Diagram illustrating synthesis of a polypeptide with a sequence of amino acids corresponding to a sequence of nucleotide triplets in the DNA. A glutamic acid (glu) is about to be attached to the growing end. Substituting A for T, as in the bracket, would change glu to val, as in sickle cell hemoglobin.

into the polypeptide) and the biochemistry of the following process are well-known, but beyond the scope of this text.

As the ribosome moves along the messenger RNA strand in a 5′ to 3′ direction, each codon in turn is brought into a position where it can (with the aid of appropriate enzymes, RNA polymerases) combine with the anticodon on a molecule of the corresponding tRNA so that the amino acid is brought into position to be attached to the growing polypeptide chain. Thus if the codon is a GAA triplet on the messenger RNA (see Fig. 5–2), it will combine with a tRNA having the anticodon CUU, which brings a glutamic acid into position to be attached to the growing polypeptide chain. If the next codon triplet is a GUA, it will combine with a tRNA that has a CAU anticodon, and a valine will be brought into

position and attached to the chain. In this way the amino acids are lined up on the template in an order specified by the sequence of triplets of the mRNA, which in turn is specified by the sequence of triplets in the DNA. The code for all 20 amino acids is now known (Table 5–1). Because there are 64 possible triplets from four bases and only 20 amino acids, the code is redundant. For example, both UUU and UUC code for phenylalanine, and leucine is coded for by six different codons. Because the chromosomal DNA is a long strand, there must be a signal to start "reading" at the beginning of a gene and to stop at the end. The "stop" RNA codons appear to be UAA, UAG, and UGA in bacteria, and evidence from the human hemoglobins confirms that UAA is a termination codon in man.

Table 5–1. The Genetic Code*

First Base (5' end)	Second Base				Third Base (3' end)
	U	C	A	G	
U	Phe	Ser	Tyr	Cys	U
	Phe	Ser	Tyr	Cys	C
	Leu	Ser	Term	Term	A
	Leu	Ser	Term	Trp	G
C	Leu	Pro	His	Arg	U
	Leu	Pro	His	Arg	C
	Leu	Pro	GluN	Arg	A
	Leu	Pro	GluN	Arg	G
A	Ileu	Thr	AspN	Ser	U
	Ileu	Thr	AspN	Ser	C
	Ileu	Thr	Lys	Arg	A
	Met	Thr	Lys	Arg	G
G	Val	Ala	Asp	Gly	U
	Val	Ala	Asp	Gly	C
	Val	Ala	Glu	Gly	A
	Val	Ala	Glu	Gly	G

*Each triplet of three bases (codon) in the messenger RNA codes for a specific amino acid or else a "termination" signal. Note the redundancy: each amino acid is coded for by two or more codons with the exception of Trp. AUG appears to be an initiation codon, as well as specifying methionine.

The mutation from the gene for normal hemoglobin beta chains to sickle beta chains presumably involves a change in the sixth triplet of the gene from CTT to CAT, so that the mRNA would carry GUA instead of GAA and would therefore place valine instead of glutamic acid in the sixth amino acid position.

To recapitulate, the information coded in the DNA sequence of the gene is *transcribed* to the messenger RNA, which carries the information to the ribosome site, where it is *translated* into a specified amino acid sequence in the corresponding polypeptide (Fig. 5–2).

The foregoing description is considerably oversimplified, and rapid progress is being made in understanding the structure of mammalian chromosomes and the regulation of gene activity, which will undoubtedly have important implications for man. The ultrastructural relationships of the chromosomal proteins to the DNA and their role in the regulation of gene activity are beginning to emerge (Chapter 2). The rapid advances in molecular genetics and their application to mapping the human genome are discussed in Chapter 7.

REGULATION OF GENE ACTIVITY

Because not all genes are active in all cells, there must be a way of suppressing the activity of certain genes and initiating that of others; the changes may be permanent, as in embryonic differentiation, or intermittent, as in cyclical production of a specific protein by a certain cell type.

Much of the regulation of gene activity occurs at the level of transcription. The first understanding of how this may occur came from bacterial genetics, with the formulation of the *"operon"* concept by Jacob and Monod. The operon is a group of genes, arranged in linear order, that produce a series of enzymes all concerned with the same biosynthetic pathway. The first gene in the series contains the *operator*, which initiates the activity of the whole group. The operator can be activated or suppressed by another gene, the *regulator*, elsewhere on the genome. The product of the regulator gene can be modified by specific molecules in the cytoplasm, so that it will activate or suppress, as the case may be, its own operon. This provides a control mechanism whereby the group of genes responsible for a group of enzymes that metabolize a sugar, for instance, will produce the enzymes only when the sugar is present in the environment, thus making the cell more efficient.

In eukaryotes the situation is somewhat different and less well understood. A region 30 base-pairs upstream from the gene, called the TATA box (for the base-pair sequence at that point) determines the site of initiation of transcription, and a CCAT (cat box) sequence 80 base-pairs upstream also exerts an influence, as do other positions still farther upstream.

Regulation is a matter of great importance, because some genetic diseases and defects may result from faulty gene regulation rather than from the production of abnormal proteins, and this suggests an approach to treatment. A disease resulting from inactivity, rather than structural abnormality, of a gene may be cured by treatment that leads to reactivation of the gene. Further details will be found in Chapter 11.

Recent advances in DNA technology have shown that the organization of genes in higher organisms (eukaryotes) is far more complex than it is in bacteria, in which the first major insights into gene structure and function were found. In higher organisms, the DNA sequences of the gene that code for the amino acid sequences of the corresponding protein are interspersed with base-pair sequences that are not represented in the corresponding proteins. The former sequences are called *exons*, and the latter *introns*. The globin genes, for example, have three exons, which code for the amino acid sequences of the globin molecule, separated by two long base-pair sequences (plus one on either end) which are called introns and are not represented in the globin molecule. Other vertebrate genes may have as many as 50 exons.

At transcription, the messenger RNA synthesized by the RNA polymerase has base-pair sequences complementary to those of the whole gene, both exons and introns. These strands of long RNA in the nucleus are referred to as heterogeneous nuclear RNA. Before leaving the nucleus, the introns are excised and the exons spliced together, to form the mature messenger RNA from which the polypeptide is translated (Fig. 5–3).

It is still not clear why the introns are there. In some genes, at least, the exons code for parts of the molecule with different functions. In the case of globin, for example, the middle exon codes for the part of the molecule that surrounds the heme, and the other two exons code for parts of the protein that wrap around and stabilize the protein. Possibly the excised

introns serve as signals that activate or suppress other genes, to coordinate their activity as the cell becomes differentiated.

Introns may also be important in evolutionary dynamics because their presence increases the rate at which the exons will be shuffled and reassorted to make new combinations. The farther apart regions of the molecule are, the more chance for recombination and new arrangements to "try out" evolutionarily.

SINGLE MUTANT GENES

A gene may be altered by mutation, which changes one of its nucleotide bases, resulting in a corresponding change in its mRNA and the polypeptide for which it codes. Thus a given gene can exist in one of several different states. Alternative forms of the same gene are called *alleles*. Each individual carries two sets of genes, one from the mother and one from the father. If the two members of a pair of genes are alike, the individual is said to be *homozygous* for this allele; if they are different, the individual is *heterozygous*. A heterozygous individual will make two kinds of mRNA for that gene, and therefore two kinds of the corresponding polypeptide.

Consider what happens in the case of a gene that codes for an enzymatic protein and a mutation that renders the protein enzymatically inactive. If an individual inherits the inactive allele from both parents, he or she will not make any active enzyme, the corresponding reaction will not occur, and thus the homo-

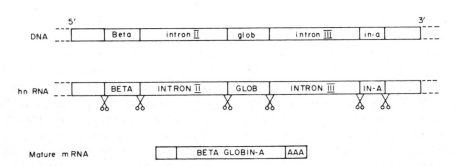

Fig. 5–3.   Fine structure of the beta-globin gene. The coding sequences are interspersed with introns. Transcription produces a messenger RNA, known as heterogeneous nuclear RNA, complementary to the DNA (represented by change from lower case letters to capitals.) The RNA is then processed by enzymes that excise the introns and add a string of adenines at the 3′ end (poly A), and is "capped" by a methylated guanosine at the 5′ end.

zygous mutant individual will be abnormal. On the other hand, an individual who is heterozygous will usually make about half as much enzyme as one who is homozygous for the normal allele. Reducing the amount of enzyme by half is usually not enough to reduce the rate of the corresponding reaction, and so the heterozygote will function normally. In this case, the trait determined by the mutant allele is said to be *recessive* to the normal trait, since the mutant allele does not produce any outward effect in the presence of the normal allele. A recessively inherited disease, then, is one that is caused only by homozygosity for a mutant gene.

If the mutant gene can produce a trait or defect in the heterozygote, the corresponding trait is said to show *dominant* inheritance. This may be because the mutant gene results in the production of an abnormal protein, such as keratin (the main protein of our hair and nails), that, even in the presence of the normal protein produced by the normal allele, results in an abnormal structure. In such cases, an individual homozygous for the mutant gene would probably be much more severely affected than the heterozygote, since there would be none of the normal protein. When the heterozygote is intermediate between the two homozygotes, with respect to the trait in question, dominance is said to be *intermediate,* and if the heterozygote resembles the mutant homozygote, the mutant is said to show *complete* dominance.

Most deleterious dominant genes in man are so rare that homozygous mutants are rarely observed, since mating between heterozygotes almost never occurs, so there is no opportunity to decide whether the given gene shows intermediate or complete dominance. An exception is Huntington disease, in which the mutant homozygote is indistinguishable from the heterozygote. In medical genetics, therefore, the term *dominant* is used for *any trait that is outwardly expressed in the heterozygote*, regardless of whether dominance is intermediate or complete.

Finally, the heterozygote may express the phenotype of both genes. For instance, a person of the AB blood group is heterozygous for

an allele that produces antigen A and an allele that produces antigen B. When each allele is expressed, irrespective of the other, they are said to be *codominant.*

Models other than a mixture of normal and abnormal structural proteins also account for the dominance of some mutant genes. For instance, a mutation may render an enzyme insensitive to feedback inhibition, or make an operator gene that is normally suppressed by some cytoplasmic regulator insensitive to the regulator. In either case, there is excessive activity of the corresponding enzyme(s). Acute intermittent porphyria and certain forms of gout may be examples of this kind. Another possibility is that the mutant gene alters the specificity of the enzyme, allowing it to attack a different substrate or to assemble macromolecular material in the wrong way. Much remains to be found out about the biochemical basis of dominance.

Note that the concept of dominance is an operational one and does not reflect any intrinsic property of the gene. Take, for example, the mutant gene for sickle cell hemoglobin. At the *clinical level*, the homozygote has a severe anemia, but the heterozygous individual is not anemic under normal circumstances, so the mutant trait would be considered recessive. However, when the red blood cells from a heterozygote are put under reduced oxygen tension, they become sickle-shaped. Thus, at the *cellular level,* the mutant gene can express itself when heterozygous, though not as strongly as when homozygous. This would be considered intermediate dominance. Finally, at the *molecular level,* the red cell from a heterozygote contains both normal and sickle hemoglobin, so the alleles are codominant. Whether a gene is considered dominant or recessive may therefore depend on the level at which one looks for its effect.

The fact that a mutant gene can be recessive and not produce any outward effect in the heterozygote means that two outwardly similar persons may be genetically different. If we consider a gene a^D and mutant form a^r, which is recessive, both homozygous a^Da^D and heterozygous a^Da^r individuals are outwardly normal but genetically different. The outward ap-

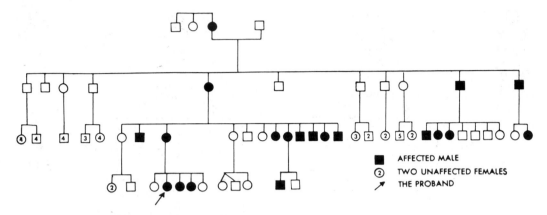

Fig. 5–4. Pedigree of hereditary "cold urticaria" illustrating autosomal dominant inheritance. There are approximately equal numbers of males and females (8:12) and among the offspring of affected individuals there are 19 affected and 20 unaffected (excluding the proband), which is close to the expected 1:1 ratio.

pearance is referred to as the *phenotype*, and the underlying genetic constitution as the *genotype*. Because of recessive genes and other irregularities to be mentioned later, one cannot always deduce the genotype from the phenotype.

MENDELIAN PEDIGREE PATTERNS

Autosomal Dominant Inheritance

As we have seen, a dominant trait is considered to be one that manifests itself in every individual who inherits the underlying gene irrespective of the state of the other allele. Thus the transmission of a dominantly inherited disease in a family is a direct reflection of the transmission of the gene. Each individual who inherits the gene will have the disease. Because each affected individual inherits the gene from an affected parent, the first characteristic of autosomal dominant inheritance is that *every affected individual has an affected parent*, except for cases presumed to have arisen by fresh mutation.

As deleterious mutant genes for dominant traits are rare (because of selection against them), the affected individual almost always inherits the mutant gene from one parent only and a normal allele from the other parent; that is, he or she (let us assume it is he) will be heterozygous. He will probably marry an unaffected woman. His children will therefore inherit a normal allele from his spouse and either the normal or the mutant allele from him. This, then, is the second rule of mendelian dominant inheritance: If the spouse is normal, *the affected individual's children will each have a 1:1 chance of inheriting the mutant gene and having the disease.*

Figure 5–4 is a pedigree of hereditary "cold urticaria," illustrating the autosomal dominant pedigree pattern (see inside front cover for a description of pedigree symbols). Carriers of the gene may have episodes of skin blotches, chills, and weakness on exposure to cold. Note that from any affected individual the disease can be traced to an affected parent, grandparent, and so on as far back as information is reliable, up to the point of first appearance in the family. Second, the ratio of affected to unaffected offspring of affected individuals is 19:20, which is compatible with a 1:1 expectation for each individual. The proband, for instance, inherited the mutant gene, which we will call a^D, from her mother and a normal allele a^r from her father. Figure 5–5 (left) shows the expectation for her children: each son and each daughter has a 1:1 chance of being affected.

If two heterozygotes mate, the offspring can draw either the normal or the mutant allele from each parent and will be homozygous normal (1 chance in 4), heterozygous (2 in 4), or homozygous mutant (1 in 4); that is, they have 3 chances in 4 of being affected (Fig. 5–5) (right).

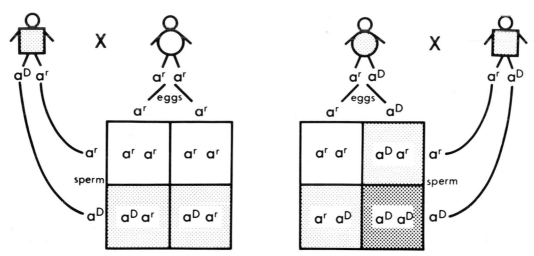

Fig. 5–5. Segregation of the gene for an autosomal dominant gene in a mating of heterozygous and homozygous normal individuals (left), and between two heterozygotes (right).

Finally, in the rare cases in which an affected person was homozygous for the mutant gene, the mate being homozygous for the normal allele, all the offspring would inherit the mutant gene and would be affected.

In summary, the pedigree pattern of autosomal dominant inheritance is characterized by the following features:

1. Each affected individual has an affected parent, to the point in the ancestry where the mutant gene arose by fresh mutation.

2. Each offspring of an affected person (with one affected and one unaffected parent) and a normal mate will have a 50:50 chance of being affected.
3. Unaffected relatives of affected persons will not have affected offspring.

Autosomal Recessive Inheritance

Because a recessive deleterious gene produces its disease only in the homozygote, affected individuals must receive one mutant

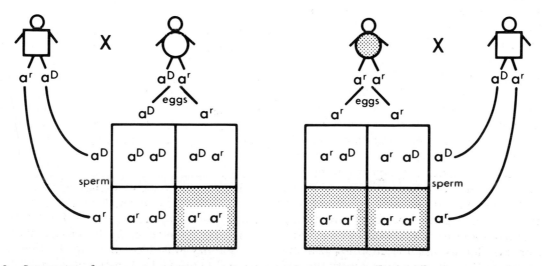

Fig. 5–6. Segregation of autosomal recessive genes in a mating between two heterozygotes (left) and between a heterozygote and a homozygous affected individual (right). The shaded symbols represent the mutant genotypes and phenotypes.

gene from each parent. Because recessively inherited diseases are usually rare in the population, almost all homozygous affected individuals arise from a mating of two heterozygous unaffected parents. Figure 5–6 (left) illustrates the types of offspring to be expected from a mating of two heterozygotes. The offspring may get the normal allele from both parents and be unaffected, a normal allele from the father and a mutant allele from the mother and be unaffected but heterozygous, a mutant allele from the father and a normal allele from the mother, also an unaffected heterozygote, or the mutant allele from both parents and be affected with the disease. Thus *each child of parents who are both heterozygous for a mutant gene has 1 chance in 4 of being homozygous and having the mutant phenotype.* There is 1 chance in 2 that the child will be heterozygous for the mutant gene. Thus, if the child is not affected, he has 2 chances in 3 of being heterozygous.

Because the average family size in most populations is less than 4 and the recurrence risk for siblings is 1 in 4, most cases of recessively inherited disease will be "sporadic." That is, the majority of cases will not have affected siblings even though the disease is inherited.

Occasionally, an affected individual may marry a heterozygote, in which case the offspring will have an equal chance of being heterozygous unaffected or homozygous affected, thus simulating dominant inheritance (Fig. 5–6) (right). This phenomenon is known as "pseudo-dominance."

Because affected individuals almost always arise from matings between heterozygotes, a recessive mutant may be transmitted through many generations without becoming homozygous. Thus it is characteristic of recessively inherited diseases that *they usually do not appear in the ancestors or collateral relatives of affected individuals.*

The chances of two parents being heterozygous for a mutant allele are increased if they are related (consanguineous)—i.e., they have a common ancestry from which they may inherit the same recessive mutant gene. If such a gene is carried by, say, 1 of every 50 in-

dividuals in the population, the chance that a heterozygote will marry an unrelated heterozygote will be 1 in 50, but if a heterozygote marries his first cousin, the chance that she will also carry it will be 1 in 8, a considerably higher risk (Fig. 5–7). It follows that *children with a recessively inherited disease are more likely to have related parents.*

Furthermore, the rarer the disease, the more likely it is that the diseased individuals will have consanguineous parents because the chance of a heterozygote marrying an unrelated heterozygote diminishes as the gene frequency decreases, whereas the probability that a given near relative will carry the gene does not change appreciably, and the *proportion* of homozygotes resulting from consanguineous matings therefore increases. Indeed, shortly after Mendel's laws were rediscovered, Garrod was led to infer that inborn errors of metabolism (Chap. 6) were autosomal recessive

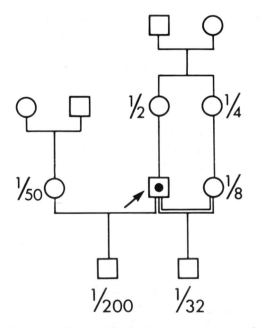

Fig. 5–7. Significance of parental consanguinity. If the proband is heterozygous for a recessive gene carried by 1 in every 50 people, the chance that his first child by an unrelated spouse will be affected is $\frac{1}{4} \times \frac{1}{50} = \frac{1}{200}$. The chance of being heterozygous for the mutant gene is $\frac{1}{2}$ for his mother (since he got the gene either from her or his father). The risk that his mother's sister would also have it is $\frac{1}{2} \times \frac{1}{2} = \frac{1}{4}$ and that the sister's daughter (the proband's cousin) would also inherit it is $\frac{1}{2} \times \frac{1}{4} = \frac{1}{8}$; the risk of the first child by his cousin being homozygous for the gene is $\frac{1}{4} \times \frac{1}{8} = \frac{1}{32}$.

phenotypes from, among other observations, the fact that most of the parents of individuals with these conditions were first cousins.[7]

Certain human groups are genetically isolated, with considerable distant consanguinity among population members (see Chap. 10). Such distant consanguinity can cause exceptions to the rule that recessive disease does not appear in collateral relatives. Figure 5–8, a pedigree of cystic fibrosis of the pancreas (see Chap. 8) in a French Canadian kindred, illustrates this. The gene must have been carried by one of the parents of the three sibs in generation I. Its descendants were transmitted to the four individuals in generation IV (IV–4 × IV–5 and IV–8 × IV–9) who (unwittingly) married their third cousins, and the disease appeared in the two first-cousin sibships in generation V.

In summary, the autosomal recessive pedigree pattern is characterized by the following features:

1. Almost never (if the gene is rare) is the disease present in the parents, ancestry, or collateral relatives.
2. The sibs of an affected child with normal parents have 1 chance in 4 of being affected, irrespective of sex.
3. The parents of affected children are more likely to be related to each other (consanguineous) than are parents of normal children; the rarer the disease, the

greater the frequency of parental consanguinity.
4. In small sibships, the majority of cases are "sporadic," i.e., the only one in the family.

Sex Linkage

X-Linked Recessive Inheritance. Genes on the X chromosomes can be dominant or recessive just as those on the autosomes, but the fact that females have two X chromosomes and males only one X and a Y leads to characteristic differences in the pedigree patterns of diseases caused by X-linked genes. In females the dominance relations of mutant and normal alleles are just as they are on the autosomes (with certain exceptions related to Lyonization, as discussed in Chapter 4). But the Y chromosome, for the most part, is not homologous to the X; that is, most genes on the X chromosome do not have a corresponding locus on the Y. (Such genes on the X chromosome are said to be *hemizygous* in the male, rather than heterozygous or homozygous.) A mutant gene on the X chromosome will therefore always be expressed in the male, even though it may behave as a recessive in the female. This accounts for the characteristic pedigree pattern of diseases showing X-linked inheritance, the gene usually being

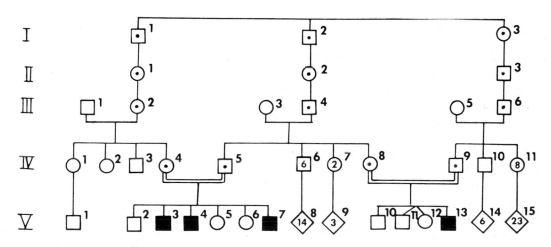

Fig. 5–8.   A pedigree of cystic fibrosis of the pancreas illustrating the effect of parental consanguinity in bringing recessive mutant genes together.

transmitted by unaffected females and producing the disease in males.

The most characteristic mating (Fig. 5–9) is that of a female heterozygous for a recessive mutant gene on the X chromosome (X^R) and its normal allele (X^D), mated to a normal male (X^DY). She will give either X^D or X^R to each of her daughters, who will also receive a normal X from the father and will each therefore have a 50:50 chance of being an outwardly normal carrier (X^DX^R) or a normal homozygote (X^DX^D). The sons will get a Y chomosome from the father and will have a 50:50 chance of being X^DY (normal) or X^RY (affected).

An affected male mated to a normal female will transmit a Y chromosome to his sons, who will be unaffected, and the X chromosome carrying the mutant gene to all his daughters, who will be unaffected, but carriers (Fig. 5–9).

In the unlikely event that an affected male (X^RY) marries a carrier female (X^DX^R), the daughters will all inherit the mutant gene from their father and will inherit from the mother either the normal allele and be carriers (X^DX^R), or the mutant allele and be affected (X^RX^R).

In summary, diseases showing X-linked recessive inheritance show the following pedigree characteristics, provided the gene concerned is rare and ignoring mutation:

1. The disease appears almost always in males, whose mothers are unaffected but heterozygous carriers of the mutant gene.
2. Each son of a carrier female has a 1:1 chance of being affected.
3. Each daughter of a carrier female has a 1:1 chance of being a carrier.
4. Affected males never transmit the gene to their sons, but they transmit it to all their daughters, who will be carriers.
5. Unaffected males never transmit the gene.

Thus the trait is usually transmitted through unaffected female ancestors and appears in their male relatives. Therefore one may expect to see it in the patient's brothers, the mother's brothers, the sons of the mother's sisters, or the mother's father. Figure 5–10 is a representative pedigree. In many families, however, the disease may be "sporadic," i.e., it may occur in only one person, either because the eligible male relatives are few and by chance have not inherited the gene or because the patient's disease has arisen by fresh mutation (see section on recurrence risks, page 84, for a more detailed discussion).

X-linked recessive traits that are lethal (such as Duchenne muscular dystrophy) or that sterilize the affected male (such as testicular feminization) are difficult to distinguish from autosomal traits that are recessive in females and dominant in males. The only difference in pedigree pattern between the two types of inheritance is transmission by affected males to their sons, which cannot happen anyway if the trait does not permit reproduction. In this case, a distinction can be made only if Lyonization (Chapter 4) can be demonstrated for the trait in carrier females, or if linkage to an X-linked marker can be shown (Chap. 9).

X-linked Dominant Inheritance. The pedigree pattern of X-linked dominant traits differs from that of autosomal dominance only in that all the daughters and none of the sons of affected males will be affected, because a male gives his X-chromosome only to his daughters. There are few examples, one being hypophosphatemic rickets.

Independent Segregation

Mendel was fortunate that the traits he chose to study were controlled by genes on different chromosomes, so that he was able to discover the law of independent segregation. This states that genes (on different chromosomes) segregate independently of one another. Thus if there are two mendelian mutant genes segregating in a family, the risks for a given individual inheriting either or both diseases can be calculated from the law of independent probability. Suppose a couple had had a child with cystic fibrosis of the pancreas, so that each child has a 1 in 4 chance of inheriting this autosomal recessive disease. Suppose one parent also has neurofibromatosis (coffee-colored skin spots, tumors of the nerve sheath, and sometimes more serious complications), so that each child has 1 chance in 2 of inheriting this

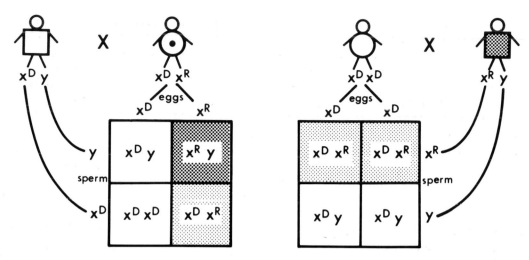

Fig. 5–9. Segregation of an X-linked recessive gene in a mating of a heterozygous female by a normal male (left) and in a mating of affected male and normal female (right)

autosomal dominant disease. Provided that the genes are on separate chromosomes, we can say that the chance of the child inheriting both diseases is $\frac{1}{2} \times \frac{1}{4} = \frac{1}{8}$; there is a $\frac{1}{2} \times \frac{3}{4} = \frac{3}{8}$ chance of inheriting neither disease, a $\frac{1}{2} \times \frac{1}{4} = \frac{1}{8}$ chance of inheriting only cystic fibrosis, and a $\frac{1}{2} \times \frac{3}{4} = \frac{3}{8}$ chance of inheriting only neurofibromatosis.

Linkage and Crossing-over

Up until recently linkage, where two genes are on the same chromosome, has been a much less important subject in human, than in other, branches of genetics. The study of linkage was crucial, for example, to formulating the chromosome theory of heredity in the early days of genetics and to the brilliant experiments of microbial genetics that elucidated the fine structure of the gene. But in humans, apart from the X-chromosome, there were too few examples of linkage to generate much interest. With the recent rapid advances in mapping (Chapter 7) and its application in prenatal diagnosis (Chapter 15), linkage has become much more relevant to medical genetics. This topic is elaborated in Chapter 9.

Irregularities in Mendelian Pedigree Patterns

Unfortunately, not all mutant genes in man display the regularity of transmission and expression shown by the characters of the garden pea that Mendel chose to demonstrate his laws. Neither, as a matter of fact, did some of the other characters that Mendel studied in the pea.

Expressivity. It is well recognized that infection by the same strain of virus or bacteria can produce wide variations in severity of disease in different patients. The same is true of genes. *Variable expressivity* is the term used for the variation in severity of effects produced by the same gene in different individuals. For instance, the dominant gene for multiple exostoses, which causes large numbers of disfiguring bone tumors in one person, may produce only a few small exostoses, detectable only by x-ray studies, in a near relative.

Penetrance. To carry the argument one step further, a gene that expresses itself clinically in one person may produce no detectable effect in another. This failure to reach the "clinical surface" is referred to as *reduced penetrance*. In statistical terms, penetrance is the % frequency with which a dominant gene in the heterozygote or a recessive gene in the homozygote produces a detectable effect. In medical genetics, reduced penetrance is most easily detected in the case of dominant genes, when an individual who must, on genetic grounds, carry the mutant gene does not show the mutant phenotype. Figure 5–11 illustrates

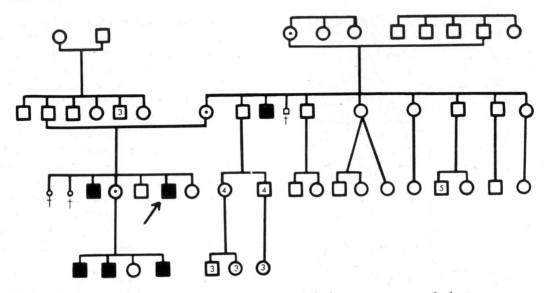

Fig. 5–10. Pedigree of hemophilia illustrating X-linked recessive pattern of inheritance.

a pedigree of the "lip-pit" syndrome in which an autosomal dominant gene results in two small pits on the lower lip in most, but not all, heterozygotes (Fig. 5–12). Less frequently, the gene may also cause cleft lip or cleft palate, or both. Thus the gene shows both reduced penetrance (II–7 carried the gene but did not show any signs of it) and variable expressivity (IV–1 has cleft lip and lip pits; III–4 has cleft lip and palate).

When penetrance is close to 100%, the autosomal dominant pedigree pattern with occasional skips is easy to identify, but the lower the penetrance, the more difficult it is to distinguish between dominant inheritance with reduced penetrance and more complicated

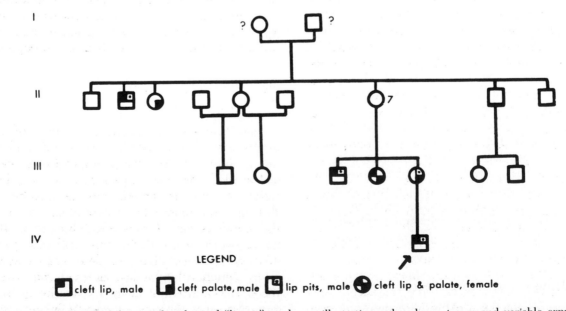

LEGEND

🔲 cleft lip, male   🔲 cleft palate, male   🔲 lip pits, male   🔴 cleft lip & palate, female

Fig. 5–11. Pedigree of dominantly inherited "lip-pit" syndrome illustrating reduced penetrance and variable expressivity (see text).

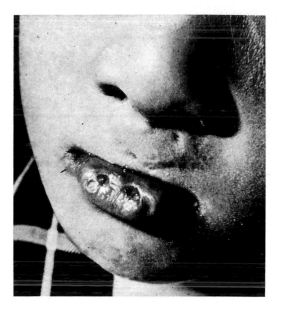

Fig. 5-12. Girl with (repaired) cleft lip and lip-pits.

modes of inheritance. The concept of reduced penetrance has sometimes been used as an "excuse" for the fact that many familial diseases do not fit the expectation for regular mendelian behavior. Nevertheless, there is no doubt that reduced penetrance is a fact of life and often poses problems for the counselor.

Failure of a gene to express itself phenotypically may occur for a variety of reasons. If the disease caused by the gene has a variable age of onset, for instance, a person who carries the gene may die before the disease becomes manifest and will appear as a "skip" in the pedigree. In other cases, the gene may involve some process with a developmental or biochemical threshold, and whether the mutant phenotype is produced will depend on whether the mutant gene has an effect severe enough to prevent the individual from reaching the threshold (see Chapter 11, Fig. 11-2). In this sense variable expressivity and penetrance are closely related phenomena.

As with dominance, the degree of penetrance of a mutant gene may also depend on how hard the observer looks for signs of its presence. The X-linked dominant gene for hypophosphatemic rickets, for instance, may produce full-blown rickets in some, but only a low blood phosphorus level in other cases.

Little is known about what makes the difference. In some cases, the effects of the mutant dominant gene in an unaffected carrier cannot be detected by any known means. Presumably, the number of such cases will decrease as our biochemical skills increase.

Phenocopies. Sometimes the effect of a mutant gene can be simulated by that of an environmental agent in a genetically nonmutant individual. For instance, congenital deafness can be caused by a recessive gene or by an environmental agent such as the drug streptomycin. This is not really an example of an irregularity in mendelian pedigree patterns, but if phenocopies are unwittingly mixed in with cases of recessive deafness, the segregation ratio will deviate from mendelian expectation. Phenocopies also cause problems for genetic counselors who sometimes have to decide whether a particular child represents a genetic type or a phenocopy.

Genetic Heterogeneity. Another source of possible confusion is the fact that different mutant genes may produce similar phenotypes, but may have different modes of inheritance. For example, congenital deafness can be caused by autosomal dominant, autosomal recessive, and X-linked recessive mutant genes, and it is important for the genetic counselor to be aware of this. As our knowledge increases, genetic heterogeneity is recognized in more and more diseases and appears to be the rule, rather than the exception.

CALCULATION OF THE SEGREGATION RATIO

In estimating the genetic component of any disease, the first question to be asked is likely to be, "What is the frequency of the disease in the near relatives of patients?" Family histories are then collected, and the number of affected and unaffected relatives is counted. However, certain biases are inherent in the collection of such data in man. To begin with, there are the problems of determining accurately which relatives are affected and which are not. We will not discuss these here. Second, the more striking the family history, the more likely it is to come to the attention of the investigator if care is not taken to avoid this bias. This is particularly true if one is using cases from the literature, but may also result from the efforts of well-meaning colleagues to refer "interesting" families. Furthermore, if one is ascertaining families by identifying an affected individual, families with more than one affected member may be more likely to be ascertained than families with only one. We will return to the question of ascertainment bias shortly.

The basic question is this: In a group of individuals of a given relationship to an affected person what proportion are themselves affected? If the relation is anything other than sib, the situation is reasonably straightforward. In a group of children ascertained through one affected parent, for instance, one simply counts the number of affected and unaffected children. If, on the other hand, one is interested in the *sibs* of affected persons, the situation is more complicated.

If we are measuring the frequency of the condition in the sibs of the proband, we must *omit the proband* from the calculation since, by definition, the probability of the proband being affected is 100%. If one were measuring the risk of contracting tuberculosis in the sibs of tuberculous patients, for instance, one might ascertain 20 tuberculous patients, the probands, and find that they had a total of 60 sibs, none of whom was affected. The frequency of tuberculosis in the whole group is $20/80 = 1$ in 4, but this does not support mendelian inheritance—the recurrence risk in the *sibs* of the probands is 0/60; the probands must be omitted since they were selected *because* they were affected. This seems almost too obvious to mention, but nevertheless the mistake does appear in the literature from time to time, leading to gross overestimations of recurrence risk for poliomyelitis, asthma, and congenital heart disease, to cite three examples.

Complete Ascertainment

Second, there is the question of ascertainment bias. If every affected case in the given population is recorded and that family is thereby included in the study, this is called *complete ascertainment*. If so, every case is a

proband. (By definition, the proband is an affected individual through whom the family is ascertained. In complete ascertainment, the family is ascertained once for each affected case, because every affected case is a proband.) We wish to estimate the frequency of the disease in the sibs of probands, so for each family we omit one proband and count the family as many times as there are probands. Thus a sibship in which there were 3 affected and 5 normal children would be scored as 2 affected out of 7, three times, or 6 out of 21. This method also applies in other situations where each family has an equal probability of being ascertained.

Table 5–2 presents a hypothetic example in which there are 5 families of 4 siblings each. In the column headed "complete ascertainment," each family is counted as many times as there are affected individuals, omitting one affected each time. This method estimates the probability of an affected sib as 8/24, or 33%. If ascertainment is, in fact, *not* complete, this method will overestimate the recurrence risk.

Single Ascertainment

At the other extreme, single ascertainment, the probands are chosen in such a way that each family is ascertained only once. Thus, every family will have one proband, and there will be some affected who are not probands but secondary cases. The more affected individuals there are in the family, the more likely the family is to be ascertained, and families with more than one affected will be over-represented in the sample as compared to their frequency in the population. In single ascertainment, this bias is exactly compensated for by omitting the proband from the calculation and counting only the sibs (Table 5–2). This estimates the probability of an affected sib as 3/15 or 20%. If, in fact, ascertainment is not single, this method will underestimate the recurrence risk.

Incomplete Multiple Ascertainment

In practice, the situation is usually somewhere between complete and single ascertain-

Table 5–2.   Methods of Counting the Proportion of Affected to Unaffected Sibs with Different Assumptions about the Mode of Ascertainment of Probands*

Family	Assumed Ascertainment Method					
	Complete Aff.	Complete T	Single Aff.	Single T	Incomplete Aff.	Incomplete T
1. ○ ○ ○ ●	0	3	0	3	0	3
2. ○ ● ● ○	2	6	1	3	1	3
3. ● ○ ○ ○	0	3	0	3	0	3
4. ● ● ● ○	6	9	2	3	4	6
5. ○ ○ ● ○	0	3	0	3	0	3
Ratio	8	24	3	15	5	18
% affected		33.3		20.0		27.8

*The probands in incomplete ascertainment are indicated by arrows. The left and middle pairs of columns represent the limiting assumptions, counting every affected case as a proband and one case per family as a proband, respectively.

ment. Some families with several affected sibs may be ascertained by only one proband, the other affected sibs being identified secondarily. Other families may be ascertained separately and independently by each affected sib, i.e., all sibs are probands; in still others some affected sibs may be ascertained independently (probands) and others discovered only secondarily. In this case, the same rule is followed: count the family once for each proband, omitting the proband each time. Table 5–2 demonstrates the procedure in the column headed "incomplete ascertainment," more properly called "incomplete multiple ascertainment." The probability of a sib being affected is estimated by this method as 5/18 or 28%.

Sometimes, particularly with data from the literature, it is not clear which affected individuals are probands and which are secondary cases. In this case, one can at least get a rough estimate by making the limiting assumptions. Assuming single ascertainment, calculate the frequency in sibs, which will underestimate the real value if ascertainment is not single. Then calculate the value assuming complete ascertainment which will overestimate the real value if ascertainment is incomplete. The true value should lie somewhere between the two.

A method that avoids the ascertainment bias is to calculate the recurrence risk only on children born after the proband, but this has the disadvantage of losing about half the data. Do *not* use children born after the first *affected* individual. Unless ascertainment is complete, this method will grossly overestimate the real value (3/9, or 33.3% for the data in Table 5–2).

The *a priori* Method

If the data are being tested for goodness of fit to a mendelian ratio, an *a priori* method can be used. In families of parents who are both heterozygous for an autosomal recessive gene, for instance, some will have several affected, some one affected, and some none affected, just on the basis of chance. If the families are ascertained by an affected child, the families in which there are no affected children will not be included in the data. (This is known as "truncate" selection—the normal families are "cut off.") It is possible to calculate, from the binomial distribution, for any family size, the expected number of families omitted because they contain no affected children, and the data can be tested to see if, when due allowance is made for these families, a satisfactory fit to a 1 in 4 ratio is obtained. Details can be found in many textbooks of human genetics. However, the method is relatively insensitive and can be

Table 5–3. Probability that a Healthy Offspring of a Patient with Huntington Disease Carries the HD Gene at Various Ages.*

Age	Risk	Age	Risk
22.0	49.6	47.5	34.8
22.5	49.3	50.0	31.5
25.0	49.0	52.5	27.8
27.5	48.4	55.0	24.8
30.0	47.6	57.5	22.1
32.5	46.6	60.0	18.7
35.0	45.5	62.5	15.2
37.5	44.2	65.0	12.8
40.0	42.5	67.5	10.8
42.5	40.3	70.0	6.2
45.0	37.8	72.5	4.6

*Reproduced with permission from Harper, P.S., and Newcombe, R.G.: Age at onset life table risks in genetic counselling for Huntington's disease. J. Med. Genet. 29:239, 1992.

misleading unless a fairly large sample size is available.

Other Methods of Segregation Analysis

Several more sophisticated methods of analyzing segregation ratios have been developed,[5,11] but are beyond the scope of this book. Again, they are most useful when a large amount of data is available.

CALCULATING RECURRENCE RISKS

Mendelian Inheritance and Bayes' Theorem

Calculating recurrence risks is simple when the disease in question shows a regular mendelian inheritance and the genotypes of the parents are known. Predictions are then made on the basis of the segregation ratios already described.

It may be, however, that the genotypes of the parents are not known but must be estimated from the family data at hand. To do this, use is often made of calculations based on Bayes' theorem, which provides a way of combining the likelihood derived from the mendelian laws (prior probability) with additional information derived from the individual family (conditional probabilities).

The product of the prior and conditional probabilities is called the joint probability. The posterior probability is defined as the joint probability of an event occurring divided by the sum of all probabilities (i.e., the joint probability of a gene or trait being inherited plus the joint probability of a gene or trait not being inherited by a given individual). The reader is referred to Table 5–4 and asked to follow along with the illustration in the next section. More detailed explanations of the use of the Bayes' theorem may be found elsewhere.[9,11]

Dominant Inheritance

Variable Age of Onset. Consider a man whose father has Huntington disease (HD). This degenerative brain disease shows autosomal dominant inheritance and has a highly variable age of onset. Our consultand (i.e., the person whose genotype we are evaluating) is unaffected at age 42. On the basis of the mendelian law, the probability that he inherited the gene from his father is $1/2$, and the probability that he did not is $1/2$. This is the prior probability based only on his antecedents. But we have another source of information. He has reached age 42 without developing the disease. We can see intuitively that the longer he lives, unaffected, the greater the probability that he did not inherit the gene. Thus, living to his age, still unaffected, contributes additional information about the probability that he carries the gene. Previous studies[8] have shown that about one third of those who inherit the gene have developed signs of the disease by this age (Table 5–3), so there is a $2/3$ probability that, if he inherited the gene, he will still be unaffected at age 42. This is the *conditional* probability. What, then, is his overall (posterior) probability?

The answer will be derived from first principles, and then by use of the formula of Bayes' theorem. There are three possible outcomes:

1. He did not inherit the gene—probability $1/2$.
2. He did inherit the gene but is unaffected at age 42—probability $1/2 \times 2/3 = 1/3$.
3. He inherited the gene and is affected at age 42—probability $1/2 \times 1/3 = 1/6$.

We exclude the third outcome, because he is unaffected. So the chance that he is a carrier ($\frac{1}{3}$) compared to the chance that he is not is as $\frac{1}{3}$ to $\frac{1}{2}$, or $\frac{2}{6}$ to $\frac{3}{6}$, which is 2 to 3, or 2 out of 5 = 40%.

That is, by surviving, unaffected, to age 42, he has reduced his chance of having inherited the gene from 50% to 40%.

A more formal approach, using Bayes' formula, is outlined in Table 5–4. The prior probability of having or not having the gene is $\frac{1}{2}$. This information is put into each of the two columns (titled "did inherit" and "did not inherit"). The conditional probability from the age of onset curve as the cumulative percentage age of onset of Huntington disease. There is a 33% probability that a person with the gene will have signs of the disease at age 42. Conversely, this means that the conditional probability that the consultand could carry the gene and still be unaffected at age 42 is 0.67 (1 − 0.33). The joint probability, in the next line of the table, that he did inherit or did not inherit the gene is the product of the prior and conditional probabilities. The probability that he is normal although he has still inherited the gene is shown in the left column as 0.5 × 0.67, or 0.33, and that he is normal because he did not inherit the gene is shown in the right column as 0.5 × 1 or 0.50. (1 because there is a 100% probability that if he does not have the gene he will not have Huntington disease.)

Now we calculate the posterior probabilities, using the joint probability in each column as the numerator and the sum of both of the joint probabilities the denominator in each column. The probability that the consultand carries the gene for HD, even though he is free of symptoms at age 42, is 0.33/0.33 + 0.50 or 0.40. Thus, there is still a 40% chance that the consultand did inherit the gene. You may check your calculation by the addition rule of probability. The posterior probability that he did not inherit the gene is 0.60 as shown in the right-hand column— and, of course, if your calculations are correct, the sum of the posterior probabilities should be 1.

Reduced Penetrance. A similar line of reasoning can be used in the case of a dominant gene with reduced penetrance. Suppose an affected father has an unaffected daughter who wants to know whether she may pass the gene on to her children. Assume that the gene shows 90% ($\frac{9}{10}$) penetrance. There are the following possible outcomes:

1. The daughter did not inherit the gene— prior probability $\frac{1}{2}$.
2. The daughter inherited the gene but does not show the phenotype—probability $\frac{1}{2}$ × $\frac{1}{10}$ = $\frac{1}{20}$ (prior probability × conditional probability = joint probability).
3. The daughter inherited the gene and shows the phenotype—probability $\frac{1}{2}$ × $\frac{9}{10}$ = $\frac{9}{20}$.

We can exclude the third outcome; the probability of outcome 2, out of the two remaining outcomes, is the posterior probability of her being a carrier:

$$\frac{\frac{1}{20}}{\frac{1}{20} + \frac{1}{2}} = \frac{1}{11}$$

Table 5–4. Bayesian Calculation of Probability That the Son of a Patient with Huntington Disease Is a Carrier, Given That He is Unaffected at Age 30

Either he:	did inherit	or	did not inherit
Probability (prior)	0.5		0.5
Probability (conditional) at age 42	1 − 0.33 = 0.67		1
Joint probability	0.5 × 0.67 = 0.33		0.5 × 1 = 0.50
Probability (posterior)	$\frac{0.33}{0.33 + 0.50} = 0.40$		$\frac{0.50}{0.33 + 0.50} = 0.60$
Risk of being a carrier		0.40	

Therefore the daughter has 1 chance in 11 of being a carrier, and the chance of her first child being affected is $^1/_{11} \times {}^1/_2 \times {}^9/_{10} = {}^9/_{220}$, or about 4%.

X-Linked Recessive Inheritance

Female with Carrier Mother and Normal Sons. This kind of reasoning is useful when a female relative of a male with an X-linked recessive disease wants to know the chances that she is a carrier. Consider the situation in Fig. 5–13. Female A is almost certainly heterozygous for the gene since she transmitted it to two children.

The prior probability of female B inheriting the gene is $^1/_2$, but each normal son she has makes it less likely that she is a carrier, and she has three normal sons. The probability that she is a carrier and has three normal sons is

$$^1/_2 \times (^1/_2)^3 = {}^1/_{16}.$$

So of the following possible outcomes:
1. She did not inherit the gene ($^1/_2$).
2. She did inherit the gene and has three normal sons ($^1/_{16}$).

The probability of outcome two is

$$\frac{^1/_{16}}{^1/_{16} + {}^1/_2} = {}^1/_9.$$

The Sporadic Case. An appreciable number of cases of X-linked recessive diseases have a negative family history. Consider, for instance,

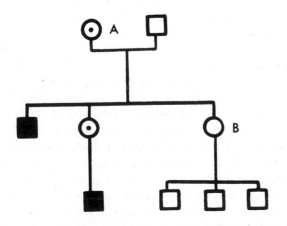

Fig. 5–13.   Hypothetical pedigree of an X-linked recessive condition.

the family of a boy with Duchenne-type muscular dystrophy with no brothers, no maternal uncles, and a negative family history (Fig. 5–14). If he represents a fresh mutation, the risk for subsequent brothers is negligible, but if his mother is heterozygous, his brothers have a 50:50 chance. What is the probability that his mother is heterozygous? We can calculate the proportion of mutant to nonmutant cases by starting from the equation (Chapter 10):

$$m = \frac{1-f}{3} x \text{ or } x = \frac{3m}{1-f},$$

where x is the disease frequency in males, m is the mutation rate, and f the fitness of the mutant phenotype (in this case 0). Therefore, in the case of a single affected male, with no affected male maternal relatives, it may be that either:
1. The son's X chromosome received a fresh mutation—probability m.
2. The mother carried the mutant gene and passed it on to her son. The probability that she carries the gene on one X is twice the disease frequency

$$\frac{3m}{1-f} \times 2$$

(because she has 2 X chromosomes) minus the probability that one of her X chromosomes carries a fresh mutation ($2m$). The probability of the mother passing it to her son is $^1/_2$.

So the posterior probability that the mother is heterozygous is

$$\frac{^1/_2 \left(\dfrac{6m}{1-f} - 2m \right)}{^1/_2 \left(\dfrac{6m}{1-f} - 2m \right) + m} = \frac{f+2}{3}.$$

For a lethal gene, where $f = 0$, this works out to $^2/_3$. That is, the chances are 2 to 1 that the mother is heterozygous for the gene, with a 1 in 2 risk for each subsequent male child. Thus the total risk for the brother of a sporadic case will be $^2/_3 \times {}^1/_2 = {}^1/_3$.

This risk will be modified downwards the more unaffected sons, brothers, mother's

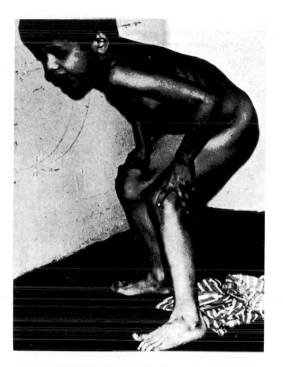

Fig. 5–14. Patient with Duchenne muscular dystrophy "climbing up himself."

brothers, and so on, there are, and upwards if the gene is not lethal and therefore more common, with proportionately fewer cases due to mutation. For example, suppose the mother of a sporadic case of Duchenne muscular dystrophy has, in addition, two normal sons. Her prior probability of being a carrier is $2/3$, and the joint probability of being a carrier and having two normal sons is $2/3 \times 1/4 = 1/6$. The probability of being a non-carrier and having 2 normal sons is $1/3$ or $2/6$. So the final (posterior) probability that she is a carrier is $1/6 : 2/6$ or 1:2 or $1/3$, instead of the original $2/3$. Table 5–5 summarizes the risks after varying numbers of unaffected sons for a lethal disease (frequency 1/100,000) and for diseases with increasing degrees of fitness (and therefore frequency). For more complex situations, the reader is advised to consult one of several expositions on the subject.[9,11]

AUTOSOMAL RECESSIVE INHERITANCE

In the great majority of cases, when the disease involved shows autosomal recessive inheritance, the parents have identified themselves as being heterozygous by the fact that they have had an affected child. The risk for each subsequent child is therefore 1 in 4. Other questions may arise, however, that usually involve the question of whether near relatives of the affected person might have affected children.

Children of Near Relatives of Affected Persons. The sib (B) of an affected person (A), married to an unrelated spouse (C), wants to know the risk that his children will get the disease. The risk depends on both B and C being heterozygous. The risk of B being heterozygous is $2/3$. C's risk can be calculated from the Hardy-Weinberg Law (Chapter 10). For cystic fibrosis of the pancreas, for instance, if the disease frequency is 1 in 2000, then

1. The frequency q of the cf gene will be $\sqrt{1/2,000}$ or $1/45$.
2. The frequency of the heterozygote, $2pq$, will be about $1/22$.
3. The frequency that B and C will both be heterozygous is

$$2/3 \times 1/22 = 1/33.$$

4. The probability of the first child being affected is:

$$1/4 \times 1/33 = 1/132.$$

As before, this probability will decrease with each unaffected child born to these parents, and an affected child will, of course, raise the risk to 1 in 4.

Matings between Affected Persons. In matings between two affected individuals who are homozygous for mutants at the same locus, all the offspring will be affected. However, the situation may be complicated by genetic heterogeneity. In a number of cases, e.g., congenital deafness and albinism, the same phenotype can be caused by mutations at different loci. If a couple who are both congenitally deaf carry mutations at different loci, their children will be unaffected. Counseling in this situation depends on the relative frequencies of mutations at the various loci, which is usually not known for a given population. In Northern Ireland, it has been shown that in two out of three matings between congenitally deaf partners (excluding those that have a known syndrome or evironmental cause), none of the children is deaf; in 1 out of 6 all the children are deaf; and in 1 out of 6 some are deaf and some are not. The data suggest that there must be several fairly common recessive genes leading to congenital deafness and that some of the sporadic cases (perhaps half) are phenocopies.

Matings between Consanguineous Partners. The question of marriage between cousins is one that the counselor meets from time to time. The issue has two aspects, genetic and social. In many societies, particularly Judaeo-Christian ones, consanguineous marriages tend to draw strong disapproval. There are widely held misapprehensions that severe inherited disorder is extremely likely, or inevitable, in the offspring of such matings. On the other hand, in some Asian and African societies, consanguineous marriages are favored, and account for a large fraction of matings.[2] What are the implications of consanguineous matings, for risk of single-gene disorders and other developmental defects?

The degree of consanguinity can be expressed as Sewall Wright's coefficient of inbreeding, F, which is defined as the probability that an individual receives, at a given locus, two genes that are identical by descent.[3] Thus F for the offspring of first cousins would be $\frac{1}{16}$. For the cousin marriage in Figure 5–7, for example, the probability that the child would receive a given allele from both his paternal and his maternal grandmother is $(\frac{1}{2})^3 \times (\frac{1}{2})^3 = \frac{1}{64}$. But the two great-grandparents have a total of 4 alleles, and the prob-

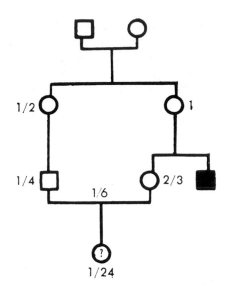

Fig. 5–15. Hypothetical pedigree of an autosomal recessive condition.

ability that the child is homozygous for any one of them is 4 times this, or $\frac{1}{16}$. Another way to calculate F is to count n, the number of connecting paths between the offspring and a common ancestor (in this case n = 6; 3 through the mother and 3 through the father), calculate $\frac{1}{2}^{n-1}$ (= $\frac{1}{2}^5$ = $\frac{1}{32}$), and sum this value for all common ancestors (in this case 2).

If there is a recessively inherited disease in the family, the risk of that disease occurring in the children of the cousin mating can be calculated from mendelian principles. For example, in Figure 5–15, if III–2's brother, III–3, had Tay-Sachs disease (see Chapter 6), III–2 would have a $\frac{2}{3}$ chance of being heterozygous, and the other probabilities can be calculated as shown. The chance of the first child being affected would be $\frac{1}{24}$.

Table 5–5. Probability That the Mother of an Isolated Case of an X-linked Trait is Heterozygous (Assume $m = \frac{1}{10}^5$)*

Disease Frequency	Number of Unaffected Sons					
	0	1	2	3	4	5
1/100,000	0.67	0.50	0.33	0.20	0.11	0.06
1/10,000	0.92	0.85	0.73	0.58	0.40	0.26
1/5,000	0.98	0.96	0.92	0.86	0.76	0.61
1/1,000	0.99	0.98	0.96	0.93	0.86	0.76

*Modified from Murphy and Chase.[9]

If there are no recessive diseases in the family, the estimate becomes much less precise. If, in Figure 5–15, one of the common grandparents carried a recessive mutant gene, then II–1 and II–2 each have a 1 in 2 chance of inheriting it, III–1 and III–2 have a 1 in 4 chance, and the chance that they are both heterozygous for the gene is $^1/_4 \times {}^1/_4 = {}^1/_{16}$. The chance that their first child will be affected is $^1/_4 \times {}^1/_{16} = {}^1/_{64}$. Because there are two common grandparents, the risk for the child is twice this, or $^1/_{32}$. But we do not know the probability that the grandparent carries a recessive mutant gene. The available data on offspring of consanguineous matings record a rather low frequency of diseases known to show mendelian recessive inheritance, probably less than 1%.[6,10]

In addition to the risks of homozygosity for specific recessive alleles, there is a general increase in homozygosity in the offspring of consanguineous matings. Thus there are significant, but small, effects of inbreeding on infant mortality, IQ, stature, and other multifactorial traits,[10] but these are not large enough to be much of a deterrent to the individual couple.

In groups that favor consanguineous marriages, an increased incidence of autosomal recessive disorders is seen, resulting in increased perinatal and neonatal mortality.[1] But in general, in countries where consanguinity is favored, fertility of consanguineous matings is higher than that of nonconsanguineous matings, indicating that social factors can outweigh the genetic risks.[2]

For incestuous matings, between first-degree relatives, the theoretical risk will be considerably greater than for first-cousin matings, and the limited amount of data available suggests that this is indeed so.[1]

In summary, the facts suggest that genetic counseling for cousins contemplating marriage should be more optimistic than the advice they often get from their church, friends, families, and, alas, some genetic counselors. Their risk of having a child with a recognizable recessively inherited disease is increased perhaps a hundredfold, but in absolute terms is still small, being of the order of 1%.[6]

SUMMARY

The genetic material is DNA, and a gene is that portion of the DNA responsible for the primary structure of a particular polypeptide. DNA consists of a double helix, which may be visualized as a rope ladder made up of paired ropes of alternating deoxyribose and phosphate molecules and rungs of purine and pyrimidine bases. Protein is produced from DNA-synthesized messenger RNA, which migrates to the cytoplasm where it becomes associated with ribosomes and transfer RNA and is translated into a polypeptide chain having the sequence of amino acids corresponding to the sequence of nucleotide triplets (codons) in the DNA.

Alternative forms of the same gene (alleles) may exist. Each individual carries two sets of genes (one from the mother and one from the father). If both members of the pair of genes are alike, the individual is homozygous for the locus; if the genes are different, he is heterozygous. A gene (of a gene pair) that is outwardly expressed in the heterozygote is dominant; if it is not expressed in the heterozygote, it is recessive; if both alleles at a locus are expressed in the heterozygote, they are codominant.

In autosomal dominant inheritance, the mutant gene produces the trait or disease in the heterozygote; each offspring has an equal chance of inheriting the mutant gene and being affected, or of inheriting the normal allele and being unaffected. In autosomal recessive inheritance, both parents are usually heterozygotes, and unaffected; one fourth of their offspring will be homozygous and have the trait or disease. X-linked recessive disorders are manifest mainly in males who receive the gene from carrier mothers (who are unaffected or minimally affected) and who transmit the gene to half of their sons, who will have the disease, and to half of their daughters, who will be carriers. An affected son will not transmit the gene to his sons, but will transmit it to all of his daughters, who will be carriers. Mutant genes close together on the same chromosome tend to segregate together and are said to be linked.

A mutant gene may express itself differently in different individuals (variable expressivity) or may not produce any effect where it would be expected to (reduced penetrance). Methods are described for calculating segregation ratios and recurrence risks that take into account the special problems of human pedigree data, including ascertainment bias, variable age of onset, reduced penetrance, mutations, and consanguinity.

REFERENCES

1. Adams, M.S.: Children of related parents. *In* Advances in Teratology, edited by D.M.H. Woollam. London, Logos Press, 1970.
2. Bittles, A.H., Mason, W.M., Green, J., and Rao, N.A.: Reproductive behaviour and health in consanguineous marriages. Science 252:789, 1991.
3. Bodmer, W.F., and Cavalli-Sforza, L.L.: Genetics, Evolution and Man. San Francisco, W.H. Freeman, 1976.
4. Bundey, S., Alam, H., Kaur, A., Mir, S., and Lancashire, R.: Why do UK-born Pakistani babies have high perinatal and neonatal mortality rates? Paediatric and Perinatal Epidemiology 5:101, 1991.
5. Emery, A.E.H.: Methodology in Medical Genetics, 2nd ed. Edinburgh, Churchill Livingstone, 1986.
6. Fraser, F.C., and Biddle, C.J.: Estimating the risk of offspring of first-cousin matings. An approach. Am. J. Hum. Gen. 28:522, 1976.
7. Garrod, A.E.: The incidence of alkaptonuria: A study in chemical individuality. Lancet ii: 1616, 1902.
8. Harper, P.S., and Newcombe, R.G.: Age at onset life table risks in genetic counselling for Huntington's disease. J. Med. Genet. 29:239, 1992.
9. Murphy, E.A., and Chase, G.A.: Principles of Genetic Counselling. Chicago, Year Book Medical Publishers, Inc., 1975.
10. Schull, W.J., and Neel, J.V.: The Effects of Inbreeding in Japanese Children. New York, Harper & Row, 1965.
11. Vogel, F., and Motulsky, A.G.: Human Genetics. Problems and Approaches, 2nd ed. New York, Springer-Verlag, 1986.
12. Weatherall, D.J.: The New Genetics and Clinical Practice. Oxford University Press, Oxford, 3rd edition, 1991.

Chapter *6*

Biochemical Genetics

Genes control the structure of polypeptides and their corresponding proteins. A gene mutation, in which a single nucleotide base is changed to another, leads to a change in an amino acid in the corresponding polypeptide and protein. Depending on the nature of this amino acid substitution, and its position in the molecule, the function of the corresponding protein may be altered. Biochemical genetics deals with the biochemical changes resulting from substituting mutant for normal proteins and—by inference—with the functions of the normal proteins. Genetic defects in enzymes (which may cause "inborn errors" of metabolism or transport) will be considered first, and those in other proteins, such as hemoglobins, subsequently. Molecular genetics at the DNA level will be reviewed in Chapter 7.

INBORN ERRORS OF METABOLISM

Biochemical genetics began when the concept of the inborn error of metabolism appeared, thanks to the insight of the English physician Sir Archibald Garrod. In 1909, through his studies of alkaptonuria, he defined the characteristics of a group of diseases resulting from inactivity of an enzyme that carries out a particular step in a chain of metabolic reactions. Thus Garrod was far ahead of his time in describing the essence of the "one gene—one enzyme" hypothesis so elegantly demonstrated experimentally by Beadle and Tatum in the bread-mold, Neurospora, some 30 years later.

The characteristics Garrod specified were that diseases resulting from inborn errors of metabolism had an increased frequency of parental consanguinity, tended to recur in sibs (in fact, alkaptonuria was the first human trait shown to fit the expectation for a mendelian autosomal recessive trait), appeared early in life, showed marked deviations from normal, and were not subject to marked fluctuations in severity. The rapid growth of biochemical knowledge, and particularly enzymology, since then has led to the identification of over 200 inborn errors and to rational means of treatment for dozens[9, 20–22] (Table 6–1).

Inborn errors of metabolism result from lack of a functional enzyme. Several mechanisms can account for this reduction in enzymatic activity. When the gene coding for a particular enzyme polypeptide is changed by a mutation, this can lead to a functional deficiency of the enzyme in several ways. In homozy-

Table 6–1. Some Treatable Inborn Errors of Metabolism

Method of treatment	Disorder	Efficacy of treatment
Dietary restriction of substrate		
Fructose	Fructosemia	Good, if started in early infancy
Galactose	Galactosemia	Good, if started in neonatal period
Lactose	Lactase deficiency	Good
Leucine, isoleucine, valine	Maple syrup urine disease	Fair, if started in neonatal period
Neutral fats	Lipoprotein lipase deficiency	Good
Phytanic acid (dairy products)	Refsum disease	Good, except for auditory and visual
Phenylalanine	Phenylketonuria	Good, if started early
Protein	Urea-cycle, e.g., citrullinemia	Limited experience
Tyrosine	Tyrosinemia	Poor
Replacement of end product		
Copper	Menkes (kinky hair) syndrome	Poor
Pancreatic enzymes (plus)	Cystic fibrosis	Improved life span
Vitamin D and phosphate	Hypophosphatemic rickets	Fair to good
Cortisol ± mineralocorticoids	Adrenogenital syndromes	Good
Thyroxine	Familial goiters	Good
Uridine	Orotic aciduria	Fair to good, if started early
Carnitine	1° and 2° carnitine deficiency	Good, but depends on underlying disorders
Depletion of storage substance		
Alkali, fluids, D-penicillamine	Cystinuria	Good, for kidney stone prevention
Copper removal by D-penicillamine	Wilson's disease	Good, if treatment before damage
Bile-acid binding resins	Hypercholesterolemia, heterozygote	Fair
Iron removed by bleeding, desferioxamine	Hemochromatosis	Fair
Uric acid depletion by uricosuric drugs	Gout	Good
Cysteamine	Cystinosis	Good, if started early
Sodium benzoate	Urea cycle disorders	Good
Sodium phenylacetate	Urea cycle disorders	Good
Amplification of mutant protein		
Vitamin B$_{12}$, protein restriction	Methylmalonicaciduria (some)	Fair to good in some types
Phenobarbital stimulation of glucuronyl transferase	Crigler-Najjar hyperbilirubinemia	Good
Replacement of mutant protein		
Gamma globulin	Agammaglobulinemia	Good
Antihemophiliac factor	Hemophilia	Good
Irradiated red cells containing adenosine deaminase	Combined immunodeficiency	Fair in some patients
Glucocerebrosidase	Type I Gaucher	Excellent
PEG-AGA	Adenosine deaminase deficiency	Clinical benefit demonstration
Biotin	Biotinidase deficiency	Excellent
Organ transplant		
Kidney	Fabry disease, cystinosis, Alport disease, polycystic kidney disease (adult)	Good, if graft survives
Bone marrow (allogenic)	Combined immunodeficiency	Successful
	Wiskott-Aldrich syndrome	Successful
Bone marrow	Mucopolysaccharidoses	Good in some types
Bone marrow	X-Linked adrenoleukodystrophy	Good, if early enough; experience limited
Liver	Urea cycle disorders	Good, experience limited
Liver	Hereditary tyrosinemia	Good
Surgical removal		
Spleen	Hereditary spherocytosis	Good
Portacaval shunt	Glycogen storage disease, type I	Fair
Colon	Multiple polyposis of colon	Good
Thyroid	Medullary thyroid carcinoma syndrome	Good

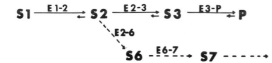

Fig. 6–1. Hypothetical metabolic pathway converting substrate S1 to end product P through the successive actions of enzymes E1–2, E2–3, and E3–P. An alternative minor pathway is indicated.

gotes for the mutant gene, the enzyme coded for by that gene may not be produced at all or be produced in an abnormal form with reduced activity. Third, the mutation may involve a gene that regulates the rate of production of the enzyme, leading to an inadequate amount of normal enzyme. So far, there are no known examples of this type in man. Fourth, the enzyme may be degraded at an excessive rate leading to a deficiency of active enzyme, as in the case of certain types of G6PD deficiency (Chapter 24). Fifth, optimal activity may depend on association with a cofactor, and mutations that interfere with absorption or biosynthesis of the cofactor, or alter the binding site on the enzyme to impair binding with the cofactor, may reduce the activity of the enzyme. The vitamin dependencies are outstanding examples of the last two types. Finally, if the enzyme consists of two or more polypeptides, each coded for by a separate gene, a mutation of any one of these genes could cause inactivity of the enzyme, and different mutant loci could have the same end result. Thus one might expect that the activity of a particular enzyme can be reduced in several different ways. This is one basis for the *genetic heterogeneity* so well recognized in many inborn errors of metabolism and elsewhere.

One useful way of classifying the diseases resulting from inborn errors of metabolism is according to the pathologic effects of the block in the metabolic pathway. Consider a prototype metabolic pathway converting substrate S1 through a series of enzyme reactions to an end product P (Fig. 6–1). Disease may result from absence of end product, pileup of substrates in the pathway proximal to the block, presence of excessive amounts of metabolites, and secondary effects of the above metabolic distortions on regulatory mechanisms in the

same or other pathways. Although many inborn errors show several of these results, one of them usually accounts for the major features of the child's disease. It must be admitted, however, that the precise mechanisms by which enzyme defects produce clinical defects are often unknown.

Defects in membrane transport present such special features that they will be considered separately from inborn errors of intermediary metabolism.

Diseases Resulting from Absence of End Product

One of the original inborn errors of metabolism, albinism is a good example of a disease in which the major clinical problems result from absence of the end product of a metabolic pathway. In our archetypical diagram (Fig. 6–2), enzyme E2–3 is indicated as missing, or inactive. All substrates beyond the block are therefore absent, including P.

In the classic type of albinism, lack of tyrosinase in the melanocyte blocks the pathway leading from tyrosine through DOPA (3,4,-dihydroxyphenylalanine) to the dark pigment melanin, so there is no pigment in the hair, skin, or iris (Fig. 6–3, block C). Note that the mutant gene affects only tyrosinase of the pigment-producing cells (melanocytes), and not that in the liver and elsewhere, showing that there must be at least two separate loci for this enzyme. Furthermore, genetic heterogeneity exists, since there are several other ways of blocking the pathway. There are at least 10 genetically different forms of albinism.[30]

Other examples of this class of disease include the various types of recessively inherited goitrous cretinism (dwarfism, mental retardation, coarse features) (Fig. 8–51) in which the pathologic effects result from a lack of thyroid hormone (Fig. 6–3, block D), pitressin-sensitive diabetes insipidus (drinking and excreting excessive amounts of water) in which

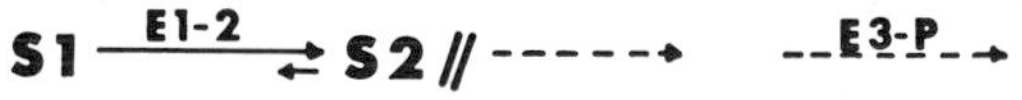

$$S1 \xrightarrow{\text{E1-2}} S2 \mathbin{/\!/} \text{------}\rightarrow \quad \text{--}\,\text{E3-P}\,\text{--}\rightarrow$$

Fig. 6–2. Pathway shown in Figure 6–1 blocked by the absence of enzyme E2–3.

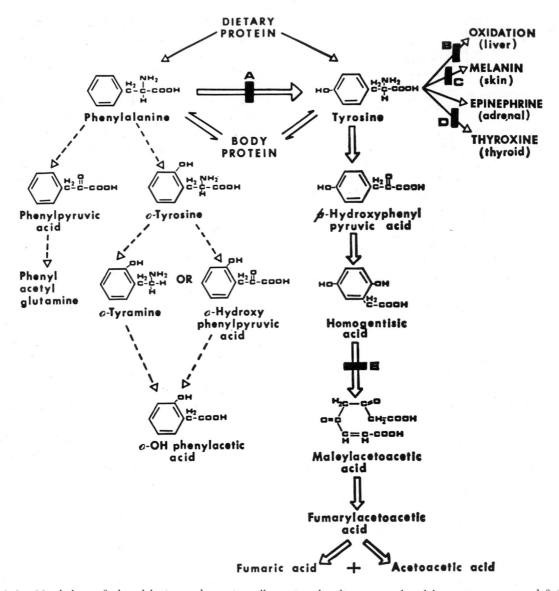

Fig. 6–3.   Metabolism of phenylalanine and tyrosine, illustrating the diseases produced by various enzyme deficiencies (see text).

the pituitary does not produce antidiuretic hormone, and the adrenogenital syndromes, in which part of the trouble results from a deficiency of cortisol. The latter syndrome will be considered later as an example of interference with regulatory mechanisms.

Diseases Resulting from Pileup of Substrate(s)

In some cases the substrate just before the block, in this case substrate S2, not being con-

verted to substrate S3, will increase in concentration and may appear in abnormal quantities in blood and urine. Because most enzymatic reactions are reversible, substrate S1 may also pile up and be excreted (Fig. 6–4).

An example is galactosemia, in which the defective enzyme is galactose-1-phosphate uridyl transferase, which normally converts galactose-1-phosphate to glucose-1-phosphate (Fig. 6–5). In the mutant homozygote this step cannot occur, and galactose-1-phosphate ac-

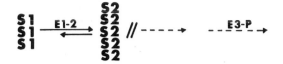

Fig. 6-4. Hypothetical pathway of Figure 6-1 showing pileup of precursor S2 when enzyme E2 3 is lacking.

cumulates in the blood cells, liver, and other tissues, damaging the liver, brain, and kidney.

Alkaptonuria is another example. The homogentisic acid accumulates in the blood (Fig. 6-3, block E) and, in polymerized form, is deposited in cartilages, leading to degeneration and arthritis. It also forms a polymer in the urine, which turns black on exposure to air. Some storage diseases in which the excess material accumulates in the lysosomes also fit into this class, but they will be considered in a later section.

Diseases Resulting from Excessive Amounts of Metabolites

In this category, the damage is done not so much by the excessive amounts of precursors behind the block as by excessive amounts of metabolites produced by the breakdown of these precursors through alternate pathways that are normally used only slightly, but are called upon to deal with the abnormal situation (Fig. 6-6).

Phenylketonuria, a Classic Inborn Error. Phenylketonuria (PKU) was not one of the five inborn errors of metabolism to which Garrod first applied the term, but it has contributed so much to our understanding that this is the classic example.[25] In 1934, a Norwegian chemist, Følling, first recognized the condition as a specific type of mental retardation by the excessive amount of phenylpyruvic acid in the urine of 2 retarded siblings. Affected children were normal at birth but became progressively retarded and were hyperactive, irritable, and spastic; many had seizures. They tended to be blue-eyed and blonde.

As the word spread, and more cases were identified, autosomal recessive inheritance was demonstrated, and a high level of phenylalanine was found in the blood (hyperphenylalaninemia). An American physician, Jervis, deduced from his metabolic data that the block was caused by a lack of the enzyme phenylalanine hydroxylase in the liver and, in 1953, demonstrated that the liver of a PKU patient did not oxidize phenylalanine to tyrosine (Fig. 6-3, block A). In the absence of the enzyme, phenylalanine accumulates in the blood and is broken down to phenylpyruvic, phenylacetic, and phenyllactic acids, which may be toxic. For instance, they may inhibit the enzyme tyrosinase, and this inhibition would account for the decreased pigmentation. The exact cause of the mental retardation is still not understood. One likely hypothesis is that the increased phenylalanine competes with other amino acids for transport into the nerve cells; the resulting imbalance of amino acids in the cell inhibits the synthesis of proteins necessary for myelin and synapse formation.

The frequency of PKU varies widely among populations; for Caucasians incidences of 1 in 10,000 to 1 in 20,000 are reported: the rates are higher in Irish in Eire, much lower in

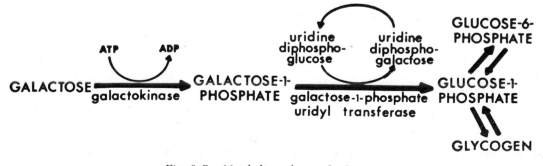

Fig. 6-5. Metabolic pathway of galactose.

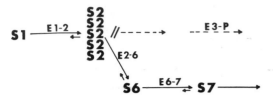

Fig. 6–6. Hypothetical pathway of Figure 6–1 showing increased use of an alternate pathway.

Ashkenazi Jews and African-Americans, and very low in Finland. As expected, heterozygotes have intermediate levels of liver phenylalanine hydroxylase activity and can be detected by measuring the ratio of phenylalanine to tyrosine in the serum under standard conditions.

The rational treatment would be to restrict the dietary intake of phenylalanine. This was first tried in the early 1950s, and the response was dramatic. The children were described as seeming to wake up, recognize their parents, and become less irritable. Their seizures disappeared and their biochemical findings returned to normal. Great was the excitement, and great the disappointment when, after a few days or weeks, the improvement ceased and the patients relapsed to their former states. Then it was realized that, if the children got no phenylalanine in the diet, they would break down their own body proteins and flood their tissues with phenylalanine. Successful treatment therefore requires careful regulation of the patient's diet to provide just enough phenylalanine, but not too much. This is not as easy as it sounds. Several commercial diets low in phenylalanine are now available, and with careful dietary management and monitoring of the levels, excellent metabolic control can be achieved.

The Collaborative Study of Children Treated for Phenylketonuria has demonstrated the undisputed value of a phenylalanine-restricted diet in the prevention of mental retardation without compromising a child's growth. During the 1960s and 1970s, it was accepted medical practice to discontinue diet therapy after a few years. In the 1980s, data suggested that there was a decline in cognitive and behavioral scores in children who had discontin-

ued their phenylalanine-restricted diets. Continued use of the special diet is now recommended, not only throughout school years but indefinitely. This is of particular relevance to women with PKU who, when not on such a diet during pregnancy, may have children with significant microcephaly, congenital anomalies, and developmental delay. The Maternal PKU Collaborative Study is now locating women with PKU in the child-bearing age bracket, informing them of the concerns of maternal PKU effects, and encouraging them to maintain or to resume their phenylalanine-restricted diet before embarking on a pregnancy, thereby reducing the risk of damage to their unborn children.

The treatment must begin early in life, before brain damage has occurred. In utero, neither the normal nor the PKU fetal liver makes phenylalanine hydroxylase. After birth, the baby is offered phenylalanine in the milk, and the enzyme is induced in the normal but not the PKU liver. It takes several days for the biochemical abnormalities to appear and several weeks for irreversible damage to occur. This is an advantage because it allows time for detection and early treatment, but also a disadvantage, because the hyperphenylalaninemia cannot be detected at birth.

The development of a successful treatment meant that it was important to detect babies with PKU early enough to prevent brain damage, and this led to the development of programs aimed at screening all babies early in life for hyperphenylalaninemia.[23] Population-wide neonatal screening was a worthy objective, but the first programs to be set up ran into unexpected trouble—genetic heterogeneity.

It is now recognized that genetic heterogeneity—different mutant genes producing similar phenotypes—is more often the rule than the exception, and PKU is a good example. At first the biochemical error seems simple; activity of the enzyme is absent in the mutant homozygote. More refined analysis has shown that there is in fact a small amount of activity (about 0.3%) but not enough to protect the patient. One might predict, therefore, that there are other mutant alleles re-

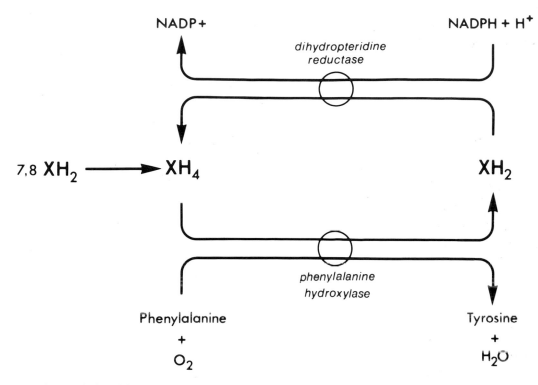

Fig. 6–7. Oxidation of phenylalanine to tyrosine: the phenylalanine hydroxylase requires a cofactor, tetrahydropterin (XH_4), which is oxidized to dihydropterin (XH_2). The enzyme dihydropteridine reductase reduces XH_2 back to XH_4 so it can be used again. A mutant hydroxylase leads to "classic" PKU; a mutant reductase leads to the "lethal" form of PKU.

sulting in mutant enzymes and other levels of activity. And indeed there are now several hyperphenylalaninemias. "Classical" PKU is type I. Type II is a "benign hyperphenylalaninemia" in which the hydroxylase enzyme has about 5% of the normal activity, the blood hyperphenylalanine level is only modestly elevated, and there is no need for the special diet. There is also a "transient" hyperphenylalaninemia, type III, in which deficiency of the liver hydroxylase activity lasts only for a few weeks or months, after which the special diet becomes unnecessary. It is essential to distinguish these types of hyperphenylalaninemia from "classic" PKU because putting these patients permanently on PKU diet would be (and was) very harmful.

To complicate matters even more, the hydroxylation of phenylalanine to tyrosine is a process much more complex than previously recognized. It is a coupled oxidative reaction. The phenylalanine hydroxylase requires a coenzyme, tetrahydropterin. This is oxidized

to dihydropterin in the reaction and then reduced again by another enzyme, a pteridine reductase, so it can participate in another oxidative reaction, i.e., act as a catalyst to the hydroxylase (Fig. 6–7).

A rare form of PKU, called "lethal PKU" because of its fatal course, has now been identified (type IV). The mutation involves the dihydropterin reductase enzyme. This enzyme is normally present in the liver, fibroblasts, and brain tissue. In the mutant homozygote the lack of reductase leads to a deficiency of coenzyme for the hydroxylase, which therefore does not act, and PKU results. Furthermore, tetrahydropterin also acts as a coenzyme for the tyrosine and tryptophan hydroxylases, which are important in the synthesis of norepinephrine and serotonin, two important neurotransmitters. Such a patient has, in addition to PKU, more direct adverse effects on brain biochemistry. Lethal PKU does not respond to the simple dietary treatment. The fact that diagnosis can be made by demonstrating the enzyme deficiency in fibro-blasts raises the possibility of prenatal diagnosis.

Still another type of PKU (type V) results from a deficiency of an enzyme, dihydrobiopterin synthetase, involved in the synthesis of dihydrobiopterin. Promising results for both these types are being obtained by oral treatment with tetrahydrobiopterin, supplemented with neurotransmitter precursors, as well as control of phenylalanine levels. Clearly, correct early diagnosis of the type of PKU is crucial. The broad spectrum of biochemical and clinical phenotypes seen in PKU and the hyperphenylalaninemias has been complemented by detailed molecular analysis. More than 50 different mutations—mostly point mutations—have now been identified, confirming the hypothesis that molecular heterogeneity underlies the phenotypic heterogeneity seen[4] (Fig. 6–8). Of the 13 exons in the PAH gene, the central region surrounding exon 7 is marked by a clustering of mutations reflecting the catalytic importance and the cofactor binding domain within this region.

In summary, elevated blood phenylalanine can occur for a variety of reasons, and the sorting out of the underlying genetic heterogeneity has taught us many lessons about biochemical pathways, about the importance of recognizing genetic heterogeneity, and about the necessity of providing the facilities to diagnose precisely the hyperphenylalaninemic babies detected in mass screening programs.

Diseases Resulting from Interference with Regulatory Mechanisms

A fourth category of pathologic effects resulting from genetic blocks in metabolic pathways are those in which lack of the end product, or too much substrate, interferes with feedback or other regulatory mechanisms.

In the *adrenogenital* syndromes, for instance, there is a block at one of several steps in the biosynthesis of cortisol by the adrenal cortex. This deficiency stimulates excessive production of ACTH by the pituitary, because the level of cortisol normally regulates the output of ACTH by a negative-feedback mechanism. The increased ACTH levels, in turn, stimulate the adrenal cortex to increase synthesis of the cortisol precursors but, of course, only as far as the block. Breakdown of the accumulated precursors by alternative pathways leads to the androgenic effects.[15] In a female fetus, this may result in masculinization of the external genitalia (Fig. 6–9). Affected boys show early virilization. Both sexes may show metabolic upset, depending on the nature and degree of deficiency.

Orotic aciduria is another example of an inborn error of metabolism resulting in a regulatory mechanism defect, and the only one, so far, in which a single mutant gene results in the absence of two sequential enzymes.[5] The pathway leads from aspartic acid and carbamyl phosphate through a series of steps to uridine monophosphate (UMP). In homozygotes for orotic aciduria, two enzymes—orotidylic acid pyrophosphorylase and decarboxylase—are absent, and the proximal precursor piles up and appears in the urine. The end product, UMP, is a feedback inhibitor of the first enzyme in the pathway. In its absence, the reaction appears to proceed more rapidly, leading to a great excess of orotic acid. Adding uridine to the diet inhibits the first enzyme and leads to a sharp decrease in the production of orotic acid.

The means by which a single mutant gene affects two different enzymes is not yet clear. Possibly a regulatory gene is involved, the mutant gene may affect a polypeptide common to the two enzymes, or the two enzymatic functions may be carried by a multifunctional protein complex.

Hereditary hypercholesterolemia is an exciting example of a relatively common disorder of metabolic regulation that has recently thrown much light on the metabolism of cholesterol.[7] This subject will be discussed in Chapter 23, Cardiovascular Disease.

The Storage Diseases

In many inborn errors of metabolism, one of the substrates that accumulates is deposited in abnormal quantities in the cells and may cause damage merely by its presence.

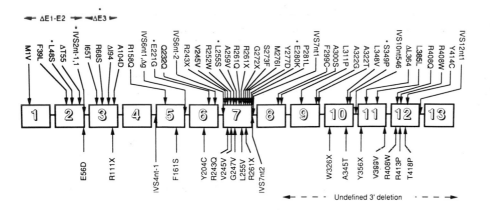
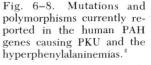

Fig. 6–8. Mutations and polymorphisms currently reported in the human PAH genes causing PKU and the hyperphenylalaninemias.[4]

The *glycogen storage diseases* are classic examples.[10] Glycogen is a polymer of alpha-D-glucose, assembled into a multibranched tree-like structure. The glycogen molecules are constantly being degraded and resynthesized to meet the varying metabolic demands of the individual. Errors can occur at various steps of mobilization or synthesis. For instance, cleavage of the outer branches of the glycogen molecule, when glucose is to be mobilized, is done by a phosphorylase. Absence of this enzyme in muscle cells results in accumulation of glycogen in muscle, causing painful muscle cramps on exercise (glycogen storage disease type V).

Many storage diseases fit into a special category, the *lysosomal diseases*. The lysosomes are intracellular organelles consisting of a lipid membrane enclosing a variety of acid hydrolytic enzymes. If a special lysosomal enzyme is missing, the corresponding substrate may accumulate in the lysosome, and the cell becomes laden with the resulting storage vacuoles. The first example to be discovered was Pompe disease, one of the glycogen storage diseases (type II). Homozygotes are deficient in α-1,4-glucosidase, a lysosomal enzyme that can hydrolyze the outer chains of glycogen to give glucose. Apparently, fragments of glycogen are constantly being taken up by the lysosomes and degraded. In Pompe disease, uptake goes on, but degradation does not; the lysosomes become swollen with glycogen in the cells of the heart, muscle, liver, and other tissues. The heart and liver enlarge, and the child usually dies within the first 6 months of life.[10]

Another well-known example of a lysosomal disease is Tay-Sachs disease, or G_{M2} gangliosidosis.[16] An autosomal recessive gene, particularly frequent in Ashkenazi Jews, causes a deficiency of an enzyme, hexoseaminidase A, that is involved in the metabolism of a class of nervous system lipids called gangliosides. In the absence of the enzyme, one of the gangliosides, G_{M2}, accumulates in the ganglion cells of the brain (and other organs and tissues) leading to progressive retardation in development, paralysis, dementia, blindness, and death by the age of 3 to 4 years. The enzyme is normally present in leukocytes and cultured fibroblasts, diminished in heterozygotes, and almost absent in homozygotes, so that the disease is a suitable candidate for population screening and prenatal diagnosis.

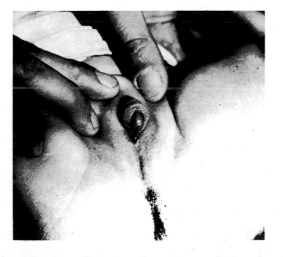

Fig. 6–9. Masculinization of a patient with the adrenogenital syndrome (female pseudohermaphrodite). The small hole at the base of the phallus leads into a vagina.

The mucopolysaccharidoses are another group of lysosomal storage disorders that are attracting considerable interest.[13] Hurler syndrome, or gargoylism, is the classic example. The defective enzyme is α-L-iduronidase, a lysosomal enzyme that cleaves the side chains from the acid mucopolysaccharides (or glycosamino-glycuronoglycans—GAG—in the modern terminology), an important component of connective tissue ground substance. Storage of mucopolysaccharide in various tissues leads to progressive mental retardation, coarsening of features, stiff joints, coronary artery insufficiency and heart valve thickening, and death, usually by the age of 10 years. A clinically milder and distinct disorder called Scheie syndrome is now known to be an allelic disorder.

Another clinically similar but less severe type is the X-linked recessive Hunter syndrome, in which the missing enzyme is sulfoiduronide sulfatase. Sanfilippo syndrome also has a similar phenotype, but in fact can result from four distinct enzyme mutations. Altogether there are 10 groups of mutants, each involving an enzyme needed for the degradation of mucopolysaccharides, resulting in at least 7 types of mucopolysaccharidoses.

Studies on cultures of somatic cells have shown that the enzyme missing in the mutant cell is secreted by normal cells or, for that matter, by cells affected by another mutant, not involving the same enzyme. Thus, if cells from a Hurler patient are cultured with those from a Hunter patient in complementation tests, each will correct the deficiency in the other and neither will store mucopolysaccharide (metabolic cooperation). This explains why females heterozygous for the Hunter mutant are not a mosaic of cells storing mucopolysaccharides and normal cells, as one would predict from the Lyon hypothesis. The normal cells correct the defect in the abnormal cells.

A final example of lysosomal storage disease has an unexpected twist—it turns out to be a receptor defect. Patients with *I-cell disease* (mucolipidosis II) resemble those with Hurler syndrome, but with an earlier onset of the physical abnormalities.[14] Several acid hydrolases (e.g. β-hexosaminidase, iduronate sulfa-

tase) are elevated in the serum. In a mixture of ML II and normal cells in culture, the ML II cells take up these enzymes released from the normal cells (endocytosis), but the normal cells will not take up the enzymes from the mutant cells. The explanation is that after these hydrolases are synthesized, they are glycosylated and phosphorylated. The mannose-6 phosphate termini are recognized by receptors, which bind them and deliver them to the lysosomes. In ML cells, the enzyme that does the phosphorylation is missing, or inactive. The enzymes do not bind to the receptors, so they cannot get into the lysosomes, and the substances they normally process there accumulate.

Because the biochemical defect is present in amniocytes, prenatal diagnosis is possible.

INBORN ERRORS OF TRANSPORT

Our increasing understanding of diseases resulting from genetically determined errors of membrane transport is a good example of how specific mutations can be used as tools to probe the biology of the normal organism.

Inborn Errors of Amino Acid Transport

Cystinuria was first classified (erroneously) as an inborn error of metabolism of cystine, but the fact that blood levels of cystine are not elevated in patients with the disease suggested that the condition was an inborn error of membrane transport rather than of intermediary metabolism. That is, the cystine was not being reabsorbed by the renal tubule from the glomerular filtrate and therefore appeared in abnormal amounts in the urine. This implied a specific transport mechanism across the tubule membrane, which was defective in the cystinuria patients. The cystine, being relatively insoluble, may form "stones" in the kidney. The discovery that not only cystine, but the structurally similar dibasic amino acids, lysine, arginine, and ornithine, were being excreted in abnormally large quantities led to the idea that there was a membrane transport system that would accept all four of these amino acids, but not the others.

Harris demonstrated genetic heterogeneity for the disease when he showed that, in some families, the heterozygotes had mild degrees of the relevant aminoacidurias, but in other families they did not.[9] It was then found that some cystinuria homozygotes had the same defect in transport across the *intestinal* membrane, and this led to further definition of genetic heterogeneity. All homozygotes have similar urinary findings, but some (type I) have greatly impaired transport of cystine and the dibasic amino acids from the intestine into plasma; others (type II) have only moderate impairment of intestinal membrane transport, and a third group (type III) have mild impairment.

Heterozygotes for the type I mutant have normal urinary amino acids—that is, the gene is "completely recessive"—whereas those of types II and III have an excess of the relevant amino acids in the urine, somewhat more marked in type II. Matings between heterozygotes of different types produce offspring with the full-blown homozygous urinary phenotype, showing that the three mutants are allelic.

The hereditary *iminoglycinurias* provide another example of genetic determination of a specific transport mechanism and of genetic heterogeneity. Homozygotes have decreased tubular resorption of proline, hydroxyproline, and glycine, with normal plasma levels. This suggests a renal tubular transport mechanism specific to these substances. As with cystinuria, there is heterogeneity when intestinal transport is examined; in some homozygotes it is impaired and in others it is not. Again, family studies suggest allelism. The condition is probably harmless.

Hartnup disease is characterized by defective transport of the neutral amino acids (other than the iminoacids and glycine), suggesting a membrane site specific to the transport of these molecules. The relation to the clinical manifestations (intermittent attacks of ataxia and a pellagra-like skin rash) remains unknown.

Finally, there are mutant genes that interfere with membrane transport of a wide variety of amino acids and other substances. The *Fanconi syndromes* (rickets, glucosuria, and aminoaciduria) are well-documented examples. In some cases, this may be secondary to impairment by some toxic metabolite of the energy supply necessary for transport; in others, there may be a defective component in the transfer mechanism beyond the binding site. Perhaps further study of mutant phenotypes will throw more light on the nature of the binding sites.

Why is it that these mutant genes produce only partial defects in tubular transport of the affected amino acids? In the iminoglycinuria homozygote, for instance, about 80% of the ability to reabsorb proline, hydroxyproline, and glycine is retained. Kinetic studies, both in vitro and in vivo, suggest that at least two kinds of system are involved in amino acid tubular transport. One type is represented by the mutant phenotypes we have been describing. They have "group" specificity, high capacity, and low affinity; they appear to operate at concentrations that exceed the usual physiological range. Another type of transport site is characterized by low capacity, high affinity, and specificity to a particular amino acid. If so, one would expect to find mutant phenotypes involving failure to transport specific amino acids, and this is so. Siblings have been reported with excessive amounts of cystine, but not of the dibasic amino acids in the urine. There are also gene-determined hyperdibasic amino-acidurias in which the transport of dibasic amino acids, but not of cystine, is impaired. Similarly, there is a "blue diaper" syndrome that involves defective intestinal transport of tryptophan, and there is a methionine malabsorption syndrome.

These mutant phenotypes have thus been beautifully specific probes with which to dissect the biology of membrane transport.

Inborn Errors of Transport of Other Than Amino Acids

Site specificity of transport is not limited to the amino acids. Genetically determined defects of membrane transport have been found for many other substances, and, again, study of the disorder has often been the first evidence that there is a specific site for the transport of that particular substance. These include the following:

Renal glucosuria—failure to reabsorb glucose; harmless (except when misdiagnosed as diabetes); pattern of inheritance varies from family to family.

Glucose-galactose malabsorption—diarrhea after ingestion of these sugars or disaccharides and polysaccharides that give rise to them; autosomal recessive.

Hypophosphatemic rickets—failure to reabsorb phosphate leads to rickets; X-linked dominant. See below.

Renal tubular acidosis—increased permeability of distal tubule cells to hydrogen; autosomal dominant in some families.

Chloridorrhea, congenital—chloride lost in intestine; autosomal recessive.

Hereditary spherocytosis—impaired transport of sodium across the blood cell membrane; autosomal dominant.

Diabetes insipidus, nephrogenic—impaired tubular resorption of water; X-linked recessive.

THE VITAMIN-RESPONSIVE INBORN ERRORS OF METABOLISM

The vitamins are a diverse class of organic compounds required in minute amounts for normal growth and function. They may act as hormones (vitamin D), antioxidants (E), neurotransmitters (A), and coenzymes (B complex).

Until recently, most vitamin-deficiency diseases resulted from a lack in the diet of the vitamin concerned. As nutrition improved, a new class of inborn errors of metabolism was recognized—those resulting from genetic defects in the metabolism of vitamins—so that the vitamin had to be given either in increased amounts or by a different route. These are known as the vitamin-responsive or vitamin-dependent disorders.[20] They result from the fact that vitamins, like other compounds, are metabolized in a series of steps, each subject to interference from the effects of mutant genes. They fit, therefore, into many

of the classes of inborn errors described in this chapter and illustrate strikingly the fact of genetic heterogeneity.

Inborn Errors of Vitamin B_{12}

One of the most thoroughly investigated groups of vitamin-responsive conditions involves vitamin B_{12} or cobalamin, and we will use it as the prototype of the group.[5] Deficiency of this vitamin leads to the features of "pernicious anemia" in which there is a megaloblastic anemia (the red blood cells are too big but too few), degenerative neurological changes, and increased excretion of methylmalonate and homocystine. Figure 6–10 outlines its metabolism and indicates some of the steps at which mutant genes are known to interfere. The legend should be read as part of the text at this point.

Three disorders, all probably autosomal recessive, give rise to a kind of juvenile pernicious anemia. In one of them, because no intrinsic factor is produced, the cobalamin-IF complex cannot attach to the ileal wall and is not absorbed. In another, the IF is present, but its capacity to bind to the ileal receptors is much reduced. In the third, the ileal transport system is defective. All three respond dramatically to normal amounts of B_{12} provided it is injected, bypassing the absorption defect.

Another B_{12}-responsive disorder, infantile megaloblastic anemia, results from a deficiency of the plasma binding-protein (TC), so that the transport of B_{12} into the cell is diminished. Treatment requires large amounts of B_{12} given indefinitely. Presumably, if the B_{12} concentration is high enough, it will get into the cell by passive diffusion or by some other route not requiring TC.

Finally, there is a group of inborn errors, the methylmalonic acidurias, in which there are large amounts of methylmalonic acid in urine and blood, leading to acidosis, coma, and death. One type (with two subgroups) involves defective synthesis of the active coenzyme, Ado-Cbl. Another type results from a defect in synthesis of some precursor of the

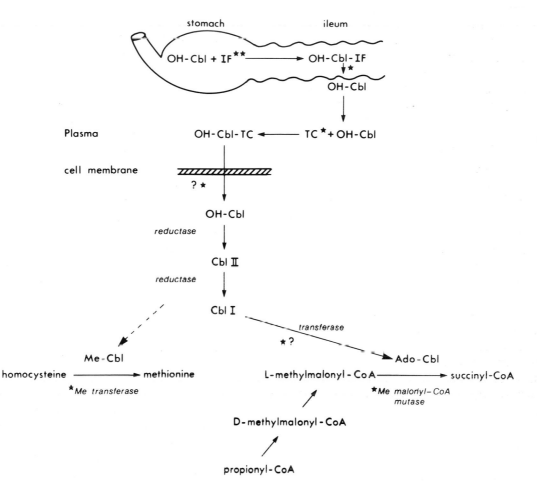

Fig. 6–10.   Metabolism of vitamin B_{12} (cobalamin). Dietary hydroxycobalamin (OH-Cbl) combines with intrinsic factor (IF) in the stomach. The complex attaches to specific receptor sites in the ileum, and OH-Cbl is transported across the intestinal wall into the blood plasma, where it binds to a transport protein (transcobalamin, TC) that carries it to the cell. The complex is admitted across the cell membrane, and cobalamin is converted to its coenzyme forms by a series of enzyme reactions. One active form, 5'-deoxyadenosylcobalamin (Ado-Cbl), is a coenzyme for the mitochondrial enzyme methyl-malonyl-CoA mutase, inactivity of which leads to methylmalonicaciduria. The other active form, methylcobalamin (Me-Cbl), is involved in folate metabolism, acting as a coenzyme for the cytoplasmic enzyme homocysteine-methyltetrahydrofolate methyltransferase, which converts homocysteine to methionine. The arrow is broken, as the exact pathway is uncertain. Its inactivation leads to one form of homocystinuria. The asterisks indicate sites of mutant action.[12]

two active coenzymes; these patients have both methylmalonic aciduria and homocystinuria. Both types respond to large amounts of B_{12}, which presumably allows the rate of the enzyme reaction to reach an effective level.

A third type has a primary defect of the mutase apoenzyme and does not respond to therapy with B_{12}.

The reader may wonder why defects involving defective transport of B_{12} do not result in methylmalonic aciduria severe enough

to cause acidosis, as do the defects involving coenzyme synthesis. At this point, so do the biochemists.

Folic Acid

At least five inborn errors of folate metabolism have been identified: one involves intestinal absorption and four concern coenzyme formation and interconversion.[20] These may cause megaloblastic anemia and a variety of neurologic problems. One of them causes homocystinuria, apparently as a result of impaired synthesis of N^5-methyltetrahydrofolate which, as well as methylcobalamin (see the previous section), is a cofactor for the methyl transferase that converts homocysteine to methionine. Therefore, we have genetic heterogeneity of homocystinuria; one of the forms responds to vitamin B_{12} and another to folate. The latter form has occurred in association with schizophrenia. As one would predict, some forms do not respond to replacement therapy.

Vitamin D (Calciferol)[11]

As with vitamin B_{12}, the activity of vitamin D depends on its proper absorption and metabolism, which have recently been found to be unexpectedly complex. A precursor is synthesized in skin exposed to ultraviolet light, but in environments where exposure is inadequate it must be supplied in the diet. In children, a deficiency leads to rickets—decreased serum calcium and phosphorus, and a softening and deformation of the growing bones caused by inadequate calcification.

A precursor of vitamin D is absorbed from the intestine or skin, bound to serum proteins, carried to the liver, hydroxylated to 25-hydroxycholecalciferol, and then carried to the kidney, where enzymatic addition of another hydroxyl group converts it to 1,25-dihydroxy-cholecalciferol, the active form. This acts on the intestine to stimulate absorption of calcium and phosphorus and can also mobilize calcium from previously formed bone.

A generation ago, rickets was an all-too-common disease, almost always resulting from nutritional deficiency. When improved nutrition virtually removed this disease (primarily by adding the vitamin to milk), a new type of rickets became apparent—inborn errors of vitamin D metabolism.[18,20] One form, autosomal recessive vitamin D-dependent rickets, could be successfully treated with massive doses of vitamin D (although the effective dose was often dangerously near the toxic dose). Then the site of the block was discovered: the enzyme that adds the second hydroxyl group was defective. When the block

was bypassed by giving 1,25-dihydroxycholecalciferol, the patient could be successfully treated with physiologic doses.

In another form of vitamin D-resistant rickets, showing X-linked dominant inheritance, the serum phosphorus is low. For some reason, females carrying the gene may have low levels of serum phosphorus but escape the overt bone disease. It was also treated with massive doses of vitamin D, but although this therapy healed the rickets, it did not permit normal growth of the long bones. The cause appears to be not in the metabolism of vitamin D, but in failure of the intestinal epithelium and renal tubule to transport phosphorus, and it is now called hypophosphatemic rickets (Fig. 6–11). The rickets appear to result directly from the deficiency in phosphorus. Thus the appropriate treatment is large amounts of phosphate to increase the level of serum phosphorus. Vitamin D is also given to correct the disturbance in intestinal calcium transport caused by the increased phosphorus concentration (Fig. 6–11). Strictly speaking, therefore, X-linked hypophosphatemic rickets should no longer be considered a vitamin-responsive disorder because the inborn error involves phosphorus, not vitamin D.

Pyridoxine (Vitamin B₆)

Another group of vitamin-dependent diseases results not from defective transport or synthesis of coenzyme but from mutations that alter the apoenzymes in a way that impairs their interaction with the coenzyme. These conditions respond, in varying degrees, to treatment with large doses of the vitamin.

Pyridoxine is an interesting example. The active form of this vitamin, pyridoxal-5'-phosphate (PLP), acts as a coenzyme for a large number of apoenzymes, which regulate the catabolism of amino acids, glycogen, and short-chain fatty acids. Thus, mutations affecting these apoenzymes can cause a variety of metabolic diseases, depending on which enzyme is affected, each of which may be responsive to large amounts of pyridoxine, although otherwise they appear quite unrelated.[20] These include infantile convulsions resulting from a

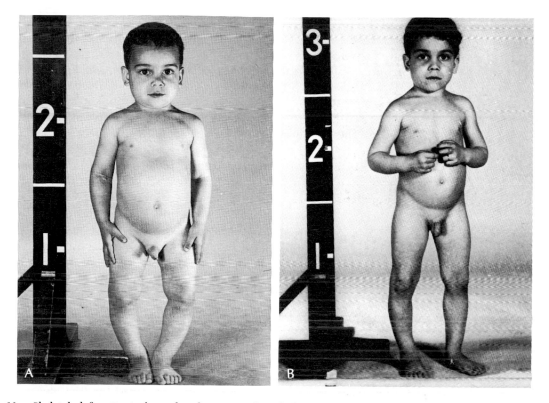

Fig. 6–11. Skeletal deformity in hypophosphatemic rickets before treatment (A) and after two years of treatment (B). (Courtesy of Dr. C.R. Scriver in Nora & Fraser, Medical Genetics, 2nd Ed. Philadelphia, Lea & Febiger, 1981.)

mutant glutamic acid decarboxylase, cystathioninuria, xanthurenic aciduria, homocystinuria (yet another form, caused by a mutant cystathionine synthase), and hyperoxaluria (Fig. 6–12).

Similar groups of diseases involving various apoenzymes of biotin and thiamine are known. The clinical and biochemical aspects of these diseases are reviewed elsewhere.[10] Altogether, there are more than 25 different

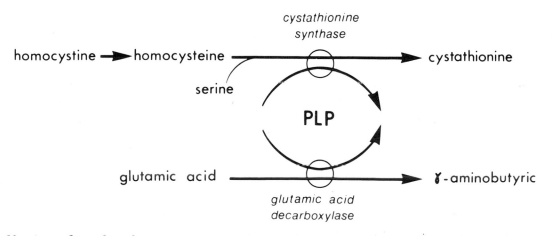

Fig. 6–12. Active form of pyridoxine, PLP, acts as a coenzyme for many enzymes. A mutation that alters the structure of glutamic acid decarboxylase so that its interaction with PLP is impaired will lead to a deficiency of γ-aminobutyric acid and convulsions. Large amounts of pyridoxine may increase the rate of the reaction and correct the deficiency. Similarly, a mutant form of cystathionine synthase can produce homocystinuria, responsive to pyridoxine treatment.

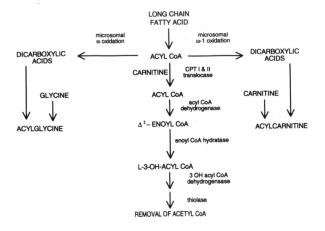

Fig. 6–13. Metabolic pathways of fatty acid oxidation.

vitamin-responsive metabolic disorders, and the list continues to grow.

ORGANIC ACID DISORDERS

Organic acid disorders are a heterogeneous group of disorders in which the common denominator is a diagnostically important elevation of organic acids or related compounds. Organic acids are carboxylic acids that are water-soluble end products of metabolism of amino acids, sugars, lipids, biogenic amines, steroids, and other compounds. By definition, organic acids exclude amino acids and have in common features of high water solubility, acidity, and ninhydrin-negativity. Although organic acids occur as physiologic intermediates of normal metabolic pathways, the number of clinically important inborn errors of organic acid metabolism is rapidly increasing, and there is accumulating evidence that some of these disorders remain undiagnosed.

Most organic acids are rapidly cleared from the circulation by the kidney, and their concentrations in the urine greatly exceed those in the plasma. Their identification and analysis depend on increasingly sophisticated detection systems including gas chromatography-mass spectrometry in which mass spectral analysis of the partitioned volatile organic acid derivatives produce a "chemical fingerprint" that allows the absolute and unambiguous identification of each organic acid.

Numerous disorders of organic acid metabolism have been identified over the past two decades. Many represent well-known disorders involving metabolic blocks in amino acid degradative pathways. These include disorders of leucine metabolism (e.g., isovaleryl aciduria), disorders of isoleucine and valine metabolism (e.g., propionic aciduria), and disorders of lysine and tryptophan metabolism (e.g., glutaric aciduria type 1) plus many others. The newest class of organic acid disorders are the fatty acid oxidation defects with, to date, 14 hereditary disorders of fatty acid catabolism discovered.[8] These involve defects in fatty acid uptake and activation, entry into the mitochondria, and mitochondrial beta-oxidation and ketone body formation.

The metabolic pathways involved are shown in Figure 6–13. Common features of fatty acid oxidation defects are metabolic decompensation during periods of prolonged fasting with hypoglycemia, absence of ketone bodies, alterations in carnitine, which functions in the pivotal role of transporting fatty acids into the mitochondria, and fatty livers. The best characterized of these disorders is medium chain acyl-coA dehydrogenase (MCAD) deficiency, an autosomal recessive disorder with an estimated frequency of ~1 in 20,000. This disorder presents in the first 2 years of life as either sudden death or an acute life threatening Reye syndrome-like episode.[27] Mortality may be as high as 60% for the first metabolic crisis. In addition to the features described above, a characteristic abnormal dicarboxylic organic profile is seen in the urine (Fig. 6–14). This disorder is particularly important clinically because the signs and symptoms are preventable if a high-risk child is identified, and if dietary treatment consisting of a low-fat, high-carbohydrate formula and avoidance of prolonged fasting is instituted. Genetic analysis of the MCAD cDNA has revealed that a single nucleotide substitution of an adenine to guanine at cDNA position 985 resulting in a lysine (K) to glutamate (E) replacement at position 329 in the mature MCAD polypeptide accounts for ~90% of MCAD mutations.[31] This is demonstrated in Chapter 7. Thus, because of its unique bio-

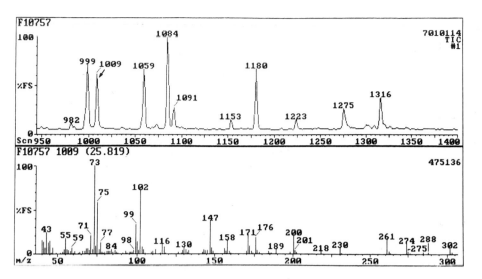

Fig. 6–14. Typical GC-MS profile of a patient with MCAD, a fatty acid oxidation defect.

chemical, molecular, and clinical characteristics, pilot programs are studying the feasibility of introducing mass neonatal screening for MCAD deficiency.

Fatty acid oxidation defects, as a subclass of organic acid disorders, may present as acute life threatening episodes in newborns and infants. Some older children with developmental delay and adults with unexplained metabolic disease may also have organic acid disorders. It is likely that in the next decade, with increasingly sophisticated analytic tools to study organic acid profiles in physiologic fluids, inborn errors of organic acid metabolism will assume as important a role in biochemical genetics and clinical medicine as amino acid disorders.

DISORDERS OF STRUCTURAL PROTEINS

In addition to enzymatic proteins, mutations in nonenzymatic proteins such as receptors, carrier proteins, and structural proteins form important classes of inborn errors of metabolism. Unlike enzymatic disorders, which are often inherited in an autosomal recessive manner, mutations in nonenzymatic proteins can cause disease in a heterozygous state and thus follow an autosomal dominant pattern of inheritance. In addition to common disorders of receptors such as the LDL receptor resulting in familial hypercholesterolemia, dis-

orders of structural proteins—the connective tissue disorders—are the best known.

Collagen is the most abundant structural protein in the body. At least 12 different types of collagens have been described, encoded by genes distributed throughout the genome. The most abundant and best studied to date are collagen types I, II, and III, with their main tissue distribution being bone, tendon, skin (type I), cartilage and vitreous (type II), and skin, arteries, uterus, and intestines (type III). The collagen molecule is a triple helical molecule with each polypeptide consisting of repeats of an amino acid sequence (glycine-X-Y)$_n$ where X is often proline and Y is the position where proline and lysine are hydroxylated to hydroxyproline and hydroxylysine respectively.[2] The schematic structure of a collagen molecule and its procollagen precursors are shown in Figure 6–15.

Several heritable disorders of connective tissues are now known to result from mutations in type I collagen. The best characterized are osteogenesis imperfecta and various forms of Ehlers-Danlos syndromes (EDS). Their clinical features and their current clinical classification are summarized in Figure 6–16. To date, more than 50 mutations affecting the synthesis and structure of Type I collagen have been found in the osteogenesis imperfectas. This is leading to a greater understanding of the pathogenesis of these disorders and how phenotypic expression depends not only

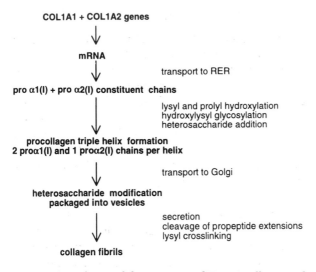

Fig. 6–15.   Schema of the structure of Type 1 collagen and its biosynthesis.

Type	Inheritance	Clinical Signs	Biochemical Defect
Osteogenesis Imperfecta			
Type I	AD	fragile bones (types I-IV) blue sclerae, hearing loss teeth abnormalities	
Type II	AD (new mutation) AR	perinatal lethal	"non-functional" COL1A1 allele or
Type III	AD AR	progressively deforming growth failure	heterogeneous mutations in COL1A1 or COL1A2
Type IV	AD	normal sclerae variable short stature hearing loss, teeth abn. bony deformity variable	
Ehlers Danlos Syndromes			
I Gravis	AD	hyperextensible skin hypermobile joints scarring, bruising	not known
II Mtis	AD	similar to EDS I but milder	not known
III Familial Hypermobility	AD	no scarring, benign	not known
IV Arterial	AD	thin skin arterial rupture	abnormal type III collagen
V X-Linked	XLR	similar to EDS II	not known
VI Ocular	AR	hypermobile joints scoliosis hyperextensible skin myopia	lysyl hydroxylase deficiency
VII Arthrochalasis multiplex congenita	AD	congenital hip dislocation hypermobile joints soft skin normal scarring	cleavage site abnormality of procollagen 1N-1 proteinase
VIII Periodontal	AD	generalized periodontitis	not known
IX Cutis Laxa	XLR	lax skin skeletal abnormalities	lysyl oxidase
X Fibronectin defect	AR	similar to EDS II	fibronectin
Marfan Syndrome	AD	Marfanoid habitus lens dislocation aortic root dilatation and rupture	fibrillin mutations in some patients

Fig. 6–16.   Clinical classification of the most common connective tissue disorders.

on the type and position of the mutation but also on its effect on triple helix assembly, its stability, and the stoichiometry of normal and mutant polypeptides. Abnormal type III collagen synthesis has been shown in EDS IV, but the biochemical basis for the other forms of EDS remains largely undefined. A third connective tissue disorder, Marfan syndrome, characterized by a Marfanoid habitus, ectopia lentis, and aortic dilation, has recently been mapped to chromosome 15q21.1, and evidence has accumulated that mutations in the FBN1 gene encoding the noncollagenous protein fibrillin result in this disorder.[3]

The three connective tissue disorders just discussed are of interest not only because of their medical importance, but also because of the lessons they teach us. These disorders, although distinct, have many phenotypical features that overlap, and the phenotypic heterogeneity seen is a consequence of marked genetic and molecular heterogeneity. The concept of "protein suicide" seen in dominant disorders where one mutant subunit can disrupt an entire multimeric protein will probably prove to be important in other disorders. Last, given the abundance of the collagen proteins, more common disorders, such as some forms of osteoarthritis, are already proving to have underlying collagen mutations.

PRINCIPLES OF TREATMENT OF INBORN ERRORS OF METABOLISM[21,22,25]

Rational methods of treating the disorders resulting from the inborn errors of metabolism depend on understanding the biochemical nature of the error and of the resulting disease processes. Correction of the end results of a genetic defect has been termed *environmental engineering*, as opposed to *genetic engineering*, which attempts to modify the genetic material itself.[22] An increasing number of genetically determined metabolic diseases are now susceptible to treatment.

Part of the problem is the organization of medical resources to get the patient with a (usually rare) genetic disease to a source of expert diagnosis and treatment, or better still, in some cases, to get the management to the patient.[23]

Approaches to therapy include avoidance, substrate restriction, removal of toxic products, product replacement, and cofactor supplementation.

Avoidance

Many genetic diseases make us particularly prone to specific environmental factors. The first approach to treatment is to avoid the agent in question. Examples include mechanical stress in persons with osteogenesis imperfecta, sunlight in albinos and those affected by xeroderma pigmentosa, ragweed pollen in those with ragweed hay fever, cigarettes in those with alpha-1 antitrypsin deficiency, flights in unpressurized aircraft in sickle-cell carriers, and certain drugs in individuals with pharmacogenetic conditions that make them respond abnormally to the drug in question (Chapter 24).

Substrate Restriction

Diseases in which the metabolites proximal to the enzyme block interfere with development or function can logically be treated by restricting the supply of substrate. This approach has been quite successful when the substrate comes primarily from the diet. Thus, reduction of dietary phenylalanine in phenylketonuria, of lactose and galactose in galactosemia, and of fructose in fructosemia are relatively effective in preventing the pathologic consequences of the genetic defect.

When the substrate is synthesized endogenously, it may be much more difficult to control its accumulation by simple dietary restriction. Sometimes it is possible to impose a block elsewhere in the pathway, where the results may be less harmful. For instance, the accumulation of oxalate in oxalosis can be reduced by treatment with calcium carbamide, which inhibits aldehyde oxidase and thereby reduces the synthesis of glycolate and its conversion to glyoxalate and oxalate.

Removal of Toxic Products

An alternative to restricting substrate would be to remove the accumulating toxic product. This approach is taken in the treatment of Wilson disease by removing excess copper with penicillamine and of hemochromatosis by bloodletting and desferioxamine, for example. In babies with urea cycle disorders, sodium benzoate and sodium phenylacetyl supplements are successful in eliminating toxic accumulations of ammonia.

One might also place in this category the prevention of hemolytic disease of the newborn due to Rh-isoimmunization by treating Rh-negative mothers of Rh-positive babies with anti-RH antibody (RhoGAM), which neutralizes any Rh antigen the mother may have received from the baby (see Chapter 19). This approach has brought about a dramatic decrease in the frequency of "Rh disease," a condition that threatened about 1 in 170 babies in Caucasian populations.

One might also include protection of individuals with pharmacogenetic conditions (see Chapter 24) that alter their responses to environmental agents, such as drugs, by avoidance of the particular agent to which they react abnormally.

Product Replacement

When the pathologic condition results from lack of a product in the metabolic pathway distal to the block, it would seem logical to replace the product. This is the rationale for treating inherited defects of thyroid hormone synthesis with thyroxin, the adrenogenital syndromes with cortisol, orotic aciduria with uridine, hemophilia with antihemophiliac globulin, and cystic fibrosis of the pancreas with pancreatic enzymes. However, replacement of the product may present technical difficulties, particularly if the product is intracellular, as in albinism, for instance.

In some diseases, product replacement is used together with substrate restriction. In homocystinuria, for instance, methionine is restricted, but cystine must be added because the homozygote cannot synthesize it from methionine.

Cofactor Supplementation

The section on vitamin-responsive disorders provides examples of treatment by cofactor supplementation, by either short circuiting a transport defect or flooding the system.

TREATMENT OF INBORN ERRORS OF TRANSPORT

Most hereditary transport defects of man are rather benign, and treatment is often limited to what might be called second-order clinical manifestations. For instance, cystinuria is a serious disorder only when urinary stones are formed. Keeping the urine diluted prevents stone formation (all that is needed is a glass of water and an alarm clock to wake the patient at the appropriate hour), and solubilization of cystine with penicillamine reduces cystine excretion and causes stones to dissolve, though, unfortunately, there are problems with toxicity.

In nephrogenic diabetes insipidus, the logical approach is to replace the water lost by inadequate tubular resorption. In renal tubular acidosis (Butler-Albright disease), in which hydrogen ion clearance is inadequate, leading to excessive excretion of bicarbonate, sodium, potassium, and calcium, treatment with alkali adjusts the imbalance quite well.

NEW TREATMENT APPROACHES[4,21,22]

In theory, the best way to treat a disease resulting from an enzyme deficiency would seem to be replacement of the enzyme, and this is already true for such conditions as congenital trypsinogen deficiency and some of the clotting disorders. This approach seems promising when the deficiency involves an extracellular enzyme and is already being used in the treatment of hemophilia and pancreatic cystic fibrosis. Intracellular enzymes, however, present problems. Rapid inactivation, failure to reach the site of reaction with the substrate, and the development of antibodies to the "naked" enzyme are some of the problems that complicate this approach. For instance, attempts to treat metachromatic leukodystrophy (a degenerative brain disease) with arylsulfatase A infusion failed, because there was no increase in enzyme in the brain, and infusion of alpha-glucosidase in patients with type II glycogenosis led to severe immunologic intolerance.[22] Enzyme replacement therapy has been successfully accomplished for one lysosomal disorder, Gaucher disease,[1] and still holds great promise for the treatment of many metabolic disorders once basic pathogenetic questions are addressed and animal models of human disease are better characterized.

Perhaps inclusion of the enzyme in a semipermeable, inert microcapsule may avoid some of these problems, and this approach has already achieved temporary correction of the biochemical phenotype of acatalasemic mice.

One intriguing development is in the treatment of mucopolysaccharidoses. We have referred previously to the fact that mixtures of normal and mutant cells show metabolic cooperation. Enzyme produced by the normal cells corrects the defect in the mutant cells. The active factors are the missing enzymes, each mutant cell supplying the enzyme for the other. Application of this work to therapy led to the discovery that injection of normal serum results in striking improvement in patients with Hunter and Hurler syndromes. Injection of white cells from nonmutant donors may be an even better approach. However, there has been trouble with antibody formation against the "foreign" protein factor, and long-term results are not as promising as anticipated.[13]

In some cases, it may be possible to induce synthesis of the missing enzymes; for example, treatment with phenobarbital induces synthesis of glucuronyl transferase and lowers the bilirubin level in the Crigler-Najjar syndrome (congenital nonhemolytic unconjugated hyperbilirubinemia). Stabilization of a defective enzyme by the addition of an appropriate compound is another possibility. The stabilization of hemoglobin S (see following section) by cyanate is an example, though unfortunately there are problems with toxicity. Because the necessary amount of enzyme activity is often far below the normal amount, a relatively small increase in activity may be therapeutic. For many disorders, however, organ or bone marrow transplantation and gene replacement therapy (Chap. 7) provide hopeful alternatives.[12]

Organ transplantation is another way of correcting an enzyme deficiency. This is complicated by the problem of graft rejection, but progress is being made. Transplantation of bone marrow and thymus has been successful in some of the immune deficiency syndromes. Liver transplantation has been performed in Wilson disease, urea cycle disorders, tyrosinemia, thalassemias, and hemophilia with promising success, and is being attempted in many other diseases involving hepatic enzymes. In the recessively inherited severe combined immunodeficiency, for example, there is a deficiency of adenosine deaminase, and the resulting accumulation of adenosine impairs the production of lymphocytes, leading to the immune defect. Promising results have been obtained by the injection of fetal liver or bone marrow cells to restore a source of enzyme. In addition, bone marrow transplantation has been attempted in more than 200 patients with various storage diseases and successful grafts have been achieved in many.[28]

Looking further into the future, directed gene change appears as a way of providing the missing enzyme in a mutant individual. This is more fully discussed in Chapter 7 on molecular genetics.

FETAL THERAPY[6,19]

One advantage of prenatal diagnosis is the possibility of treating the disorder in question before birth, but progress so far has not been encouraging.

One success story in this area is the treatment, or prevention, of hemolytic disease of the newborn caused by maternal Rh immunization (Chapter 19). One type of *fetal thrombocytopenia* is also caused by maternal immunization, in this case by fetal platelets. It can be treated by transfusion of platelets into the fetus.

A small group of *inborn errors of metabolism* can be treated by supplying a missing product *in utero* much as they are treated after birth. They are so rare that reports of prenatal treatment are anecdotal. They include treatment of vitamin B_{12}-responsive *methylmalonic acidemia* with large doses of vitamin B_{12} (there is no evidence that results are any better than those of postnatal treatment), treatment of multiple carboxylase deficiency with biotin, maternal treatment with dexamethasone to prevent masculinization of female external genitalia in congenital adrenal hyperplasia (variable results), and (theoretically) treatment of *galactosemia* by maternal dietary galactose restriction.[6]

Injection of genetically normal fetal stem cells into the affected fetus is a promising approach. These primitive cells from bone marrow or liver are not rejected immunologically by the fetus as adult stem cells would be, and may colonize the marrow or liver, where they may produce the missing product. Theoretically, this approach should apply to any of the disorders now treated by postnatal marrow or liver stem cell transplants. Trials with thalassemia are in progress.

Methods of treatment are being developed for a number of *anatomic disorders*, mostly nongenetic, that can cause fetal damage, e.g., by blocking circulation of fluids or pressing on developing organs. These include hydrocephalus, hydronephrosis, diaphragmatic hernia, pleural effusions and cardiac arrhythmias. Results have been disappointing so far. Risks are high, and the potential for harm is great. Much more work is needed in defining risks for mother and fetus, refining techniques, and learning how to select cases that will benefit.[19]

In this discussion of principles of treatment of the inborn errors of metabolism and transport, we have shown how an understanding of the nature of the basic error, and of the mechanism by which the error leads to the specific features of the disease, leads to rational methods of treatment. We have also shown how imaginative applications of new advances in modern biology hold promise of further exciting advances in therapy. The future—in this respect—looks bright.[21]

THE GENETICS OF PROTEIN STRUCTURE

Inborn errors of metabolism may reflect enzymatic quantitative variation. Hemoglobinopathies represent examples of disorders of qualitative variation. We have said that mutation of a gene results in the substitution of one amino acid for another in the corresponding polypeptide chain. This is not always true. The genetic code is redundant, and a mutation that changes one triplet to another coding for the same amino acid will not produce any change in the structure of the protein—though it may change its rate of synthesis. Nevertheless, the majority of mutations in genes coding for polypeptides would be expected to result in an amino acid substitution.

The Hemoglobins

Hemoglobin was the first molecule in which an association was shown between a mutant gene—for sickle-cell disease—and a specific amino acid substitution. Sickle-cell disease is a form of chronic hemolytic anemia characterized by the presence of elongated filiform or crescent-shaped red blood cells. Family studies in the 1940s showed that (with certain exceptions that later proved the rule) the disease fitted the segregation ratio expected for autosomal recessive inheritance. Heterozygotes showed the sickle-cell trait—sickle cells were not normally present in blood smears, but when the red cells were made hypoxic—by incubation or treatment with sodium metabisulfite—sickling would occur.

The disease has an extraordinarily high frequency in populations of West African origin, occurring in about 1 in 400 African-Americans. In addition to the effects of chronic anemia, the patients may suffer from intravascular sickling resulting in thrombi and local infarcts in the intestine (sometimes mistaken for appendicitis), lungs, kidneys, or brain.

After Pauling's discovery that the disease resulted from a physicochemical difference in the hemoglobin molecule (the first "molecular disease") and Ingram's demonstration that sickle-cell hemoglobin differed from normal hemoglobin by a single amino acid—a valine substituted for a glutamic acid—progress was rapid. The molecule, already known to be a tetramer, was shown to consist of four polypeptide chains, two alpha and two beta chains. The sickle-cell substitution involved the sixth amino acid from the N-terminal of the beta chain. The high frequency in West Africans appears to result from an increased resistance of heterozygotes to falciparum malaria—heterozygote advantage.

By electrophoretic and chromatographic procedures, a large number of other "mutant" hemoglobins have been identified—over 290 affecting the beta chain and 175 the alpha chain. Almost all are associated with a single amino acid substitution. By convention, the normal molecule is assigned the formula $alpha_2^A$ $beta_2^A$, and the mutant forms are designated according to the amino acid substitution. For instance, sickle-cell hemoglobin is $alpha_2^A$ $beta_2^{4Glu-Val}$, or $alpha_2^A$ $beta_2^S$ for short.

One of the triumphs of molecular biology has been the use of these amino acid substitutions in specific regions of the molecule, and the resulting alteration of charge and bonding, to elucidate the functional properties of the molecule in physicochemical terms.[26,28,29]

Each chain is coiled and folded in a complex but characteristic manner and has a pocket that contains a heme group—a porphyrin ring with an iron atom at its center that combines with oxygen (Fig. 6–17). The molecule is *allosteric* with respect to its affinity for oxygen; as a molecule of deoxyhemoglobin moves into a region of increasing oxygen tension, an oxygen atom will bind to an iron atom in the heme group of one chain, causing the iron atom to move slightly, which results in a slight twist in the chain where the heme group is attached to it. This, in turn, causes a change in the conformation of the other chains in the tetramere that increases the affinity of their heme groups for oxygen and decreases the affinity for carbon dioxide. As the next heme group combines with oxygen, the affinity of the other two changes still more, and so on. Thus, when the hemoglobin arrives in the lung,

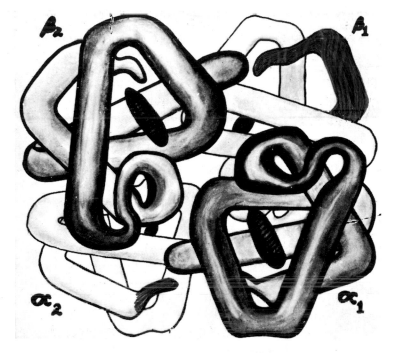

Fig. 6–17.   Hemoglobin molecule.

where the oxygen tension is high, its affinity for oxygen increases, and it readily picks up oxygen, but as it moves to the periphery, where the oxygen tension is low, it begins to lose oxygen, and its affinity decreases so that it more easily releases the oxygen where it is needed.

The alpha chain has 141 amino acids, and the beta chain 146. The amino acid sequence is similar, though not identical, in the two chains. The sequence of amino acids is the *primary structure* of the polypeptide chain. Much of the chain is in the form of a helix, named by the protein chemists the alpha helix (not the same alpha as the chain), but some segments are not coiled. The helical coiling is the *secondary structure*. The (mostly) coiled chain is folded in a complex way (Fig. 6–18), forming a pocket for the heme group and surfaces for relating to the other three chains of the tetramere. This is referred to as its *tertiary structure*. This tertiary structure is similar in the two chains. Figure 6–18 indicates that there are eight helical segments, designated alphabetically from A to H, with non-helical portions at the bends, designated by

the letters of the segments they join. Specific amino acids can be numbered consecutively from the N-terminal, or by their position in the segment. For instance, the sickle-cell substitution involves amino acid 6 from the N-

BETA CHAIN

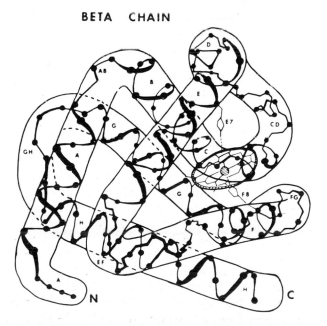

Fig. 6–18.   Diagram of the beta chain of hemoglobin.

terminal, or A3, since the first three amino acids are nonhelical. (The advantage of the helical nomenclature is that it allows more meaningful comparisons between corresponding amino acids in different chains. Thus, the histidine F8 is linked to the heme group in the alpha chain, the beta chain, and myoglobin.) Finally, the four chains are associated to form a more or less globular molecule, and this association is the *quaternary structure* of the molecule.

It is now clear that the primary structure of the chain determines its secondary, tertiary, and quaternary substructures. It does so by means of the side chains on the amino acids, which form bonds with other side chains; the sequence of amino acids determines the positions of the bonds, and thus the folding. The nature of the folding determines the way in which it associates with other chains. The short side chains such as oxygen and nitrogen tend to be polar, or hydrophilic, and the longer radicals, such as phenyl rings, tend to be nonpolar, or hydrophobic, or "greasy." It appears that the internally situated side chains, those lining the heme pockets or binding one helical segment to another, are hydrophobic, whereas external side chains can be either hydrophilic or hydrophobic.

The normal structure and function of the hemoglobin molecule depends on the collective forces of four factors: a large alpha-helical content (at least 75%) of each chain; the firm binding of the heme group in its pocket; the internal siting of the nonpolar amino acids that determine the folding of the chain; and the stability of the contacts holding the alpha and beta chains together.

THE HEMOGLOBINOPATHIES

Mutations giving rise to amino acid substitutions can produce *hemoglobinopathies* (hemoglobins with abnormal functions) by interfering with any of these.[29] They can be classified into four groups: unstable hemoglobins, hemoglobins with increased oxygen affinity, hemoglobins with reduced oxygen affinity, and methemoglobin.

The Unstable Hemoglobins. In this group, the amino acid substitution leads to changes that make the molecule tend to undergo spontaneous oxidation and precipitate to form insoluble inclusions, resulting in a hemolytic anemia (premature breakdown of red blood cells). Examples are:

—Hemoglobin Köln (beta 98 FG5 Val → Met). The larger side chain of methionine distorts the tight interhelical FG segment, breaking several contacts with the heme, resulting in loss of the heme group, exposure of the hydrophobic side chains to water, and precipitation.

—Hemoglobin Hammersmith (beta 42 CD1 Phe → Ser). The serine side chain is too short to reach the heme group that normally binds with the Phe.

—Hemoglobin Bristol (beta 67 E11 Val → Asp). The Val side chain is nonpolar and the Asp polar, resulting in gross distortion of the E segment to neutralize its charge.

—Hemoglobin Gun Hill (Beta 91–95 F7-FG2 → O). A deletion of part of the FG segment results in loss of heme contacts.

Hemoglobins with Increased Oxygen Affinity. Amino acid substitutions resulting in increased oxygen affinity create a relative oxygen deficit in the periphery and a compensatory increase in red cells (polycythemia). There is little, if any, danger to health (except the possible hazards of unnecessary treatment). One example is:

—Hemoglobin Chesapeake (alpha 92 FG4 Arg → Leu). The arginine forms part of the bridge from alpha 1 to beta 2. The change to a Leu changes the spatial relations and the oxygen affinity is increased.

Hemoglobins with Reduced Oxygen Affinity. Some amino acid substitutions reduce oxygen affinity, so that oxygen is given up more readily in the periphery. This may reduce the stimulus to produce red cells (erythropoietin) and lead to a mild anemia. An example is:

—Hemoglobin Kansas (beta 102 G4 Asn → Thr).

Methemoglobin. The iron atom in the globin chain is in the ferrous state. It is oxidized slowly to the ferric state (nothing to do with oxygen-binding for transport), forming methemoglobin, which is blue, but an enzyme, methemoglobin, reductase, quickly reduces it again. Certain amino acid substitutions affect the microenvironment of the heme group, resulting in an inability of the ferrous iron to remain reduced. The methemoglobin causes cyanosis, a bluish discoloration of the skin, but heterozygotes have no ill effects other than those resulting from unnecessary cardiovascular investigations because of the cyanosis. Examples are:

—Hemoglobin M Boston (alpha 58 E7 His → Tyr). This histidine is adjacent to the heme group; the tyrosine forms an ionic bond with the Fe, changing it to ferric.
—Hemoglobin M Saskatoon (beta 63 E7 His → Tyr). This is the beta chain counterpart.

SICKLE CELL HEMOGLOBIN

Ironically, the nature of the defect in the hemoglobinopathy that initiated all this progress is still unclear. The beta 6A3 Glu → Val substitutes a nonpolar valine for a charged glutamic acid on the surface of the beta chain. Most substitutions involving a surface amino acid are silent, but this one changes the physicochemical properties in a way that leads to the formation of polymers, which increases the deformability of the red cell, and results in blockage at the terminal arterioles with consequent peripheral oxygen deficit. This occurs particularly during the "crises," precipitated by causes still not understood, in which signs and symptoms become acute.

HEMOGLOBIN F

Hemoglobin F is the normal major hemoglobin found in the fetus. It consists of two alpha chains and two gamma (γ) chains which are similar to beta chains but differ from them at 39 sites. The switch from hemoglobin F to A is an interesting problem of gene regulation. Several weeks before birth, the level of hemoglobin A begins to increase and that of F to decrease, so that the newborn has about equal amounts of each, and by the end of the first year, only about 2% of the hemoglobin is F. This means that in the young blood cells (reticulocytes) of the embryo, the gamma chain gene is active and the beta chain gene is suppressed, whereas in adult reticulocytes the converse is the case, with the switch occurring over a period of months, before and after the birth. That this switch is under genetic control is shown by the existence of a dominant gene for *hereditary persistence of fetal hemoglobin* (HPFH). The gene is closely linked to the gamma-delta-beta locus (see section on mapping the hemoglobin loci) and suppresses the switch to activity of the beta chain gene on the same chromosome; the normal concurrent suppression of the gamma chain gene does not occur. Thus the adult heterozygote has diminished amounts of A and increased amounts of F, and the homozygote has no A and almost all F, as in the embryo. Fortunately, hemoglobin F seems to work effectively in the adult, and there are no ill effects. Because the mutant gene results in failure of the switch, it follows that there must be a normal gene (sometimes called Y^1) that is responsible for the switch. There are now several different HPFH mutants, which will be discussed further in the section on the thalassemias.

MAPPING THE HEMOGLOBIN LOCI

The fine structure of the hemoglobin loci is now known in some detail, and it is interesting to consider the train of events leading to our knowledge of the map.[26,29] When it was found that hemoglobin S differed from hemoglobin A by a single amino acid, little was known of the structure of hemoglobin. The second mutant hemoglobin to be discovered was hemoglobin C, which (by an extraordinary coincidence) involved the same amino acid as S—6 Glu → Lys. Family studies showed that these were alleles, since S/C heterozygotes with normal mates had either A/S or A/C children but not S/C or A/A children.

This was confirmed by the biochemical evidence—S/C heterozygotes produced no hemoglobin A. In the light of our present knowledge of gene structure and function, they had to be alleles, of course, but at the time this was not obvious, because the idea that genes act by controlling amino acid sequences of polypeptides was just beginning to emerge.

Then a family was described in which another mutant hemoglobin, Hopkins II, and S were both present. The Ho/S "heterozygote" did have large amounts of A as well, which showed that these mutant genes were not allelic, and therefore that hemoglobin is specified by at least 2 loci. Furthermore, the double heterozygote produced an entirely new hemoglobin—$\alpha_2^{Ho}\beta_2^{S}$. Concurrently, the biochemists were finding that hemoglobin is a tetramere made up of two pairs of chains, alpha and beta; presumably the two loci were for the two chains.

Meanwhile, hemoglobin A_2, which constitutes about 2% of normal adult hemoglobin, was found to consist of alpha chains combined with a new type of chain, called delta (δ), which is similar to the beta chain and differs at no more than 10 amino acid sites. Thus there are three sites coding for the adult hemoglobins. Later, fetal hemoglobin (F) was discovered and shown to consist of alpha and gamma (γ) chains.

A puzzling feature was that, whereas an A/S heterozygote has about 50% Hb S, as do other β chain mutants, most of the α chain heterozygotes, e.g., A/G, have only about 25% mutant Hb. Why? A possible answer would be that there are 2 α loci, so that an individual carries 4 α chain genes; if one of them is mutant, 3 will be making normal α chains, and the mutant Hb would only be $1/4$ of the total. This prediction was confirmed by a Hungarian family in which 3 members each had 2 mutant hemoglobins—Hb Buda (α 61 Lys $\rightarrow$ Asn) and Hb Pest (α 74 Asp $\rightarrow$ Asn)—and each also had 50% Hb A. Because their children had either Buda or Pest, they must have been heterozygotes with one mutant (and one normal) α chain gene on each chromosome. There are now several such examples. However, in some populations (mostly African), there appears to be only one α locus. Perhaps the second locus arose by duplication relatively recently, evolutionarily speaking, and has not yet spread through the entire population.

The γ chain gene has also been duplicated, and in this case the 2 genes differ by one nucleotide. Because normal fetuses always have two types of γ chains, differing at position 136, which is either Gly or Ala, there must be two loci, one for $^G\gamma$ and one for $^A\gamma$.

Insight into the fine structure map of the Hb loci began with Hb Lepore, an abnormal Hb found in small quantities in some β-thalassemia patients. Amino acid sequencing showed that it begins with a stretch of δ sequences and ends with a stretch of β sequences. The explanation invokes the phenomenon of *unequal crossing over*. The δ and β sequences are similar enough that when the chromosomes pair in meiosis, a δ gene may mispair with a β gene; if crossing over occurs, one of the resulting strands will have a deletion (Hb Lepore) and the other a duplication (Fig. 6–19).

An example of the duplication (Hb Miyada) has since been found. It begins with a β and ends with a δ sequence. These findings *prove that the δ chain gene must be adjacent to and precede the β chain gene.*

Another example of unequal crossing over provides further information. Hb Kenya begins with γ sequences and ends with β sequences, and the only γ Hb produced is $^G\gamma$. This can be explained by unequal crossing over after mispairing of the $^A\gamma$ with the β gene. (Draw it out for yourself.) An individual with Hb Kenya also behaves like a person with hereditary persistence of fetal hemoglobin mutant (HPFH), suggesting that this gene (Y) lies between $^A\gamma$ and δ.

See the end of the chapter for further exciting developments.

UNIVERSALITY OF THE CODE

All of the amino acid substitutions so far are compatible with the Escherichia coli code—e.g., it would be impossible to get from Met (AUG) to Trp (UGG) by a single base substitution, and no such mutation is known. Conversely, a change from Glu to Val requires

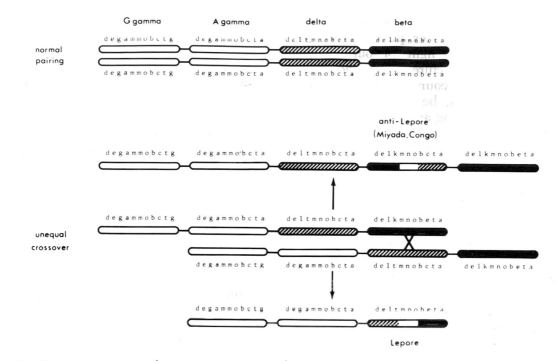

Fig. 6 19.   Diagram representing how new genes can arise by unequal crossing over. The two gamma genes, G_γ and A_γ, are represented by the letters "degammobctg" and "degammobcta," respectively (identical except for g and a). The delta locus is represented as "deltmnobcta"[11] and beta as "delkmnobeta," similar but not identical. If, at meiosis, the delta gene pairs with the beta gene, and a cross-over occurs, two recombinant chromosomes will arise. One will lack the delta and beta genes and have a "new" gene beginning with delta sequences and ending with beta sequences—deltmnobeta—hemoglobin Lepore. The other will have an "extra" gene that begins with beta and ends with delta sequences—delkmnobcta—hemoglobin Miyada.

changing GAA to GUA or CAG to CUG, a single base substitution, and a number of these are known.

This kind of analysis of the known mutants and the necessary base substitutions can provide further information about the code in man.[26,28] For example, there are several Val → Met mutations; of the four codons for Val (GUU, GUC, GUA, GUG), only the last converts to AUG by a single step, so this must be the codon that is used in man. Still further information about the $\gamma\ \delta\ \beta$ region is provided by other types of mutation.

TERMINATION CODON MUTATIONS[28]

Hb Constant Spring has 31 extra amino acids on the end of an otherwise normal α chain. The first extra amino acid (142) is Gln (CAA or CAG); UAA and UAG are termination codons, so presumably the U has mutated to a C and transcription therefore does not stop

there but goes on "reading" the DNA until the next termination codon. If this is so, there should be six other mutant hemoglobins iden tical to Constant Spring, except for amino acid 142, and three such are known—Hb Icaria α 142 Lys (UAA → AAA), Hb Koya Dora, 142 Ser (UAA → UCA), and Hb Seal Rock, 142 Glu (UAA → GAA).

Conversely, Hb McKees Rock lacks the last two amino acids of the β chain. The next-to-last amino acid is Tyr (UAU), which has presumably mutated to UAA (term). Perhaps similar mutations nearer the other end of the gene account for some of the thalassemia mutations.

Frame Shift Mutations. If only a single nucleotide, or any nonmultiple of 3, is deleted, there will be a "frame-shift," and a new sequence of AAs will be read out. Hb Wayne is an example. Note that Wayne code is α^A code shifted one to the left; this shift "mutates" the termination codon, so extra AAs are

α^A	Ser	Lys	Tyr	Arg	(Term)					
Wayne	Ser	Asn	Thr	Val	Lys	Leu	Glu	Pro	arg	(Term)
α^A		AAA	UAC	CGU	AAA	GCU	GGA	GCC	UCG	GUA
Wayne		AAU	ACC	GUA	AAG	CUG	GAG	CCU	CGG	UAG

added until a new term codon appears. This interpretation is confirmed by the fact that the post-terminal sequences deduced from Hb Wayne are consistent with those seen in Constant Spring.

The preceding studies are an elegant example of the fruitful interaction between genetics and biochemistry. Family studies identify gene mutations affecting the molecule, and these can be used by the protein biochemist to elucidate the relation between the structure of the molecule and its function.

The Thalassemias

The thalassemias are another large and important group of hereditary anemias characterized by diminished production of hemoglobin.[26] The first to be recognized was Cooley's anemia, alias thalassemia major, target cell anemia, microcythemia, or Mediterranean anemia. Because the amount of hemoglobin in the red cell is diminished, the cell tends to be small and irregular in shape and to have a "target" appearance. Anemia, spleen enlargement, growth retardation, marrow hypertrophy with resulting bone changes, and death in childhood are the usual course, which can be improved somewhat only by repeated transfusions and the use of chelating agents to get rid of excess iron. Thalassemia major was thought to result from the homozygous state of a gene that caused thalassemia minor (a mild anemia) in the heterozygote. This turned out to be a great oversimplification.

The more information accumulated, the more variability became apparent. The degree of hemoglobin deficiency varied widely from family to family. Then two groups were recognized—those that "interacted" with the sickle-cell gene (which turned out to be those involving suppression of beta chain synthesis) and those that did not (those in which alpha chain synthesis was suppressed).

The Alpha Thalassemias. The variability in severity among different families with α-thalassemia became more understandable when it was discovered that there are two alpha chain loci-4 genes per individual. Then two major groups emerged.

The α-thalassemia 1 mutation results from deletion of both α loci. This was proven by the following method. Reticulocytes (pre-red blood cells) are synthesizing almost exclusively messenger RNA for globin chains. It was possible to isolate mRNA for the α chain and, using the enzyme reverse transcriptase, to synthesize a complementary DNA (cDNA) that had sequences identical to those of the α chain gene. When this cDNA was annealed with DNA from a normal person, it combined with it, showing that those sequences were present in the normal DNA. But this cDNA would not anneal with DNA from an α-thalassemia 1 homozygote, showing that these sequences were absent. Heterozygotes annealed only 50% of the DNA. More recently, this has been confirmed by sequencing of the DNA.

Because homozygous α-thalassemia 1 mutants make no α chains, the fetus makes only gamma chains, and these form an unstable tetramer γ^4, or hemoglobin Barts. Hydrops fetalis develops (hydrops means excessive fluid in the tissues), and the fetus dies. Heterozygotes have thalassemia minor, and make some (5 to 10%) hemoglobin Barts at birth.

The α-thalassemia 2 mutant is a deletion of 1 α chain locus. The homozygote therefore has α-thalassemia minor, just as the α-thalassemia 1 heterozygote, because both are missing two loci A compound heterozygote—α-thal 1/α-thal 2—has only one active α chain gene, and this causes hemoglobin H disease, more severe than α-thalassemia minor. Hemoglobin H is a tetramer of β chains, which form because of the lack of α chains to make hemoglobin A.

Hb Constant Spring behaves like an α-thalassemia 2 mutant; in combination with α-thal-

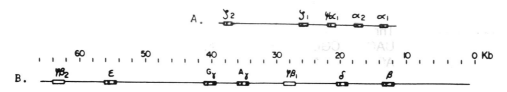

Fig. 6–20.   Fine structure of the alpha-globin (A) and beta-globin (B) gene families. See text.

assemia 1 it causes Hb H disease, plus a small amount of Hb Constant Spring. Probably the Hb Constant Spring mRNA is unstable.

Beta Thalassemias. The *beta thalassemias* are also heterogeneous. In most of this group, the beta gene is not deleted. In the β^+ mutants suppression of activity is incomplete and results from reduced amounts of mRNA synthesis. In the β^O mutants mRNA is either not produced or not functional. In the $\delta\beta^O$ type, the β gene is deleted. The β gene is also partially deleted in Hb Lepore, so this also acts as a β Thal mutant.

The *HPFH (hereditary persistence of fetal hemoglobin)* genes are also β-thalassemias in the sense that they suppress β chain synthesis but have the compensating feature that hemoglobin F continues to be produced. In the Negro type the β gene is deleted, along with the HPFH$^+$ (Y$^+$) region. In the Greek type, less Hb F is produced and what there is only $^A\gamma$, so presumably there has been a deletion that involves the $^G\gamma$ locus. Finally, Hb Kenya is an HPFH gene, since the delta gene (and presumably the Y$^+$ locus) is deleted.

All of the above HPFH mutants belong to the "homogeneous" type, since every red cell has increased Hb F production. However, the Swiss type (and some others) are called the "heterogeneous" type, since Hb F is present in only some cells. The reason is not entirely clear. It seems that normally there are a small number of red cell precursor cells that produce Hb F in the fetus, and this proportion is increased in the heterogeneous HPFHs. Thus, the proportion of such cells must be under genetic control. The proportion of cells making Hb F can also be increased somewhat in the β-thalassemias as a compensatory response to the lack of beta chains.

Modern methods of DNA analysis have led to further rapid advances in mapping the fine structure of the globin genes (Fig. 6–20A).[26,28]

The alpha globin gene complex has been mapped to near the end of chromosome 16q. An embryonic equivalent to the gamma locus has been found for the alpha complex and labeled zeta (ζ). There are two zeta genes. Another locus has a sequence identical to that of the alpha-1 gene, except for a mutation resulting in a termination codon, so that it is not transcribed. This is considered to be a *pseudogene*, on its way to evolutionary oblivion, and designated psi alpha ($\psi\alpha$).

The beta complex is located in chromosome 11p (Fig. 6–20B). There is an epsilon locus (ϵ) that produces a chain before the gamma chains appear. Before the epsilon locus and after the two gamma loci, there is a pseudo-beta gene. The second one (psi-beta-1) is followed by the delta and beta loci.

Study of the thalassemias at the molecular level has led to a better understanding of their pathogenesis on the one hand, and of the functions of the globin gene on the other. The β^O thalassemias (in which β-globin chains are completely absent) are heterogeneous. Some result from deletions, but in most the β-globin genes are structurally normal. In about half of these β-globin mRNA is present, but not translated because of nonsense mutations (most) or frame shift mutations. Those in which there is no messenger may involve a mutation in an intervening sequence that interferes with splicing, or in the TATA box or the CCATT box sequence, which are involved in control of transcription.

The β^+-thalassemia (normal β-globin produced in reduced amounts) involve abnormal processing, stability or transport of the messenger. In one type (common in Mediterraneans) an intervening sequence mutation leads to anomalous splicing. Another has a base substitution that creates an alternative splice-site, causing abnormal processing of the messenger.

Most α-thalassemia genotypes involve deletion of one (α-thalassemia 2) or two (α-thalassemia 1) α-globin genes. Several non-deletion mutants occur, involving mutations at splice-sites or more complex alterations.

The use of restriction enzyme and molecular analysis in the prenatal diagnosis of hemoglobinopathies and other disorders is dealt with in Chapter 7.

Understanding of the thalassemias has progressed rapidly in the past few years. The molecular biology of hemoglobin synthesis and its regulation is one of the most productive areas contributing to our understanding of the gene regulation in eukaryotic cells.

SUMMARY

Biochemical genetics deals with the biochemical changes resulting from substituting mutant for normal proteins. If the abnormal protein is an enzyme, an inborn error of metabolism may result. Diseases caused by abnormal enzymes may result from (1) absence of end product, (2) pileup of substrate, (3) excessive amounts of metabolites, (4) interference with regulatory mechanisms, and (5) abnormal storage. Other genetic defects of enzymes may result in inborn errors of membrane transport of amino acids and a variety of other substances such as glucose and phosphorus.

Treatment of inborn errors of metabolism and transport include (1) avoidance, (2) substrate restriction, (3) removal of toxic products, (4) product replacement, (5) cofactor supplementation, (6) organ transplantation, and (7) general supportive measures. New approaches include enzyme replacement, induction of synthesis, and incorporation of the missing genetic information into mutant cells using devices such as bacteriophage transduction.

Genetic defects of protein structure have been extensively studied in the hemoglobinopathies, with sickle cell disease as the prototype. A single amino acid substitution results in a mutant polypeptide. The changes in the primary structure may lead to alteration of secondary, tertiary, and quaternary structures, with consequent changes in function. Much has been learned about the structure and function of proteins by the study of the effects of specific amino acid substitutions.

Normal, adult hemoglobin A consists of alpha and beta chains; a normal minor component of adult hemoglobin consists of alpha and delta chains, and normal fetal hemoglobin consists of alpha and gamma chains, so at least 4 genes must be responsible for the production of globin chains. A mechanism by which "new" genes may arise is demonstrated by hemoglobin Lepore which arose by "unequal crossing over" between two similar but not identical genes, those for the beta and delta chains. Family and biochemical studies of mutant hemoglobins have allowed mapping of the loci. There are 2 adjacent identical genes for alpha chains and an unlinked complex including two gamma loci, delta and beta, in that order.

The thalassemias are hereditary anemias resulting from varying degrees of suppression of alpha or beta chain synthesis. They can result from deletion of the locus involved or abnormalities of transcription or translation. Much has been learned about the molecular biology of gene regulation from their study.

REFERENCES

1. Brady, R.O. and Barton, N.W.: Enzyme replacement therapy for Type I Gaucher disease. *In* Treatment of Genetic Diseases, edited by R.J. Desnick, New York, Churchill Livingstone, 1991.
2. Byers, P.H.: Brittle bones-fragile molecules: Disorders of collagen gene structure and expression. Trends Genet. 6:293, 1990.
3. Dietz, H.C., et al.: Marfan syndrome caused by a recurrent de novo missense mutation in the fibrillan gene. Nature (London) 352:337, 1991.
4. Eisensmith, R.C. and Woo, S.L.C.: Molecular basis of phenylketonuria and related hyperphenylalaninemias: Mutations and polymorphisms in the human phenylalanine hydroxylase gene. Human Mutation 1:13, 1992.
5. Fenton, W.A. and Rosenberg, L.E.: Inherited disorders of cobalamin transport and metabolism. *In* The

Metabolic Basis of Inherited Disease, 6th ed., edited by C.R. Scriver et al., New York, McGraw-Hill Book Co., 1989, Chapter 82.

6. Goldberg, J.D. and Golbus, M.S.: In utero therapy for genetic diseases. *In* Treatment of Genetic Diseases. Edited by R. J. Desnick, New York, Churchill Livingstone, 1991.

7. Goldstein, J.L., and Brown, M.S.: Familial hypercholesterolemia. *In* The Metabolic Basis of Inherited Diseases, 6th ed., edited by C.R. Scriver et al., New York, McGraw-Hill Book Co., 1989, Chapter 48.

8. Hale, D.E. and Bennett, M.J.: Fatty acid oxidation disorders: A new class of metabolic diseases. J. Pediatr. 121:1, 1992.

9. Harris, H.: The Principles of Human Biochemical Genetics, 2nd ed., New York, Elsevier, 1975.

10. Hers, H.-G. et al.: The glycogen storage diseases. *In* The Metabolic Basis of Inherited Disease, 6th ed., edited by C.R. Scriver et al., New York, McGraw-Hill Book Co., 1989, Chapter 12.

11. Kelley, W.N.: Hereditary orotic aciduria. *In* The Metabolic Basis of Inherited Disease, 5th ed., edited by J.B. Stanbury et al., New York, McGraw-Hill Book Co., 1983.

12. Krivit, W. and Shapiro, E.G.: Bone marrow transplantation for storage diseases. *In* Treatment of Genetic Diseases, edited by R.J. Desnick, New York, Churchill Livingstone, 1991.

13. Neufeld, E.F. and Muenzer, J.: The mucopolysaccharidoses. *In* The Metabolic Basis of Inherited Disease, 6th ed., edited by C.R. Scriver et al., New York, McGraw-Hill Book Co., 1989, Chapter 61.

14. Neufeld, E.F., and McKusick, V.A.: Disorders of lysosomal enzyme synthesis. *In* The Metabolic Basis of Inherited Disease, edited by J.B. Stanbury et al., New York, McGraw-Hill Book Co., 1983.

15. New, M.I., et al.: The adrenal hyperplasias and related conditions. *In* The Metabolic Basis of Inherited Disease, 6th ed., edited by C.R. Scriver et al., New York, McGraw-Hill Book Co., 1989, Chapter 74.

16. O'Brien, J.S.: B-galactosidase deficiency. *In* The Metabolic Basis of Inherited Disease, 6th ed., edited by C.R. Scriver et al., New York, McGraw-Hill Book Co., 1989, Chapter 71.

17. Palmiter, R.D., et al.: Metallothionein—human GH fusion genes stimulate growth of mice. Science 222:809, 1983.

18. Rasmussen, H., and Tenenhouse, H.S.: Hypophosphatemias. *In* The Metabolic Basis of Inherited Disease, 6th ed., edited by C.R. Scriver et al., New York, McGraw-Hill Book Co., 1989, Chapter 105.

19. Rodick, C.H. and Fisk, N.M. Intrauterine therapy. *In* Antenatal Diagnosis of Fetal Abnormalities, edited by J.O. Drife and D. Donnai, New York, Springer-Verlag, 1991.

20. Rosenblatt, D.S.: Inherited disorders of folate transport and metabolism. *In* The Metabolic Basis of Inherited Disease, 6th ed., edited by C.R. Scriver et al., New York, McGraw-Hill Book Co., 1989, Chapter 81.

21. Schweitzer, L.B. and Desnick, R.J.: Inherited metabolic diseases: advances in delineation, diagnosis, and treatment. Birth Defects: Original Article Series 19(5):39, 1983.

22. Scriver, C.R.: Treatment of inborn errors of metabolism. *In* Advances in Treatment of Inborn Errors of Metabolism, edited by M.d'A. Crawford, et al., John Wiley and Sons, New York, 1982.

23. Scriver, C.R., Laberge, C., Clow, C., and Fraser, F.C.: Genetics and Medicine. An evolving relationship. Science 200:964, 1978.

24. Scriver, C.R., Beaudet, A.L., Sly, W. and Valee, D.L. (eds): The Metabolic Basis of Inherited Disease, 6th ed., New York, McGraw-Hill Book Co., 1989.

25. Scriver, C.R., and Woo, S.L.: The phenylalanine hydroxylating system. *In* The Metabolic Basis of Inherited Disease, 6th ed., edited by C.R. Scriver, et al., New York, McGraw-Hill Book Co., 1989, Chapter 15.

26. Spritz, R.A., and Forget, B.B.: The thalassemias: molecular mechanisms of human genetic disease. Am. J. Hum. Genet. 35:333, 1983.

27. Touma, E.H. and Charpentier, C.: Medium chain acyl-CoA dehydrogenase deficiency. Arch. Dis. Child. 67.142, 1992.

28. Weatherall, D.J.: The New Genetics and Clinical Practice. 3rd ed., Oxford, Oxford University Press, 1991.

29. Weatherall, D.J., et al.: The Hemoglobinopathies. *In* The Metabolic Basis of Inherited Disease, 6th ed., edited by C.R. Scriver, et al., New York, McGraw-Hill Book Co., 1989, Chapter 93.

30. Witkop, C., et al.: Albinism and other disorders of pigment metabolism. *In* The Metabolic Basis of Inherited Disease, 6th ed., edited by C.R. Scriver et al., New York, McGraw-Hill Book Co., 1989, Chapter 119.

31. Yokota, I. et al.: Molecular survey of a prevalent mutation, 985A-to-G transition and identification of five infrequent mutations in the MCAD gene in 55 patients with MCAD deficiency. Am. J. Hum. Genet. 49:1280, 1991.

Chapter 7

Molecular Genetics

I GROW OLD LEARNING SOMETHING NEW EVERY DAY.

SOLON

There have been spectacular advances in the field of molecular genetics since Watson and Crick published their observations on the structure of DNA in 1953. The technologic advances in our ability to analyze the human genome have led to increased understanding of the organization and regulation of gene structure and function, to the isolation and characterization of genes and the nature of their gene products, and to the elucidation of diverse classes of mutations underlying human genetic diseases.

This chapter will focus on updating the reader on the laboratory tools that have revolutionized our ability to analyze human genetic disorders at the molecular level. With concrete examples illustrating the application of molecular genetics to the study of genetic disorders, the reader will become familiar with how molecular genetics has revolutionized the practice of medical genetics.

At the same time, there is increased hope that successful treatment of many heritable disorders can be accomplished. The chapter will conclude with an introduction to the current steps being taken in **gene therapy**. The most difficult challenge lies in integrating the use of such powerful techniques in biology with day-to-day ethically and socially responsible clinical medicine.

THE TECHNIQUES

Cloning

Understanding the techniques of molecular biology requires understanding the principles of molecular cloning. Cloning refers to replicating selected segments of DNA in an organism that can multiply. This ability to generate innumerable exact copies (clones) of a sequence of interest is the basis of recombinant DNA technology. One technique of cloning is summarized in Figure 7–1. Essentially, the process involves generating a **library** (a collection of clones including the sequence of interest) by splicing segments of human DNA into **vectors** (DNA molecules that can replicate autonomously in a host cell) and then propagating these vectors containing the cloned pieces of DNA in specially selected host cells.

First, the target piece of DNA is cleaved with a specific **restriction endonuclease** (Fig. 7–2). Restriction endonucleases are bacterial enzymes that recognize specific double stranded sequences of DNA. In bacteria, these

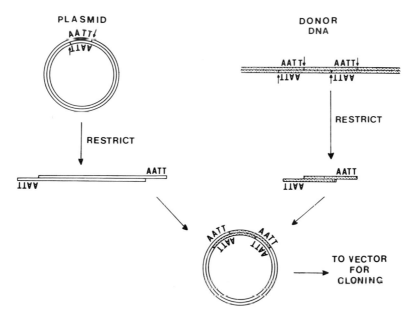

Fig. 7–1. Schema of Cloning.

enzymes protect the host cell from invasion by foreign DNA by cutting the latter DNA at specific base sequences. For example, the restriction endonuclease EcoR1 recognizes and cuts between the G and A of the sequence GAATTC. Note that the complementary strand of double stranded DNA, CTTAAG, has the same base sequence in the opposite direction, i.e., it is palindromic. Thus, when the enzyme cuts between the G and A of both strands, each DNA strand will have a "sticky"

EcoRI	5´- GAATTC - 3´ 3´- CTTAAG - 5´
Hind II	5´- GTPyPuAC - 3´ 3´- CAPuPyTG - 5´
Hind III	5´- AAGCTT - 3´ 3´- TTCGAA - 5´
Hinf I	5´- GANTC - 3´ 3´- CTNAG - 5´
Hpa I	5´- GTTAAC - 3´ 3´- CAATTG - 5´

Fig. 7–2. Some typical restriction endonucleases.

tail with a 4 base pair overhang that is complementary to the other.

Thus:

$$\begin{array}{ccc}
& \text{EcoR1} & \\
\downarrow & \text{restriction} & \\
\text{---NNGAATTCNN---} & \rightarrow & \text{---NNG} \qquad \text{AATTCNN---} \\
\text{---NNCTTAAGNN---} & & \text{---NNCTTAA} \qquad \text{GNN---} \\
\uparrow & &
\end{array}$$

In the human genome consisting of 3×10^9 nucleotides, there are recognition sites nonrandomly distributed every 4^6 base pairs for 6-cutter enzymes such as EcoR1. Thus EcoR1 digested total genomic human DNA is a series of double stranded fragments of variable lengths with identical single stranded sticky tails. All DNA molecules, human or otherwise, when digested with EcoR1 will contain two types of identical sticky tails that are complementary. Vector DNA digested with EcoR1 and mixed with EcoR1 digested human DNA can be joined together at random under appropriate conditions by the enzyme DNA **ligase** through interaction between the complementary four-base tails and repair of the breaks in the DNA strands through the completion of the phosphodiesterase backbones. Thus, by chance, the human DNA sequence can be incorporated into the vector DNA.

Vectors are pieces of extrachromosomal DNA such as bacteriophages (bacterial viruses with a large ~45 kb. double-stranded DNA molecule) or plasmids (circular double-stranded DNA molecules that replicate in bacteria or in yeast). A recircularized plasmid containing an inserted (cloned) fragment of human DNA can be introduced into bacterial hosts, usually Escherichia coli, which are grown on a selective medium that permits the growth only of those bacteria that contain a plasmid. The result is a **library** of bacterial clones, each containing a plasmid that has a distinct segment of donor DNA from which the clone of choice can be selected. Cloning into plasmids is a standard procedure for the selection and growth of large amounts of the cloned insert for molecular analysis. Methods for selecting the plasmid containing the particular recombinant fragment of interest include splicing in a biochemical marker, such as drug resistance, or using a labeled antibody to identify the product of the cloned gene. Newer vectors for cloning large fragments of DNA include **cosmids** and most recently **yeast artificial chromosomes (YACs)**. Cosmids are essentially plasmids with features of bacteriophage lambda into which can be inserted as much as 50 kb of linear DNA, which after infection into bacteria recircularizes and replicates as plasmids. YACs are vectors that allow cloning and replication of DNA fragments up to 1000 kb. into the yeast host, Saccharomyces cerevisiae. The latter vectors currently represent the largest cloning vehicles available.

The purpose of creating a library is to isolate large quantities of DNA fragments or genes for further analysis. The two most common types of libraries are **genomic** and **complementary** DNA libraries. Genomic libraries can be constructed with total genomic DNA (with up to 10 million clones representing the entire human genome) or with DNA from either a specific chromosome or a specific region of a chromosome (chromosome specific library) generated by isolating a chromosomal region of interest by fluorescent-activated flow sort-

ing, or most recently with laser dissection, of human chromosomes. Complementary DNA (cDNA) libraries represent copies of the population of mRNA present in the cells or tissue of interest. Such libraries have the advantage of containing clones of coding regions of genes without the noncoding introns present in genomic DNA. In addition, a specific single-copy DNA sequence of interest may be represented only infrequently in a genomic DNA library, and it may be much easier to select for that expressed sequence by screening a cDNA library built from a tissue that is enriched for the mRNA of interest, e.g., a liver cDNA library to isolate genes that are expressed in the liver. Construction of cDNA libraries involves first isolating total or polyA+ RNA from the tissue of interest, synthesizing a DNA complementary copy of this template RNA using the enzyme **reverse transcriptase**, an RNA-dependent DNA polymerase, removing the RNA template and synthesizing a second- strand yielding double-stranded cDNA. This double-stranded cDNA can then be cloned directly. Construction of a cDNA library into a plasmid vector is summarized in Figure 7–3.

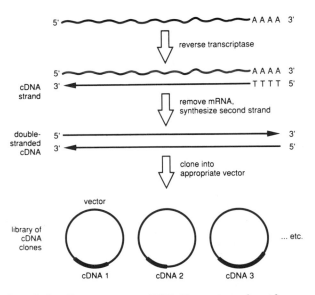

Fig. 7–3.   Constructing a cDNA library in a plasmid vector. Starting with RNA from a tissue of interest, RNA is copied into first-strand cDNA using the enzyme reverse transcriptase. Following second-strand synthesis, the double-stranded cDNA can be subcloned into the appropriate vector.

Detecting DNA and RNA Sequences

This section reviews traditional ways of analyzing DNA and RNA and explores revolutionary new techniques. The principle of detecting a sequence of interest involves using a **probe** to find its complementary sequence of interest among a DNA or RNA sample that contains millions of DNA fragments or thousands of RNA transcripts. This is accomplished by means of nucleic acid hybridization using **Southern** or **Northern blotting** for DNA and RNA hybridization respectively. More recently, the DNA sequence of interest can be amplified using the innovative technique of **polymerase chain reaction** (PCR) amplification to allow it to be studied without the need for molecular hybridization.

Southern blotting was developed in the mid 1970's by E. M. Southern and is illustrated in

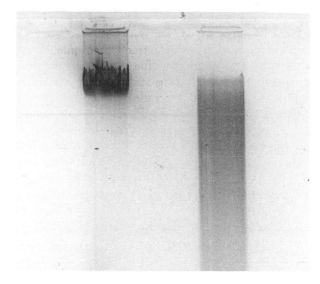

Fig. 7–5. Ethidium bromide-stained agarose gel showing undigested high molecular weight DNA (on left) and a smear of digested genomic DNA (on right).

Figure 7–4.[22] Genomic DNA is isolated from any tissue source such as white blood cells or cultured skin fibroblasts and appears as a high molecular weight band when electrophoresed on an agarose gel that has been stained with ethidium bromide, a fluorescent DNA dye (Fig. 7–5). The DNA is digested with a restriction endonuclease into a million or so double-stranded fragments of various lengths. The fragments are separated according to size by electrophoresis on an agarose gel in which the fragments migrate according to length with the smaller fragments migrating further than larger fragments. The double-stranded fragments are then converted into single strands by exposure to alkali and transferred by blotting onto a cellulose nitrate or nylon filter paper to which the fragments adhere. This technique creates a "Southern" blot. (A similar transfer of RNA is called a "Northern" blot).

If the starting DNA comes from a simple organism, and thus contains relatively few fragments of DNA, staining the DNA on the gel will reveal a number of distinct bands. However, with human DNA there are so many fragments that no one fragment is distinct in the overall "smear" (Fig. 7–5).

To identify the fragment of interest a specific labelled **probe** is used. A probe is a piece

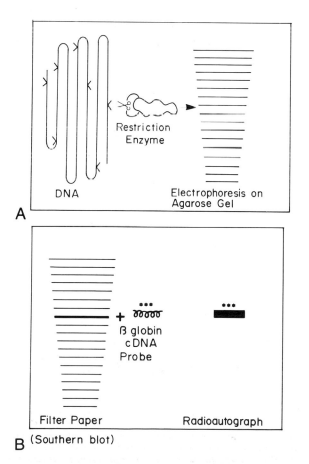

Fig. 7–4. Schema of Southern blotting.

Family F

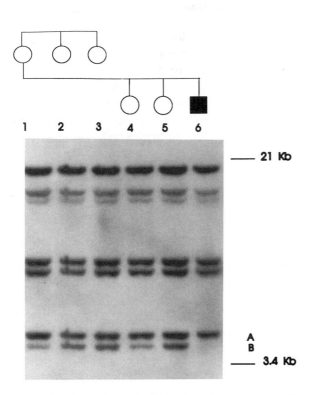

Fig. 7–6. Autoradiograph of Southern blot of Family F.'s Hind III digested DNA hybridized with a dystrophin cDNA probe. Lane 6 shows a DNA sample from a boy affected with DMD, with no hybridization seen with one Hind III fragment B. This represents a molecular deletion within the dystrophin gene. Lanes 1 and 4 contain samples from the boy's mother and sister, respectively. The signal intensity of fragment B in lanes 1 and 4 is less than in lanes 2, 3, and 5. Densitometric analysis of B/A identifies the individuals in lanes 1 and 4 as high-probability DMD carriers, whereas the remaining females studied are low-probability carriers. These results can then be confirmed by quantitative PCR.

(see Fig. 7–4). When the probe is a genomic, unique-sequence, cloned piece of DNA, usually only one or two bands appear following hybridization to restricted genomic DNA. With a cDNA probe (containing DNA sequences complementary only to the coding regions), hybridization occurs with genomic fragments of many different sizes because of the presence of introns. This is demonstrated in Figure 7–6.

Polymerase chain reaction (PCR)[13,20] is a technique that allows the selective amplification of a specific fragment of DNA out of a background of total DNA (Fig. 7–7). Two short stretches of synthetic DNA known as oligonucleotide primers that flank the region of interest are synthesized. The primer at one end is complementary to the coding strand, and the other primer is complementary to the noncoding strand at the other end. During a

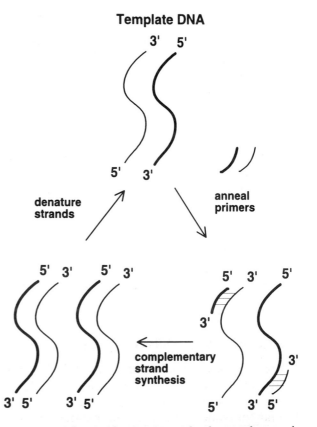

Fig. 7–7. Schema of one PCR cycle showing how each cycle doubles the amount of target DNA. Using a heat-stable Taq polymerase and on-average 25 to 30 temperature cycles, a target sequence can be amplified 10^6-fold.

of genomic or complementary DNA that has been cloned and radioactively labeled, made single-stranded by denaturation, and then applied to the filter containing the electrophoresed DNA fragments. Under appropriate conditions of hybridization and given the specificity of the labeled probe, the single-stranded probe will anneal only to its complementary sequence on the filter. After washing to remove excess probe, the filter is exposed to x-ray film and distinct bands labeled by the probes will now be demonstrable in each lane of DNA by autoradiography

PCR reaction, the double stranded DNA is denatured at 95°C, and the temperature is reduced to allow the primers to anneal to their single-stranded complement. Then synthesis of the complementary strands of the selected region will proceed in the presence of the thermostable enzyme Taq DNA polymerase (isolated from the thermophilic bacterium Thermus aquaticus) and deoxynucleotides. With each repeated cycle of denaturation, annealing of primers, and synthesis of the complementary strand, the number of target DNA sequences doubles. After approximately 30 cycles, the target DNA sequence can be exponentially amplified 10^5- to 10^6-fold.

The technique of PCR is now one of the most widely applied in genetic diagnosis and counseling as well as for research in molecular biology. Samples of relatively poor-quality DNA and *as small as those from single cells* can be used to amplify DNA sequences. This means that noninvasive techniques can be employed for sample collection, e.g., from mouthwash swabs or hair root analysis. Exponential amplification of specific sequences permits rapid cloning and characterization of genes. PCR greatly facilitates the preparation of cDNA libraries, because one can start with minute quantities of RNA, synthesize a single-stranded cDNA from the mRNA using **reverse transcriptase** as described, then synthesize the second strand of cDNA using a PCR primer. Thus a double stranded template is formed that then acts as a template for subsequent PCR cycles. In addition, because the target PCR fragment is now present in excess relative to the rest of the patient's DNA, the gene of interest can be analyzed directly for mutations. This is described in further detail in the next section.

The Nature and Identification of Gene Mutations

Protein work in the past identified much naturally occurring variation and predicted enormous naturally occurring variability in the human genome. The tools of molecular biology have allowed us to explore and analyze these differences at the level of the nucleotide sequence in the genome. With these new tools

at hand, one can ask (and begin to answer) the following questions about genetic disorders:

1. Is the disorder of concern caused by a specific error (mutation) in the patient's genetic makeup?
2. What is the precise error?
3. Is the mutation disease-causing and not a naturally occurring non-deleterious variation (polymorphism)?
4. If a mutation that co-segregates with the disorder is found how do we know it and how can the mutation be best detected?
5. Where has it arisen?
6. Why has it occurred?
7. Can it be fixed?

Two approaches are used to address the issue of the genetic basis of human disease. One is the candidate gene approach; the second is positional cloning (Fig. 7–8).

Since the advent of recombinant DNA technology, several hundred disease genes have been cloned using the **candidate gene** ap-

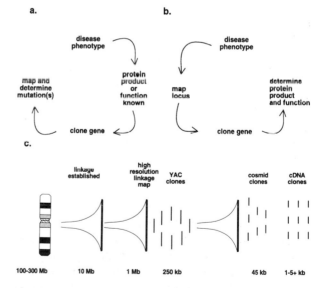

Fig. 7–8. The two main methods of identifying genes are shown in a and b. Functional cloning (a) depends on prior information about the underlying biochemical defect, whereas in positional cloning (b), the protein product and its function are determined only after the gene is cloned. In c, a graphic representation and scale of the positional cloning schema leading to the cloning of a cDNA of interest and ultimate mutation detection are depicted. Adapted with permission from Collins, F.S.: Cystic fibrosis: molecular biology and therapeutic implications. Science 256:774, 1992.

proach, also known as functional cloning. This approach depends on knowing the biochemical or biologic basis for the disorder. A candidate gene for a particular disorder is one whose product has properties to suggest that it may prove to be the disease gene of concern. A candidate gene may be isolated in two ways. First, prior knowledge of the amino acid sequence of the wild type protein product permits isolation of the relevant cDNA encoding that protein from the appropriate library expressing this transcript. For example, the synthesis of beta globin cDNA depended on the isolation of beta globin mRNA from reticulocytes (young red blood cells that are still synthesizing hemoglobin); and the cDNA encoding phenylalanine hydroxylase (the enzyme that is faulty in classical phenylketonuria) was isolated from a human liver cDNA library. The second way depends on a genetic disorder being assigned by mapping strategies to a particular chromosome (see positional cloning, below). In the physical interval identified by gene mapping, a gene or cDNA may be located whose product may have properties to suggest that it may in fact be a gene responsible for the disease in question. A search for mutations in that candidate gene may then proceed.

For disorders with no potential candidate genes to guide the molecular search, a **positional cloning**[5] approach is followed. Positional cloning of a gene in which mutations are subsequently identified to be disease-causing proceeds without prior information about the biologic defect. Positional cloning is initiated by first mapping the responsible gene to a particular chromosomal location (see Chap. 9). Fine genetic mapping subsequently narrows down the region of interest, usually to a region of approximately a million base pairs. Transcripts in this region are then isolated from a variety of tissues and a search for mutations ultimately by sequence analysis ensues. Examples of loci isolated by a positional cloning approach are listed in Figure 7–9. These are all single-gene mendelian disorders, but similar molecular strategies are being applied for complex genetic disorders such as Type 2 diabetes and hypertension for which mapping

DISEASE	LOCUS
cystic fibrosis	CFTR
chronic granulomatous disease	CGD
familial adenomatous polyposis	APC
retinoblastoma	RB
Duchenne muscular dystrophy	DYS
Neurofibromatosis - 1	NF-1
myotonic dystrophy	MT-PK
fragile X syndrome	FMR-1

Fig. 7–9.   A list of selected human diseases whose genes have been cloned by positional cloning and in which mutations produce changes in phenotype.

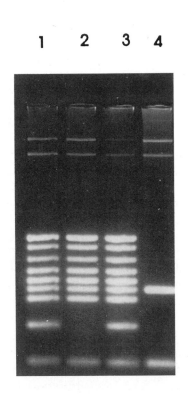

DMD Multiplex PCR

Fig. 7–10.   Deletions in the dystrophin gene causing DMD can be detected either by Southern blotting, as shown in Figure 7–6, or by multiplex PCR analysis, as shown here. Multiple exons are coamplified in one PCR reaction and following electrophoresis in an agarose gel, deletions of differing exons are detected in lanes 2 and 4. Multiplex PCR has been applied to other mendelian disorders, e.g., cystic fibrosis, in which heterogeneous mutations have been identified.

Table 7–1. Classes of Mutations*

Class	Example	Locus	Protein
1. Large deletions	β-thalassemia Duchenne/Becker muscular dystrophy (DMD/BMD)	HBB DYS	β-globin dystrophin
	Hemophilia A	F8C	factor VIIIc
	Hypercholesterolemia	LDLR	LDL receptor
2. Large duplications	DMD/BMD	DYS	Dystrophin
	Charcot-Marie-Tooth	CMT1a	?
	Hypercholesterolemia	LDLR	LDL receptor
3. Insertions	Hemophilia A	F8C	Factor VIIIc
	Gyrate atrophy of retina	OAT	ornithine-d- amino-transferase
4. Point mutations causing a. defective mRNA synthesis	β-thalassemia e.g., Promoter mutants RNA splicing errors mRNA capping or tailing mutants	HBB	β-globin
	Lesch-Nyhan syndrome	HPRT	Hypoxanthine guanine phosphorib transf.
b. non-functional mRNA	Nonsense and frameshift mutations Numerous examples:		
	-Cystic fibrosis	CFTR	CFTR protein
	-β-thalassemia	HBB	β globin
c. decreased protein function	Missense mutations Numerous examples:		
	-Cystic fibrosis	CFTR	CFTR protein
	-Hemoglobinopathies	HBB	β-globin
	-Hemophilia B	F9	Factor IX
	-Antitrypsin deficiency	PI	protease inhibitor (antitrypsin, alpha 1)
5. Unstable heritable elements	Fragile X syndrome	FMR-1	FMR-1 product
	Myotonic dystrophy	MT-PK	protein kinase
	Kennedy disease	SBMA	androgen receptor
	Huntington disease	HD	identification pending
6. mitochondrial DNA mutations	Leber's optic atrophy		10 mt DNA pt mutations especially at nt 11778
	MELAS		mt tRNA mutation
	MERRF		mt tRNA mutation
	Kearns-Sayre syndrome		mt DNA deletion

studies and analysis of candidate susceptibility genes are currently in progress.

Mutations underlying genetic disorders are, not surprisingly, very diverse given the numerous complex steps required from transcription of a gene through to its translation into protein.[15] The hemoglobinopathies have historically served as models to illustrate the molecular heterogeneity underlying disease, with more than 80 single base substitutions alone identified in the beta-thalassemias (see Chap. 6). Such heterogeneity has proven to be the rule as more and more disease genes are cloned. In addition, new classes of mutations involving expanding trinucleotide repeats[3] correlating with disease expression have been identified in four genetic disorders,

suggesting that this phenomenon may be responsible for a significant proportion of genetic disease. Classes of mutations involving both nuclear genes and the mitochondrial genome with illustrative examples are summarized in Table 7–1, with specific details available in the references.

With the advent of recombinant DNA technology in the late 1970s, it became apparent that point mutations or large DNA alterations are the cause of numerous genetic disorders. This is now well recognized. Representative examples are given in Figure 7–10. Expansion of trinucleotide repeats, which are highly polymorphic in the general population, is the basis of four known heritable disorders and is a newly recognized phenomenon.

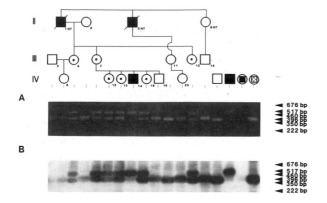

A

B

Fig. 7–11. Expansion of the androgen receptor CAG repeat in X-linked spinal and bulbar muscular atrophy (SBMA). Analysis of the PCR products obtained by amplification of the CAG repeat region is shown in the individuals of this SBMA kindred. A. The PCR products are electrophoresed in an agarose gel and stained with ethidium bromide. B. Southern analysis of the gel shown in A is probed with an androgen receptor cDNA probe. Individual IV-14 is affected with SBMA and has one ~500 bp band which contains 51 CAG repeats by sequence analysis (not shown). The normal allele is an ~400 bp band with 23 repeats by sequence analysis (not shown). High-probability carrier status can be established in the six females on the basis of detecting normal and expanded alleles. Positive and negative controls are shown to the right of the family study. The control lane with no hybridization signal is from a patient with a complete deletion of the androgen receptor gene. Reproduced with permission from Belsham, D.D., Greenberg, C., et al.: J. Neurol. Sci. 112:133, 1992.

Kennedy disease (spinal and bulbar muscular atrophy, SBMA) is an X-linked recessive adult-onset genetic disorder characterized by slowly progressive muscle weakness and wasting caused by neurogenic loss of anterior horn cells. Affected males may have reduced fertility or enlargement of the mammary glands (gynecomastia). The mapping of the SBMA gene to chromosome Xq11-12 in the region of the androgen receptor gene led to the discovery of a highly polymorphic CAG repeat in exon one of the androgen receptor gene. All affected SBMA individuals have been shown to have at least twice the number of CAG repeats seen in the general population. This has allowed accurate disease diagnosis in males and carrier assignment of females in high-risk families (Fig. 7–11).

Fragile X syndrome is also an X-linked recessive disorder, but with incomplete penetrance. The estimated incidence of this disorder is 1 in 1250 males and 1 in 2500 females.

Affected males can be identified clinically by moderate to severe mental retardation, a characteristic behavioral profile with autistic-like features, and a recognizable phenotype of a large head, long facies, large ears, and large testicles (Figs. 7–12, 7–13). One third of female carriers may have cognitive and behavioral difficulties, but often without distinguishing physical characteristics. The cytogenetic detection in the late 1970s of a constriction at the end of the long arm of the X chromosome, known as a fragile-X site (Fig. 7–14), not only led to its diagnostic use in clinical genetics but ultimately to the cloning of the FMR-1 gene.

The FMR-1 gene encodes a protein of 592 amino acids with a molecular weight of 67,000 daltons. A CGG repeat is present in the 5' untranslated region. Normally, between 6 and 60 CGG repeats are present, but expansion of this region to >200 repeats (600 to 5000 base pairs) is seen in affected, fully expressing males. Carrier, phenotypically normal males, who are referred to as "transmitting males," have an increased number of CGG repeats in the range between 60 and 200. Daughters of transmitting males, who are obligate carriers of this

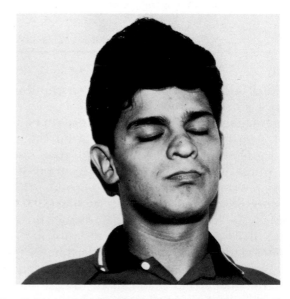

Fig. 7–12. A patient with the fragile X syndrome. The face was long and narrow, the mandible prominent, and the ears relatively prominent. Courtesy of Dr. James Moscarella, Children's Hospital and Health Center, San Diego, California.)

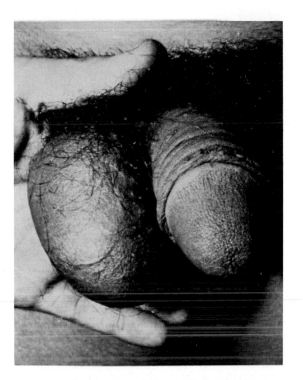

Fig. 7–13. The macro-orchidism of the fragile X syndrome. (Courtesy of Dr. J. M. Cantú, Instituto Mexicano del Seguro Social, I.M.S.S., Guadalajara, Mexico. The report of this family was published in Hum. Genet., 33:23, 1976.)

mildly expanded FMR-1 gene, are known as premutation carriers, are cytogenetically negative, and are always phenotypically normal.

However, premutations are unstable meiotically, and can undergo either expansion resulting in offspring with an increase in repeat number or reduction to normal size. There is a direct correlation between copy number and phenotype with severely affected fragile-X males having a fully expanded FMR-1 mutation. Expansion to full mutation occurs only from a premutation, but premutations can remain meiotically stable for many generations before expanding. The risk of repeat expansion to the full mutation appears to correlate with the size of the premutation, but it is currently unknown what causes the repeat to become unstable.

Although there are many unanswered questions, our understanding of the molecular basis for the fragile X has now facilitated accurate diagnosis, carrier assignment, and risk

assessment in families and DNA-based methods of diagnosis have largely superseded the cytogenetic-based approach. Fragile-X syndrome represents the first instance in which there is a molecular explanation for the "variable expressivity" so characteristic of mendelian disorders.

A similar phenomenon of molecular expansion of a CTG repeat in the 3′ untranslated region of the MT-PK gene on chromosome 19 is seen in the autosomal dominant disorder, **myotonic dystrophy** (also see Chap. 8). This is a multisystem disorder characterized by myotonia (failure of muscle relaxation), muscle weakness, cataracts, cardiac arrhythmias, occasionally male infertility and other endocrine dysfunction, and occasionally cognitive impairment. The congenital form of myotonic dystrophy is associated with profound neonatal hypotonia, severe morbidity, and increased mortality. Neonates with congenital myotonic dystrophy are invariably born to affected mothers. Such infants have dramatic CTG repeat expansions in the range of 1000 repeats, often 25-fold larger than those of their mothers, who have premutations and are often asymptomatic. This increase in clinical severity with successive generations is known as "anticipation." As in fragile X, there is a positive correlation between degree of CTG re-

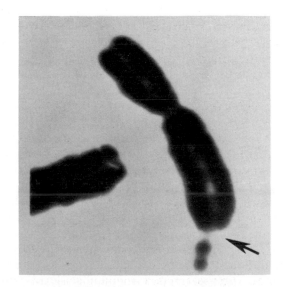

Fig. 7–14.   Fragile X chromosome.

DM - EcoR1

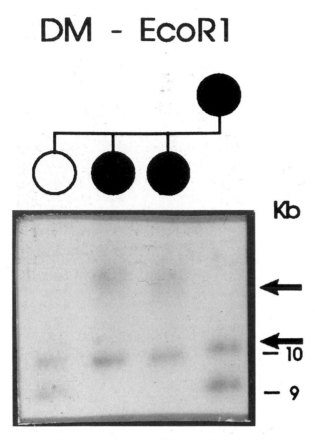

Kb

←

← — 10

— 9

Fig. 7–15. Expansion of MT-PK CTG repeat in a two generation D.M. family shown in this autoradiograph of a Southern analysis of EcoR1-digested DNA probed with a MT-PK probe. The usual polymorphic bands seen are 9 kb and 10 kb. The mother in lane 4 is clinically asymptomatic but has mild facial weakness and shows one normal 9 kb allele and one mildly expanded allele seen above 10 kb. The daughters in lanes 2 and 3 are severely affected and show one 10 kb allele (inferred to be paternal in origin) and one greatly expanded allele seen as a smear of DNA (top arrow). The daughter in lane 1 is asymptomatic and clinically normal, and based on the normal 9 and 10 kb alleles seen would be predicted not to be a carrier of the mutation causing myotonic dystrophy. Courtesy of Dr. R. Korneluk, University of Ottawa.

peat length and clinical severity. However, the correlation in myotonic dystrophy is not absolute, and extreme care must be exercised in using molecular data in disease prediction. An example of a family study of myotonic dystrophy and the MT-PK genotypes is shown in Figure 7–15. Most recently, expansion of a CAG repeat on chromosome 4p has been determined to be the molecular basis for Huntingdon disease (an autosomal disease of neurodegenerative movement disorder), with the

most severely affected individuals having the largest number of repeats (also see Chap. 8). Little is known yet as to whether this is an absolute phenomenon in all patients or what the normal gene product of the Huntingdon locus is.

Mutation Detection. The diversity of mutation types described above requires the use of various detection systems. The technique used will clearly depend not only on the type of mutation anticipated but also on how common any given disease allele is in a given population. A disease that results from a single predominant mutation, e.g., sickle cell anemia, in which sickle hemoglobin always results from a single nucleotide change (A to T) in the sixth codon of beta-globin,[18,19] lends itself to one direct detection system. However, a disease in which each affected family may have a different mutation (e.g., Lesch-Nyhan syndrome, beta-thalassemia, hemophilia A and B) has to be approached differently, either directly or indirectly.

The **direct methods** for mutation detection include Southern blotting using conventional cloned DNA probes for the detection of gross deletions, duplications, unstable repeats, or point mutations that create or destroy a specific restriction endonuclease. PCR amplification of a target DNA fragment of interest, followed by mutation detection is also used. PCR-based methods encompass the following: direct gel visualization for the detection of deletions or the sizing of unstable repeats; restriction enzyme digest and gel electrophoresis of the restricted fragment (Fig. 7–16); or allele-specific oligonucleotide (ASO) analysis (Fig. 7–17), in which a single point mutation can be identified using selective hybridization of short, synthetic, wild-type and mutant probes that differ only in the one nucleotide of interest.

Other methods of direct mutation detection include: PCR followed by direct sequencing of the amplified product; competitive oligonucleotide priming (allele specific PCR), in which a wild-type PCR primer cannot anneal in the presence of the mutation in question and thus no PCR product is made; and the ligase chain reaction, in which the PCR re-

A

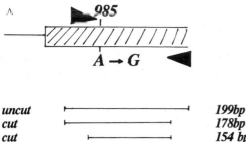

uncut	199bp
cut	178bp wild type
cut	154 bp mutant

Nco1 site C'CATGG

Fig. 7–16. In A, direct detection of the common A to G point mutation at position 985 in the MCAD gene causing MCAD deficiency by Nco1 digestion of a 199 bp PCR amplified target DNA fragment is shown schematically. In B, agarose gel electrophoresis shows in the cut lane of the affected child only a 154 bp fragment following Nco1 digestion, heterozygotes show 2 bands at 154 and 178 bp, whereas a homozygous normal control shows only a 178 bp band

B

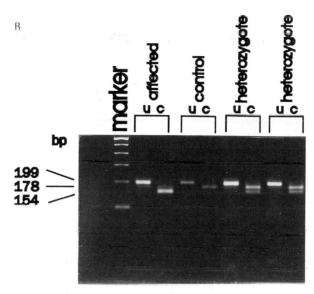

action will proceed and the product will be formed only when an enzymatic ligase reaction can join two halves of the fragment of interest. A review of the various methods of mutation detection is found in Rossiter and Caskey.[17]

Polymorphism Analysis and Its Role in Genetic Disease Prediction

The mutational heterogeneity that underlies most human genetic disorders provides the basis for the study of how gene structure is related to gene function and for the specifying which sequences are essential for gene func-

tion. However, the precise molecular abnormalities underlying most genetic disorders are mutationally too diverse to allow their diagnosis by direct DNA tests. The approach to the diagnosis of such disorders is often met by indirect tests making use of closely linked polymorphisms (see Chap. 9). This strategy of indirect testing can also be exploited for those disorders whose metabolic basis is not known or whose map location is known, but where the responsible gene has not yet been cloned.

Indirect diagnosis is achieved by screening for and analyzing sequence differences e.g., point mutations between homologous segments of DNA. These sequence differences

ASO HYBRIDIZATION ANALYSIS OF gly^{317}→asp MUTATION

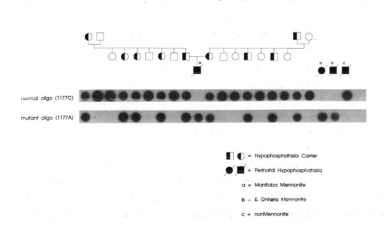

Fig. 7–17. Allele-specific-oligonucleotide (ASO) hybridization analysis of a unique single G to A single-base substitution at position 1177 in the cDNA encoding the liver\bone\kidney form of alkaline phosphatase causing a lethal form of hypophosphatasia, a disorder of bone mineralization, in Canadian individuals of Mennonite descent. All individuals who were felt to be carriers biochemically are heterozygous for this mutation, whereas all noncarriers are homozygous for the normal sequence. Only the deceased affected Mennonite babies are homozygous for this mutation, which changes a glycine to an aspartate residue at amino acid position 317 of the mature protein.

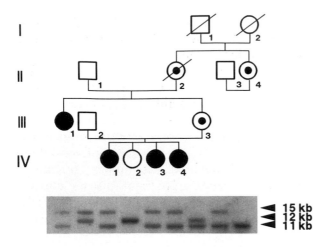

Fig. 7–18.   Tracking RFLPs in the anonymous locus DXYS1 flanking the androgen receptor gene in a family with complete androgen insensitivity syndrome (CAIS). The polymorphic X-specific alleles are 11 and 12 kb. The Y-specific allele is 15 kb. All individuals with a 15 kb allele have an XY karyotype. Individuals III-1, IV-1, IV-3, and IV-4 who are phenotypically female with 46, XY karyotypes are affected with CAIS, and thus the maternally inherited 11 kb DXYS1 allele is segregating with the mutant CAIS allele. Individual IV-2 would be predicted to be a noncarrier, having inherited the alternate maternal 12 kb allele.

are often neutral *polymorphisms* and not true *mutations*. Given the genetic diversity in the human genome, it should not be surprising to find numerous classes of polymorphisms. Polymorphisms are very useful as genetic markers in that they follow mendelian codominant inheritance and can be used to follow the inheritance of a small region of DNA through a pedigree.

To be useful, a genetic marker must fulfill the following criteria: (1) it must have a known chromosomal location; (2) it must be informative (i.e., existing in two forms) within the family of interest; (3) the genetic distance between the disease locus in question and the marker locus must be known. In a pedigree with a known genetic disease that is mapped to a known chromosomal location, the segregation of the disease-causing mutation can be indirectly inferred or predicted by analyzing the co-segregation of polymorphisms that are present either intragenically or in flanking loci (see Chap. 9). The 1980s saw the utilization of two main classes of polymorphisms: (1) restriction fragment length polymorphisms

(**RFLPs**);[2] and (2) variable number of tandem repeated DNA sequences (**VNTR**). These classes of polymorphisms changed the face of genetics, and the 1990s have seen the elucidation of a useful newer class of polymorphisms known as **microsatellites**.

Restriction Fragment Length Polymorphism (RFLP). When genomic DNA from different individuals is analyzed by Southern blot analysis with a DNA probe, often the same pattern of bands is observed. Sometimes a differing pattern of fragments known as RFLPs are observed as a result of a gross DNA alteration, such as a deletion or duplication, but usually from single nucleotide changes that either create or destroy a particular restriction enzyme site. This nucleotide substitution can be the actual site of the disease-causing mutation as in the case of sickle cell anemia, or more commonly they reflect innocuous DNA variation that is often intronic or, if within exons, causes no significant amino acid shift (Fig. 7–18). RFLPs are thus "homologous segments of restriction endonuclease-cleaved DNA of differing lengths." Given the fact that there are hundreds of restriction endonucleases and that it is estimated that nucleotide substitutions occur in 1 in 100 to 1 in 500 bases, RFLPs are abundantly distributed throughout the human genome and have been used for disease prediction in many genetic disorders. Such RFLPs, however, are usually diallelic and often limited in their usefulness if they are not informative in a particular family of interest (see Fig. 9–4).

Variable Number Tandem Repeat (VNTR). A second category of DNA markers has been developed called VNTRs. This represents a particular subtype of **satellite DNA** in the human genome, so named because many of the original tandem repeats were isolated by density centrifugation as a separate "satellite" fraction of DNA. The VNTRs are sequences of 11 to 60 base pairs that are repeated in a head-to tail fashion several times. The number of repeats at any one locus is heritable, but variable. In this class of polymorphism, the restriction sites for a particular enzyme stay the same, but fragment length in the interval between the restriction sites differs as deter-

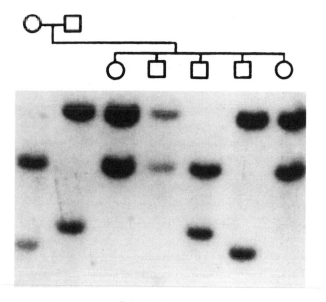

Probe: 3'HVR

Enzyme: PvuII

Fig. 7–19. Southern blot showing mendelian codominant segregation of a highly polymorphic VNTR polymorphism near the PKD1 locus on chromosome 16. Courtesy of Drs. D. Rosenblatt and E. Lamothe, McGill University.

mined by the number of tandemly repeated sequences. The number of repeats varies among people because of unequal crossing over (see Fig. 6–19). VNTRs (also known as **minisatellites**)[11] are better markers than RFLPs because there are usually many differing alleles, so that homologous chromosomes are readily distinguishable and thus are extremely useful in family studies (Fig. 7–19).[23] VNTRs are also very useful in forensic medicine and paternity testing using "DNA fingerprinting."

Microsatellites, also known as simple sequence repeats (SSR), represent the newest class of genomic sequences with an unusually high polymorphic content. A microsatellite consists of a mono-, di-, tri-, and tetranucleotide that is repeated in tandemly arranged copies similar to VNTRs. The most common class of microsatellite is the dinucleotide CA.GT dimer and is referred to as a (CA) or (GT) repeat. First demonstrated only a decade ago, it is now known that microsatellite loci are abundant throughout the human ge-

nome, estimated to be found on an average of every 18 to 28 kb. This means that there is a very high chance that any disease locus or cloned gene will have a microsatellite nearby. Microsatellites can be easily typed with PCR. Given their highly polymorphic nature, they are very useful as genetic markers to follow the segregation of a disease in an at-risk family (Fig. 7–20). A panel of microsatellites dispersed throughout the human genome is also an enormously powerful tool for efficient and rapid gene mapping, reflecting an order of magnitude improvement over RFLP-based

Family W

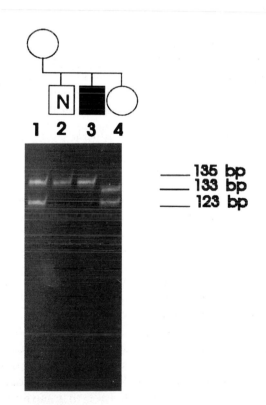

Fig. 7–20. Ethidium bromide-stained polyacrylamide gel demonstrating segregation of a polymorphic (AC)n repeat in the 3' end of the dystrophin gene in a family with Duchenne muscular dystrophy. The affected boy shown in lane 3 probably represents a new mutation (barring germ-line mosaicism in the mother) because his unaffected brother inherited the same 135 bp (AC)n allele as his affected brother. The sister shown in lane 4 has a very low probability of being a DMD carrier, having inherited the opposite 123 bp maternal allele. Her 133 bp allele is inferred to be paternal in origin.

approaches. They are also highly useful in the study of mating systems and the genetic structure of different populations.

Single-strand Conformation Polymorphism (SSCP).[14] Lastly, a spectrum of techniques exist to screen DNA segments for sequence variation, particularly single base pair changes. These methods are particularly valuable for diseases with high mutational diversity where it is impractical to sequence the entire gene, or where standard polymorphism analysis does not suffice or is not useful, as in the index case of a family representing a new mutation. Most of these methods are PCR-based and can rapidly screen large genes for the presence of new mutations. One of the commonly used methods for scanning regions of genes for mutations is the SSCP method. This refers to the detection of single strand conformation polymorphisms utilizing the fact that the electrophoretic mobility of single stranded nucleic acid fragments that are up to ~400 bases in length and differ by a single nucleotide will be different under denaturing gel conditions. This technique has been valuable as a strategy for mutation screening in a variety of genetic diseases with a representative example given in Fig. 7–21.

Human Genome Initiative

The technologic advances we have witnessed have led to the creation of a major research project, international in scope, which aims to map and sequence the entire human genome. This formidable task will result in the identification of all the genes in our genome and the listing in precise order of its 3 billion base pairs. With the advent of automated DNA sequencing technology and a huge, worldwide, coordinated effort, it is estimated that the human genome project can realize its goals in 15 years. The elucidation of thousands of genes will lead to advances in our understanding of normal and abnormal growth and development. Although better knowledge of the genome may speed development of new approaches to disease prevention and treatment including gene therapy (discussed next),

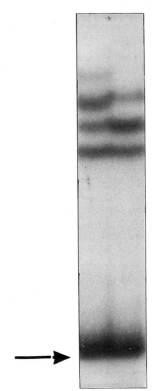

Fig. 7–21.   SSCP of exon 3 of the *HEXA* gene. Lane 1 contains a sample from a carrier of Tay-Sachs disease with one normal copy of exon 3 and one copy of exon 3 containing a C409-to-T mutation (Akli, S. et al., Genomics 11:124, 1991) that creates a termination codon. The mutation causes a shift in mobility of the mutant DNA strand seen as a slower migrating band at the top of lane 1. Lane 2 contains a sample from a noncarrier with two normal copies of exon 3. The arrow at the bottom denotes the double-stranded, i.e., nondenatured form of the sample. Courtesy of Dr. B. Triggs-Raine, University of Manitoba.

we will be faced with unprecedented moral, ethical, and social challenges; how to integrate rapid advances into our knowledge base to the benefit of patients, and at the same time maintain their right to privacy and confidentiality.

GENE THERAPY

The most dramatic approach to the treatment of genetic disease is gene therapy—the manipulation of genes to correct the inherited defect.

Somatic gene therapy involves correcting the defect in the patient's somatic cells. This involves putting the normal gene into the patient's mutant cells in a way that will restore the normal function of those cells and correct the patient's disorder. This can be done by putting the normal gene into a vector that can be targeted to the cells of the appropriate organ in the patient or (the usual approach at present) introducing the normal gene into the patient's cells in culture, and then returning the "corrected" cells to a site in the patient where they can function to supply the missing product.

There are many ingenious methods for getting the "therapeutic" DNA into the mutant cells, the most practical ones being by way of a viral vector,[7] often a retrovirus. These are simple RNA viruses with only three structural genes, which can be removed and replaced by the gene to be transferred. Retroviruses have been referred to as the Trojan horse of somatic cell gene therapy. Integration is highly efficient, in dividing cells, and the viruses can be engineered so that they will not produce further infectious particles.

The next problem is incorporating the normal DNA into the mutant cell's genome. Possible approaches are:

1. to cut out the mutant gene and replace it with the normal one. This is not technically feasible, as yet.
2. to alter the mutant gene back to the normal state. This has been done in experimental animals by homologous recombination—the normal gene, with appropriate flanking sequences to direct it to the appropriate site, is incorporated into the mutant cell's genome by recombination during mitosis. Recombination is rare, but techniques for selecting recombinant cells are improving. If "targeting" became efficient, this would be the desirable method, but at present it is not practical for human gene therapy.
3. to introduce the normal gene into the mutant cells where it becomes incorporated into the cells' genome at random. This is referred to as **gene augmentation**, and is at present the only feasible

method of gene transfer for use in humans.

The third problem is how to get the genetically "corrected" cells into the patient, at a site where they can correct the patient's deficit. The standard approach is to take cells from the patient, expose them to the vector carrying the therapeutic gene, select the corrected cells, grow them in culture, and put them back in the patient.

After extensive experiments in animals to demonstrate efficacy and safety, and intensive bioethical review, the first clinical trials were begun in September, 1990.[1] The disease chosen was **adenosine deaminase (ADA) deficiency**, a recessively inherited inborn error leading to failure of the immune system so that patients can not resist bacterial and viral infections. Treatment with bone marrow replacement was possible, but had many drawbacks, and treatment with enzyme replacement was expensive and not very satisfactory. The first children, treated with their own lymphocytes into which the normal ADA gene had been introduced, are doing well at the time of writing, and prospects are promising. Treatment has to be repeated every few months as the treated cells have a finite life span. It would be better to treat the hematopoietic stem cells, the primitive cells that are the source of the hematopoietic cells, and to replace them in the marrow or liver, where they would produce a permanent supply of "corrected" cells. Progress is being made in methods to extract the rare stem cells from the patient's marrow for genetic manipulation.

This approach is suitable only for diseases in which the missing product can be supplied in cells derived from the hematopoietic system stem cells, that is, diseases now treatable by marrow transplantation. Furthermore, retroviruses will only deliver the curative DNA to dividing cells. But in some conditions, the site of the defect cannot be reached by this method, for instance in diseases where the product is missing in the central nervous or respiratory system. Imaginative new approaches are being developed to get around these logistical problems. The hepatocytes of the *liver* are not usually susceptible to retroviruses, but are so during a transient period of dedifferentiation in culture. This has opened the way to introducing the gene for the LDL receptor into hepatocytes from a patient with familial hypercholesterolemia (in this case a rabbit patient), which are then transferred back into the patient's liver. Significant lowering of cholesterol was achieved, and a clinical protocol has been approved.

Skin fibroblasts and keratinocytes are easily accessible for culture, manipulation, and return to the skin. A protocol for the treatment of hemophilia B by supplying factor IX this way is under way in China. A similar approach has been taken with endothelial cells cultured from and returned to the *vascular system.*

Cells of the *respiratory system* are not so easily accessible for culture, and retroviruses will not infect these non-dividing cells. But adenoviruses will, and the normal allele of the gene for cystic fibrosis has been transferred to the airway epithelium of cotton rats by introducing a genetically engineered replication-deficient adenovirus into the trachea. Clinical trials are contemplated as soon as concerns about safety have been satisfied.[16]

The inaccessibility of the central nervous system is being approached in two ways. One is to use a vector that will infect neurons, such as the herpes viruses. Another is to put the required gene into fibroblasts, and implant these into the patient's brain, to supply the missing product. These methods may have some promise for disorders (not necessarily genetic) such as Alzheimer and Parkinson disease.[8]

A promising new way of getting the patient's corrected cells back to an effective site is the use of myoblasts, immature muscle cells. The patient's engineered myoblasts are replaced in the muscle where they become incorporated, and produce the needed protein. The gene for human growth factor has been transferred into mouse muscles, and produced human growth hormone for at least several months.

Another field in which gene therapy may have a bright future is **cancer**. The rapid advances in understanding of the molecular basis of cancer is opening the way to therapeutic approaches. In vitro reversion of the malignant morphology of tumor cells has been achieved by introducing normal versions of mutant oncogenes or tumor suppressor genes, including the WTp53, RB, WT1 and NF genes.[9] The problem is to get the vector into the tumor cells. Other approaches include the use of antisense oligodeoxynucleotides that selectively inhibit the mRNA for the oncogene in question, and genetic immunomodulation to enhance the antitumor response of the host's immune system.[9] The first approved gene therapy protocol for cancer adds the gene for tumor necrosis factor (TNF) to tumor-infiltrating lymphocytes (TIL). The TILs invade tumors and attack the tumor cells, and TNF is a powerful anticancer agent, but very toxic. Using the TIL cells to bring the TNF directly to the tumor cells may make it much more effective, without toxicity. Several patients are under treatment.

Drug targeting is another approach that is beginning to show promise. A gene is introduced into the tumor cells that make them, but not the normal cells, susceptible to an anticancer drug.[9] The main obstacle to this approach is how to deliver genes effectively to the tumors in vivo.

One approach to somatic gene therapy is to introduce genetically engineered cells or vectors carrying "corrective" DNA into the fetus, where they might become incorporated into the fetal tissues and prevent prenatal effects of the genetic disorder. This possibility raises serious concerns, particularly about the eugenic implications. Such concerns seem to be based on the assumption that there would be high efficiency and that the procedure would be widespread. Neither is likely to be the case. Fetal therapy cannot be done until after the gonads have differentiated, or there could be germ cell alteration, which is unacceptable. The technical difficulties of obtaining fetal tissue for gene alteration and getting the altered cells back into an effective fetal site are so formidable that postnatal gene therapy and (more probably) prenatal diagnosis are likely to be preferable alternatives for some time to come.

Germ line gene therapy refers to directed genetic change in gametes or cells that give rise to gametes. There is great public concern about manipulating the gene pool in this way, not only because of possible unforeseen dangers (cancer, developmental disturbance, eugenic misuse), but because of a nonspecific revulsion to the idea of "playing God" by tampering with the secrets of life. Virtually all bodies that have pronounced judgment on the subject have considered germ line therapy ethically unacceptable and not to be allowed.

In fact, it is highly unlikely that anyone will seriously suggest germ line gene therapy in the foreseeable future, for at least the following reasons. Germ line therapy would require 100% targeting, otherwise each offspring of the treated individual would require prenatal diagnosis, and we would be no better off than we are now. Furthermore, there would have to be gene replacement, rather than insertion or modification, or the mutant gene would still be there and could be passed on. Gene replacement is not feasible in humans with present technology. Genes have been introduced into the germ cells of mice and transmitted to the next generation—putting the human growth hormone gene into mice with pituitary dwarfism, for example. But the technique is not suitable for use in people. Uptake is very inefficient, and the few first-generation offspring that incorporate the "therapeutic" gene are mosaic, so that animals that carry the gene in every body cell appear only in the second generation. Finally, because the unforeseen risks cannot be evaluated without doing the procedure (assuming it ever became feasible) and observing the results over a long period, no germ line gene therapy is likely to get through the ethical review process.

The ethics of somatic gene therapy are not essentially different from those of other therapies. Due regard must be given to safety, informed decision making, and the wise allocation of resources.

Even germ line gene therapy does not raise questions that have not been raised before, although, if it became feasible, it would give such questions a new urgency. Apart from the question of safety, the main concerns center around our responsibility to future generations, and particularly the possibility that we might create deleterious mutations that would be passed on to "generations of their descendants." But mutations are happening all the time and, if they are harmful, get removed by selection; only if germ line therapy were widely applied and obviously mutagenic would there be serious effects on our germ plasm.

As for its application for eugenic purposes, again, it would have to be widely applied to have appreciable effects on gene frequencies. Of course we would abhor the use of gene manipulation for eugenic purposes—that is, to discriminate against certain groups of people. Society must guard against it by regulating the use of this, and other, genetic technologies, not by shunning them.

If it ever came to pass that a simple, inexpensive, safe, method of gene therapy was developed, with 100% targeting, it would be necessary to rethink the question.

REFERENCES

1. Anderson, W.F.: Human gene therapy. Science 256:808, 1992.
2. Botstein, D., White, R.L., Skolnick, M., and Davies, R.W.: Construction of a genetic linkage map in man using restriction fragment length polymorphisms. Am. J. Hum. Genet. 32:314, 1980.
3. Caskey, C.T., Pizutti, A., Fu, Y.-H., et al.: Triplet repeat mutations in human disease. Science 256:784, 1992.
4. Collins, F.S.: Cystic fibrosis: Molecular biology and therapeutic implications. Science 256:774, 1992.
5. Collins, F.S.: Positional cloning: Let's not call it reverse anymore. Nature Genetics 1:3, 1992.
6. Cystic Fibrosis Genetic Analysis Consortium: Worldwide survey of the delta F508 mutation. Am. J. Hum. Genet. 47:354, 1990.
7. Desnick, R.J. and Schuchman, E.H.: Human gene therapy: Strategies and prospects for inborn errors of metabolism. In Treatment of Genetic Diseases. Edited by R.J. Desnick. New York, Churchill Livingstone, 1991.
8. Friedmann, T.: Gene therapy. In Therapy for Genetic Disease. Edited by T. Friedmann. New York, Oxford University Press, 1991.
9. Gutierrez, A.A., Lemoine, N.R. and Sikora, K.: Gene therapy for cancer. Lancet 339:715, 1992.
10. Human Gene Mapping International Workshop Reports: Cytogenetics. Cell Genet. 1987–1991 (supplements).
11. Jeffries, A.J., Wilson, V. and Thein, S.L.: Hypervariable minisatellite regions in human DNA. Nature 314:67, 1985.
12. McKusick, V.A.: Mendelian inheritance in man; Catalogs of autosomal dominant, autosomal recessive, and

X-linked phenotypes. 10th ed. Baltimore, Johns Hopkins University Press, 1992.

13. Mullis, K.B., and Faloona, F.A.: Specific synthesis of DNA in vitro via a polymerase-catalysed chain reaction. Methods Enzymol. 155:335, 1987.
14. Orita, M., Iwahana, H., Kanazawa, H., et al.: Detection of polymorphisms of human DNA by gel electrophoresis as single strand conformation polymorphisms. Proc. Nat. Acad. Sci. USA 86:2766, 1989.
15. Richards, R.I. and Sutherland, G.R.: Heritable unstable DNA sequences Nature Genetics 1:7, 1992.
16. Rosenfeld, M.A., Yoshimura, K., Trapnell, B.C., et al.: In vivo transfer of the human cystic fibrosis transmembrane conductance regulator gene to the airway epithelium. Cell 68:143, 1992.
17. Rossiter, B.J.F. and Caskey, C.T.: Molecular studies of human genetic disease. FASEB J. 5:21, 1991.
18. Saiki, R.K., Scharf, S., Faloona, F., et al. Enzymatic amplification of beta-globin genomic sequences and re-striction analysis for the diagnosis of sickle cell anemia. Science 230:1350, 1985.
19. Saiki, R.K., Bugawan, T.L., Horn, G.T., et al.: Analysis of enzymatically amplified Beta-globin and HLA-DQ alpha DNA with allele-specific oligonucleotide probes. Nature 324:163, 1986.
20. Saiki, R.K., Gelfand, D.H., Stoffel, S., et al.: Primer-mediated enzymatic amplification of DNA with a thermostable DNA polymerase. Science 239:487, 1988.
21. Scriver, C.R., Beaudet, A.L., Sly, W.S. and Valle, D. (eds.): The Metabolic Basis of Inherited Disease. 6th ed. New York, McGraw-Hill, 1989.
22. Southern, E.R.: Detection of specific sequences among DNA fragments separated by gel electrophoresis. J. Mol. Biol. 98:503, 1975.
23. Weber, J.L. and May, P.E. Abundant class of DNA polymorphisms which can be typed using the polymerase chain reaction. Am. J. Hum. Genet. 44:388, 1989.

Chapter 8
Selected Mendelian Diseases

HOMO SUM, HUMANI NIL A ME ALIENUM PUTO.

TERENCE

We stated in the preface that we lack the space and no longer find it possible to provide clinical descriptions of many diseases of genetic interest, but must refer the reader to other texts. Of particular value as a resource for this chapter are McKusick's Mendelian Inheritance in Man and the Birth Defects Encyclopedia. A more detailed selection of such references is provided in Appendix B. For this chapter on mendelian disorders, we have tried to limit our discussion to approximately 100 of the most common or informative clinical problems, with the full recognition that conditions commonly seen in one genetics center may be less common in another because of the interest and expertise of the respective staffs.

As in previous editions, we shall subgroup the diseases according to modes of inheritance, which will, of course, take into consideration disorders that are inherited by more than one mode. We will also describe diseases that may be common in some populations, but not in others (e.g., Tay-Sachs), and uncommon diseases of historic interest (e.g., alkaptonuria). What has been surprising to us is how many of the diseases selected by these criteria have already been mapped within the human genome.

Finally, in this chapter, we shall reference relevant entries in recent monographs and secondary sources much more extensively than original articles.

AUTOSOMAL DOMINANT DISEASES

In Chapter 5, the principles of dominant inheritance are discussed. A dominant disease is one that is expressed in the heterozygote; that is, only a single dose of a mutant gene is required to produce the disease. Every affected individual has an affected parent unless the disease has arisen as a fresh mutation. Each offspring of an affected parent has a 50:50 chance of having the disease, but unaffected relatives of affected persons will *not* have affected children. Because these diseases are rare, it is highly unusual in a random-mating population for more than one parent to have the disease. In the following discussion of diseases, space does not permit clinical descriptions in the detail needed for precise diagnosis. We offer, rather, a guide, indicating the kinds of diagnostic and prognostic problems and some of the genetic pitfalls of which the counselor must be aware.

Achondroplasia[1,2]

History. True achondroplasia has emerged as a distinct entity from the broader category of dysplastic dwarfs which has been recognized throughout medical history. Numerous chondrodystrophies, some recessive and some nonrecurrent, have been misclassified as "classic" achondroplasia in the past, so care should be taken to secure the diagnosis before genetic counseling (Fig. 8–1).

Diagnostic Features. *General.* Equal sex distribution. Severely dwarfed. Early motor progress may be slow but intelligence is normal.

Head. Large head, prominent forehead, saddle nose with midfacial hypoplasia, small foramen magnum (occasionally producing hydrocephalus). Megalocephaly may occur.

Vertebrae. Lumbar lordosis with anterior beaking of upper lumbar vertebrae; progressive narrowing of lumbar interpeduncular spaces, small cuboid vertebral bodies with short pedicles.

Extremities. Rhizomelic limbs (shortening more pronounced proximally) with epiphyseal ossification centers inserted into metaphyseal ends of bones, producing ball-and-socket appearance; short trident-shaped hand.

Pelvis. Small iliac wings and reduced sacroiliac curve with narrow greater sciatic notch.

Prevalence. 1:10,000, about 85% being fresh mutations—these show an increased mean paternal age. The mutation rate is estimated as 1.4×10^{-5}. Hypochondroplasia, a milder form also showing autosomal dominant inheritance, may be an allelic mutant.

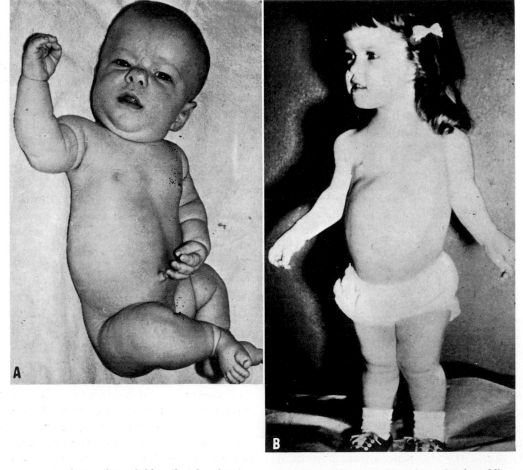

Fig. 8–1. A. Infant and B. child with achondroplasia. Note rhizomelic extremities, large head, saddle-nose.

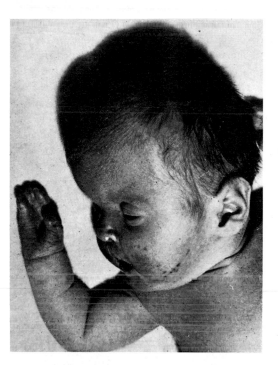

Fig. 8–2. Characteristic appearance of head and hands in Apert syndrome.

Clinical Course. Hydrocephalus may occur because of the narrow foramen magnum. Recurrent otitis media, possibly caused by short eustachian tubes, should be treated aggressively. Lumbar lordosis often appears during weight bearing, leading to hip flexion contractures that should be treated with stretching exercises. Bowing of the legs may result from overgrowth of the fibula and requires orthopedic treatment. The small maxilla may create orthodontic problems. Food intake should conform to body size, to avoid obesity. The disproportionate body size may lead to problems of social adjustment, with which lay groups such as the Little People of America can be helpful.

Spinal cord compression is not uncommon, especially in the second and third decades, because of bony impingement or herniated intervertebral discs; neurologic disabilities, such as paraplegia, may result. Early signs should be watched for and treated aggressively.

Treatment. Symptomatic and supportive; relief of spinal cord compression, should it occur.

Acrocephalosyndactyly (ACS Type I: Includes Apert, Apert-Crouzon ACSII, Vogt Cephalodactyly)[1,2]

History. Apert receives the credit for describing this syndrome in 1906. Because the skull abnormality in this condition caused mental retardation, few patients had children, and almost all cases were sporadic. An increased mean paternal age was the main evidence for autosomal dominant inheritance.

Diagnostic Features. *General.* Severe mental deficiency may or may not occur. Some shortness of stature.

Head. High forehead, flat occiput, short anteroposterior diameter, irregular craniosynostosis, midfacial hypoplasia, hypertelorism, antimongoloid slant, strabismus (Fig. 8–2).

Ears. Often low-set.

Mouth. Narrow, high-arched palate; occasional cleft palate.

Skeleton. Osseous and/or cutaneous syndactyly of hands and feet, most often involving digits 2 to 4 ("mitten-hand"). Variable fusion of nails. Syndactyly of all toes. Occasional limitation of joint mobility, radioulnar synostosis, fused vertebrae.

Cardiovascular. Rare congenital lesions, including coarctation of the aorta.

Gastrointestinal. Occasional esophageal atresia, pyloric stenosis.

Genitourinary. Occasional polycystic kidney, hydronephrosis.

X ray. Osseous syndactyly; occasional radioulnar synostosis, vertebral fusion, and diastasis of the symphysis pubis.

Prevalence. 1:160,000, with the majority of patients representing fresh mutations.

Clinical Course. Intellectual impairment may progress with increased intracranial pressure. Evaluation (and treatment) of the many possible associated anomalies must be considered.

Treatment. Early surgical relief of the craniosynostosis if it is accompanied by increased intracranial pressure. Surgical mobilization of the thumb (when indicated) and separation of cutaneous syndactyly. Surgical intervention in congenital cardiovascular and genitourinary malformations. Special schooling for the retarded.

Differential Diagnosis. Several genetically determined disorders have craniosynostosis associated with syndactyly as a feature, mostly inherited as autosomal dominants. Among these are the following:

1. *Crouzon craniofacial dysostosis* is not associated with syndactyly.
2. Acrocephalosyndactyly Type III, Saethre-Chotzen syndrome, is characterized by facial asymmetry, low-set frontal hairline, ptosis, variable brachydactyly, and cutaneous syndactyly.
3. Acrocephalosyndactyly Type V, acrocephalopolysyndactyly Type I (Noack syndrome). This syndrome has preaxial polysyndactyly and no mental retardation.
4. *Acrocephalopolysyndactyly Type II (Carpenter syndrome)* is similar to Noack syndrome except that it shows autosomal recessive inheritance. Obesity may be quite pronounced and retardation is common.
5. Other autosomal dominant acrocephalosyndactylies may be distinguished by certain features of the hand malformation. They may well be clinical variants of the same mutant gene, but until treatment allows propagation and family studies, the question remains open.

Alpha-1-Antitrypsin Deficiency[2,4]

During the past decade, a severe obstructive lung disease in young and middle-aged adults and a cholestatic or cirrhotic liver disease in children have been found to be associated with a decreased plasma level of the protease inhibitor (Pi) alpha-1-antitrypsin (α-1-AT).

Population studies of electrophoretic variants have revealed 30 codominant alleles for what is now called the Pi system. The homozygous PiZZ phenotype is associated with less than 20% α-1-AT activity, a 10% risk of cholestasis or cirrhosis in childhood, and a 60 to 70% risk of lung disease in adult life. Heterozygotes have intermediate levels of activity of α-1-AT (PiSZ = 38% and PiMZ = 58%) as opposed to 100% activity for the PiMM phenotype. Cigarette smoking and other air pollutants contribute to the progression of the lung disease in homozygotes and even in heterozygotes (e.g., PiSZ). A few observations have been reported of children with lung disease in the presence of a severe deficiency of α-1-AT.

The prevalence of α-1-AT deficiency (<20% of the normal plasma level of 2.0 to 2.2 g/l) in Swedish neonates is 1:1400. A simple screening test for the PiZZ phenotype is now available and may be considered in the context of early detection and environmental counseling.

AORTIC SUPRAVALVULAR STENOSIS WITH OR WITHOUT ELFIN FACIES (WILLIAMS-BEUREN SYNDROME)[1,2,8]

"Elfin" facies and other noncardiovascular features of this syndrome were recognized in patients having infantile hypercalcemia during the 1950s. The disease was particularly prevalent in England, where excessively large doses of vitamin D supplementation were used during this period, and the frequency fell dramatically when the supplement was reduced. In 1961, a syndrome of elfin facies and supravalvular aortic stenosis was described, and in 1963, it was appreciated that patients with infantile hypercalcemia and those with supravalvular aortic stenosis suffered from the same disease. Beuren in 1972, described familial cases of supravalvular aortic stenosis with and without elfin facies. Familial supravalvular aortic stenosis without elfin facies has been considered by some to be a separate disease entity to which the term Eisenberg type has been ascribed.

Diagnostic Features. *General.* Mild to moderate mental and growth retardation; low birth weight.

Facies. "Elfin" facies, i.e., full face, wide mouth and full upper lip without a cupid's bow, and pouting lower lip; hypertelorism, retroussé nose, small mandible, and prominent ears, sometimes pointed (Fig. 8–3).

Cardiovascular. Supravalvular aortic stenosis, multiple peripheral pulmonary artery

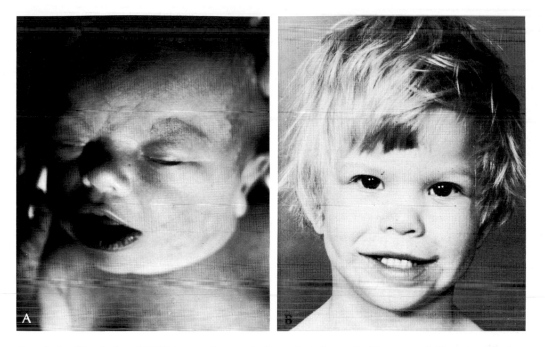

Fig. 8–3. The facies of Williams syndrome. A. In early infancy. B. The same child at age 3 years.

branch stenoses, supravalvular pulmonic stenosis.

Renal. Nephrocalcinosis in some cases.

Laboratory. Hypercalcemia is usually not detectable in the newborn and is more often discovered after about 3 months of age, throughout infancy, and sometimes as late as 3 years of age. Most patients with Williams-Beuren syndrome are never detected as having hypercalcemia.

Clinical Course. In general, patients who develop the aortic disease have fewer or insignificant manifestations of renal disease and ectopic calcification. Whether the vascular lesions are produced in utero or during infancy has been questioned: the answer is probably both. We have seen newborns with aortic disease as well as patients of reliable observers who asserted that no clinical evidence of vascular disease existed in early infancy and that the findings became manifest later. Patients with supravalvular aortic stenosis and elfin facies may be expected to be somewhat retarded; those with aortic disease and without elfin facies generally are not retarded.

Counseling. Patients with the full-blown syndrome of supravalvular aortic stenosis,

mental retardation, and elfin facies are frequently sporadic; however, families compatible with autosomal dominant transmission of the full syndrome have been recognized, as have families with supravalvular aortic stenosis without retardation or elfin facies. We have seen families in which variations of the disorder existed in different family members. Some patients had elfin facies with cardiovascular disease. Others had elfin facies without cardiovascular disease, and still others had cardiovascular disease without elfin facies. The counselor should be guarded in offering the projection of sporadic occurrence, when so many autosomal dominant cases clearly exist.

Treatment. Because of the probability of progression of the disease and the possible relationship of this disorder to the patient's ability to handle vitamin D, it seems prudent to restrict this vitamin. Furthermore, because of the possibility of an antenatal teratogenic effect of vitamin D on the developing cardiovascular system, it seems equally prudent to suggest the avoidance of vitamin D supplements during future pregnancies by any mother who has had a child with this syndrome. Surgical intervention may be required for the su-

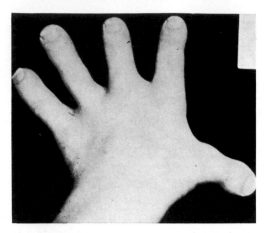

Fig. 8–4.   Brachydactyly, Fitch type II (brachydactyly C).

pravalvular aortic stenosis or for supravalvular pulmonic stenosis unaccompanied by peripheral pulmonary branch stenosis. Surgery is not possible for multiple pulmonary artery branch stenoses.

Brachydactyly[7]

Brachydactyly occurs in several syndromes or by itself (Fig. 8–4). Several dominant mutant genes cause shortening of specific phalanges and/or metacarpals and metatarsals. These are summarized in Table 8–1 according to a classification proposed by Fitch,[6] which removes much of the previously existing confusion. Cross-references to other classifications are included. The first seven types refer to mutant genes affecting single bones. The

Table 8–1.   The Dominantly Inherited Brachydactylies

Nomenclature			Hand Brachyphalangy			Short		Short Stature	Other Features
Fitch*	Bell[†]	Other	Distal	Middle	Prox	Metacarp	Metatars		
1	D	Stub thumb	1						Broad distal phalanx, thumb, and big toe
2	A-2	Brachy-mesopha-langy 2	2						Short middle phalanx in toe 2
3	A-3	Brachy-mesopha-langy 5	5						
4	E					2			
5	E					4			
6	E						4		
7	E					4	4		
8	B (A-5)	Apical dystrophy	2–5 small or absent	2–5 small or absent					Broad or bifid thumb in 50% maybe absence of nails, syndactyly. Same abnormalities in toes.
9	A-1 A-4?	Farrabee		2–5	1 often 2–5	some cases	some cases	+	Distal-middle fusions, radial clinodactyly digit 4
10	E		1	5		4,5	4,5	+	Other metacarpals and phalanges may be short
11	C	Brahy-mesopha-langy 2, 3,5		2,3,5	2 and some-times 3	often 1		some cases	Proximal 2 may be double or have radial projection. Other skeletal anomalies—a chondro-osseous dystrophy

*Fitch, N.: Classification and identification of inherited brachydactylies. J. Med. Genet. 16:36, 1979.
[†]Bell, J.: On brachydactyly and symphalangism. In Treasury of Human Inheritance, Vol. 5. London, Cambridge University Press, 1951.

remainder have more general effects. Some include short stature. Because short children have short hands, it is worthwhile to look for brachydactyly radiologically to obtain information that may explain a child's short stature.

Branchio-Oto-Renal Dysplasia (Bor Syndrome)[1,2]

Preauricular pits and branchial clefts may show dominant inheritance, either separately or together (Fig. 8–5). In association with deafness and renal anomalies, they constitute the BOR syndrome, in which patients may have hearing loss (80%), either neurosensory, conductive, or mixed; preauricular pits (80%); branchial fistulas or cysts (60%); anomalous ear pinnae, lachrymal duct stenosis, and renal anomalies. The latter may range from mild asymptomatic dysplasia to absence. Roughly 5 to 10% of gene carriers have major renal findings. Penetrance is about 90%. Four of 8 probands with pits in a school for the deaf had the BOR syndrome. The existence of a separate mutant gene producing pits, clefts, and deafness without renal anomalies has not been convincingly demonstrated. Any child with

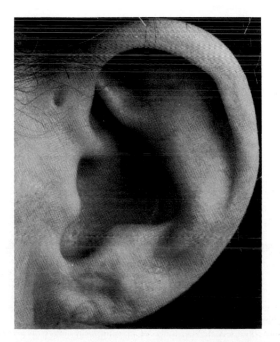

Fig. 8–5.   Preauricular pit in child with BOR syndrome.

deafness and preauricular pits deserves renal investigation.

Cleft Lip With Lip Pits[1,2]

This dominantly inherited disorder has, as its sentinel lesion, pits in the vermilion of the lower lip that are the openings of accessory salivary glands (see Figs. 5–12 and 5–13). Mucous discharge from these pits may be distressing enough to warrant excision of the fistulas. From the point of view of genetic counseling, the more important consideration is that over half of patients with familial lip pits have a cleft lip and/or palate. Therefore, when counseling for cleft lip or cleft palate, the physician should look carefully at the lips of the patient (and of the parents) before giving the usual low recurrence risk. Penetrance is high if a careful search is made for minor expressions such as submucous cleft palate. If lip pits are present in a parent, the child's risk for lip pits is about 50% and for cleft lip and/or palate about 25%.

Cleidocranial Dysplasia (Cleidocranial Dysostosis, CCD)[1,2]

History. Marie and Sainton reported the first clinical observation of this disorder in a father and son. The antiquity of this malformation is illustrated by the fact that it has been observed in a Neanderthal skull by Grieg. Penetrance is high, although expressivity may be low, requiring careful radiologic examination to establish the diagnosis. About one third of cases appear to be fresh mutations.

Diagnostic Features. *General.* Normal intelligence. Equal sex distribution. Moderately reduced stature. Variable severity.

Head. Open cranial sutures or late mineralization with bulging calvaria and frontal and parietal bossing.

Mouth. High-arched palate, late dentition, abnormal dysplastic teeth.

Thorax. Partial to complete aplasia of clavicles, which allows the patient to appose the shoulders (Fig. 8–6).

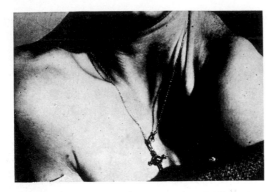

Fig. 8–6. Ability to appose shoulders in cleidocranial dysostosis.

Hands. Asymmetric length of fingers (short middle phalanx, fifth finger; long second metacarpal).

Skeletal. In addition to skull and clavicle defects, a wide symphysis pubis, vertebral malformations.

X-ray. Late mineralization of cranial sutures and pubic rami, absent or hypoplastic clavicles, pseudoepiphyses of metacarpals (Fig. 8–7).

Clinical Course. Closure of the cranial sutures may be delayed for many years. The eruption of permanent teeth may also be significantly delayed, and when they appear, the teeth are usually abnormal—enamel hypoplasia, retention cysts, supernumerary teeth, and malformed roots (which complicate extraction). The narrow pelvis in the female may make normal delivery impossible.

Treatment. Supportive.

Crouzon Craniofacial Dysostosis (Crouzon Disease)[1,2]

The characteristic facies of the patient with craniofacial dysostosis is associated with premature synostosis of the cranial sutures of varying degree and age of onset (Fig. 8–8). There may be acro- or brachydactyly, shallow orbits leading to exophthalmos and liability to optic nerve damage, hypertelorism, hypoplasia of the maxilla, beaked nose, short upper lip, high-arched short palate, malocclusion, and mandibular prognathism. Mental retardation is an occasional feature, as are coarctation of

the aorta and aortic stenosis. Progressive visual impairment occurs in many patients, and neurosurgery may be indicated. About 25% of cases result from fresh mutations. This syndrome includes pseudo-Crouzon disease, which does not have prognathism.

Craniostenosis (The Craniosynostoses, CRS)[1,2]

The genetics of premature synostosis of the cranial sutures is unclear. The frequency is roughly 1/2000 live births, although an unusual clustering of cases in Colorado has produced a higher rate and an active search for environmental influences. A few well-known dominantly inherited syndromes involve craniosynostosis, for example, acrocephalosyndactyly and craniofacial dysostosis. Cohen lists over 70 syndromes in which craniosynostosis is a feature. Most are autosomal recessive, somewhat fewer are autosomal dominant, or

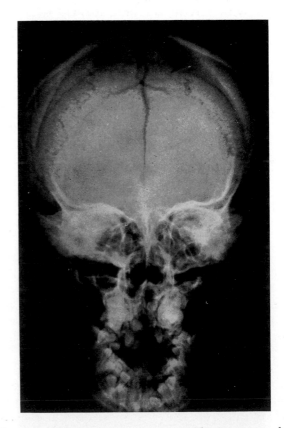

Fig. 8–7. X-ray evidence of open sagittal suture in an adult with cleidocranial dysostosis.

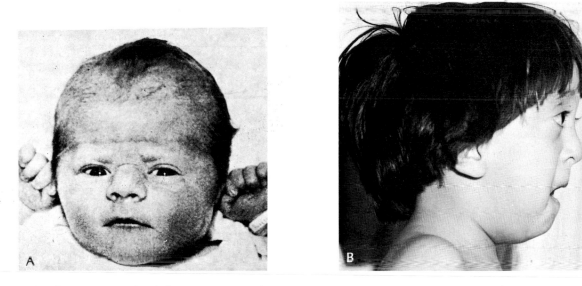

Fig. 8-8. Crouzon Craniofacial dysostosis. A. Newborn. Note that the hands are normal (as contrasted with the Apert syndrome). B. Five-year-old Note exophthalmos.

X-linked, a few are chromosomal, (deletion 7p21.3-p21.2), and about one third are of unknown etiology. Occasional families show mendelian inheritance of non-syndromic craniosynostosis. Several studies of patients coming to medical attention for craniosynostosis can be summarized as follows. The majority (about 57%) have sagittal synostosis, about 10% of these having involvement of other sutures. About 25% of those with sagittal synostosis have associated malformations, particularly cardiac (5%). About 10% are retarded, but about one half of these have a reasonable explanation for retardation unrelated to the synostosis. Only about 2% have a positive family history, occasionally dominant but more often in sibs; in the latter group the rate of recurrence is about 2%.

Of those with coronal involvement, about 10% have Crouzon disease. About 40% have associated malformations. Hydrocephaly presents a significant risk (5%). About 15% have complex malformation syndromes. About 15 to 20% are retarded, the rate being higher for bilateral (25%) than for unilateral (10%) cases and for those with other malformations or a complicated medical history. About 10% have a positive family history, usually with vertical transmission, suggesting autosomal dominant inheritance. A minority have affected sibs with normal parents. The rate of recurrence in sibs of affected patients with unaffected parents is about 3%.

Deafness, Dominant Forms[2,8]

Several of genetically determined forms of deafness, with and without associated abnormalities, follow an autosomal dominant mode of inheritance. The following list is extracted from the useful review by Konigsmark and Gorlin. These include syndromes discussed in this chapter (BOR, Waardenburg, and Treacher-Collins syndromes), as well as the following:

A. Deafness without associated anomalies
  1. Congenital severe sensorineural deafness
  2. Progressive nerve deafness, childhood onset
  3. Unilateral sensorineural deafness
  4. Low-frequency sensorineural hearing loss
  5. Midfrequency sensorineural hearing loss
  6. High-frequency sensorineural hearing loss
  7. Otosclerosis (penetrance of 25 to 40%)

B. Deafness with external ear malformations
   8. Deafness with preauricular pits (BOR syndrome)
   9. Incudostapedial abnormality, thickened ears
  10. Conductive hearing loss and deformed ears
C. Deafness with defects of the integument
  11. Waardenburg syndrome
  12. Congenital deafness with albinism
  13. Leopard syndrome
  14. Progressive hearing loss with anhidrosis
  15. Deafness with keratopachyderma, digital constrictions
  16. Hearing loss with knuckle pads, leuconychia
D. Deafness with eye defect
  17. Hearing loss, myopia, cataract, saddle nose (Marshall & Stickler syndrome)
E. Deafness with nervous system disease
  18. Acoustic neuroma
  19. Sensory radicular neuropathy
F. Deafness with skeletal defects
  20. Hearing loss, proximal symphalangism
  21. Craniofacial dysostosis
  22. Mandibulofacial dysostosis
  23. Osteogenesis imperfecta
  24. Deafness, bony fusions, shortness, mitral insufficiency, freckles (Forney syndrome).

See McKusick's catalogue for a more extensive list.

Ectodermal Dysplasia[1,2]

Ectodermal dysplasia exists in several forms, which may show autosomal dominant, autosomal recessive, or X-linked inheritance. Dominant forms include the Basan syndrome and the Rapp-Hodgkin syndrome.

Ectodermal Dysplasia, Hidrotic (Clouston Type). These patients have alopecia that is often total, severe dystrophy of the nails, hyperpigmentation of the skin, especially over joints, and palmar dyskeratosis (Fig. 8–9).

Cataracts, mental subnormality, and shortness of stature have occasionally been described. In this syndrome, the teeth and the sweat and sebaceous glands are normal. Clouston reported a pedigree of 119 individuals in a French-Canadian family.

Ehlers-Danlos Syndrome[2,4]

History. Ehlers in 1901 and Danlos in 1908 described features of this syndrome. However, many observers before the twentieth century had also provided clinical descriptions, perhaps the earliest of which was the case of van Meekeren, reported in 1682.

Recognition of genetic heterogeneity has led to a profusion of types and subtypes.

Type I—Gravis

Diagnostic Features. *General.* Normal intelligence and growth. Equal sex distribution. Variable in severity.

Skin. Strikingly hyperextensible, velvety, fragile, and prone to laceration from minor trauma (Fig. 8–10). "Cigarette-paper" scars and molluscoid pseudotumors at pressure points. Subcutaneous bleeding. Increase in number of elastic fibers, but no pathologic features by EM or light microscopy. Surgical healing often presents a difficult problem in management.

Eyes. Epicanthic folds, blue sclerae, strabismus, keratoconus, retinal detachment, and subluxation of the lens.

Ears. Hypermobile, tendency to "lop ears."

Musculoskeletal. Hyperextensibility of joints with tendency to dislocation, kyphoscoliosis, and inguinal and diaphragmatic hernias.

Cardiovascular. Risk of cystic medial necrosis and dissection of medium-sized arteries (e.g., subclavian, renal) and occasionally dissecting aneurysm of the aorta. Atrioventricular valve regurgitation.

Lungs. Risk of rupture of lung, mediastinal emphysema, and pneumothorax.

Abdomen. Risk of gastrointestinal diverticulae and friability of the bowel with spontaneous rupture.

Clinical Course. Patients with hyperelastosis cutis, like those with Marfan syndrome, may lead reasonably normal lives or may be seriously debilitated. They are likely to be born

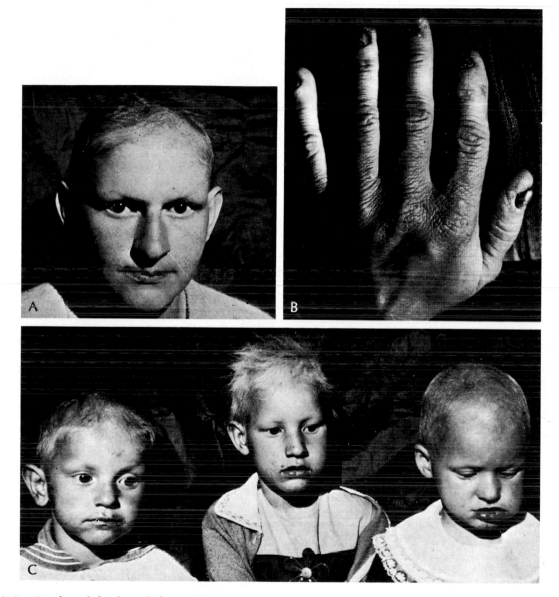

Fig. 8–9. Ectodermal dysplasia, hidrotic (Clouston type). A. Mother of children in C. B. Nail dysplasia in patient shown in A. C. Siblings.

prematurely because of premature rupture of the fetal membrane. These patients are at risk of vascular accidents and sudden death. Ruptured aneurysms of the cerebral arteries, dissection and rupture of subclavian, carotid, femoral, and other medium-sized arteries, as well as dissecting aneurysms of the aorta, can all lead rapidly to death in children and adults. Rupture of lungs and abdominal viscera has

also been reported to produce fatalities in this syndrome. Unfortunately, the magnitude of the risk is not known. Frequent lacerations from minor injuries, which are not easily sutured because of the fragility of the skin, result in excessive scarring and skin ulcerations.

Type II—Mitis—resembles the classic type, but the features are mild, and autosomal dominant inheritance is not fully established.

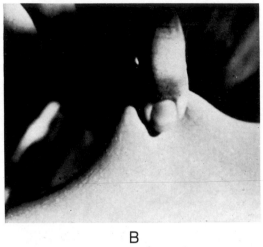

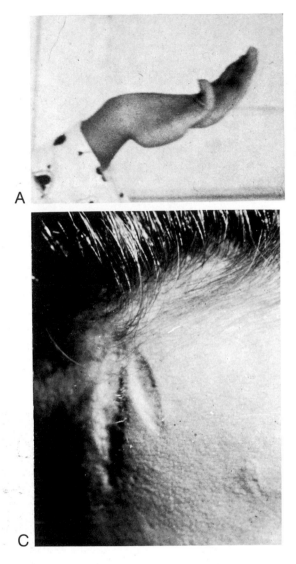

Fig. 8–10.   Ehlers-Danlos syndrome. A. Joint laxity. B. Distensibility of skin. C. Scarring of laceration-prone skin.

cated at 17q21.31-22.05) with two or more clinical forms of osteogenesis imperfecta. VII A2 (collagen 1, alpha-2 polypeptide) is located at 7q21.3-22.1) with two or more clinical forms of osteogenesis imperfecta.

Other types through XI are not clearly defined as to mode of inheritance.

Treatment. Symptomatic and supportive. Surgical intervention for vascular and visceral accidents.

Epidermolysis Bullosa[1,2]

There are several (perhaps 11) genetic forms of this disease. The common forms are dominant, and the uncommon and more debilitating forms, which may be lethal, are recessive. The *simple* dominant form may be observed at birth as superficial blisters (Fig. 8–11) or may not be noted until produced by mild trauma, such as that associated with crawling. The lesions are intraepidermal and are not followed by scarring. There are at least two non-allelic forms, in one of which the gene is linked (5 cm) to the red cell soluble glutamate-pyruvate transaminase locus. The *dystrophic* dominant form in which the nails are affected may lead to scarring and contractures. Ankles and fingers are particularly vulnerable.

Type III—Benign Hypermobile—has minimal skin features but generalized joint laxity.

Type VIII—Periodontosis Type—is not well characterized yet. Patients have fragile, bruisable skin, cigarette-paper scars, and loose joints, in addition to marfanoid features and extensive periodontal destruction.

Type IV—Arterial Type may be dominant or recessive.

Type V—is X-linked.

Type VI—is recessive.

Type VII—may be dominant or recessive. VII A1 (collagen 1, alpha-1 polypeptide is lo-

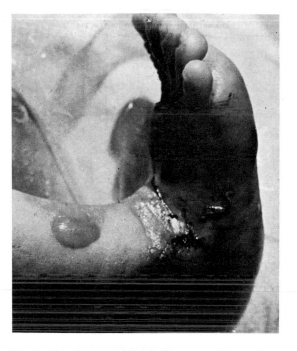

Fig. 8–11. Epidermolysis bullosa in newborn infant.

There are several different types, with variable expressivity both within and between types. A defect in the anchoring fibril protein has been postulated.

Holt-Oram (Heart and Hand) Syndrome[1,2,9]

In this syndrome a cardiac anomaly, commonly atrial septal defect or ventricular septal defect, is associated with a skeletal malformation involving the radial aspect of the upper limb (Fig. 8–12). Most often the thumb is finger-like (digitalization of the thumb), but it may be hypoplastic or absent. The radius and the forearm are variably involved and, in the severest forms, phocomelia may occur. The clinician should be alert to the possibility of coexisting gastrointestinal anomalies such as tracheoesophageal fistula in patients with thumb abnormalities or radial dysplasia with or without cardiac involvement. Anal atresia is also occasionally encountered in patients with limb and cardiac anomalies.

Huntington Disease[2,7]

Huntington disease (HD) may become manifest in childhood, but is usually recognized in the third or fourth decades. The initial manifestation is often emotional disturbance followed by choreic movements, seizures, and progressive dementia. Death usually occurs between 4 and 20 years after the onset of symptoms. Huntington disease is an example of a serious and disabling autosomal dominant disease that continues to be transmitted through successive generations because its late onset results in a relatively small reduction in reproductive fitness. The late onset of the disease also makes genetic counseling difficult.

Now that it is possible to diagnose in the asymptomatic offspring of an affected parent the presence of the HD gene on the short arm of chromosome 4 (4p16.3) using probes and the techniques of recombinant DNA technology, one might predict that the majority of the patients at risk would seek to learn if they carry the gene. This has not been the case, however, and only about half of such patients wish to know.

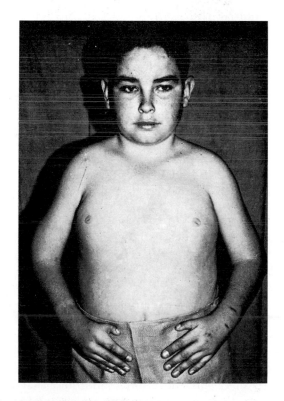

Fig. 8–12. Patient with Holt-Oram syndrome (with VSD and ASD). Note severe dysplasia of thumbs.

The gene has now been identified and the defect has been traced to a cytosine-adenine-guanine (CAG) repeat that recurs at least 42 times instead of the 11 to 34 times found in patients without the disease. This finding will immediately permit even more accurate screening of patients at risk and should lead to understanding the mechanism of the disease and eventually to the development of strategies of medical intervention.

HD has a frequency of about 4 to 7 per 100,000, and new mutations are rare.

Idiopathic Hypertrophic Subaortic Stenosis (IHSS) [Asymmetric Septal Hypertrophy (ASH), Obstructive Cardiomyopathy][1,2,9]

This highly penetrant dominant disorder is characterized by variable expressivity ranging from an abnormality detectable only by echocardiography (ECHO) to severe disability or, most strikingly, unexpected sudden death. The pathophysiologic key to the disease is hypertrophy of the interventricular septum with obstruction of the outflow tract of the left ventricle. ECHO is extremely useful, not only in the diagnosis of the disorder, but in the surveillance of the preclinical family members at risk and the noninvasive monitoring of progression of the disease. Figure 8–13A reveals typical echocardiographic findings of IHSS, including the systolic anterior motion (SAM) of the mitral valve which contributes in a major way to obstructing the subaortic outflow. Figure 8–13B shows how strikingly the left ventricular cavity may be obliterated during systole.

Mandibulofacial Dysostosis (MFDI; Treacher Collins Syndrome; Franceschetti-Klein Syndrome)[1,2]

History. In 1900, Treacher Collins reported a patient with this pattern of anomalies and has since been accorded the eponym. A more extensive treatment of the problem was presented in 1949, by Franceschetti and Klein, who called the condition mandibulofacial dysostosis; they are also sometimes credited with the eponym. The possibility has been raised that the MFDI locus is on 5q.

Diagnostic Features. *General.* Usually normal intelligence. Equal sex distribution. Normal growth in stature. Features of the syndrome vary and may be minimal; there is reduced penetrance.

Head. Mandibular and malar hypoplasia, depression of the temple, extension of scalp hair to cheeks, occasional skin tags and fistulas between ear and mouth, occasional cleft palate.

Eyes. Antimongoloid slant, notches at junction of outer and middle third of lower lids, absence of eyelashes (partial or complete), occasional microphthalmia (Fig. 8–14).

Ears. Malformed auricles and defects of the external ear canal; conductive deafness.

Nose. Occasional choanal atresia.

Skeletal. Occasional cervical vertebral anomalies.

Cardiovascular. Occasional congenital heart disease.

Genitourinary. Occasional cryptorchism.

Prevalence. Figure unavailable. The disorder is relatively common for a single mutant gene syndrome. About 60% of patients do not have affected parents, but it may be impossible to distinguish between fresh mutation and reduced penetrance in a particular case, making counseling difficult.

Clinical Course. The growth of the facial bones in childhood, especially during adolescence, produces considerable cosmetic improvement. An awareness of the high frequency of hearing deficit is necessary to ensure prompt recognition and treatment.

Treatment. Plastic surgery and hearing aids as indicated.

Differential Diagnosis.

1. *Robin syndrome.* Mandibular hypoplasia, glossoptosis, and posterior cleft palate. Although familial cases have been seen, they are rare, and this syndrome does not fit a simple mendelian pattern.
2. *Goldenhar syndrome* (see oculo-auriculo-vertebral dysplasia) shares many features of mandibulofacial dysostosis, but in addition there are epibulbar dermoids

and notching (usually unilateral) of the upper, rather than the lower, lid. A few familial cases have been reported. *Hemifacial microsomia* (unilateral microtia, macrostomia, and failure of formation of the mandibular ramus and condyles) may be a variant of the same syndrome.

3. *Nager acrofacial dysostosis* has the additional findings of limb anomalies.

Marfan Syndrome (MFS, Arachnodactyly, Dolichostenomelia)[1,2,9]

History. Antoine Marfan, a professor of pediatrics in Paris, reported the skeletal manifestations of this syndrome in 1896. He originally called the condition dolichostenomelia (long, thin extremities). Achard renamed the disorder arachnodactyly (spider fingers) in 1902. It was not until 1931 that the inheritance of

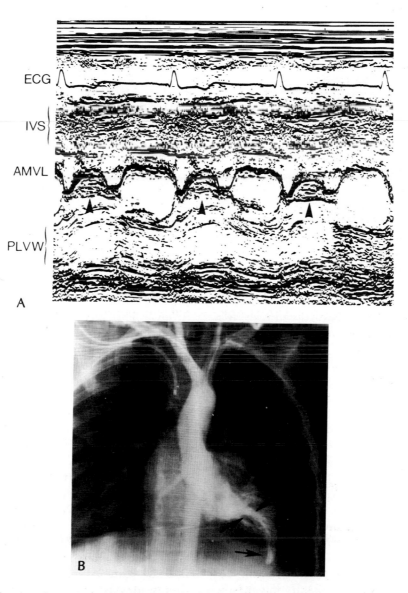

Fig. 8–13.   Echocardiogram showing greatly increased septal-free wall ratio (>1.3/1), septal hypertrophy, and systolic anterior motion of mitral valve (arrows) in IHSS. B, Angiocardiogram demonstrating left ventricular chamber obliteration during systole.

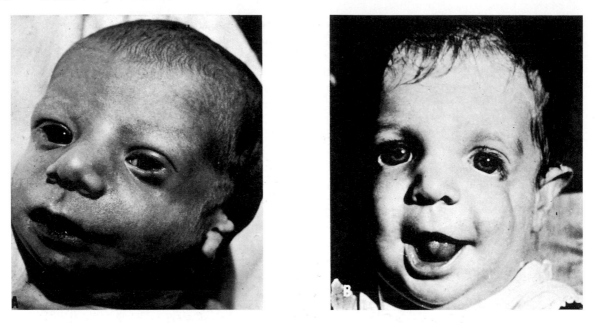

Fig. 8–14.   Mandibulofacial dysostosis in infant and young child. Note eye and ear anomalies.

the syndrome, as a dominant trait, was demonstrated by Weve. Penetrance is high, but expressivity is variable. About 15% of cases have normal parents; in these the increased mean paternal age suggests that they are new mutations.

Diagnostic Features. The diagnostic features are not invariable, and carriers of the gene may have anything from virtually no signs of the disease to the full-blown syndrome (Figs. 8–15 to 8–17).

General. Taller than unaffected sibs. Normal intelligence. Equal sex distribution. Variable expressivity and reduced penetrance complicate the diagnosis and counseling.

Head. Dolichocephaly (long head).

Eyes. Superior-temporal subluxation of lens and iridodonesis, myopia, spontaneous retinal detachment, blue sclerae.

Musculoskeletal. Frequent hypotonia and muscular underdevelopment. Long, thin extremities, kyphoscoliosis, and joint laxity. Pectus excavatum or carinatum. Ratio of upper segment (vertex to pubis) to lower segment (pubis to sole) less than normal for age (e.g., 0.85 instead of 0.93 in white adult males). Arm span greater than height. Hand-height ratio greater than 11%; foot-height ratio greater than 15%. Increased metacarpal index (length/width). Frequent inguinal and femoral hernias.

Cardiovascular. Cardiovascular disease is present in 60 to 80% of patients with the syndrome. The most frequent problem is mitral dysfunction, which may be as mild as an apical systolic click with minimal mitral prolapse by echocardiography to as severe as ruptured chordae with florid mitral regurgitation and acute death. Aortic cystic medial necrosis with dissecting aneurysm; aortic dilatation with aortic valvular insufficiency; aneurysms (with rupture) of sinuses of Valsalva. Echocardiography is a useful method of monitoring preclinical changes in the mitral valve and aorta (Figs. 8–16A, B). Medial degeneration of pulmonary arteries with dissection. Progressive dilatation of pulmonary arteries.

Prevalence. 1:60,000.

Clinical Course. As with some other single mutant gene syndromes, the Marfan syndrome may be regarded as an **abiotrophy**. That is, many of the features may not be present at birth, but may become manifest over a period of years. This is particularly true of the

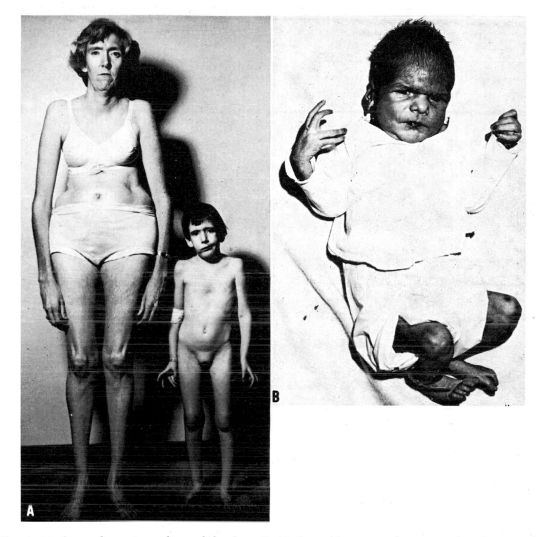

Fig. 8–15. A. Marfan syndrome in mother and daughter. B. Marfan syndrome in infancy. Note long fingers and toes as early expression of the syndrome.

cardiovascular abnormalities, which are usually responsible for the premature deaths of these patients. Death may occur in infancy or childhood, or in early or later adult life, depending on the rate of progression of the cardiovascular disease. The average age at death was 32 years (±16.4), and a cardiovascular etiology was implicated in 52 of 56 deaths of known cause in one series (Table 8–2). Feared complications often responsible for rapid deterioration are dissecting aneurysms of the aorta, ruptured sinus of Valsalva, and ruptured mitral chordae tendineae. More gradual deterioration may be found in patients who

have progressive aortic or mitral regurgitation. It is interesting to note that the cardiovascular complication tends to be similar within a given family.

Treatment. Symptomatic and supportive. Surgical intervention for aortic aneurysm and aortic and mitral valvular disease. Propranolol may be useful.

Differential Diagnosis. *Homocystinuria.* Differentiating points found in homocystinuria are presence of homocystine in the urine, the high frequency of mental retardation, inferior nasal subluxation of the lens, thrombosis of medium-sized arteries, and osteoporosis.

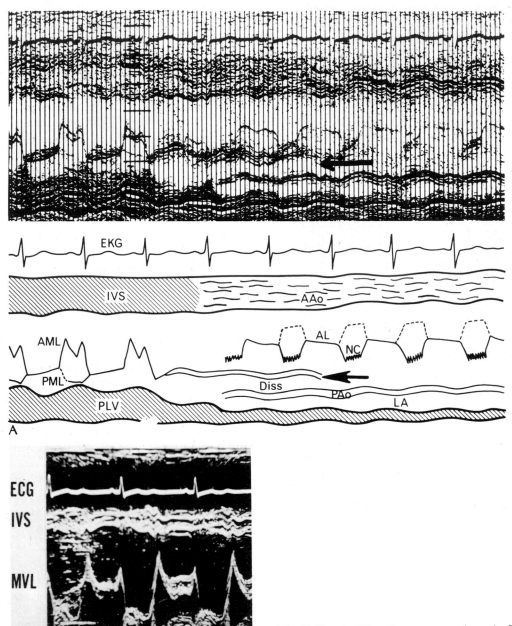

Fig. 8–16. A. Dissecting aneurysm (arrow) of aorta in patient with Marfan syndrome as shown by echocardiography and line drawing. B. Echocardiographic demonstration of severe prolapse and invagination (arrow) of posterior leaflet of mitral valve in patient with Marfan syndrome.

Muscular Dystrophy, Dominant[1,2]

Facioscapulohumoral, Landouzy-Dejérine Dystrophy. Onset is in the teens or early adulthood but may be much later. Facial and shoulder muscles are affected.

Oculopharyngeal Muscular Dystrophy. This disorder also comes on in later life and is characterized by ptosis and dysphagia and, in some families, wasting of various muscle groups.

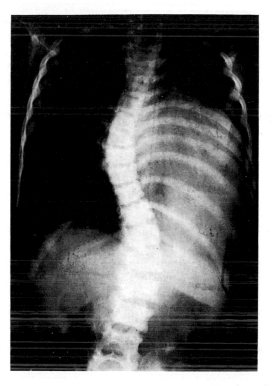

Fig. 8–17. Prominent scoliosis in 4-year-old girl with Marfan syndrome.

Myotonia

Two myotonic disorders that are inherited as autosomal dominant diseases deserve mention. Only one of these, myotonic dystrophy, is progressive and severely disabling.

Myotonic Dystrophy (DM, Steinert Disease).[1,2,6] This illness may occur in childhood, but is more likely to be recognized in early adult life. The congenital type with severe mental retardation occurs only if the gene is transmitted through the mother. There is difficulty in relaxing contracted muscles, often first noticed in the jaw or hand (Fig. 8–18A). Muscle wasting and weakness follow. Involvement of the facial muscles produces the expressionless facies of myotonic dystrophy (Fig. 8–18B). Cataracts develop, which may be detected initially as iridescent flecks. Frontal baldness is characteristic in males. This disorder, which affects males and females equally, produces hypogonadism in both sexes. The male has testicular atrophy, and the female has amenorrhea, dysmenorrhea, and ovarian

cysts. Cardiac arrhythmias, conduction defects, and congestive heart failure are common. Mental deterioration is also a feature. Death occurs in the fourth, fifth, or sixth decades and is often related to pneumonia or congestive heart failure. Corticosteroids, quinine, and procaine amide may provide symptomatic improvement. The DM gene has been localized to band 19q13.3, identified, and the molecular basis has been defined as an expansion of a trinucleotide (CTG) repeat at the 3' end of a transcript encoding a protein kinase. Unaffected individuals have between 5 and 27 copies, whereas severely affected patients have many hundreds of repeats.[6] Penetrance is high; about 55% of cases represent new mutations; expressivity is variable. Slit lamp and EMG examinations are useful in detecting subclinical cases.

Myotonia Congenita (Thomsen Disease)[1,2]

This disorder is more of an annoyance than a serious disability. Symptoms (difficulty in relaxing contracted muscles) begin in childhood. The voluntary muscles, especially of the limbs and trunk, hypertrophy. The myotonia, which is most severe on the first contraction, diminishes after a period of "warming up." The affected individual learns to avoid sudden movement, fatigue, chills, and excitement, which exacerbate the myotonia. The disease may be distinguished from myotonic dystrophy by its lack of progression, the absence of

Table 8–2. Probability of Surviving X Additional Years at a Given Age for Patients with Marfan Syndrome

Present Age (yr.)	Probability (%)					
	Additional Years, Males			Additional Years, Females		
	6	10	20	6	10	20
10	97	93	78	95	95	85
20	90	84	55	92	90	81
30	72	66	38	94	90	74
40	86	58	32	82	67	—

Modified from Murdoch, J. L., et al.: Life expectancy and causes of death in Marfan syndrome. N. Engl. J. Med. 286:804, 1972.

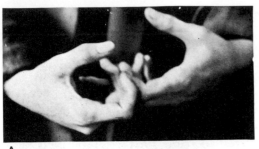

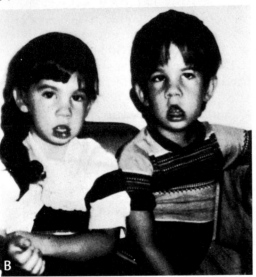

Fig. 8–18.   Myotonic dystrophy. A. Difficulty in relaxing contracted muscles of hands. B. Expressionless facies.

cataracts, hypogonadism, mental deterioration, and frontal baldness and the presence of muscle hypertrophy. Life expectancy is normal. Symptomatic improvement has been gained by treatment with corticosteroids, chlorothiazides (potassium depletion), quinine, and procaine amide.

Nail-Patella Syndrome (NPS1)[1,2]

The nails, especially on the thumb, are hypoplastic or sometimes absent; the patellae are hypoplastic or absent (Fig. 8–19). There may be hypoplasia of the fibular head, lateral condyle, elbows, and scapulae. Iliac spurs are common. Cloverleaf pigmentation of the inner iris margin occurs in about half the patients; occasionally keratoconus, cataracts, and ptosis occur. Nephropathy resulting in proteinuria

or in overt renal disease (30%) with glomerulonephritic pathology may be fatal. The major disabilities are the limitation in joint mobility and the complicating osteoarthritis. The nail-patella locus is at 9q34, closely linked to the ABO blood group locus and adenylate kinase-1.

Nephropathy With Deafness (Alport Syndrome)[1,2]

Hereditary nephropathy with deafness is the most common form of familial nephritis. The disease shows autosomal dominant inheritance and X-linked inheritance. An individual carrying the gene may be asymptomatic, have mild intermittent hematuria and/or albuminuria, or have severe kidney disease with the clinical picture of acute or chronic glomerular nephritis, pyelonephritis, or nephrosis. About one third of the affected individuals have neurosensory deafness with onset usually in the second decade. Ocular defects such as spherophakia and cataracts occur less frequently.

Neurofibromatosis (Von Recklinghausen Disease NF 1)[2,3]

This disorder, first recognized by von Recklinghausen in 1882, is one of the most common mendelian diseases. The gene is located at 17q11.2.

Diagnostic Features. *General.* Variable manifestations. Intellectual impairment in 10%. Usually a mild disease, but occasionally severely debilitating.

Skin. Café-au-lait spots; 75% of patients have six or more spots more than 1.5 cm across (Fig.

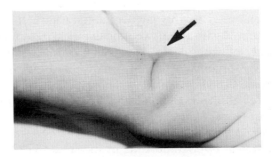

Fig. 8–19.   External appearance of absent patella in nail-patella syndrome.

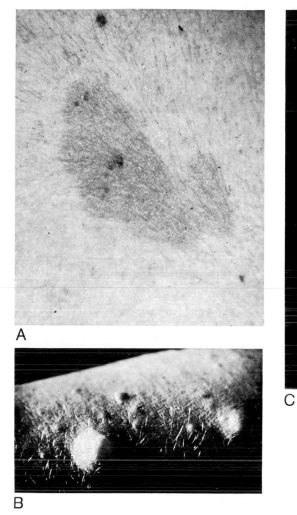

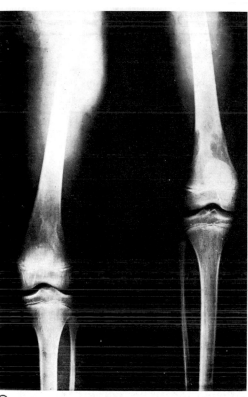

Fig. 8–20.   Neurofibromatosis. A. Café-au-lait spot. B. Skin tumors. C. Lesions of long bones.

8–20A). Neurofibromatous tumors occur sub-cutaneously along nerves (Fig. 8–20B). Molluscum fibrosum; axillary freckles; occasionally lipomata, angiomata. Malignant degeneration occurs in 3 to 15% of the neurofibromata.

Eyes. Rarely tumors of the eyelid, optic disc; retinal detachment, buphthalmos, exophthalmos, glaucoma, corneal opacity, Lisch nodules of the iris.

CNS. Tumors of brain, cranial nerves, and spinal cord—gliomas and cysts. Seizures in 12%. Mental retardation in 5%.

Skeletal. Subperiosteal cysts (Fig. 8–20C), scoliosis, bowing of lower leg, rib fusion, local overgrowth.

Cardiovascular. Rarely, hypertension secondary to pheochromocytoma; neurofibroma of heart and pulmonic stenosis.

Other. Occasional neurofibroma of kidney, stomach, tongue; acromegaly; sexual precocity.

X-ray. Subperiosteal cysts, scoliosis, scalloping of vertebral bodies, rib fusion.

Prevalence. 1:3000. About 50% of patients represent fresh mutations.

Clinical Course. Café-au-lait spots are frequently the first clue to the presence of this disorder. Subcutaneous tumors may be noted later. Some of the patients eventually experience neurologic problems. Nerve compres-

Table 8–3.   Features of the Noonan Syndrome*

Area	Findings
General	Female or male, normal life expectancy except as modified by cardiovascular disease, small stature not invariable; **chromatin-positive female**. Factor XI deficiency, Von Willebrand disease, and platelet dysfunction underlie various bleeding abnormalities.
Neurologic	Intellectual development is fair to good but usually below that of siblings; occasional hearing loss.
Head	Characteristic facies; narrow maxilla, small mandible.
Eyes	Frequent epicanthic folds, **ptosis**, and **hypertelorism**.
Ears	Usually prominent, fleshy, **posteriorly rotated, and low-set**.
Neck	Webbed in about 50% of patients; low posterior hairline.
Chest	Shield-shaped; widely spaced hypoplastic nipples; breast development variable in females.
Cardiovascular	Anomalies in approximately 50%: **pulmonic stenosis** is most common, often with atrial septal defect; coarctation of aorta rarely occurs. Left ventricular disease similar to IHSS and **pulmonary branch stenosis** frequently found.
Extremities	Cubitus valgus; lymphedema of dorsum of hands and feet in infancy; dystrophic nails; short fifth finger with clinodactyly.
Urogenital	Variable fertility. Ovarian dysgenesis and infertility in some females, **normal fertility in others**. Cryptorchism in the usually infertile male.
Skeletal	Pectus excavatum frequent; scoliosis, kyphosis in about 20%, sometimes Klippel-Feil syndrome.
Skin and Nails	Pigmented nevi frequent; marked **tendency to keloid formation** (beware if correcting webs or ptosis); nails dystrophic, short, wide, not convex.
Dermatoglyphics	Distal axial triradius; ridge count not increased.
Incidence	Undetermined but estimated to be between 1:1,000 and 1:2,500.

*Many findings are similar or identical to those observed in the Turner syndrome. Features that help to distinguish between the syndromes are in **bold face**.

sion involving the optic nerve may lead to blindness. If the transmitting parent is the mother, the disease is more severe in the child, which presumably represents genomic imprinting (see Chap. 14, Nontraditional Inheritance).

Treatment. Surgical relief of tumor compression, excision of pheochromocytoma, and general supportive care.

Differential Diagnosis. Neurofibromatosis 2 (NF 2, acoustic neuroma) is characterized by eight-nerve masses and at least two of the following: neurofibroma, meningioma, glioma, schwannoma, juvenile lenticular opacity. Gene locus 22q11.21-q13.1. The gene has been identified.

Noonan Syndrome (XX and XY Turner Phenotype; Ullrich, Bonnevie-Ullrich, Pterygium Colli Syndrome)[1,2,9]

Noonan syndrome shares many features of the Turner syndrome (Table 8–3), although after infancy the facies may be different. Noonan syndrome is estimated to have a population frequency between 1:1,000 and 1:2,500.

In our series, about three fourths of the patients had evidence of direct transmission of the phenotype and about one fourth were "sporadic." Features that are useful in distinguishing the syndromes will be emphasized. First, female patients with the Noonan syndrome are chromatin-positive, but this does not rule out Turner syndrome resulting from mosaicism or structural anomalies of the X chromosome (discussed in Chapter 4).

Small stature, webbing of the neck, cubitus valgus, lymphedema and other classic Turner stigmata are found in the Noonan syndrome (see Figs. 8–21 and 8–22). Some female patients having Noonan syndrome may be over 60 inches tall, but they are often significantly shorter than their sibs. The males are often between 66 and 70 inches in height, but again they are usually significantly shorter than their male sibs. Ptosis and ocular hypertelorism are perhaps more common in the Noonan than in the Turner syndrome.

Cardiovascular anomalies are useful differentiating findings. The Noonan patient has pulmonic stenosis and, rarely, coarctation of the aorta, which is just the opposite of the

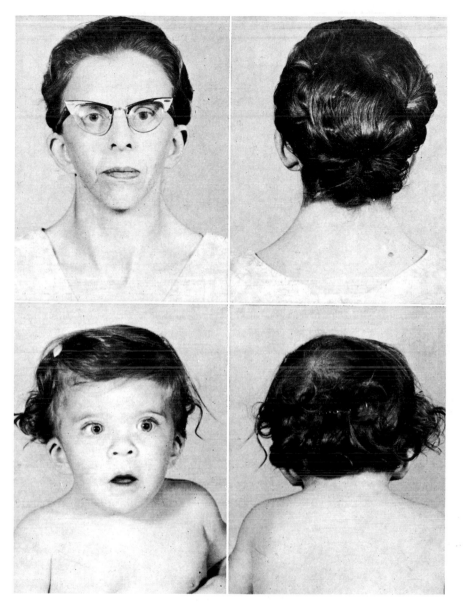

Fig. 8–21. Characteristic facial features of Noonan syndrome in mother and daughter. (From Nora, J. J., and Sinha, A. K.: Am. J. Dis. Child., 116:345, 1968. Copyright 1968, American Medical Association.)

patient with Turner syndrome. However, Turner mosaics may have pulmonic stenosis. Several other heart lesions may be found in either type of patient, but there is almost no overlap with respect to pulmonic stenosis and coarctation of the aorta. One important heart lesion recognized in Noonan patients is left ventricular disease, echocardiographically similar to idiopathic hypertrophic subaortic stenosis (IHSS), which may be missed because it

is obscured by pulmonic stenosis. A clue to the presence of ventricular disease is the electrocardiographic finding of left axis deviation. The echocardiogram is useful in diagnosing and monitoring this left ventricular disease. Pulmonary artery branch stenosis is also common in Noonan syndrome.

Prenatal diagnosis of Noonan syndrome has been achieved by sonographic recognition of hydrops, ascites, and cystic hygroma, which

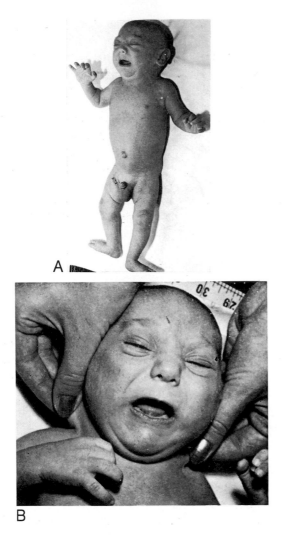

Fig. 8–22.   Noonan syndrome. A. Full-length view of male infant. B. Webbing of neck of infant in A.

portend a poor prognosis, but which may also resolve spontaneously.

In regard to fertility, although some female patients with Noonan syndrome have streak gonads, most do not. They may develop secondary sexual characteristics and reproduce. Cryptorchism is a characteristic finding in the males, most of whom are infertile. The authors have now seen 7 males with many stigmata of the Noonan syndrome who have transmitted these features to a male and a female offspring. Orchiopexy has been attempted in a number of males with this syndrome and has been mostly unsuccessful. The infertility of the male, however, is not asso-

ciated with lack of virilization. Many of these males are heavily muscled.

Intellectual achievement in patients with the Noonan syndrome is variable, as it is in the Turner syndrome, in both cases being compatible with high intelligence or moderate mental retardation. We have the clinical impression that the mean for patients with Noonan syndrome falls slightly to moderately below the midparent IQ.

The clinical course is influenced to a great extent by the presence or absence of cardiovascular disease. In its absence normal life expectancy can be predicted. Counseling of individuals with Noonan syndrome must approach the questions of fertility and transmission of the disease. For the female, the probability that she is fertile appears to be reasonably good. The male is most likely to be infertile. In addition to overlap of features with Turner syndrome, there are similarities to the X-linked Aarskog-Scott syndrome, the autosomal-dominant LEOPARD and Watson syndromes, neurofibromatosis, and the Klippel-Feil syndrome.

OCULO-AURICULO-VERTEBRAL SYNDROME (GOLDENHAR SYNDROME)[1,2]

This syndrome is similar in many ways to the Treacher Collins syndrome and has a prevalence on the order of 1:15,000. Malformed ears, frequent deafness, and mandibular and malar hypoplasia are common to both syndromes. The Goldenhar syndrome has the additional features of epibulbar dermoids and notching of the upper, rather than the lower lid (Fig. 8–23), and there is a higher frequency of vertebral anomalies (cervical and thoracic vertebral fusions and hemivertebrae). Dental malocclusion is frequent; cleft lip and palate and congenital heart diseases (transposition of the great vessels and tetralogy of Fallot) are occasionally encountered. Intelligence is usually normal, and if development of speech is delayed, hearing loss should be the first etiological consideration. Although the facial defects may be profound, plastic surgery provides reasonably satisfactory restoration.

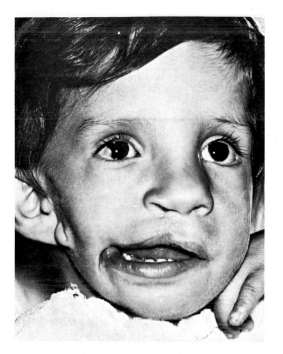

Fig. 8–23. Facies in oculo-auriculo-vertebral syndrome. Note the epibulbar dermoid in right eye.

OSTEOGENESIS IMPERFECTA (OI)[2,4]

History. In 1788, Ekman reported the occurrence of brittle bones in three generations. Since then, numerous reports stressing various aspects of the syndrome—brittle bones, blue sclerae, and deafness—have cluttered the literature with many alternative eponyms and descriptive names.

Four major types of the disease are proposed, and within each of these types there may heterogeneity of clinical findings, and phenotypes caused by mutations in two or more genes and accompanied by more than one form of inheritance. Gene loci of some of the underlying defects in collagen have been mapped to chromosomes 17 and 7. The four types are: a dominant progressive form with blue sclerae (OI type I or OI tarda); a dominant neonatal lethal form (OI type II, dominant); a recessive perinatal lethal form (OI type II recessive); a progressively deforming recessive type with normal sclerae (OI type III); and dominant form with normal sclerae (OI type IV). The clinical features of the common OI type I will be discussed below.

Diagnostic Features. *General.* Normal intelligence. Equal sex distribution. Stature short to severely malformed and dwarfed. Increased metabolic rate, hyperthermia, excessive sweating. Cultured fibroblasts have a characteristic morphology and secrete abnormal collagen.

Head. Thin, bulging calvaria, open fontanelles, overhanging occiput and temporal areas (helmet-head). Multiple wormian bones. Translucent teeth, predisposition to caries.

Eyes. Blue sclerae, occasional keratoconus, megalocornea, embryotoxon.

Ears. Deafness, otosclerotic, usually not beginning until adulthood.

Teeth. Normal, group A; opalescent dentin, group B.

Musculoskeletal. Frequent fractures with normal healing rate, leading to bowing of the legs, pseudoarthroses, "hourglass" vertebrae, kyphoscoliosis (Fig. 8–24). Pectus excavatum and carinatum, hyperextensible joints. Long bones have thin cortex, slender shaft, abrupt widening at epiphyses, osteoporosis.

Cardiovascular. Premature arteriosclerosis. Mucoid, valvular changes, aortic insufficiency, and mitral regurgitation.

Skin. Thin, translucent; capillary fragility.

Prevalence. 1:60,000.

Clinical Course. In *osteogenesis imperfecta tarda,* fractures may be present at birth or begin in infancy or childhood. The patient may have had dozens of fractures by puberty, when there is a trend to improvement. Frequent fractures may result in severe dwarfing. Some carriers of the gene may have only blue sclerae, and some may have no signs (incomplete penetrance). OI type IV without blue sclerae, also dominant, may be progressively deforming; *Osteogenesis imperfecta congenita (OIC or OI type II) lethalis* is much more severe than the tarda type, involving numerous fractures in utero, deformed long bones, and a skull that crackles on pressure. Counseling of a person with a sporadic case of osteogenesis imperfecta is therefore difficult. If there are fractures at birth, one must decide between an early onset tarda type or the true congenita

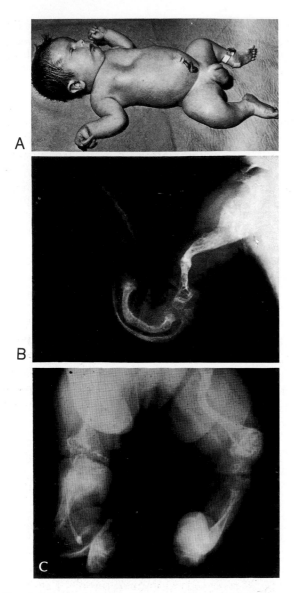

Fig. 8–24. A. newborn with osteogenesis imperfecta congenita (OIC) and deformities of multiple fractures at birth. B. Fracture deformities of arm. C. Deformities of lower extremities.

type. In the tarda type, the long bones are usually thin or of normal caliber. In the lethal type, the bones are broad or "crumpled." If it is the tarda type, it may be a fresh mutation (low recurrence risk), or there may be reduced penetrance in a parent. We counsel a fairly low but not negligible risk if there are no other cases of blue sclerae or bone fragility in the family. If the baby has the congenita type, recessive inheritance is likely. Under-

lying collagen defects, prenatal diagnosis, and RFLP studies are areas of active investigation at this time. Two or more clinical forms of the disease are each located at 7q21.3-q22.1 (collagen 1, alpha-2 polypeptide) with Ehlers-Danlos type VIIA2; and at 17q21.31-q22.05 (collagen 1, alpha-1 polypeptide) with Ehlers-Danlos, type VIIA1.

Treatment. Symptomatic and supportive.

Differential Diagnosis. A difficult disorder to distinguish from osteogenesis imperfecta is pycnodysostosis. On the basis of absence of blue sclerae, recessive inheritance, and micrognathia, Maroteaux and Lamy have suggested that Toulouse-Lautrec suffered from pycnodysostosis rather than osteogenesis imperfecta.

Peroneal Muscular Atrophy (Charcot-Marie-Tooth Disease)[2]

This relatively common genetic disease manifests itself as weakness and atrophy of the peroneal muscles and advances insidiously to involve other muscles in the leg and arm. Deep tendon reflexes are diminished; pes cavus is common. Sensory and trophic changes occur. In some families there is reduced peripheral nerve conduction velocity and demyelinization. In other families, there appears to be neuronal degeneration affecting anterior horn cells and dorsal root ganglia. Genetic heterogeneity occurs; in addition to the autosomal dominant disease there are also autosomal recessive and X-linked forms. This, and the variable age of onset, make genetic counseling difficult. The gene locus of the autosomal dominant slow nerve conduction type 1b is 1q21.2-q23.

Polycystic Kidneys (Adult Form)[1,2]

This topic will be discussed in greater detail in the section on recessively inherited disease. The adult forms have a population frequency of about 1:1000. The usual dominant type of polycystic kidney disease consists of bilateral cysts in kidney, frequently in liver, and often associated with cerebrovascular berry aneurysm. Hematuria, flank pain, progressive

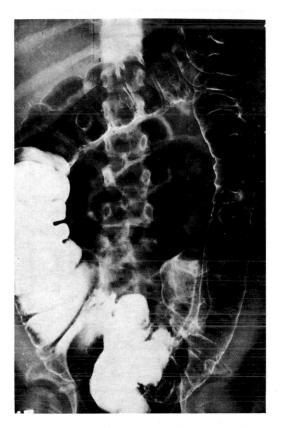

Fig. 8–25. Radiographic evidence of polyps in colon of patient with polyposis I.

renal failure, hypertension, and stroke are common in the natural history. About 70% of patients have renal failure by the age of 70. Ultrasound is a useful noninvasive diagnostic aid in the study of this disease. The penetrance appears to be high, especially if ultrasound is used in family studies. The gene locus is 16p13.31-p13.12. An autosomal dominant medullary type has also been described.

Polyposis of the Colon (Familial Adenomatous Polyposis Coli, APC, Includes Gardner Syndrome)[1,2,11]

Syndromes that were formerly called polyposis I and Gardner syndrome appear to be allelic disorders determined by mutations at 5q21-q22, the APC gene locus. Figure 8–25 illustrates the polyps.

Malignant change may occur as early as the second decade. Gastrointestinal bleeding and diarrhea may be presenting complaints. Colectomy is required. First degree relatives of affected individuals should have regular examinations.

In Gardner syndrome, sebaceous and epidermal inclusion cysts of the face, scalp, and back and osteomata of face, jaw, and calvaria are the lesions associated with intestinal polyps. The adenomatous polyps are usually present in the colon or rectum but may occasionally be found in the stomach or small intestine. Carcinoma develops in almost half of the individuals with this syndrome.

Polyposis, Hamartomatous Intestinal (Peutz-Jeghers Syndrome)[1,2]

Pigmented spots (blue-gray or brown) appear in infancy or early childhood and have a tendency to fade in the adult. These spots, which are located on the lips, perioral area, buccal mucous membranes, and fingers, serve as sentinel signs of the syndrome (Fig. 8–26). Benign polyps are located mainly in the je-

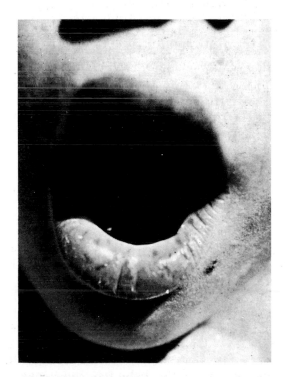

Fig. 8–26. Pigmented spots on lips of child with polyposis II (Peutz-Jeghers syndrome).

junum but occasionally elsewhere in the intestine, bladder, and respiratory tract. Colicky abdominal pain, gastrointestinal bleeding and intussusception, which are complications of the disease, usually appear in childhood. Malignant transformation of the polyps occurs less commonly in this type than in the familial polyposis described in the preceding text. The gene is mapped to 5q2.

Porphyrias, Hepatic[2,4]

In *acute intermittent porphyria* (known as the "Swedish type," but not restricted to Swedes), there are no skin lesions. Acute colicky abdominal pain and neuropathic attacks occur, which may be precipitated by barbiturates and other drugs. Porphobilinogen is always present in the urine and uroporphyrin may appear later in the attack, turning the urine burgundy red.

The biochemical defect in intermittent acute porphyria is an interesting example of how an enzymatic defect can show dominant inheritance. Succinate and glycine are the precursors for the porphyrias from which heme is synthesized. They are synthesized to δ-aminolevulinic acid (ALA) by the enzyme ALA synthetase, which is the rate-limiting enzyme for heme synthesis. ALA is converted to porphobilinogen (PBG), which is metabolized to uroporphyrinogen 1 (URO) by URO synthetase, and then is converted to coproporphyrinogen, to protoporphyrinogen, to heme. Hence it acts as a negative feedback regulator of ALA synthetase. In heterozygotes for intermittent acute porphyria, the level of URO synthetase is reduced to 50% of normal. This reduces the synthesis of heme, which increases the activity of ALA synthetase, leading to compensatory overproduction of ALA and PBG and their excretion in the urine. How this results in the drug sensitivity is still not clear—perhaps the limitation of heme synthesis impedes the synthesis of the cytochrome P 450 (for which heme is required) and this is necessary for drug biotransformation. The URO synthetase defect can be detected in the red blood cells, which can be useful for family

studies. The gene for uroporphyrinogen 1 synthase has been assigned to 11q23.2-11qter.

In *porphyria variegata* (the "South African" type, but worldwide in distribution), in addition to the acute visceral and neurologic attacks, photosensitivity with cutaneous lesions develops on exposure to the sun. The enzyme block is probably between protoporphyrinogen and heme. Again, ALA synthetase levels are elevated. In *porphyria cutaneous tarda*, the manifestations are most striking in the skin. The gene locus is confirmed at 1p34. These three types almost always become symptomatic after puberty. The nature of the metabolic defect is still not clear. Liver and red cells show reduced URO decarboxylase activity.

Hereditary coproporphyria resembles acute intermittent porphyria except that symptoms may begin in childhood and coproporphyrin III is present in large amounts in the feces. The probable primary defect is a deficiency of coproporphyrinogen oxidase.

Avoidance of precipitating factors such as barbiturates, alcohol, and sunlight is an important aspect of the treatment. The acute episode may terminate fatally with neurologic damage and water and electrolyte imbalance. Personality changes, "hysteria," and "neurosis" are described in patients having visceral attacks. Needless to say, the diagnosis must be made correctly to avoid the disaster of sedating such a "hysterical" patient with barbiturates.

Sickle Cell Trait[2,4]

Sickle cell trait, the heterozygous manifestation of the gene for sickle cell disease, is inherited as a dominant and produces relatively little disability when compared with the homozygous form. The trait is present in about 1 of 11 North Americans of African descent, most of whom are asymptomatic but may exhibit a mild chronic anemia. Certain stress situations may be fatal, however, as illustrated by the deaths of four African-American heterozygote army recruits at Fort Bliss, Texas, in 1970. Under lowered oxygen tension, as experienced in unpressurized aircraft or parachute drops, heterozygotes may have symptoms similar to homozygotes or even infarction of the spleen. Sickledex and dithionite tests appear to be useful for screening, and confirmation is made by hemoglobin electrophoresis. Some researchers in sickle cell disease feel that sickle cell screening tests should be made widely available, so that heterozygous couples should be advised of their high risk of having children with sickle cell disease. The hemoglobin beta locus is at 11p15.5.

Spherocytosis, Hereditary

Hereditary spherocytosis (HS) is a chronic hemolytic anemia in which the red blood cells are spheroid and have increased osmotic fragility (Fig. 8–27). The disorder is highly variable and appears clinically shortly after birth in some individuals and not until adulthood, if at all, in others. Splenomegaly is usually present. Infections can lead to crises associated with more severe anemia, weakness, pallor, and other symptoms, depending upon the degree of anemia. These crises result from temporary bone marrow aplasia with no new red blood cell production. Diagnosis depends on demonstration of spherocytes in the peripheral blood and increased osmotic fragility, sometimes demonstrable only after incubation at 37°C for 24 hours. Treatment by splenectomy lengthens the red cell life span but carries the risk of increased susceptibility to infection. Splenectomy should be approached with considerable reservation. Immunization against the pneumococcus is currently advo-

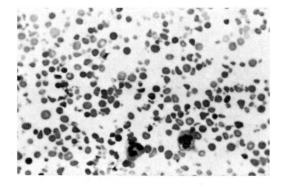

Fig. 8–27.   Spherocytosis.

cated for patients requiring splenectomy for any reason. Spherocytosis and increased osmotic fragility persist following splenectomy. Counseling is complicated by reduced penetrance; carriers may be detected only by special tests, such as autohemolysis, or sometimes not at all. About 20% of cases are sporadic, presumably representing fresh mutations. Dominant inheritance is the rule. In type I spherocytosis, the defect is in the spectrin beta chain, and in type II (which may be heterogeneous), a locus at 8p11 has been confirmed. A rare recessive form has also been reported.

Trichorhinophalangeal Syndrome Type I and Type II (Langer-Giedion Syndrome)

As the name suggests, this syndrome involves the hair, nose, and phalanges, but is not limited to these (Fig. 8–28). The hair is fine and sparse, especially in the temporal areas, and the eyebrows are sparse, being heavier medially than laterally. The facies is characteristic, with a high forehead, bulbous nose with tented alae, midfacial hypoplasia, long philtrum, an upper lip that appears thin because the vermilion is almost horizontal, small teeth, high arched palate, and large prominent ears. Slow growth of postnatal onset leads to proportionate short stature. The middle, and sometimes other, phalanges show cone-shaped epiphyses, with irregular brachydactyly and clinodactyly. The inheritance is usually dominant, although a few families compatible with autosomal recessive inheritance are known. The type II form, Langer-Giedion syndrome, has, additionally, microcephaly, mild mental retardation, and multiple exostoses and is associated in approximately half the patients with a deletion of the long arm of chromosome 8. The deletion is 8q24.11-q24.13. It has been proposed that the mutant gene in type I disease is located in the same region.

TUBEROUS SCLEROSIS[1,2]

This disorder of skin, brain, and bones, sometimes incorrectly referred to as adenoma

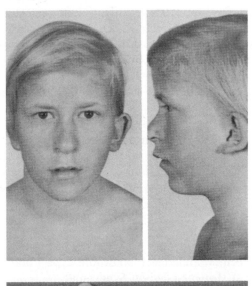

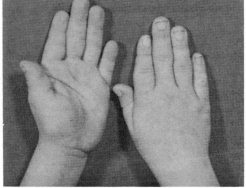

Fig. 8–28.   Facial features and brachydactyly in trichorhinophalangeal syndrome (see text).

sebaceum, has been recognized in the world literature for approximately 100 years. The prevalence is about 1:100,000. Penetrance is high but probably not complete. The majority of cases are "sporadic," but the mean paternal age is not increased.

Diagnostic Features. *General.* Mild to severe intellectual impairment. Equal sex distribution. Normal growth. Seizures beginning in childhood. The signs and symptoms are highly variable, and the condition often goes unrecognized.

Skin. Adenoma sebaceum in a "butterfly" distribution on the face (Fig. 8–29A). Shagreen (granular, untanned leather) patches on trunk, depigmented patches (Fig. 8–29B), café-au-lait spots, hemangiomas, fibromas. Black light (Wood's lamp) frequently reveals depigmented patches not visible under usual lighting.

Eyes. Retinal lesions, nodular, cystic, or phacomatous; unequal pupils may be associated with CNS lesions in some patients.

CNS. Intracranial mineralization; cortical gliomas and angiomas.

Skeletal. Bone cysts, especially in hands.

Visceral. Rhabdomyomas of the heart or kidney; tumors or hemangiomas of kidney, liver, spleen, or lung.

X ray. Intracranial calcifications. (Fig. 8–30), bone cysts of the hand, abnormal IVP. Computerized tomography (CT) may reveal the characteristic tumors.

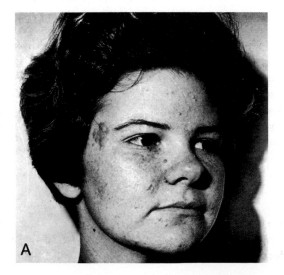

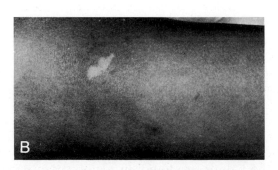

Fig. 8–29.   Tuberous sclerosis. A. Adenoma sebaceum of face. B. Depigmented area on leg as first sign in child of patient in A.

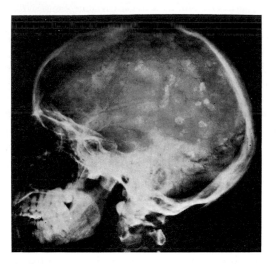

Fig. 8-30.   Intracranial calcifications in tuberous sclerosis.

Laboratory. Abnormal EEG and CT scan. The gene locus for tuberous sclerosis 1 is at 9q33-q34.

Clinical Course. The earliest manifestation of this disorder may be convulsions. In the infant having seizures, there may not yet be adenoma sebaceum, fibrous nodules of the face, or shagreen skin, but small depigmented patches of the skin should alert the physician to this diagnosis. Examination with a Wood's light is useful in detecting depigmented areas. Screening of any patient with mental retardation or seizures of unknown cause, and the parents, is recommended. Intracranial calcification may take years to become evident by x-ray studies, but CT scan in individuals at risk will produce earlier results. The seizures may become progressively harder to control, and behavioral problems and intellectual deficiencies declare themselves with increasing involvement of the brain. Over one third of the patients function at a satisfactory level in adult life maintaining homes and jobs, although requiring anticonvulsant therapy.

Cardiac arrhythmias and obstruction secondary to the rhabdomyomas of the heart present a threat to life, although not as frequent a threat as status epilepticus. Tumors of the kidney are found in many patients, and space-occupying intracranial tumors in a small percentage of individuals with this disorder.

Treatment. Anticonvulsant therapy. Antiarrhythmic therapy (for cardiac arrhythmias); surgical excision of operable tumors; custodial care for the severely affected patients.

Differential Diagnosis. Tuberous sclerosis should be considered in cases of unexplained mental retardation or seizures. A condition that has been designated tuberous sclerosis 2 may map to chromosome 11q. Other disorders associated with convulsions, skin lesions, and intracranial calcifications, such as Sturge-Weber syndrome, von Hippel-Lindau syndrome, Maffucci syndrome, and neurofibromatosis, are readily distinguishable on clinical and radiologic grounds.

VON WILLEBRAND DISEASE[7,8]

Von Willebrand disease (vWD) was initially distinguished from classic hemophilia by prolonged bleeding time. The tourniquet test is usually positive. Nosebleeds, bruising, and gastrointestinal, urinary, and uterine bleeding are common, but hemarthroses are rare. There is low factor VIII (anti-hemophiliac globulin or AHG), reduced adhesiveness of platelets, and the plasma from patients with Hemophilia A (classic hemophilia) will correct both the AHG deficiency and the vascular defect. The factor VIII-von Willebrand factor is considered to be: a complex of factor VIII:C (the deficiency in hemophilia A), the clot-promoting (procoagulant) activity; ristocetin cofactor (VIII R:RCO) for platelet agglutination; and factor VIII: Ag (factor VIII related antigen), which is usually absent or decreased in vWD, but normal in classic hemophilia. The von Willebrand factor (vWD) gene, which has been localized to chromosome 12 (12 pter-p12), is synthesized by endothelial cells that line blood vessels. Complementary DNA (cDNA) has been cloned, and there is promise that prenatal diagnosis will soon be possible.

WAARDENBURG SYNDROME[1,2]

The triad of white forelock, lateral displacement of the inner canthi (Fig. 8–31), and congenital sensorineural deafness was first described by Waardenburg, a Dutch

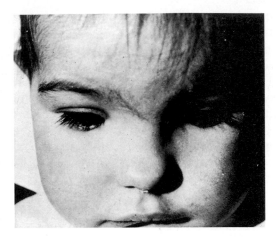

Fig. 8–31.   Child with Waardenburg syndrome. Note lateral displacement of median canthi, medial overgrowth of eyebrows, and broad nasal bridge.

opthalmologist-geneticist, in 1951. Other features also occur, and one is always present. Approximate frequencies are given in the following paragraphs.

Diagnostic Features.

General. Normal intelligence. Equal sex ratio. Normal growth.

Skin. Areas of vitiligo (20%).

Head. White forelock (30%), and early graying (20%). Synophrys is frequent (70 to 100%).

Eyes. Lateral displacement of median canthi (100% in the classic type) with lateral displacement of the inferior lacrimal puncta. Heterochromia of the irides (35%)—(higher in dark-eyed people?) and hypoplasia of the iris (10%).

Nose. Broad high bridge (80 to 100%).

Ears. Congenital nonprogressive, sensorineural hearing loss (25%).

Laboratory. The gene locus is confirmed at 2q37.3.

Prevalence. 1:40,000 in the Netherlands; 1:20,000 in Kenya. About 3% of children with profound hearing loss. About one third do not have affected parents, and these have an increased mean paternal age.

Clinical Course. The white forelock may be present at birth, appear early in childhood or not until adult life, and may even disappear.

Treatment. Early recognition and hearing aids.

A dominantly inherited combination of deafness with white forelock but without canthal displacement has been described as Waardenburg syndrome type II. About half of the heterozygotes are deaf. Because the broad nose bridge and synophrys are less frequent (25%), it may be difficult to separate these patients from those with nonsyndromal dominant hearing loss.

AUTOSOMAL RECESSIVE DISEASES

Diseases produced by single mutant genes, whether they are transmitted as dominants or recessives, autosomal or X-linked, are uncommon disorders. The dividing line between common and uncommon diseases is generally taken as 1:1000. No mendelian disease in the white North American population is more common than 1:1000, with cystic fibrosis being the closest to this incidence. Sickle cell disease in African-Americans, which generally exceeds the 1:1000 incidence and thus qualifies as a common disease, is recognized as a special case because it offers a heterozygote advantage in resistance to malaria.

An autosomal recessive disease is manifested clinically only in the homozygote. In the usual random-mating situation, both parents are free of the disease but are heterozygous for the mutant gene. The affected child often appears as a "sporadic" case, because it is unlikely that the mutant gene will become homozygous in the parental relatives (unless there is inbreeding), and with the small size of most human families, the 1 in 4 risk of recurrence is often not realized.

At the molecular level, the mutant gene results in an abnormal or deficient enzyme. This may be illustrated by classic phenylketonuria. A patient with this disease is homozygous for a mutant form of the gene that specifies phenylalanine hydroxylase and has almost none of this enzyme, which is necessary to maintain a key metabolic pathway. This deficiency allows the toxic accumulation of metabolites that damage the central nervous system. The heterozygous parents of the patient have only about half as much of this enzyme as normals, but this half dose is sufficient to perform the necessary functions, and they are clinically unaffected.

Acrodermatitis Enteropathica[1,2]

This disorder is an example of a genetic disease in more than one species that may be "cured" by the addition of a mineral supplement to the diet. Diarrhea, bullous dermatitis, and failure to thrive are the characteristic features of this disease. Thymic hypoplasia and pancreatic islet cell hyperplasia have also been described. There is a continuum of severity depending on the degree of deficiency of zinc. The absence of low molecular weight zinc-binding factor produced by the pancreas may be the underlying mechanism of the zinc deficiency. The disease is treated and essentially cured by zinc supplementation. The binding factor is present in human breast milk, which improves the clinical condition.

ADRENOCORTICAL DISORDERS OF SYNTHESIS[2,4]

The inherited adrenocortical syndromes are summarized in Table 8–4.

The syndromes carrying Roman numeral designations are the five types of adrenal hyperplasia.

Excess Androgen Secretion (Adrenogenital Syndrome)

Defect of 21-Hydroxylase (Adrenal Hyperplasia III). This is by far the most common type of adrenocortical hyperfunction (about 90% of cases). The frequency ranges from 1:500 in certain Eskimos to 1:5000 in Switzerland to 1:40,000 in the USA. The defect leads to lack of hydrocortisone, resulting in overproduction of pituitary corticotropin, which leads to adrenocortical hyperplasia with overproduction of metabolites behind the block and of androgens. This results in pseudohermaphroditism in females (see Fig. 6–7) and premature virilization in males. In some cases (about 2%), the block is not quite complete, and enough hydrocortisone is produced to maintain electrolyte balance. In the others, there is loss of sodium with anorexia, vomiting, diarrhea, and dehydration. The two types are family-specific. The myocardial effects of hyperkalemia are particularly life-threatening and may be misdiagnosed as congenital heart disease until the electrocardiogram reveals the hyperkalemic changes. Close linkage of this gene on chromosome 6(6p21.3) to the major histocompatibility complex permits confident prenatal diagnosis.

Defect of 11-Hydroxylase (Adrenal Hyperplasia IV). In this much less common form of adrenogenital syndrome, the block results in a pileup of the hydrocortisone precursor,

Table 8–4. Inherited Adrenocortical Hyperfunction Syndromes

Enzyme	Virilization	Salt	Hypertension
21-Hydroxylase* III	yes	K retention Na loss frequent	no
11-Hydroxylase IV	yes	No loss	frequent
3-Beta-hydroxysteroid II hydrogenase	mild	K retention Na loss	no
17–20 Desmolase	no	No loss	no
20–22 Desmolase I	no	Na loss	
17-Hydroxylase V	no	Na retention K loss	yes
18-Hydroxylase	no	Na loss K retention	no
18-Hydroxysteroid dehydrogenase	no	Na loss K retention	no

*HLA linkage permits prenatal diagnosis.

compound S, and desoxycortisone. The latter may result in hypertension. Virilization and masculinization of female genitalia occurs as in the common type of adrenogenital syndrome. The gene is localized to 8q21.

Defect in 3-Beta-Hydroxysteroid Dehydrogenase (Adrenogenital Hyperplasia II). This is a rare defect that occurs early in adrenal steroidogenesis and affects the mineralocorticoid, glucocorticoid, and sex steroid pathways. The patients are salt losers, and males are incompletely virilized because the testicular hormones are not synthesized. Males have hypospadias with or without cryptorchidism, and salt loss is severe, usually leading to death in infancy. The locus maps to 1p13. Treatment includes hydration, hydrocortisone, and, for the salt losers, desoxycortisone acetate.

Defect in 17–20 Desmolase. The synthetic block in this rare cause of ambiguous genitalia in genetic males involves the synthesis of testosterone from pregnenolone, progesterone, or their 17-hydroxylated equivalents. Testicles are present in affected males, who would presumably be infertile. The condition is familial, but the inheritance is not clear.

Lipoid Adrenal Hyperplasia (Adrenal Hyperplasia I)

Another rare defect results from a deficiency of one of the enzymes, 20–22 desmolase, involved in the conversion of cholesterol to pregnenolone. Lipids and cholesterol accumulate in the adrenal cortex. Patients are salt losers, and males are feminized.

Excess Mineralocorticoid Secretion

Partial Defect of 17-alpha-Hydroxylase (Adrenal Hyperplasia V). This defect prevents the formation of cortisol or any of its 17-alpha-hydroxylated precursors, as well as the sex steroids. It causes hypertension, hypokalemia, and lack of sexual maturation in the few cases (all female) reported. The locus is provisionally assigned to chromosome 10.

Defects in Mineralocorticoid Synthesis. Two conditions, in which the missing enzymes are 18-hydroxylase and 18-hydroxysteroid dehydrogenase, respectively, result in hypoaldosteronism, with dehydration, vomiting, failure to thrive, hyponatremia, and hyperkalemia, Corticosterone levels are high. Treatment with salt and mineralocorticoid corrects the problem. The need for therapy diminishes with age.

Albinism[2,4]

Albinism is a hereditary defect in the metabolism of melanin resulting in an absence or major decrease of this pigment in the skin, mucosa, hair, and eyes. Generalized "classic" oculocutaneous albinism was one of Garrod's original four inborn errors of metabolism. There are at least 7 genetically different types of generalized albinism.

Indirect evidence for genetic heterogeneity came from the observation that the frequency of albinism was higher (1:20,000) than would be expected on the basis of the observed frequency of parental consanguineous matings (about 20% first cousin marriages). More direct proof came from the observation of matings between two albino parents that resulted in nonalbino offspring.

Tyrosinase-negative Oculocutaneous Albinism. This is the "classic type" in which the hair bulb does not develop pigment when incubated with tyrosine, indicating an absence of tyrosinase activity. Melanocytes are present and contain protein structures (premelanosomes) on which melanin is normally deposited, but no melanin granules are present. The skin and hair are milk-white, and the iris color is red, or, in oblique light, translucent gray to blue (Fig. 8–32). The retina has no visible pigment, and there are severe photophobia and nystagmus.

The frequency is about 1:35,000 persons, though it may be higher in certain populations (perhaps 1:15,000 for Northern Ireland, for instance). The heterozygote, if lightly pigmented, may have a translucent iris. A rare X-linked recessive type also exists.

Albinism with Hemorrhagic Diathesis (Hermansky Pudlak Syndrome)

These albinos resemble the classic type and have a negative tyrosine-incubation test. The melanocytes contain immature melanosomes. They also have bleeding tendencies, manifested by bruising, repeated nosebleeds, and prolonged bleeding after tooth extraction. The reticuloendothelial cells in blood vessels, spleen, liver, lymph nodes, and bone marrow are packed with a black to greenish-blue pigment, possibly a ceroid. The coagulation defect may reside in the platelets.

Tyrosinase-positive Oculocutaneous Albinism

In this type, the affected child may be very blond in infancy but may gradually accumulate pigment with age, so the hair changes from white to cream, tan, yellow, light brown, or red, particularly in members of dark-skinned races. Photophobia and nystagmus are less severe than in the classic type. The frequency is about 1:14,000 in U.S. Negroes and 1:40,000 Caucasians, but reaches 1.2% in the Brandywine isolate of Maryland. The biochemical defect is not known, but the tyrosine-incubation test is positive.

Albinism with Giant Granules in Leukocytes (Chediak-Higashi Syndrome)

In this fatal disease of childhood, there is hypopigmentation, photophobia, anemia, leukopenia, thrombocytopenia, a marked susceptibility to infection, peripheral neuropathy, and frequently a lymphoma. Instead of the normal granulations, the granulocytes have a few peroxidase-positive giant granules that stain like the normal granulations for that cell type. The lymphocytes and monocytes have one or two azurophilic inclusions. They may be absent at birth but have been observed as early as 2 weeks of age.

Hypopigmentation-Microphthalmia-Oligophrenia (Cross Syndrome)

In a consanguineous Amish family, two brothers and a sister were described with white

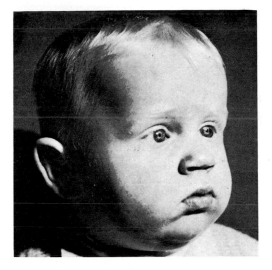

Fig. 8-32.   Albinism (classic oculocutaneous).

hair, microphthalmia, severe mental and physical retardation, spasticity, and athetoid movements. The tyrosine-incubation test was weakly positive. There is a similar mutant in the mouse, microphthalmia-white.

The Yellow-type Albino

In some albinos, the hair is white at birth but develops a bright yellow cast by the age of about one year. The tyrosine-incubation test is equivocal. Photophobia and nystagmus are less severe than in the tyrosine-positive type. The basis for the pigment defect is unclear. The condition is frequent in Amerindians, particularly the Jemez (1:140) and the Tule Cuma of the Honduras.

Amino Acid Metabolism, Inborn Errors[3,4]

This group of diseases is not only important as a fertile field for contemporary investigation, but has great historic interest. Sir Archibald Garrod, in 1902, consulting with Bateson, discovered alkaptonuria, the first disease in man that followed a recessive mendelian pattern of inheritance. From this disease he developed the concept of inborn errors of metabolism and suggested that the cause could be the absence of a special enzyme, thus

Table 8–5. Selected Inborn Errors of Amino Acid Metabolism

Amino Acid	Enzyme	Disease	Clinical Manifestations
Cystine	Defects in renal and GI transport	Cystinuria	Three types, all with progressive renal colic and GU obstruction
Cystine	?	Cystinosis	Three types, deposition of cystine crystals in reticuloendothelial system, kidney and eye; growth retardation, rickets, renal failure; death in first decade
Histidine	Histidase	Histidinemia	Impaired speech, some mental retardation
Methionine	Cystathionine β-synthase Methylenetetrahydrofolate reductase	Homocystinuria (one type)	Ectopia lentis and occasionally other Marfan-like features, coronary artery disease, frequent mental retardation
Phenylalanine	Phenylalanine hydroxylase	Phenylketonuria	Mental retardation, schizoid behavior, eczematous rash, light pigmentation, convulsions
Tryptophan	Defect in GI transport of tryptophan	Hartnup disease	Cutaneous photosensitivity with rash, cerebellar ataxia, pyramidal tract signs
Tryptophan	Defect in GI transport of tryptophan	Blue diaper syndrome	Indicanuria (causing blue diaper), hypercalcemia, nephrocalcinosis
Tyrosine	Homogentisic acid oxidase	Alkaptonuria	Black urine, black cartilage; blue ears, nose, cheeks, sclerae; arthritis
Tyrosine	Tyrosinase	Albinism	Two recessive types; fair skin, ocular problems, nystagmus, refractive errors
Tyrosine	Fumaryl-acetoacetate hydroxylase	Tyrosinemia	Failure to thrive, hepatic cirrhosis, renal tubular defects with hypophosphatemic rickets; tyrosyluria
Valine, leucine, isoleucine	Deficiency in branched chain ketoacid decarboxylase	Maple syrup urine disease	Maple syrup odor to urine; mental and neurologic deterioration; death in infancy

anticipating by decades the idea of one gene-one enzyme. Through the technology of modern biochemistry, the yield from this field is approaching bumper-crop proportions. No effort will be made to list completely the known errors (and variants) in the metabolism of amino acids. Rather, a selection of disorders that have fundamental, clinical, or historic importance will be presented. These diseases are summarized, together with additional related disorders, in Table 8–5.

Alkaptonuria

Alkaptonuria is a rare disorder with an estimated incidence in the population of about 1:200,000. The basic defect in the activity of an enzyme (which Garrod predicted in 1908) was eventually demonstrated by La Du and coworkers in 1958 to be an absence of homogentisic acid oxidase (see Fig. 6–3). An arrest occurs in the catabolism of tyrosine, and large quantities of homogentisic acid are excreted in the urine (see Fig. 6–3). The urine of affected patients turns black on standing from

alkalinization of a polymerized product of homogentisic acid, permitting diagnosis in infancy by black staining of the diaper (if left long enough). The reducing properties of the urine distinguish it from the black urine of phenol poisoning or melanotic tumors. The accumulation of the homogentisic acid polymer in mesenchymal tissue, such as cartilage, is responsible for the bluish-black discoloration of the ears, nose, cheeks, and sclerae (ochronosis). Arthritis, occurring in about half of the older patients, results from degeneration of pigmented cartilage. The patient is otherwise symptom-free. No successful treatment is known.

Cystinuria

This disorder, or rather group of disorders (there are at least three types) is also of historic interest. It is another of Garrod's four original inborn errors of metabolism. The clinical findings in the homozygotes of all three types include the excretion of large amounts of the dibasic amino acids cystine, ornithine,

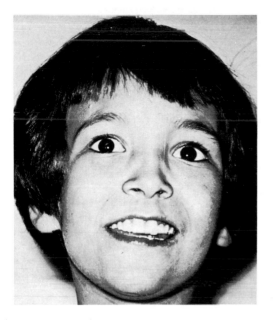

Fig. 8–33.   Inferonasal subluxation of lens may be seen in right eye of this patient with homocystinuria.

arginine, and lysine, the formation of cystine stones in the kidney, renal colic, and urinary tract obstruction. Specific enzyme abnormalities have not been discovered, since the problem seems to be localized to renal and gastrointestinal transport. For further details, see Chapter 6.

About two thirds of patients benefit from hydration therapy (2 glasses of water at bedtime and at 2 to 3 A.M.) to reduce the urinary concentration of cystine. For the rest, penicillamine may be effective, but there may be undesirable side effects.

Histidinemia

This rare metabolic error results from a deficiency of histidase and has a prevalence of about 1:20,000. The bacterial inhibition spot test, when added to a PKU screening program, provides an inexpensive means of screening. Serum histidine is elevated, and the urine contains excessive amounts of histidine and imidazole metabolites. The ferric chloride test is positive in histidinemia as it is in phenylketonuria. Over half of the patients described had defective speech, and most of these were mentally retarded. These proportions are

unduly high, because of ascertainment bias. The histidase gene has been assigned to 12q22-q23.

Homocystinuria

History. This disorder exists in three forms. The absence of cystathionine beta-synthetase was demonstrated to be the basic defect by Mudd and colleagues in 1964. The original patients were ascertained through surveys of mentally retarded populations. Other affected individuals had been originally thought to have Marfan syndrome.

Heterogeneity has been found to exist in this disease as in so many others. About half of the patients are responsive to vitamin B_6 and may be spared the complication of mental retardation if the disease is detected early and treated with large doses. Homocystinuria caused by deficiency of a different enzyme (methylene-tetra-hydrofolate reductase) is best treated with folic acid in addition to B_6 (Chapter 6). A defect in cobalamin metabolism produces a homocystinuria-megaloblastic anemia responsive to vitamin B_{12}.

The prevalence of all forms of homocystinuria appears to be in the range of 1:150,000 to 300,000.

Diagnostic Features. *General.* Frequent mental retardation. Equal sex distribution. Height varies from normal to tall.

Skin. Malar flush.

Eyes. Subluxation of lens (inferior-nasal), myopia, cataracts (Fig. 8–33).

Skeletal. Some patients resemble those with Marfan syndrome: tall; slender, long fingers and toes; pectus excavatum or carinatum; genu valgum, kyphoscoliosis; joint laxity; US/LS ratio less than normal (Fig. 8–34).

Cardiovascular. Arterial thromboses of coronary, renal, carotid, cerebral, and other medium-sized vessels, leading to myocardial infarction, renal hypertension, and stroke. Venous thromboses and pulmonary infarction. Early-onset coronary disease may also occur in the heterozygote.

Gastrointestinal. Bleeding secondary to vascular disease and infarction.

CNS. Abnormal EEG, seizures.

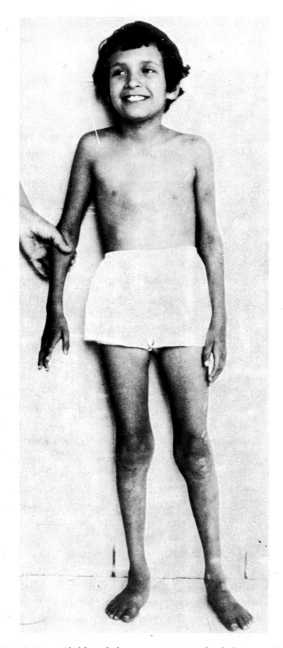

Fig. 8–34. Child with homocystinuria. The habitus is slim but barely suggestive of Marfan syndrome. The fingers and toes are not excessively long nor is the US/LS ratio abnormal.

X ray. Osteoporosis.

Laboratory. Homocystine in urine by the nitroprusside test, electrophoresis, or column chromatography; bacterial inhibition spot test. The locus for cystathionine beta-synthase is confirmed at 21q22.3.

Clinical Course. The disease may be well tolerated for several decades or be fatal in the first decade, depending, in large measure, on the vascular complications. Cerebral vascular disease may be responsible for early or late death. Myocardial infarction is more likely to occur after age 20. Although over half of the patients are retarded, some patients responsive to B_6 therapy may attend college. The visual impairment may be particularly disabling.

Treatment. Vitamin B_6 for those with the B_6-responsive form appears to have the potential to reduce most complications from retardation to vascular complications. Methionine restriction and cystine supplementation for those not responsive to B_6 may modify the complications, but to a lesser degree than in the B_6 responsive group. Folates and B_6 may reverse the schizophrenia in the methylation defect.

Differential Diagnosis. The most important diagnostic alternative is the *Marfan syndrome*, which may be distinguished by dominant inheritance, a negative nitroprusside test, superior-temporal subluxation of the lens, vascular disease of the great vessels, and absence of mental retardation and malar flush. In addition, the Marfan syndrome has more striking arachnodactyly and joint laxity.

Maple Syrup Urine Disease (Branched Chain Ketonuria)

Menkes and co-workers described, in 1954, a family in which 4 of 6 infants died in the first weeks of life with vomiting, hypertonicity, and a maple syrup odor to the urine. In 1957, Westall, Dancis, and Miller found an elevation in the urine and blood of the branched chain amino acids, valine, leucine, and isoleucine. The frequency is estimated as 1:200,000 births. The biochemical defect seems to be a deficiency in branched chain ketoacid decarboxylase. Elevation of the branched chain ketoacids is not present at birth, but can be demonstrated in the plasma on the fourth day. Death usually occurs during the first year following progressive neurologic deterioration in

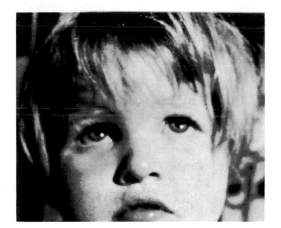

Fig. 8–35. Fair skin and hair and blue eyes are common in patients with PKU (as in this example) but far from invariable.

untreated patients. Arrest of neurologic damage has been achieved by dietary management through the exclusion of valine, leucine, and isoleucine from the diet. A special preparation lacking these amino acids is used to reduce the quantity of excess branched chain amino acids. Then foods containing these amino acids are restarted gradually in the diet and maintained at a low level to meet requirements for growth. Dietary management is much more difficult than for PKU and is done best in a center with the appropriate experience and resources.

Several variants with milder manifestations are known. Inborn errors in the metabolism of other branched-chain amino acids occur, but are so rare that they will not be included here.

Phenylketonuria (PKU)

The genetics and biochemistry of this classic example of an inborn error of metabolism are reviewed in Chapter 6. Only the type I clinical disease will be reviewed here.

Diagnostic Features and Clinical Course. Affected children appear perfectly normal at birth but, if they are not treated, the developmental milestones may be delayed within the first few months, and the delay becomes progressively more severe, including a precip-

itous loss of IQ in the first year. Seizures may begin at 6 to 12 months, and the majority have abnormal EEGs even if they have no seizures. The skin is dry and rough, and the hair and eyes tend to be lighter than expected from the family background (Fig. 8–35). They are hyperactive, irritable children with an increased muscle tone and awkward gait, who show voluntary, purposeless, repetitive motions.

The classic diagnostic test is the ferric chloride test or the Phenistix test (Ames Co.), but this may not become positive for several days. Routine screening procedures make use of the Guthrie test (a bacterial inhibition assay), paper chromatography, or fluorimetric methods. The diagnosis should always be confirmed by a quantitative measurement of plasma phenylalanine and the appropriate tests to determine the nature of the hyper-phenylalaninemia.

Treatment. Treatment consists of a low phenylalanine diet instituted as soon as possible. Some phenylalanine must be added to prevent depletion of the body's proteins. Phenylalanine levels must be monitored frequently, as the requirements decrease in the first few years. If the biochemical abnormalities are corrected, convulsions cease and growth is normal. Damage to the intelligence can be prevented with careful monitoring and control of the phenylalanine intake (see Chapter 6). A trend in many centers is to maintain a low phenylalanine intake throughout the lifetime of the patient. See Chapter 16 for the teratogenic implications of pregnancy.

Heterozygote Detection. The detection of individuals heterozygous for the PKU gene would be of value in some counseling situations, and more so as the frequency of successfully treated adults increases. Quite good discrimination is achieved by giving intravenous phenylalanine and following the kinetics of its disappearance from the blood, using the phenylalanine/tyrosine ratio. In spite of claims to the contrary, there do not seem to be any deleterious effects of the heterozygous gene to the carrier. The gene locus for phenylalanine hydroxylase has been confirmed at 12q24.1, which opens the door to the diag-

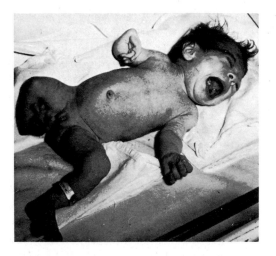

Fig. 8–36. Skeletal anomalies in newborn with Fanconi pancytopenia.

nostic possibilities of recombinant DNA technology.

Hyperphenylalaninemia. Screening programs for phenylketonuria are complicated by the presence of an occasional case of hyperphenylalaninemia without the characteristic findings of phenylketonuria. These must be distinguished, because these children will not benefit and, indeed, may suffer when put on a low phenylalanine diet. Although the situation is still unclear, there appears to be one type in which the liver phenylalanine hydroxylase is late-maturing, and which will revert to normal within a few months. Another type produces a mild hyperphenylalaninemia, usually without neurologic damage. A third type may result from a defective binding site of the cofactor.

Tyrosinemia, Type I[2,4]

This inborn error is rare except in the Lac St. Jean region of Quebec, where its frequency is about 1.5:1000, a striking example of founder effect.

The predominant clinical findings in the infant are failure to thrive, vomiting, diarrhea and hepatomegaly, severe or fatal liver failure, and in the older patients, chronic hepatic cirrhosis and renal tubular failure. Varying degrees of mental retardation may occur. The hypoglycemia, hepatomegaly, and ascites are prominent clinical manifestations. Tyrosinemia, which is defined as a plasma level greater than 0.70 mol/mL, can be detected by current screening methods for aminoacidopathies.

Treatment consisting of dietary limitation of tyrosine and phenylalanine through special formulas has been successful in producing improved liver function, reduction of ascites, and satisfactory weight gain. However, the metabolic defect may cause damage before birth.

The basic enzymatic defect is thought to be a deficiency of fumaryl-aceto-acetate hydroxylase. As with hyperphenylalaninemia, there are many conditions that produce hypertyrosinemia.

Hereditary tyrosinemia must be distinguished from acquired neonatal tyrosinemia in which an apoenzyme that can be activated is present (steroids and folic acid benefit these patients). The gene has been assigned to 15q23-24.

Tyrosinemia type II, caused by tyrosine transaminase deficiency, has a locus that maps to 16q22.1-q22.3.

Anemia[1,2,4]

To avoid repeating gene loci for each condition, the hemoglobin alpha chain locus is at 16pter-p13.3 and the beta chain locus is at 11p15.5.

Fanconi Pancytopenia. This disease is characterized by pancytopenia, bone marrow hypoplasia, and characteristic congenital anomalies, most commonly abnormalities of the thumb, absent radii, microcephaly, a patchy dark skin pigmentation, and shortness of stature. Associated anomalies may include abnormalities of the eye, heart, kidney, and skeleton, as well as mental retardation and deafness (Fig. 8–36).

The pancytopenia generally does not develop until the child is 3 to 12 years of age. The bone marrow is hypocellular with increased fat content. Hemoglobin electropho-

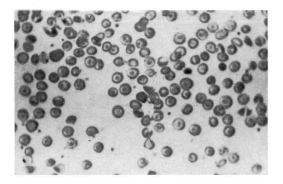

Fig. 8–37. Target cells characteristic of hemoglobin C disease.

resis reveals an increase in Hb F to 5 to 15%. Chromosomal studies show increased chromatid breaks along with unusual chromosomal alignments. The use of chromosome-breaking agents to exaggerate chromosome fragility may allow heterozygote detection and be useful in prenatal diagnosis.

Clinical complications include bleeding, infections, and anemia, which require symptomatic treatment with platelets, antibiotics, and red cells. Other therapy consists of combined corticosteroids and androgens. Patients may show hematologic response in 2 to 4 months, at which time the corticosteroids and androgens may be reduced but usually are not withdrawn completely without relapse.

Confusion in nomenclature results from the fact that four disorders bear the eponym Fanconi: Fanconi pancytopenia with multiple anomalies, type 1 and type 2, reflecting the existence of two separate loci, and Fanconi

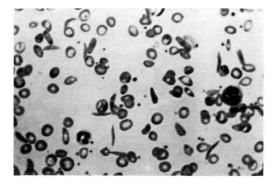

Fig. 8–38. Sickle cells in hemoglobin S disease.

renotubular syndromes I and II, which are also autosomal recessive. Fanconi syndrome I is a disorder characterized by vitamin D-resistant rickets, osteomalacia, chronic acidosis, glycosuria, and aminoaciduria without cystinosis, which becomes manifest in infancy and childhood. Fanconi syndrome II presents in adults in the fourth and fifth decades of life with findings similar to (though less severe than) those of Fanconi I.

Hemoglobin C Disease

Hemoglobin C disease is the homozygous manifestation of a beta chain abnormality that produces moderately severe hemolytic anemia. The molecular basis of the disorder is the replacement of glutamic acid by lysine in residue 6 of the beta chain. The disease is relatively common, and the usually asymptomatic heterozygote is estimated to represent about 2% of the African-American population. Because of the high gene frequencies involved, heterozygotes with hemoglobin S and hemoglobin C are not uncommon, and the compound heterozygote has a hemolytic anemia that is difficult to distinguish clinically from sickle cell disease. A clinical clue to the presence of hemoglobin C disease is the presence of target cells (frequently more than 50% of the red cells, Fig. 8–37). Electrophoresis will confirm the diagnosis.

Hemoglobin S Disease (Sickle Cell Anemia)

This beta chain disorder occupies a most important position in the development of medical genetics. Its molecular basis is discussed in Chapter 6.

Sickle cell disease is transmitted as an autosomal recessive disorder, and sickle cell trait, which is generally benign under normal conditions, is inherited as an autosomal dominant. Sickle cell disease is characterized by chronic anemia and intravascular sickling resulting from lowered oxygen tension (Fig. 8–38). The sickling of the red blood cells results in increased blood viscosity, which produces capillary stasis, vascular occlusion, thrombi, and infarction. Infection often instigates the above cycle, which is referred to as a crisis and is associated with pain. The bone marrow may temporarily cease to function during this period, resulting in more severe anemia. The homozygote often does not survive childhood, although affected adults are encountered. Growth and development are poor.

The diagnosis is made by demonstration of the sickling phenomenon on peripheral blood smear and confirmed by hemoglobin electrophoresis, which reveals hemoglobin S. Mass screening tests, such as the Sickledex and dithionite tests, are currently being emphasized.

There is no successful treatment at present. Management consists of avoiding low oxygen tension situations (such as nonpressurized aircraft) and promptly attending to infections. Crises are treated symptomatically, depending on the severity. The individual should be kept well hydrated during an episode. If the hemoglobin level drops to low levels, blood transfusion may be necessary, although patients usually tolerate hemoglobin levels of 5 to 6 g/100 mL blood very well. Prenatal diagnosis is now available (see Chapter 15).

Pyruvate Kinase Deficiency

Pyruvate kinase (PK) deficiency, a chronic hemolytic anemia, is highly variable in its severity. PK deficiency and G6PD deficiency are the two most common inherited hemolytic anemias due to enzyme defects. Diagnosis is by enzyme assay, which is also capable of detecting the asymptomatic heterozygote. Conservative management with transfusions is recommended. Splenectomy sometimes helps by decreasing transfusion requirements, but is not curative; the hemolysis persists, and hemolytic or aplastic crises may occur.

The Thalassemias

The thalassemias have been observed in most racial groups, but have a particularly high incidence in the Mediterranean region (betas), the Middle East, and the Orient (alphas).

The genetics and molecular biochemistry of the thalassemias are discussed in Chapter 6.

The Beta Thalassemias. *"True" beta thalassemia*, or Cooley anemia, occurs in homozygotes during the first few months of life, with severe anemia, frequent infections, stunting of growth, bossing of the skull, maxillary overgrowth, hepatosplenomegaly, and, if the patient survives long enough, hemochromatosis. The blood smear shows anisopoikilocytosis, hypochromia, target cells, and basophilic stippling. Fetal hemoglobin is increased, and A_2 levels are low, normal, or high, but almost always high if expressed as a proportion of hemoglobin A.

The heterozygous genes vary in expression from almost as severe as the homozygous form (thalassemia intermedia) to mild (thalassemia minor) to virtually normal (thalassemia minima). Hemoglobin A_2 is elevated, and small amounts of hemoglobin F are present.

A rare *delta-beta thalassemia* is milder than Cooley anemia. Only hemoglobin F is present in the homozygote. The heterozygote resembles thalassemia minor, with a high level of hemoglobin F.

Hemoglobin Lepore appears to have arisen by unequal crossing over (Chapter 6). Because the composite delta-beta chain is formed at a reduced rate, the gene behaves like a thalassemia gene.

The gene for *hereditary persistence of fetal hemoglobin* has a total deficiency of beta and delta chains from the genes on the chromosome upon which it is located (the cis position), but the gamma gene is normal so the homozygote continues to produce hemoglobin F and there is no clinical abnormality.

The beta-thalassemia genes interact with the beta chain structural mutants and are thus called "interacting" types. For instance, a patient with a hemoglobin S gene on one chromosome and a beta thalassemia allele on the other has a disease similar to sickle cell disease, since the majority of the hemoglobin produced is hemoglobin S.

The Alpha Thalassemias. Mutants at the alpha thalassemia locus suppress alpha chain

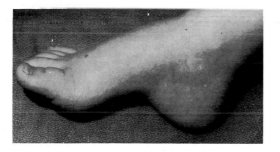

Fig. 8–39.   Pes cavus in Friedreich ataxia—a sentinel feature.

production to varying degrees. The severe type, alpha thalassemia-1, is fatal in the homozygote, causing hemoglobin Bart's hydrops fetalis syndrome. The heterozygote has a mild thalassemia with normal levels of F and A$_2$, and a decreased production of alpha chain demonstrable by isotope incorporation studies.

Hemoglobin Bart's hydrops fetalis syndrome is caused by homozygosity for the alpha thalassemia-1 mutation, resulting in absence of all 4 alpha-globin loci. Because there are no alpha chains, there is no hemoglobin A or F, but mainly hemoglobin Bart's, a tetramere of gamma chains, which is unstable. This disorder is a frequent cause of stillbirth in Southeast Asia. Prenatal diagnosis is now possible.

Hemoglobin H disease appears to result from deletion of 2 of the 4 alpha chain loci (Chapter 6). Patients have a variable course, similar to that of thalassemia major, or milder. The alpha thalassemia genes in the heterozygote produce mild abnormalities, if any.

Therapy for all the thalassemia syndromes is entirely supportive, including transfusions, folic acid, and intensive treatment of infections. However, transfusions may result in hemochromatosis. Recent results suggest that this may be overcome by the use of a chelating agent, desferrioxamine. Splenectomy is indicated only if there are indications of hypersplenism and preferably after 5 years of age because of the increased risk of infection. Prenatal diagnosis is discussed in Chapter 15.

ATAXIA, FRIEDREICH[1,2]

This degenerative disease is one of the many inherited spinocerebellar ataxias. A classifica-

tion is provided in McKusick's catalogue.[1] It is characterized by cerebellar ataxia, pes cavus (Fig. 8–39), loss of deep tendon reflexes, slowed conduction time, and scoliosis beginning in preadolescence. Clinical manifestations of the spinocerebellar disorder are incoordination of limb movements, dysarthria, and nystagmus. Average duration of life is about 15 years from the time of onset. Heart disease, an unusual myocardiopathy, frequently is responsible for death of the patient in congestive heart failure or cardiac arrhythmia. The gene locus is 9q13-q21.1. Prenatal diagnosis has been achieved.

ATAXIA TELANGIECTASIA (AT; LOUIS-BAR SYNDROME)[1,2]

The cardinal features of this disorder are ataxia, telangiectases, and an immunological deficiency of both cellular and humoral immunity. The first manifestations, progressing from infancy, are usually related to the ataxia: incoordination, often severe enough to prevent ambulation; choreoathetosis; nystagmus; dysarthric speech; and drooling.

The child has frequent infections and fails to thrive; later, respiratory infections involving the sinuses and the lungs predominate. These infections do not respond to antimicrobial therapy. This failure may be related to the absence of IgA, the secretory immunoglobulin that protects the mucous membranes. In addition to the humoral immune deficit, there is a cellular immune deficiency with the characteristic findings of lymphopenia and diminished delayed hypersensitivity and capacity for allograft rejection. Thus it is difficult to obtain karyotypes from peripheral blood. The thymus is small and dysplastic at post mortem.

Because the telangiectases may not be readily apparent until later in the course, some patients may be misdiagnosed as having Friedreich ataxia. When telangiectases appear, they are most evident in the bulbar conjunctivae (Fig. 8–40).

AT cells are very sensitive to chromosome breaking agents similar to the situation with Fanconi pancytopenia and xeroderma pigmen-

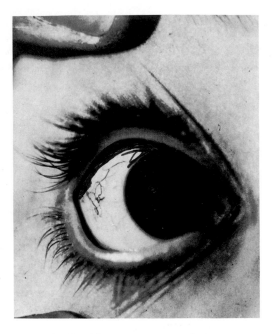

Fig. 8–40.   The eye in ataxia telangiectasia.

tosum. There is a high incidence of lympho-reticular and other neoplasms, and these are the second most frequent cause of death.

Recent evidence suggests that heterozygotes may also have an increased frequency of chromosome breaks following exposure to irradiation and an increased risk for lymphoreticular malignancy. These individuals would then constitute a special high risk group with respect to exposure to occupational or medical irradiation. The gene locus is 11q22-q23.

COLOR BLINDNESS, TOTAL[2]

This autosomal recessive form of color blindness is due to absence of the cones. The vision of affected individuals is better at night. The more common forms of color blindness are X-linked, and the general problem of color blindness and biologic variability is discussed in Chapter 25.

CYSTIC FIBROSIS (CF, MUCOVISCIDOSIS)[2,4,10]

Cystic fibrosis (CF) is the most common disease caused by a single mutant gene in Caucasian children. Estimates of the inci-dence of cystic fibrosis in the American population range from 1:1000 to 1:3700, (we now use 1:2500 in counseling, which calculates by Hardy-Weinberg to a carrier prevalence of 1:25), but it is rarely encountered in blacks and Orientals. The first comprehensive clinical and pathologic description of the disease was presented by Anderson, in 1938, and the mode of transmission was demonstrated by Lowe and co-workers, in 1949, who removed it from the various malabsorption syndromes known as sprue. The clinical course is variable. Most of the clinical problems are caused by obstruction of organ ducts by abnormally thick secretions. The basic defect relates to a polypeptide designated the CFTR (for cystic fibrosis transmembrane conductance regulator) protein.

Cystic fibrosis may present as an acute surgical emergency of the newborn as meconium ileus, or become evident in early childhood as chronic pulmonary disease and steatorrhea. Other clinical findings include cirrhosis of the liver, cor pulmonale, prolapse of the rectum, glycosuria, ocular lesions, and massive salt loss with dehydration, coma, and even death from high environmental temperatures. The disease may be diagnosed by an elevated level of sweat chloride (>60 mEq/L) and absence of pancreatic enzymes.

Treatment is directed at the control of the pulmonary infections, dietary management, and prevention and replacement of abnormal salt loss. With improving management, life expectancy is increasing, and about 75% of patients who survive infancy will live to at least 15 to 20 years of age. A new direction of therapy may be possible through the direct transfer of the CFTR gene to the airway epithelium.[10] Lung transplantation has also been proposed for the most advanced cases. Males are sterile because of testicular tubule degeneration; a few female patients have reproduced. The question has not been satisfactorily answered as to how the high incidence of such a lethal mutant gene can be maintained in the population. Heterozygote advantage and genetic heterogeneity are possible explanations.

The CF gene has now been localized to 7q31.3-q32. This advance at last makes possible the prenatal diagnosis of affected individuals. The situation is complicated by the recognition of multiple mutations with different frequencies in different populations. The delta-F508 mutation is present on average in about 70% of non-Jewish Caucasians, but is higher in Scandinavian and lower in Mediterranean populations. It is now possible to identify over 90% of cystic fibrosis carriers by testing for delta-F508 and nine other major mutations concurrently.

DEAFNESS[2,7]

Congenital deafness is often a difficult problem for the counselor who, in the sporadic case, has to decide between an environmental cause, such as kernicterus, rubella, or meningitis, or a dominant gene, either as a fresh mutation or showing reduced penetrance, or a recessive gene. About 75% of cases result from recessive genes, of which there are several different kinds, 20% are due to environmental causes, 3% to autosomal dominant genes, and 2% to X-linked genes. More recent American studies suggest a lower proportion of genetic cases.

Empiric risk rates for profound childhood deafness not associated with a syndrome have been provided by Stevenson and others (Table 8–6). Of course these risks are approximate and will change according to the number of normal or abnormal children born. For example, for normal parents with one deaf child the 1/6 risk applies to the sibs of the first child,

Table 8–6. Risk for Sib or Child of Person With Congenital Deafness

Family Situation		Risk
Parents consanguineous	sib	1/4
Two or more deaf sibs	sib	1/4
Nonconsanguineous parents, sporadic case	sib	1/6
One parent deaf, sporadic case	child	1/30
Parent deaf, with deaf relatives	child	1/10
Deaf parents, deaf child	sib	1/2.5
Both parents deaf, one with deaf relatives	child	1/7
Both parents deaf, with deaf relatives	child	1/3

and would fall to about 1/10 if there were 3 unaffected sibs. Similarly, the risk for the offspring of two deaf parents is about 10%; if the first child is deaf, the risk for the next child rises to 60%, but if the first child is normal, the risk goes down to 4%.

In addition, deafness is a part of a number of syndromes. Those showing recessive inheritance are listed.

A. Deafness with no associated anomalies
   1. Congenital severe sensorineural deafness
   2. Early onset sensorineural deafness
   3. Congenital moderate hearing loss
B. Deafness with external ear malformations
   1. Conductive hearing loss with low-set malformed ears.
   2. Microtia, meatal atresia, and conductive hearing loss
C. Deafness with integumentary system disease
   1. Neural hearing loss with atopic dermatitis
   2. Hearing loss with pili torti
   3. Onychodystrophy and deafness
D. Deafness associated with eye disease
   1. Hearing loss with myopia and mild mental retardation
   2. Congenital deafness with retinitis pigmentosa (Usher syndrome)
   3. Hearing loss with retinal degeneration and diabetes mellitus (Alström-Hallgren syndrome)
   4. Deafness, retinal changes, muscular wasting, and mental retardation
   5. Hearing loss, optic atrophy, and juvenile diabetes (DIDMOAD syndrome)
   6. Hearing loss with polyneuropathy and optic atrophy.
E. Deafness with nervous system disease
   1. Deafness with mental deficiency, ataxia, and hypogonadism (Richards-Rundel syndrome)
F. Deafness associated with skeletal disease
   1. Conductive hearing loss, cleft palate, characteristic facies, and bone dysplasia (oto-palato-digital syndrome)

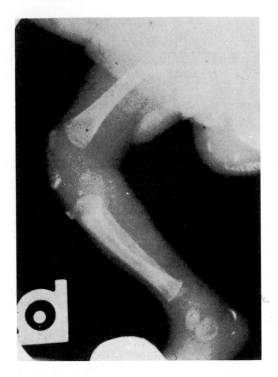

Fig. 8–41.   Punctate calcific deposits in chondrodysplasia punctata.

2. Deafness with tibial absence
3. Deafness with split hand and foot
4. Deafness with splayed long bones (Pyle disease)
G. Deafness with other abnormalities
1. Deafness with goiter (Pendred syndrome. This may account for as much as 10% of hereditary deafness. Patients may be euthyroid.)
2. Neural hearing loss with goiter, high PBI, and stippled epiphyses
3. Deafness, prolonged Q-T interval and sudden death (Jervell and Lange-Nielsen syndrome). The patient is at risk for sudden death from ventricular fibrillation. Maintenance doses of propranolol may prevent the arrhythmia.

DWARFISM[1,2]

Many genetic and chromosomal diseases are accompanied by short stature. This section refers to a selected number that do not fall into other obvious categories such as Down syndrome or Morquio disease. The reader is referred to numerous reviews for nosological classifications and clinical descriptions of the ever-growing list of short-stature syndromes.

Bloom Syndrome

This relatively rare disorder is characterized by small size at birth, short stature, dolichocephaly, a telangiectatic erythema of the face resembling lupus erythematosus, and malar hypoplasia. Sunlight exacerbates the butterfly facial lesions, and telangiectases may be found on the hands and arms. A marked increase in sister-chromatid exchanges in cultured cells, as revealed by special staining techniques, may be related to the increased risk of malignancy, most often leukemia.

Chondrodysplasia Punctata (Chondrodysplasia Calcificans Congenita, Chondrodystrophia Calcificans Punctata)

The nosology of chondrodystrophy with stippled epiphyses, formerly known as the Conradi-Hünerman syndrome, is evolving rapidly. Calcific stippling in and around the joints occurs in a number of conditions, including cretinism, trisomies 18 and 21, several chondrodysplasias, Zellweger syndrome, and maternal warfarin embryopathy. A feature of the *rhizomelic*, recessively inherited type of chondrodysplasia punctata is symmetrical proximal shortening of the upper limbs with or without shortening of the lower limbs. The metaphyses are splayed and surrounded by coarse, variable stippling (Fig. 8–41). Coronal clefts of the vertebrae are present. The facies is characteristic with a flat face, low nasal bridge, simian appearance, cataracts, and ichthyotic skin changes (Fig. 8–42). The outcome is usually fatal within the first year.

The nonrhizomelic types (Conradi-Hünerman) include a mild, dominant type with variable asymmetric shortening, often with calcification of laryngeal and tracheal cartilages, an X-linked recessive type, and an X-linked dominant type, lethal in males. Warfarin em-

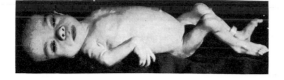

Fig. 8–42.   Note short proximal long bones (especially humerus), flexion contractures and saddle nose in patient with chondrodysplasia punctata.

bryopathy produces a phenocopy of the dominant type.

Chondroectodermal Dysplasia (Ellis-van Creveld Syndrome)

History. This clinical entity was recognized by Ellis and van Creveld in 1940. The pattern of inheritance was shown to be autosomal recessive by Metrakos and Fraser in 1954. McKusick, in 1964, reported a number of patients from an inbred Amish population that approximately equaled the number of all previously reported cases in the world literature (which illustrates the deleterious effects of in-

breeding in making manifest the effects of autosomal recessive single mutant genes).

Diagnostic Features. *General.* Intelligence is usually normal. Equal sex distribution. Moderately to severely dwarfed.

Head. Abnormalities of mouth; short upper lip bound by frenula to alveolar ridge; dental problems (dysplastic teeth, delayed eruption).

Musculoskeletal. Polydactyly, ulnar (Fig. 8–43); short extremities, more extreme distally; spondylolisthesis; fusion of hamate and capitate, inability to make a fist.

Cardiovascular. Congenital heart lesions in about 50% of patients, commonly a large atrial septal defect.

Clinical Course. In the past, many of these patients died in infancy as a consequence of their congenital heart lesions. Those without heart disease or with mild or treated cardiac lesions will survive into adult life with the major handicaps being shortness of stature and, in some, the limitation of hand function.

Treatment. Symptomatic and supportive, especially for the congenital heart defects.

Differential Diagnosis. Other disorders causing dwarfism, polydactyly, and congenital

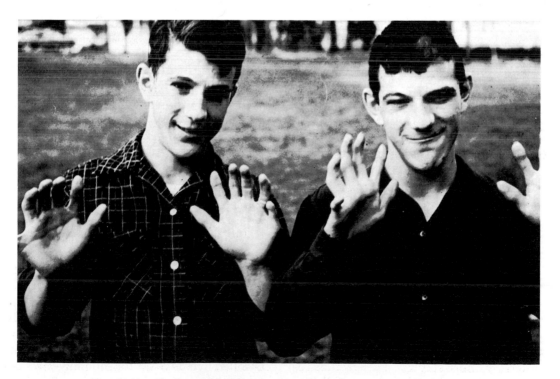

Fig. 8–43.   Brothers with Ellis-van Creveld syndrome. Note polydactyly.

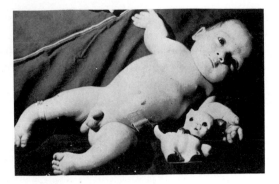

Fig. 8–44.   Infant with diastrophic dwarfism. Club feet help to distinguish the disorder from achondroplasia.

heart disease, in particular, asphyxiating thoracic dystrophy.

Diastrophic Dwarfism

Patients with this disorder may look like achondroplastic dwarfs at birth because of the

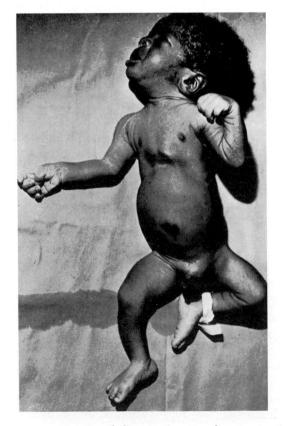

Fig. 8–45.   Constricted thoracic cage impeding respiration in Jeune syndrome.

shortness of their limbs (Fig. 8–44). However, there are classic stigmata that distinguish diastrophic dwarfism from other forms of dwarfism detectable at birth. One is the cystic swelling of the external ear, much in appearance like the "cauliflower ear" of the wrestler or boxer, followed by calcification of the lesion. Other differentiating features are club feet (varus deformity) and short first metacarpals associated with small, proximally placed thumbs. Intelligence and overall general health are satisfactory. Orthopedic correction of the foot deformity and the progressive scoliosis have not proved to be entirely satisfactory.

Thoracic Dystrophy, Asphyxiating (Jeune Syndrome)

This disease often terminates fatally in infancy. The thoracic cage is greatly constricted by shortened ribs, and the constriction impedes respiratory excursions and produces asphyxiation (Fig. 8–45). There are relatively short limbs, hypoplastic square iliac wings, deformed acetabulum, and irregular epiphyses and metaphyses. Polydactyly may be present, and the overall picture of skeletal anomalies has led some observers to consider this disease to be a variant of the Ellis-van Creveld syndrome. Patients who survive infancy have improvement in the relative growth of the rib cage and satisfactory respiration, but progressive renal disease becomes manifest.

EHLERS-DANLOS SYNDROME—RECESSIVE FORMS[2,4]

The more common dominant forms have been discussed earlier.

Type IV—Ecchymotic

This form may be recessive or dominant. Joint hypermobility may be confined to the fingers. The skin is thin, translucent, inextensible, and very prone to bruising. Patients are prone to sudden death from major arterial tears or rupture of the bowel. Type III collagen is lacking in the skin of homozygotes and diminished in heterozygotes.

Type VI—Ocular Type

There is a deficiency of the enzyme lysyl hydroxylase, leading to a lack of hydroxylysine in the collagen. The skin features are moderate; there is severe scoliosis, and patients are prone to retinal detachment or ocular rupture.

Type VII—Arthrochalasis Multiplex Congenita

Type VII may be recessive or dominant. The procollagen peptidase, or protease, is deficient. Patients have moderately stretchable skin, short stature, and severe joint laxity with congenital dislocations.

GALACTOSEMIA[2,4]

This disease results from the absence of a specific enzyme, galactose-1-phosphate (Gal 1-P) uridyl transferase (see Chapter 6). Frequency estimates range from 1:18,000 to 1:180,000, with most values in the lower ranges. Diagnosis is by the finding of nutritional failure, mental retardation, cataracts, and hepatosplenomegaly with cirrhosis. Urinalysis for reducing substances with Benedict's solution is positive, but with Clinistix (glucose oxidase) is negative, indicating that the reducing sugar is not glucose. Galactose, along with other amino acids and albumin, may be identified in the urine by chemical and chromatographic means. Blood galactose is elevated; there is an abnormal galactose tolerance test (beware of insulin shock) and a deficiency of Gal 1-P uridyl transferase in the erythrocytes.

Vomiting, diarrhea, and jaundice develop days or weeks after the first milk ingestion, followed by dehydration, poor growth, parenchymal liver damage, and in 1 to 2 months, cataract formation. These problems, plus involvement of the central nervous system, progress unless a galactose-free (milk-free) diet is given. The earlier the diet is started, the better the outcome. Impairment of mental function is least if the galactose-free diet is begun prenatally.

The gene locus has been confirmed at 9p13, the enzyme defect is present in fibroblasts, and prenatal diagnosis is possible. There are transferase variants, including a Negro variant, that retain some ability to metabolize galactose and may, as in the case of the Duarte variant, be entirely asymptomatic.

In the heterozygote carrier, Gal 1-P uridyl transferase activity in the blood is about midway between that of the normal and the homozygote. Galactosemia can also result from a deficiency of galactokinase, (galactosemia II) but symptoms do not occur in infancy. Cataracts occur at various ages and may also occur in some heterozygotes.

THE GLYCOGEN STORAGE DISEASES[2,4]

The glycogenoses are a group of diseases resulting from derangements in synthesis or degradation of glycogen. At least 15 enzyme defects of glycogen metabolism have been categorized, and there are still cases that do not fit readily into any of these categories. Some patients with combined defects have been observed. Von Gierke disease has the distinction of being the first inborn error of metabolism in which the deficiency of a known tissue enzyme was demonstrated.

In general, the glycogenoses involve disorders of the liver or muscle, alone or in combination with heart, kidney, and nervous system. The clinical manifestations of the disorders are, of course, related to the systems involved. For example, cardiomegaly may be present in any of the three entities (Pompe, limit dextrinosis, amylopectinosis) in which the heart is involved, although only in Pompe disease do the cardiac findings consistently predominate. Hepatomegaly and hypoglycemia are prominent in the types that have liver involvement, and hypotonia is prominent in those with muscle and/or nervous system involvement.

The prognosis and severity vary both among and within the type of glycogenosis. In general, von Gierke disease (type Ia) is very severe, yet there are reports of survival to adulthood. In type VIa (Hers disease), the disease is generally milder, but severe involvement has been observed in some cases.

Table 8–7 lists some of the glycogenoses with the specific enzymes demonstrated to be absent or deficient in each disorder. As with the mucopolysaccharidoses, these categories (and those omitted) must be accepted with flexibility. Revisions will continue as the heterogeneity of these diseases becomes better appreciated. Provisional gene locus assignments have been made for VII to chromosome 1 (1cen-q32) and for VIII to Xq12-q13.

HEPATOLENTICULAR DEGENERATION (WILSON DISEASE)[2,4]

The disease is usually characterized by a low amount of ceruloplasmin, which is the copper-containing plasma protein, but there is a type with normal ceruloplasmin. The basic defect, still not identified, leads to the accumulation of toxic amounts of copper in certain tissues. The clinical effects, which become manifest in childhood or adult life, are liver disease, central nervous system symptoms, and a pathognomonic Kayser-Fleischer ring, a gold discoloration around the cornea. Hepatomegaly, ascites, jaundice, cirrhosis, and abnormal liver function tests call attention to the liver disease. Tremor (sometimes "wing-flapping"), indistinct speech, staring, drooling, hypertonicity, emotional lability, and occasionally seizures are features of the central nervous system involvement. Laboratory confirmation comes from the demonstration of low plasma copper, low ceruloplasmin, high urinary copper, and aminoaciduria. Defective radioactive copper uptake identifies patients with normal ceruloplasmin. Treatment by restricting dietary copper and the use of a chelating agent, penicillamine, is effective, to the extent that irreversible damage has not occurred. Early diagnosis is therefore crucial. The gene locus for Wilson disease has been confirmed on the long arm of chromosome 13 (13q14-q21).

HYPOPHOSPHATASIA[2,4]

This disease, with skeletal abnormalities, low alkaline phosphatase, and hypercalcemia, described by Rathbun in 1948, has a spectrum of severity and can be caused by mutations in two or more genes. The infantile and childhood types are recessive and the adult type is dominant. Over half of the patients die as infants, but others appear to survive to adult life with little or no detectable problem. The skeletal abnormalities resemble those of rickets: fragile bones with bowed legs, poorly mineralized skull with late closure of fontanelles, and rachitic rosary (Fig. 8–46). Those who survive infancy have dental problems, such as defective dentin and premature loss of teeth. In the more severe cases there is respiratory insufficiency and hypotonia, failure to thrive, and nephrocalcinosis. The homozygote has low serum alkaline phosphatase and high urinary

Table 8–7. Selected Glycogenoses

Disease	Organs Affected and Clinical Manifestations	Enzyme
Ia von Gierke	Liver, kidney, intestinal mucosa; hepatomegaly, hypoglycemia, hyperlipidemia, hyperuricemia, growth retardation, bleeding diathesis.	Glucose-6-phosphatase
II Pompe (cardiac)	Heart, muscle, liver, CNS; cardiomegaly, profound hypotonia, death in infancy. There are also early childhood and adult onset forms.	Lysosomal alpha-1,4-glycosidase (acid maltase)
III Limit dextrinosis (Forbes, Cori)	Liver, muscle, heart; hepatomegaly, hypoglycemia, cardiomegaly.	Amylo-1,6-glucosidase (debrancher)
IV Amylopectinosis	Liver, kidney, heart, muscle, CNS, RE system; hepatosplenomegaly, cirrhosis.	Alpha-1,4-glucan-6-glucosyl transferase (brancher)
V McArdle	Muscle; appears in adult life as muscular fatigue and pain with exercise, myoglobinuria.	Muscle phosphorylase
VI Hers	Liver; hepatomegaly, hypoglycemia, acidosis—mild to severe	Liver phosphorylase
VII Tarui	Like V McArdle	Phosphofructokinase
VIII	Muscle weakness	Liver phosphorylase kinase

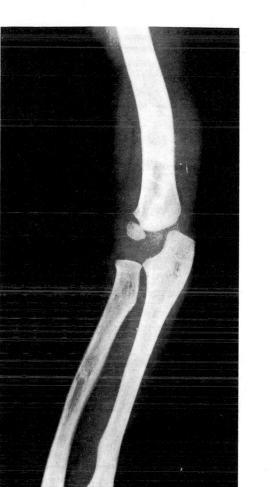

Fig. 8–46.   Metaphyseal rarefaction in hypophosphatasia.

disease. The early recognition of congenital hypothyroidism (cretinism, Fig. 8–47) is vital, so that therapy can be started and mental retardation avoided. Several recessive types have been identified, including (1) familial goiter caused by failure to transport iodine into the thyroid, (2) familial goiter, with or without cretinism, from failure to form organic iodine, (3) an incomplete organification defect, in which chlorate causes an appreciable discharge of iodide in affected individuals, who have moderate goiter and sensorineural deafness, but are only minimally hypothyroid, i.e., Pendred syndrome, (4) goitrous cretinism from defective coupling of mono- and diiodotyrosine into triiodothyronine and thyroxine, (5) goitrous cretinism from failure to deiodinate mono- and diiodotyrosine, (6) familial goiter with abnormal thyroglobulin synthesis, (7) familial pituitary hypothyroidism, either isolated TSH deficiency, panhypopituitarism, or absence of the pituitary, (8) cretinism with impaired thyroid response to thyrotropin, (9) familial disorders of thyroid binding globulin with goiter, usu-

excretion of phosphoethanolamine and inorganic pyrophosphate. The heterozygote may have low serum alkaline phosphatase or high urinary phosphoethanolamine, or both. A "pseudohypophosphatasia" has been described with the classic clinical picture but it has a normal phosphatase activity by the usual method of assay. The gene for the infantile form has been assigned to 1p36.1-p34.

HYPOTHYROIDISM[2,4]

The synthesis, storage, secretion, delivery, and utilization of the thyroid hormones involve a complex sequence of metabolic events. Interruption at any step will lead to thyroid

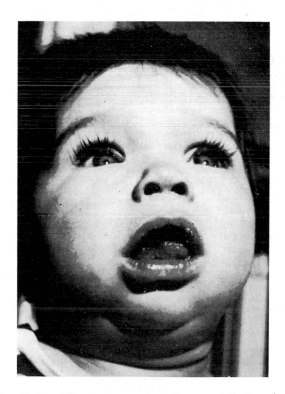

Fig. 8–47.   Characteristic coarse facies and thick protuberant tongue of cretinism.

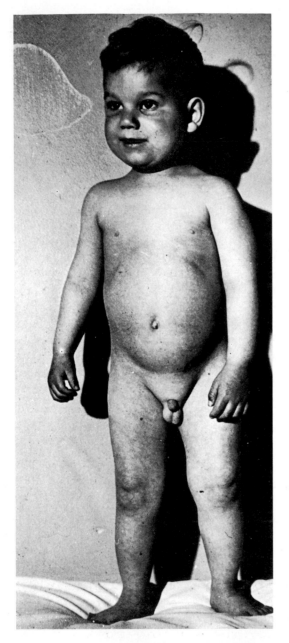

Fig. 8–48.   Laurence-Moon syndrome. The only feature of the syndrome apparent in this photo is obesity.

ally X-linked recessive, and (10) a heterogeneous group of disorders involving resistance of target organs to the thyroid hormones.

Patients with familial thyroid disease may be identified in screening programs or come to the physician's attention because of failure to thrive or other significant signs early in life or may remain undetected till much later.

Once the hypothyroid state has been diagnosed, vigorous treatment should be started, with extensive investigation to identify the site of the block being postponed until much later.

LAURENCE-MOON SYNDROME[1,2]

This syndrome was recognized for its ophthalmologic abnormality and associated defects over 100 years ago. Retinitis pigmentosa is present in about two thirds of the patients, and obesity, mental retardation, postaxial polydactyly, and syndactyly are even more common (Fig. 8–48). Hypogonadism and genital hypoplasia are found in over half of these individuals. This syndrome should be distinguished on clinical grounds from the Prader-Willi syndrome and the Biedl-Bardet syndrome.

THE LIPIDOSES[2,4]

These disorders represent a somewhat specialized area of interest, and we have elected to summarize them as a group in narrative and tabular form. Tay-Sachs disease, however, will be discussed in greater detail.

As the name of the group implies, these diseases are characterized by abnormalities of lipid metabolism with accumulation of lipids in viscera, brain, and blood vessels, producing derangements of these systems. Table 8–8 presents a selection of lipidoses (including the classic disorders—Niemann-Pick, Gaucher, and Tay-Sachs diseases) in which hepato-splenomegaly and neurologic deterioration predominate. The generalized gangliosidoses, GM (1), types I, II, III, and Farber disease have some clinical features found in the mucopolysaccharidoses, as do the mucolipidoses, which are discussed in this connection and listed in Table 8–9. The three types of gangliosidosis GM(2) have clinical findings similar to the prototype of this group, Tay-Sachs disease. All of the lipidoses selected for discussion are autosomal recessive except for Fabry disease, which is X-linked recessive.

Table 8–8 also provides the salient clinical and laboratory features. It is recognized that Niemann-Pick, Gaucher, and Tay-Sachs dis-

Table 8–8.   Selected Lipidoses

Disease	Laboratory Findings	Clinical Manifestations
Autosomal Recessive		
Niemann-Pick	Sphingomyelin accumulation; Niemann-Pick cells in bone marrow; deficiency of sphingomyelin-splitting enzyme in infantile type	Four clinical types varying from degeneration and death by 2 years of age to survival to adult life with little or no handicap; hepatosplenomegaly, mental retardation, neurologic deterioration
Gaucher	Glucocerebroside accumulation; Gaucher cells in bone marrow; deficiency of glucocerebroside-splitting enzyme	Three clinical types; spectrum ranges from acute form in infancy with hepatosplenomegaly and neurologic deterioration with death in infancy or early childhood, to chronic form with onset in childhood or adulthood with hepatosplenomegaly, hypersplenism, bone and joint and neurological involvement
Farber	Ceramide and mucopolysaccharide accumulation	Granulomatous lesions of skin; arthropathy; hoarse cry; irritability; failure to thrive
Generalized gangliosidosis GM(1), Type I	Ganglioside GM(1) accumulation in brain and viscera; cytoplasmic vacuoles; deficiency of A, B, and C isozymes of beta-galactosidase	Skeletal abnormalities suggestive of the Hurler syndrome; cherry-red macular spot; hepatosplenomegaly; death by age 2 years.
Generalized gangliosidosis GM(1), Type II	Ganglioside GM(1) accumulation in brain but not viscera; deficiency of B and C isozymes of beta-galactosidase	Similar to but later in onset than GM(1), Type 1; survival to 10 years of age
Gangliosidosis GM(2), Type I (Tay-Sachs disease; amaurotic family idiocy)	Tay-Sachs ganglioside GM(2) accumulation; component A hexosaminidase deficient	Onset in infancy of development retardation, blindness, paralysis, dementia; death by 4 years of age; cherry-red macular spot
Gangliosidosis GM(2), Type II (Sandhoff)	Ganglioside GM(2) accumulation in brain; hexosaminidase A and B deficient	Similar to Tay-Sachs; not predominantly in Jewish population
Gangliosidosis GM(2), Type III	Ganglioside GM(2) accumulation in brain; hexosaminidase A partially deficient	Later onset, non-Jewish origin; may survive to 10 years of age
X-linked Recessive		
Fabry	Cellular accumulation of ceramidetrihexoside; deficiency of ceramidetrihexosidase	Skin nodules; burning in hands and feet; progressive renal insufficiency; death of affected males in thirties or forties

eases may occur in individuals of various racial backgrounds, but that Jews are most often afflicted. It has become clear that a catastrophic course and early death of patients with Niemann-Pick and Gaucher diseases is by no means invariable. Again, the heterogeneity of types, presentations, and clinical courses appears in this group of disorders as in so many others. Gene loci have been assigned for several of these diseases. Enzyme replacement is at least a clinical "possibility." Aglucerase, a modified form of glucocerebrocidase, is now available to treat a patient with Gaucher disease for only $300,000 per year.

Tay-Sachs Disease (GM2-Gangliosidosis Type 1)

Tay-Sachs disease is characterized by the onset in infancy of severe developmental retardation progressing to dementia, blindness, paralysis, and death by age 2 to 3 years. A "cherry-red spot" on examination of the eye grounds is a hallmark of this and related disorders. The prevalence rate of Tay-Sachs disease (1:5000) among Ashkenazi Jews has prompted the offering of screening programs directed at this high-risk group. The heterozygote may be detected by enzymatic assay of serum or fibroblasts, which reveal 40 to 60% of the activity of normals. The deficient enzyme is hexosaminidase A. The prevalence rate of Tay-Sachs disease in non-Jewish populations is on the order of 1:400,000, with the exception of the French Canadians of Quebec, who have a prevalence rate approaching that of Ashkenazi Jews. The gene locus is confirmed on the long arm of chromosome 15 (15q22-q25.1).

MECKEL SYNDROME

Occipital meningoencephalocele (Fig. 8–49), polydactyly, and cystic dysplasia of the kidneys are the classic features of this triad, but many other anomalies occur. Study of the affected sibs of patients with the triad shows that the kidney dysplasia is the only constant feature. A brain defect—occipital meningocele (67%) and/or anencephaly (27%) or hydrocephaly (12%)—occurs in 90%, postaxial polydactyly in 75%, liver cysts and/or fibrosis in 70%, with lower frequencies of penile, cardiac, and splenic anomalies, cleft lip and/or cleft palate, and microphthalmia. Almost all patients have at least three of these anomalies, but not always the same ones. Only about two thirds have the classic triad. Prenatal diagnosis by ultrasound has been achieved.

THE MUCOLIPIDOSES[2,4]

Mucolipidosis I (Lipomucopolysaccharidosis)

This disease has mild Hurler-like features without excess mucopolysacchariduria, but with peculiar fibroblast inclusions. Early psychomotor development is normal. Clinical fea-

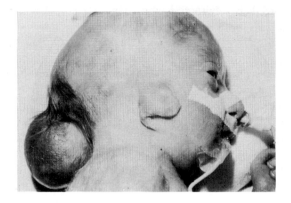

Fig. 8–49.   Occipital meningoencephalocele in infant with Meckel syndrome.

tures become apparent in the second and third years of life. Hepatosplenomegaly is inconsistent. Joint mobility may be increased initially, but becomes restricted by 4 years of age. Patients may have cherry-red macular spots and, less frequently, corneal opacities. X-ray findings are similar to those of MPS III. Mental retardation is moderate.

Mucolipidosis II (Leroy Syndrome, I-Cell Disease)

This is another disease with clinical features of Hurler syndrome with no increase in mu-

Table 8–9.   Mucopolysaccharidoses (MPS) and Mucolipidoses (ML)

Disease	Inheritance	Corneal Clouding	Mental Retardation	Other*
MPS IH (Hurler)	AR	++	++	Severe disease; heart; skeletal; dwarfing; hepatosplenomegaly
MPS IS (Scheie)	AR	++	0	Milder disease; skeletal; heart; psychosis
MPS II (Hunter)	XR	0	+/−	Milder disease; heart; skeletal; dwarfing; deafness; hepatosplenomegaly
MPS III (Sanfilippo)	AR	0	++	Severe CNS; mild somatic; skeletal
MPS IV (Morquio)	AR	+	0	Severe skeletal; heart; dwarfism
MPS VI (Maroteaux-Lamy)	AR	+	0	Milder disease; skeletal; dwarfing; hepatosplenomegaly
MPS VII (Sly)	AR	+	+/−	Hepatosplenomegaly; aortic disease
ML I (Lipomucopolysaccharidosis)	AR	+/−	+	Mild skeletal and facial manifestations
ML II (Leroy syndrome; I-cell disease)	AR	0	++	Severe disease; skeletal; CNS
ML III (Pseudo-Hurler polydystrophy)	AR	+	+	Milder disease; stiff joints; heart
ML IV	AR	+	+	Ashkenazi

*Note that there are subtypes with differences in severity, enzyme defects, and considerable heterogeneity within these broad disease categories.

copolysaccharides in the urine. It was first reported by Leroy and DeMars in 1967. Unusual cytoplasmic inclusions were noted by these authors in cultured fibroblasts, but metachromatic granules have not been observed in leukocytes. Growth and intellectual retardation, coarse Hurler-like facies, hyperplastic gums, stiff joints, congenital dislocation of the hip, kyphosis, and x-ray findings compatible with MPS I are features of this syndrome. Hepatosplenomegaly is minimal, and corneal clouding has not been noted. Prevalence and life expectancy are not known. The gene has been assigned to 4q21-q23.

Mucolipidosis III (Pseudo-Hurler Polydystrophy)

This disorder was described by Maroteaux and Lamy in 1965. It is characterized by stiff joints, corneal clouding, coarse facies, genu valgum, aortic valve disease, and mild to moderate intellectual retardation. Metachromatic granules do not appear in the leukocytes but are visible in excess in the urine. Median nerve signs, which appear in these patients as in other disorders of this group, are relieved by carpal tunnel release. Life expectancy and prevalence for this syndrome are not known. The gene locus is 4q21-q23.

Mucolipidosis IV

This condition is characterized by corneal clouding from early infancy, psychomotor retardation, and retinal degeneration. There are no skeletal or facial abnormalities. Accumulations of ganglioside and hyaluronic acid in cultured skin fibroblasts occur.

MUCOPOLYSACCHARIDOSES

Advances in the study of mucopolysaccharidoses offer a continuing educational challenge to those who are not actively involved in the field. Heterogeneity is apparent in the classification scheme that includes seven general categories (MPS I through VIII, with V remaining vacant) based on differences in enzymatic defects, urinary MPS excretion, phenotype, and genetic transmission. The types

are further subdivided on other bases: severity (MPS I, II, VI), presumably related to different alleles at the same MPS locus; similar severity and phenotype produced by different enzyme defects (MPS III); phenotypic variants and enzymatic differences (MPS IV); and, possibly, mode of inheritance (MPS II). Table 8–9 lists their distinguishing features.

Patients with mucopolysaccharidoses have many common features, but clinical as well as biochemical findings can be used to distinguish the various types. However, the clinical features may not be apparent in infants and even in young children with mucopolysaccharidoses. Secondly, some patients with classic features of Morquio syndrome do not excrete keratan sulfate in the urine. Patients with clinical signs of mucolipidoses also do not excrete mucopolysaccharides in the urine. Still other phenotypically related conditions defy classification into the major categories. It is clear that there is considerably greater heterogeneity within this group of diseases than had been previously recognized. Cell culture techniques are helping to define more clearly the individual disorders within the mucopolysaccharidoses, mucolipidoses, and gangliosidoses, and the categories presented at this time must be accepted with flexibility.

Mucopolysaccharidosis Type I (Includes Type IH and Type IS, Hurler and Scheie Syndromes, Hurler-Scheie Syndrome)

Hurler published a description of this disorder in 1919. Dorfman and Lorincz discovered mucopolysacchariduria in patients with the Hurler syndrome in 1957, establishing the nature of the disease. Scheie syndrome, formerly called MPSV, and more recently MPSIS, is a milder form of Hurler syndrome, which will be described below.

Diagnostic Features. *General.* Progressive mental retardation. Equal sex distribution. Dwarfed, hirsute. Death usually in first decade.

Head. Large, bulging, scaphocephalic. Hydrocephalus, coarse facial features (gargoyle-like) (Figs. 8–50, 8–51).

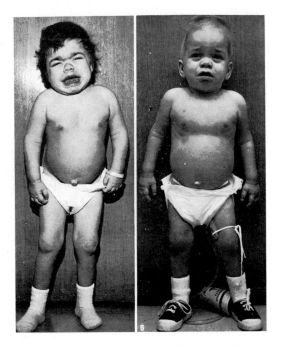

Fig. 8–50. Two- and 3-year-old siblings with Hurler syndrome. Note "gargoyle" facies, claw hands, and limitations in joint mobility.

Eyes. Cloudy corneas, retinal pigmentation, hypertelorism.

Ears. Occasional deafness.

Nose. Broad, wide nostrils, flat bridge, mucoid rhinitis.

Mouth. Full lips; enlarged tongue; teeth small, malformed; alveolar hypertrophy.

Neck. Short.

Hands. Broad, "stiff" stubby fingers—flexion contractures (claw hand).

Skeletal. Generalized limitation in extensibility of joints, broad spatulate ribs, flaring rib cage, kyphosis and thoraco-lumbar gibbus secondary to anterior beaking of vertebral bodies.

Abdomen. Protuberant, hepatosplenomegaly, diastasis recti, umbilical hernia, inguinal hernia.

Cardiovascular. Deposition of mucopolysaccharides in cardiac valves and in coronary arteries, leading to congestive heart failure and coronary occlusion.

X ray. "Shoe-shaped" sella, beaking of lumbar vertebrae, spatulate ribs, diaphyseal irregularities, short malformed phalangeal bones.

Laboratory. Dermatan sulfate and heparan sulfate in urine; metachromatic granules in leukocytes; enzyme defect in α-L-iduronidase. The gene locus is 22q11.

Prevalence. 1:40,000.

Clinical Course. The patient appears normal at birth and during early growth and intellectual development. A gibbus may be observed during the first few months of life, but evidence of mental retardation is seldom recognized before 6 months to 1 year of age. Stiff joints, protuberant abdomen, and persistent rhinitis are frequent reasons for initial medical consultation. Regression in mental and physical development becomes more apparent with increasing age. The joint stiffness becomes more generalized and involves wrists, knees, ankles, and back.

At 2 to 3 years of age, the clouding of the corneas and hepatosplenomegaly become increasingly obvious. Heart murmurs are heard and are probably related to the valvular depositions of mucopolysaccharides. The aortic and mitral valves are most often affected, but all four valves may be involved. The coronary arteries exhibit pronounced intimal thickening, which may produce coronary occlusion. The clinical course is one of progressive deterioration, with cardiac death in the first decade or early in the second decade.

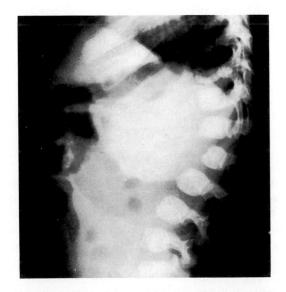

Fig. 8–51. "Beaking" of lumbar vertebrae and gibbus in MPS IH (Hurler).

Patients with the form of MPS, recognized by Scheie in 1962 have a normal to superior intellect and nearly normal height. They have stiff joints, claw hands, and striking corneal clouding. Retinitis pigmentosa, hirsutism, a broad-mouthed face, and aortic valvular disease with aortic insufficiency are also found. The corneal clouding constitutes a significant problem. Efforts at corneal transplants have resulted in opacification of the grafts. Psychotic episodes have been reported. The life expectancy and prevalence of this disorder are as yet undetermined.

Treatment. Symptomatic.

Differential Diagnosis. Although many diseases have various combinations of dwarfing, hepatosplenomegaly, and mental retardation, the major differential is from other forms of mucopolysaccharidoses, mucolipidoses, and gangliosidoses (Table 8–9).

Mucopolysaccharidosis II, or Hunter syndrome, is described in the section on X-linked diseases.

Mucopolysaccharidosis Types IIIA, B, C, and D (Sanfilippo A, B, C, and D)

In this disease, described by Sanfilippo and colleagues in 1963, the somatic manifestations are relatively mild, but the mental retardation is severe. Heparan sulfate, alone excreted in excess in the urine, differentiates this disease from MPS I and II. The intellectual deterioration, which is progressive throughout the school-age period, is accompanied by reasonably good physical strength, making these patients management problems requiring hospitalization. Dwarfing is not significant and stiffness of joints is less than in MPS I and II. Metachromatic granules are found in the lymphocytes. The corneas are clear. Patients with this syndrome generally survive several decades. Four distinct enzyme defects permit subdivision into types III A (Heparan N-sulfatase); IIIB(N-acetyl-α-D-glucosaminidase); IIIC acetyl COA-α-glucosaminide N-acetyltransferase); and IIID(N-acetylglucosamine-6-sulfate sulfatase).

Mucopolysaccharidosis Type IV A and B (Morquio Syndrome)

Morquio and Brailsford described this syndrome independently in 1929, although Osler had reported siblings in 1897 as having achondroplasia who probably had MPS IV. The severe form of the disease is now called MPS IV A or Morquio A, and the milder form of the disease (what appeared in earlier literature as the "Brailsford" type) is called Morquio B. The enzyme defect in MPS IV A is galactosamine-6-sulfate sulfatase, and in MPS IV B is β-galactosidase. Keratan sulfate is excreted in the urine of both types, and a disorder in which there is no urinary excretion of MPS but similar skeletal features has been described.

The Morquio syndrome may be difficult to distinguish from the Hurler syndrome during the first year of life on the basis of somatic features, but with increasing age the key differences become readily apparent. Patients with the Morquio syndrome are generally *not* retarded, and the skeletal features are quite distinctive. The type IV A patients are severely dwarfed; the head seems to rest on a barrel chest. There is a pigeon breast. The joints are usually not stiff, but the wrists and hands are deformed. Knock knees and changes in the femoral heads may be noted, as well as generalized osteoporosis and characteristically flat vertebrae (Fig. 8–52).

The type B patient is more susceptible to the dangerous complication of atlanto-axial dislocation because of hypoplasia of the odontoid, but otherwise has milder skeletal manifestations.

Corneal clouding may not be detectable until after the patient is 10 years of age. Patients have a broad mouth with widely spaced teeth. Heart disease, specifically aortic insufficiency, has been observed, usually in the type A form. Metachromatic granules are found in cultured fibroblasts and the mucopolysacchariduria specific for this syndrome is keratosulfate. The prevalence has been estimated at about 1:40,000. Death commonly occurs between the second and fifth decades in type A, but the type B is compatible with longer life expectancy. The gene locus for type IV B is 3p21-p14.2.

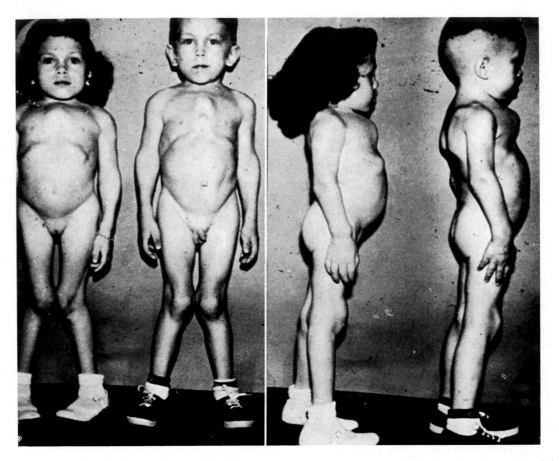

Fig. 8–52.   Severe skeletal dysplasia of MPS IV (Morquio)—head resting on barrel chest, pigeon breast, and knock-knees.

Mucopolysaccharidosis Type VI (Maroteaux-Lamy Syndrome)

Maroteaux, Lamy, and coworkers described this condition in 1963. Growth retardation, knock knees, stiff joints, and corneal clouding occur without mental retardation (Fig. 8–53). The enzyme, arylsulfatase B (the locus for which is on the long arm of chromosome 5) is deficient. Excessive dermatan sulfate is excreted in the urine. Metachromatic granules in the leukocytes are more striking in MPS VI than in any of the other mucopolysaccharidoses. The skeletal and growth abnormality is similar to that in MPS I, but the disease differs by virtue of the normal intelligence and lack of heparan sulfate in the urine. There is a range of severity from death in the teens to a mild form, which is sometimes associated with aortic stenosis. The gene locus is 5q11-q13.

Mucopolysaccharidosis Type VII (Sly Syndrome)

The characteristics of this syndrome appear in Table 8–9. Of interest in MPS VII is that the gene for the enzyme deficient in the syndrome has been located at 7q21.1-q22.

MUSCULAR ATROPHY, PROGRESSIVE SPINAL (WERDNIG-HOFFMANN SYNDROME)[1,2]

The hereditary spinal muscular atrophies include several entities listed in McKusick's catalogue. The infantile type is one of the causes of extreme hypotonia of infancy. There is often a history of diminished or absent fetal movements. The hypotonia and areflexia are noted at birth or shortly after. The infant is limp, the muscles are thin, and the only limb

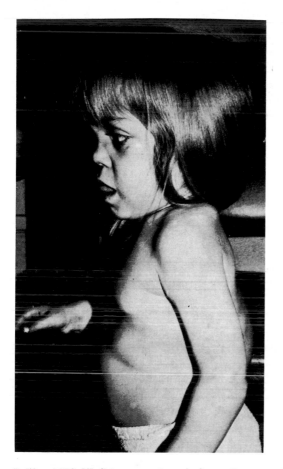

Fig. 8–53.   MPS VI (Maroteaux-Lamy) shares features of MPS IH and MPS IV. In contrast with MPS IH, there is normal intelligence.

MUSCULAR DYSTROPHY, RECESSIVE[1,2]

The category muscular dystrophy comprises the largest group of muscle diseases of childhood. Inheritance may be autosomal recessive, autosomal dominant, or X-linked recessive. The three autosomal recessive forms are: muscular dystrophy I (limb-girdle, Leyden-Möbius) (Fig. 8–54); muscular dystrophy II, which resembles the X-linked Duchenne type; and a congenital muscular dystrophy that produces arthrogryposis. In all forms of this disease, there is progressive weakness and atrophy with increasing disability and deformity. Early in the course of the Duchenne type and muscular dystrophy II, there is pseudohypertrophy. A cardiomyopathy is present in many of the nosologic types, but less commonly in the autosomal forms.

PEROXISOMAL DISORDERS[2,3,12]

This group of diseases, which includes autosomal recessive neonatal adrenoleukodystrophy, X-linked adrenoleukodystrophy, the Zellweger syndrome, and the Refsum syndrome is briefly discussed here, not because

movements may be of the fingers. Progressive paralysis of respiratory muscles leads to death (often from respiratory infection) during the first year of life. Some patients have a later onset of the disease, with weakness becoming apparent at 1 or 2 years of age. These patients may survive adolescence. Muscle biopsy reveals fascicular atrophy. The basic abnormality is degeneration of the anterior horn cells with progressive loss of motor neurons. In the juvenile form (Kugelberg-Welander), onset is usually after 2 years of age and may occur in adolescence or adulthood. The proximal muscles are affected first. The frequency is estimated as 1:24,000 live births, with a carrier frequency of about 1:80.

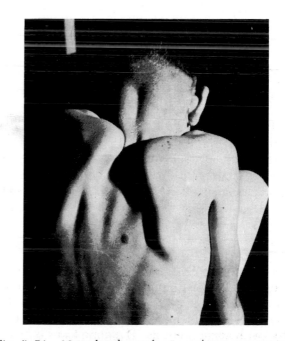

Fig. 8–54.   Muscular dystrophy I produces progressive atrophy and weakness of the limb girdle.

the disorders are common, but because they represent a recently recognized category.

Peroxisomes are membrane-bound, subcellular organelles found in the cytoplasm of many types of cells, such as brain, liver, adrenal, and kidney. They contain a variety of enzymes, such as catalase that form and utilize hydrogen peroxide. Peroxisomes also contain other oxidases (e.g. the system for beta-oxidation of long-chain fatty acids). Accumulation of very long-chain or branch-chain fatty acids is a feature common to disorders classified as peroxisomal.

The Adrenoleukodystrophies

Neonatal adrenoleukodystrophy is characterized by onset in the newborn of demyelination, severe hypotonia, seizures, adrenal atrophy, and hepatic fibrosis. There is accumulation of very long-chain fatty acids, pipecolic aciduria, and an autosomal recessive mode of inheritance. X-linked adrenoleukodystrophy (which may cause Addison disease and cerebral sclerosis) is a progressive demyelinating disease of males beginning in childhood leading to dementia and adrenal insufficiency. The gene locus is Xq28 for the X-linked form.

Zellweger (Cerebrohepatorenal) Syndrome

This condition is usually lethal in early infancy and is characterized by gross defects in brain development, unusual facies, hypotonia, hepatic dysgenesis, renal cysts, respiratory problems, and cardiovascular anomalies. Chondral calcification, most marked in the patellar areas, is similar to that seen in Conradi syndrome. Five enzymatic defects have been found in Zellweger patients, including beta-oxidation (as in adrenoleukodystrophy) and phytanic acid oxidase (as in Refsum syndrome). The gene locus has been confirmed at 7q11.23.

Refsum Syndrome

The cardinal features of this syndrome are ataxia, chronic polyneuritis, retinitis pigmentosa, cardiac conduction defects, and deafness. Atrioventricular conduction may be completely blocked, requiring pacemaker im-

plantation. The defect is a phytanic oxidase deficiency of peroxisomes leading to accumulation of branch-chain phytanic acid, which is mainly obtained exogenously through foods containing phytol. A diet free of chlorophyll and related compounds and plasmapheresis produces clinical improvement.

POLYCYSTIC DISEASE OF KIDNEYS AND LIVER WITH CHILDHOOD ONSET[1,2]

There are several forms of childhood polycystic kidney disease with liver involvement, as well as the dominantly inherited adult form. These childhood types have been classified as the perinatal, neonatal, and infantile types and the juvenile group. They are not entirely family-specific.

The Perinatal Type. Children with the perinatal type present at birth with marked abdominal distension due to huge symmetric renal masses; they die within 6 weeks. There is cystic formation, appearing as longitudinal dilatation, of 90% of the renal tubules, and ectasia of the bile ducts with minimal periportal fibrosis. A "Potter's facies," with low-set floppy ears, micrognathia, and snub nose, is often present.

The Neonatal Type. In this group, the kidney enlargement becomes manifest within the first month of life, and death occurs within one year. The kidneys are entirely cystic, with over 60% of the tubules involved. In the liver there are several diffusely scattered cystic portal areas, and dilatation of all the intrahepatic bile ducts.

The Infantile Type. Children with the infantile type of polycystic disease of the kidneys usually present in the first 6 months with enlargement of the liver, with or without palpable enlargement of kidneys and/or spleen. They may present with signs of renal failure or portal hypertension. The kidneys are cystic with involvement of about 25% of the tubules, and the liver shows dilatation and infolding of the intrahepatic bile ducts and ductules with moderate periportal fibrosis.

The Juvenile Group. In this group, the child usually presents between 1 and 5 years of age with enlargement of the liver, spleen, and kidney. The clinical picture is that of portal obstruction. The liver is hard and finely mottled with biliary dilatation and infolding and marked biliary fibrosis. The kidneys show dilatation of about 10% of tubules or less.

PORPHYRIA, ERYTHROPOIETIC, CONGENITAL[2,4]

The hepatic porphyrias are inherited as dominant traits (see dominant diseases); the rare congenital erythropoietic porphyria is autosomal recessive. Burgundy-red urine is a constant finding. Splenomegaly and cutaneous mutilation are features. Onset is in infancy. The acute visceral and neurological attacks that characterize the hepatic forms are absent in this disorder. Another point of differentiation is that porphyrins are present in the erythrocytes of erythropoietic porphyria but not in hepatic porphyria. The defect is the conversion of porphobilinogen to uroporphyrinogen in the developing erythrocyte caused by a deficiency in uroporphyrinogen III synthase.

THE PREMATURE SENILITIES[2,3]

Cockayne Syndrome

Cockayne described this syndrome of senile appearance in sibs in 1946. Growth failure and loss of adipose tissue become apparent during late infancy. Cataracts, mental retardation, hearing loss, unsteady gait, retinal degeneration, marble epiphyses, and dermal photosensitivity are observed in a child who fails to grow and has the appearance of a "little, old man" (Fig. 8–55). There is no specific treatment other than supportive and symptomatic care for the syndromes of senile appearance of Cockayne, Werner, Rothmund, and Hutchinson-Gilford (progeria).

Poikiloderma Congenitale of Rothmund

Patients with this disorder of the skin and eyes may initially appear to have an ectodermal dysplasia or a disorder of senile appearance. Between 3 to 12 months of age the skin begins to show a marbled surface pattern pro-

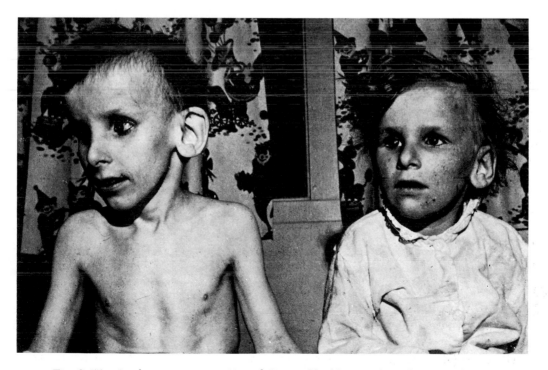

Fig. 8–55. Senile appearance in 10- and 7-year-old siblings with Cockayne syndrome.

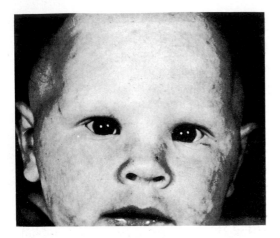

Fig. 8–56.   Alopecia and "marbled-skin" pattern in patient with Rothmund syndrome (age 6 years).

duced by an erythema that progresses to telangiectasia, scarring and atrophy (Fig. 8–56). Juvenile cataracts develop between 18 months and 10 years of age. The typical patient is short and has cataracts, sparse, prematurely gray hair, deficiencies of teeth, and dystrophy of the nails. The skin shows punctate areas of atrophy, telangiectasia, and hyperpigmentation.

Progeria (Hutchinson-Gilford Syndrome)

The autosomal recessive mode of inheritance of this rare syndrome is suspected from its occurrence in sibs, although family data are scarce. Some authors favor autosomal dominant inheritance, with most cases representing fresh mutations. As in Cockayne syndrome, the infant usually appears normal at birth, although there may be sclerodermatous skin and midfacial cyanosis, and it is not for several months to as long as 2 years that the suspicion of abnormal development occurs, often because of a progressive retardation in weight gain and growth. Unlike Cockayne syndrome, intelligence does not appear to be impaired. Baldness is early in onset. Growth reaches a plateau at about 18 months and the eventual height attainment may be that of a 5-year-old. There are loss of fat, periarticular fibrosis with joint-stiffening, and skeletal abnormalities, such as hypoplasia, dysplasia, and

a characteristic degeneration of the clavicle and distal phalanges (Fig. 8–57). Generalized atherosclerosis progresses from as early as 5 years of age to the time of death in the second decade, often of coronary artery disease.

Werner Syndrome

In this syndrome, the appearance of premature senility begins in young adult life, although the effects of the disease have had an earlier onset as manifested by moderate growth retardation with decreased height attainment. There is thin skin with loss of subcutaneous fat that is replaced by fibrous, thick subcutaneous tissue. Other findings include premature graying and balding, cataracts, atherosclerosis, osteoporosis, muscle hypoplasia, thin extremities, pinched face, reduced fertility, diabetes, and liver atrophy.

RETINITIS PIGMENTOSA (RP)[1,2]

This group of diseases results from degeneration of the retinal neuroepithelium with

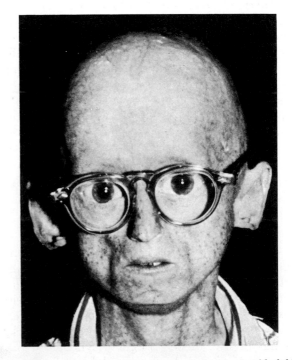

Fig. 8–57.   Appearance of advanced age in 15-year-old child with progeria.

progressive loss of rods and cones, beginning peripherally, and migration of pigment into the retina from the pigmented epithelium. This results in slowly progressive decreased night vision and restriction of visual fields, which may precede morphologic retinal changes. An electroretinogram and fluorescein angiography are diagnostically useful. There are three genetic types.

The *autosomal recessive* type is the most common, comprising about 80% of cases (if sporadic cases are included). Onset is in the first two decades, with severe visual loss by about the fifth decade or later.

The *autosomal dominant* form, RPI, appears in the first two decades, with milder symptoms and slower progression, with central vision preserved into the sixth or seventh decade. Incomplete penetrance has been reported in some families. The gene locus is 3q21-q24.

The *X-linked recessive forms* are the rarest and the most severe, with profound visual loss by the fourth decade. Female carriers may show retinal changes, but not always. Two separate RP loci have been described; RP2 is assigned to Xp11.3 and RP3 is at Xp21.

Because of the genetic heterogeneity, variable age of onset, and reduced penetrance, retinitis pigmentosa is one of the most difficult diseases for which to counsel. A sporadic case in a male, for example, may be an example of the X-linked type (check the female relatives), a new dominant mutation, dominant with reduced penetrance in a parent, or the autosomal recessive type. Estimation of recurrence risks should make use of the information provided by the pedigree and the relative frequencies of the three types.

SMITH-LEMLI-OPITZ SYNDROME[1,2]

The clinical features of this relatively common syndrome are growth deficiency of prenatal onset, failure to thrive, mental retardation, microcephaly, low-set ears, ptosis, broad nose with upturned nares, micrognathia, high palate, broad lateral palatine ridge, short neck, simian crease, flexed fingers, syndactyly between second and third toes, clubbed feet, and cryptorchism and/or hypospadias (Figs. 8–58

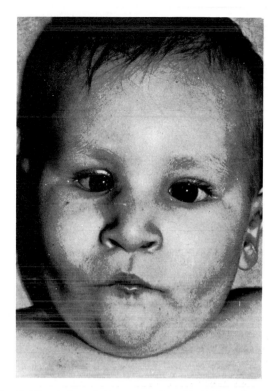

Fig. 8–58.   Anteverted nares, epicanthic folds and strabismus contribute to characteristic facies of Smith-Lemli-Opitz.

to 8–60). Other features sometimes found include breech birth, epicanthic folds, strabismus, cleft palate, heart defect, dysplasia epiphysialis punctata, and pyloric stenosis. Probably no one feature is always present.

Because of the poor prognostic outlook, one must be cautious neither to overdiagnose this syndrome in patients with syndactyly of the second and third toes and few other defects, nor to fail to recognize the associated anomalies leading to a diagnosis of Smith-Lemli-Opitz syndrome, with all that this implies.

THROMBOCYTOPENIA ABSENT RADIUS (TAR) SYNDROME[2]

The name of the syndrome reveals much of its content. It is distinguished from the Fanconi pancytopenic syndrome in that TAR selectively involves platelets, rather than extending to other blood cells, and is not accompanied by chromosomal breaks. An-

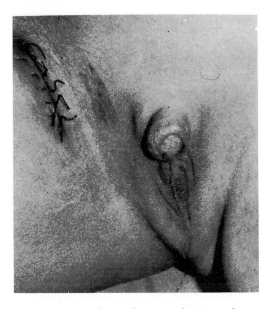

Fig. 8–59. Hypospadias and cryptorchism are features of Smith-Lemli-Opitz, and congenital heart disease is common (note stitches and incision of recent cardiac catheterization).

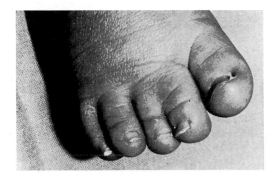

Fig. 8–60. Syndactyly between second and third toes is an important feature of Smith-Lemli-Opitz, but it is also found in otherwise normal individuals.

other point of differentiation is that the thumbs are normal in TAR (Fig. 8–61). Congenital heart disease, including atrial septal defect and tetralogy of Fallot, is found in about 30% of patients with TAR. Renal malformations are also found.

X-LINKED DISEASES

From the discussion of the Lyon hypothesis in Chapter 4, it would be expected that the heterozygote (female carrier) for a recessive X-linked single mutant gene would show variable manifestations of the mutant gene, depending on what proportion of her cells show the normal versus the mutant phenotype. In autosomal recessive diseases the heterozygote has approximately 50% of the normal gene product, which under normal circumstances is sufficient to prevent unfavorable manifestations of the mutant gene. This is quite a different matter from having about 50% mutant and 50% normal cells. Furthermore, the random inactivation of the X chromosome does not necessarily lead to 50% of the cells carrying the mutant gene being inactivated. Randomly, a 60 to 40, 75 to 25 or even 90 to 10 partition could occur. Under these circumstances, the "protective influence" of the normal gene product may be so diminished as to permit manifestations of the disease in the heterozygote. For instance, hemophilia A is a disease of males, but minor or occasionally major expression caused by Lyonizing may be found in some female carriers—presumably those in whom, by chance, a high proportion of the Xs carrying the normal allele were inactivated. Fundamental and clinical aspects of the Lyon hypothesis have been extensively investigated in G6PD deficiency, which will be discussed in Chapter 24.

The term *hemizygote* is used in the male to emphasize that the X and Y chromosomes do not represent homologous pairs as do the autosomes. An X-linked mutant gene that is transmitted as a recessive becomes manifest

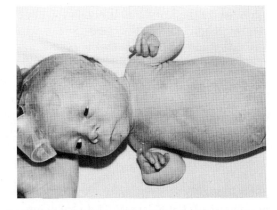

Fig. 8–61. Characteristic arm deformities in infant with TAR syndrome.

in the male because there is no "protection" from a homologous locus on the Y chromosome as there would be in an autosomal recessive.

As outlined in Chapter 5, on the average, an X-linked recessive disease, in the usual random-mating situation, is transmitted by the usually unaffected heterozygous carrier female to half of her sons. (The carrier state is transmitted to half of her daughters.) The affected male does not transmit the disease. All of his sons will be free of the disease, but *all* of his daughters will be carriers.

If the condition is lethal or causes sterility in affected males, it may be difficult to distinguish X-linked recessive inheritance from autosomal inheritance with expression of the heterozygous gene only in males (sex-limited inheritance), because there is no opportunity for male-to-male transmission. Lyonization in somatic cells or demonstration of linkage to an X chromosome locus are solutions.

The transmission of the X-linked dominant diseases is from the affected male to all of his daughters and none of his sons. The heterozygous female is, by definition, always affected in X-linked dominant diseases, but the disease is generally milder than in the affected male. Of her offspring, half would be affected irrespective of sex.

SEX-LIMITED AND SEX-CONTROLLED TRAITS

Certain genes that are present in both sexes act only in one sex. An example is milk-yield genes in cows. Beard growth, hair distribution, and possibly male-pattern baldness represent examples of **sex-limited traits** in humans.

The term *sex-controlled trait* is usually used in the context of multifactorial inheritance. Certain diseases affect one sex more than another, and it is presumed that the slight "environmental" difference provided by a difference in sex is sufficient to influence the threshold of a polygenic predisposition. Examples are the predominance of females with congenital dislocation of the hip, patent ductus arteriosus, and atrial septal defect; and the predominance of males with pyloric stenosis,

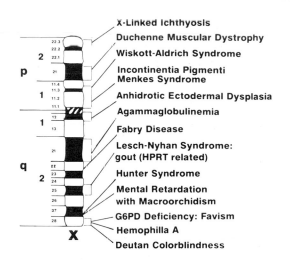

Fig. 8–62. A partial map of the X chromosome including the loci for some of the conditions discussed in this section.

coarctation of the aorta, and transposition of the great vessels.

X-LINKED RECESSIVE DISORDERS (Fig. 8–62)

Angiokeratoma, Diffuse (Fabry Disease)[3,4]

Small dark nodular lesions clustered in the umbilical area, around the buttocks, genitalia, and knees and on mucous membranes may first be noted in early childhood. Burning pain of the hands and feet associated with fever, heat, cold, or exercise is often the first symptom. Corneal opacities appear early. Progressive renal insufficiency is the critical feature and is usually responsible for the death of affected males in their thirties or forties. As in other X-linked recessive disorders, heterozygous females may be mildly affected. The biochemical defect is a deficiency of the enzyme alphagalactosidase A, which leads to a cellular accumulation of the glycophosphosphingolipids, trihexosyl and digalactosyl ceramide, in urine, plasma, and cultured fibroblasts. The carrier female has enzyme levels that fall between those of the affected male and the normal and may develop mild signs of the disease, including corneal opacities. Other findings in affected individuals may include seizures, diarrhea, hemoptysis, and nosebleeds. Renal transplantion may be beneficial. Prenatal diagnosis by enzyme assay in cultured amniotic fluid cells is possible. The gene locus is Xq22.

Diabetes Insipidus[2,4]

Two types of X-linked diabetes insipidus are known: nephrogenic and neurohypophyseal. An autosomal dominant neurohypophyseal type has also been recognized. In the nephrogenic form there is failure of renal tubular response to antidiuretic hormone (pitressin-resistant) in the male and partial defect in the female. Mental and physical retardation may occur, perhaps secondary to dehydration. Water replacement is necessary; thiazides may reduce urine flow. Partial impairment of concentration is present in some heterozygotes.

The neurohypophyseal type responds to pitressin and may follow an X-linked or occasionally an autosomal dominant pattern. Deficiency in hypothalamic nuclei has been demonstrated in some of these patients.

Ectodermal Dysplasia, Anhidrotic[2,3]

In addition to the defective hair, teeth, and sweat glands, there may be a saddle nose, frontal bossing, periorbital pigmentation, and sometimes deafness or mental retardation. The major findings are absence of teeth, hair, and sweat and mucous glands. Darwin described the "toothless men of Sind" in 1875, noting that a total of only 12 teeth was distributed among the 10 affected men in the Hindu family he observed.

Male patients with this disease suffer during hot weather because of their inability to sweat. Scalp and body hair is sparse, and complete baldness occurs early in life. They also may lack mucous glands in the upper respiratory system, a defect that increases susceptibility to infection. Some observers report a mosaic patch distribution of skin abnormalities in some mildly affected female carriers of this disorder.

Problems early in life from this disease are the not insignificant threat to life from hyperthermia and difficult respiratory infections, complicated by the absence of mucous glands. In later life, the alimentary and cosmetic problems are managed by false teeth and wigs.

The inability to sweat distinguishes this disorder clinically from the hidrotic ectodermal dysplasias that are mainly autosomal dominant. The gene locus is Xq11-q12.

Glucose 6-Phosphate Dehydrogenase (G6PD) Deficiency[2,4]

This disorder (gene locus Xq28) is one of the more informative genetic diseases. Because it also is one of the classic examples of a pharmacogenetic disease, it will be discussed in that chapter (Chap. 24).

Hemophilia A (Classic Hemophilia, AHG or Factor VIII Deficiency)[2,4]

Hemophilia shows X-linked recessive inheritance with transmission to affected males by usually asymptomatic carrier females who possess moderate to normal levels of antihemophilic globulin (AHG, factor VIII). The frequency is between 1:25,000 and 1:10,000 male births.

Clinically, the disease is characterized by recurrent episodes of bleeding that may develop spontaneously or following minor trauma. Bleeding into the joint spaces is characteristic, and repeated hemarthroses lead to thickening and destruction of articular surfaces, resulting in permanent crippling. Hemorrhage may develop in any area—mucosal, subcutaneous, intramuscular, retroperitoneal, or intraorgan. The disease may present following circumcision, although many babies have sufficient tissue thromboplastin to prevent bleeding from this procedure. Bleeding is a notorious sequel of dental extractions.

Clinical confirmation rests on demonstration of a prolonged clotting time and activated partial thromboplastin time, normal one-stage prothrombin time, and deficient factor VIII activity in the plasma. Capillary fragility and bleeding time are normal. Cross-reacting material (CRM)-positive and CRM-negative forms exist.

Treatment consists of local pressure, if possible, and temporary correction of the coagulative defect by transfusion of plasma or fractions of plasma rich in AHG. The development of concentrates of antihemophilic factor—frozen cryoprecipitates of AHG or lyophilized AHG-rich plasma fractions—has greatly simplified management and improved the outlook dramatically for hemophiliacs who formerly spent many months of childhood in hospitals. Special care for hemarthrosis to prevent permanent damage, administration of AHG before surgical procedures, and the encouragement of normal emotional and intellectual development are important aspects of medical care. Unfortunately, the benefits of AHG from human blood products have been accompanied by hepatitis and acquired immune deficiency syndrome (AIDS). With present methods of screening of donor blood, the risk of new cases of AIDS is being reduced as is hepatitis B—but non-A, non-B hepatitis cannot yet be detected. It is hoped that in the near future a recombinant DNA product will become an option.

Genetics. The gene for hemophilia A (clotting factor VIII:C) is a large segment, 186,000 nucleotides long, located at Xq28, where a number of other genes have been confirmed, such as G6PD and deutan color blindness. Recent advances in recombinant DNA technology have permitted informative carrier identification and prenatal diagnosis through the use of gene probes. The method is as follows: DNA from peripheral blood leukocytes of a potential carrier female and from affected family members are obtained to characterize patterns of restriction fragment length polymorphisms (RFLP). If the woman is heterozygous for one of the RFLP's (the DNA is cut by a restriction enzyme) and this pattern is found in an affected male, such information may be used to establish the carrier state in the female and the presence of an affected fetus. Chorionic villus sampling for fetal DNA provides first trimester diagnoses. Amniotic fluid cells may be used in the mid-trimester. Informative RFLP's may not be found in perhaps 10% of cases. In these situations, fetal plasma obtained by fetoscopy is an alternative.

Hemophilia B (Christmas Disease, PTC or Factor IX Deficiency)[2,4]

This disease, with the gene locus at Xq27.1-q27.2, is similar clinically to AHG deficiency and is $1/10$ to $1/5$ as frequent. Most cases have an immunologically detectable but inactive factor IX molecule (CRM positive), but there is also a CRM negative type. Mild and severe types exist. It is differentiated from classic hemophilia by the thromboplastin generation test, specific assay of factor IX activity and by gene probes (as in hemophilia A), which permit prenatal diagnosis. Treatment consists of concentrated specific PTC factor or banked plasma.

Ichthyosis (Steroid Sulfatase Deficiency)[2,4]

X-linked recessive, autosomal recessive and autosomal dominant forms of ichthyosis exist that may be distinguished not only by pedigree analysis, but by clinical presentation, course, and histological findings. The autosomal recessive form is the most severe, presenting at birth and often leading to death from sepsis of electrolyte imbalance in the first months of life. The X-linked form is also seen at birth, but is not as extensive, having a predilection for head, abdomen, and flexures. The dominant form (ichthyosis vulgaris), which is characterized histologically by epidermal atrophy, is not usually recognized for several months after birth and is most noticeable on palms and soles; throughout life it may be appreciated only as excessive dryness and shininess of the skin of the extremities. The X-linked form has histologic findings of hypertrophy of the epidermis and a more striking "fish-skin" appearance. Steroid sulfatase deficiency and X-linked ichthyosis illustrate the opposite of genetic heterogeneity—rather than one disease having more than one cause, that which was previously thought to be two diseases turns out to have the same cause.

The locus for X-linked ichthyosis is at Xpter-p22.32. Like Xg, this locus does not undergo Lyonization.

Kinky Hair Syndrome (Menkes Syndrome).[2,4]

This progressive brain disease, first recognized by Menkes in 1962, is characterized by pili torti, scorbutic changes in the metaphyses of the long bones, tortuosity of the cerebral and other arteries, which may lead to vascular occlusion, hypothermia, and death within 3 years, with progressive brain degeneration. The kinky hair, fragmentation of the internal elastic lamina in the arteries, and bone changes have recently been traced to a defect in the intestinal absorption of copper. The pili torti develops only after several weeks, and the disease may be more common than presently realized. At this time, there is a question as to whether the locus is at Xp11.4-p11.23 (tissue inhibitor of metalloproteinase) or at Xq12-q13.

Lesch-Nyhan Syndrome[3,4]

This disorder was first reported in 1964 by Lesch and Nyhan as a familial abnormality of uric acid metabolism and central nervous function. Self-mutilation, hyperuricemia, choreoathetosis, spastic cerebral palsy, and mental retardation are the major features. The patients described to date have been male. A deficiency of hypoxanthine-guanine phosphoribosyl-transferase and the demonstration of two populations of fibroblasts in heterozygous females (supporting the Lyon hypothesis) have been subsequently reported. The locus is assigned to Xq26-q27.2. A large number of specific point mutations (e.g., HPRT Chicago, HPRT New Haven) have been described.

Diagnostic Features and Clinical Course. The patient appears to be normal at birth, but during early infancy is observed to become hyperirritable and slow in motor development. Spasticity and choreoathetoid movements become apparent in late infancy. After teeth erupt, the patient begins to mutilate his lips and fingers by chewing them. Teeth-grinding, swinging of the arms, increasing spasticity, and mental and motor retardation are observed. Serum uric acid levels are greatly elevated. Hematuria and renal damage and failure may occur secondary to uric acid stones. Death in childhood following progressive neurologic and renal damage is common.

Treatment. Allopurinol to decrease uric acid levels. Restraints to deter self-mutilation.

Lowe Oculo-cerebro-renal Syndrome[1,2]

This syndrome of cataracts, hydrophthalmos, mental retardation, and renal tubular dysfunction was reported by Lowe and colleagues in 1952. Growth and mental development are poor. The patients are both hyperactive and hypotonic. Deep tendon reflexes are diminished. Congenital cataracts and frequently glaucoma are present (Fig. 8–63). The renal tubular dysfunction is characterized by poor ammonium production, hyperchloremic acidosis, phosphaturia with hypophosphatemia, aminoaciduria, and albuminuria. Osteoporosis and vitamin D-resistant rickets develop. Cryptorchism is common. These severe manifestations are confined to the male. The heterozygous carrier female may show some fine opacities of the lens, presumably reflecting the Lyon hypothesis and the results of random inactivation of X chromosomes. Renal insufficiency and dehydration are commonly responsible for death. Treatment with vitamin D and alkali and surgical attention to the ocular problems have been recommended. The gene locus is Xq25.

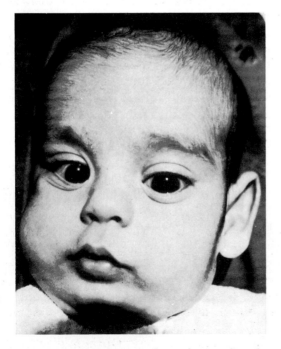

Fig. 8–63. Facies in Lowe oculo-cerebro-renal syndrome. The hydrophthalmos and cataracts may be seen in this photograph.

Mental Retardation, X-linked[2]

Mental retardation has many causes, genetic and environmental. There are nonspecific types, one at Xp22.3 and another in the region of Xq11-12. An additional hereditary, nonprogressive form associated with short stature and moderate microcephaly, is the Renpenning type. The fragile X syndrome was described in Chapter 4 because it is identified by a marker Xq27.3 chromosome produced by a mutation leading to abnormal methylation at the fragile site.

Mucopolysaccharidosis Type II A and B (Hunter Syndrome A and B)[2,4]

The autosomal recessive forms of mucopolysaccharidoses were discussed earlier. Hunter syndrome (see Fig. 8–64) has two allelic forms, a severe form (A) and a mild form (B). The enzyme defects are the same, sulfoiduronate

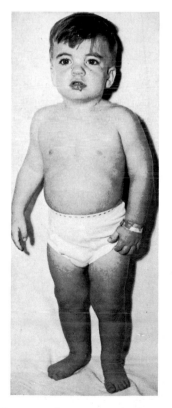

Fig. 8–64.   Hunter syndrome. Note the facies and the "claw hand."

sulfatase, and the urinary MPS excreted is dermatan sulfate and heparan sulfate.

Type A patients, although less severely affected than patients with Hurler syndrome, commonly do not survive beyond the teens. However, Type B patients may live into the fourth, fifth, and sixth decades. Mental retardation may be minimal or absent; we have investigated a type B family (Fig. 8–65), in which one affected individual was an engineer. The skeletal abnormality may not be as debilitating as in MPS I, but the features are similar—claw hand, stiff joints (Fig. 8–64). There is, however, no gibbus. The facies is coarse (gargoylism), and there is hepatosplenomegaly. Deafness is a more frequent and severe problem in MPS II than in the other diseases in this group, in all of which it may also occur. Metachromatic granules are found more readily in lymphocytes than in polymorphs and less readily in these patients than in patients with the Hurler syndrome.

A clinical differentiating point between MPS I and MPS II is the absence of corneal clouding in patients with the Hunter syndrome. However, retinal changes may occur and diminish or terminate vision. Heart disease is prominent in these patients and is similar to the cardiac disease in MPS I (coronary artery disease). A cardiac death is likely between the second and fifth decades. The prevalence is estimated at 1:200,000. The gene locus is Xq27.3.

Muscular Dystrophy[2,4]

The X-linked forms of muscular dystrophy are more frequently encountered than those in other genetic categories. The most common of the three X-linked forms is pseudohypertrophic muscular dystrophy (Duchenne type), and the less common are the tardive types of Becker and Dreifuss. Both autosomal recessive and dominant forms occur. The recessive forms were discussed earlier and the rare dominant forms may be found described in appropriate references.

The patient with the Duchenne muscular dystrophy (DMD) becomes symptomatic by the time he is 5 years old. The muscles, es-

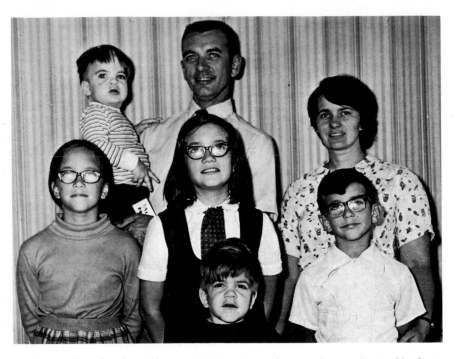

Fig. 8–65.   Family with two affected males with type II B Hunter syndrome, who may be readily distinguished from their siblings.

pecially of his lower limbs, appear to be unusually well-developed, yet he is weak and unable to walk well, pedal a tricycle, or climb stairs. From a sitting position on the floor, he characteristically "climbs up himself" (See Fig. 5–14). By the time the patient is 10 years old, he is usually confined to a chair, and death usually occurs before 20 years of age. The muscle of the heart, as well as skeletal muscle, is affected. Myocardial disease and congestive heart failure are observed. Mental retardation is present in about one third of the patients. Creatinuria accompanies the disease, and creatine phosphokinase (CPK or CK) is proving useful in the detection of female carriers, but levels tend to increase during pregnancy. The locus is Xp21.2 and the gene has been cloned, which permits prenatal diagnosis at some centers.

In Chapter 7, the molecular genetics of DMD are reviewed. In this section, we stress the clinical aspects of predictive and prenatal testing. First, one begins with the pedigree of a family under consideration. For carrier detection, creatine phosphokinase levels are obtained on three consecutive days. Although very high levels of CK are present not only in the patient with clinical DMD and in the preclinical state (e.g., the newborn), CK for carrier detection is less diagnostic. Not only is pregnancy a confounding variable, but exercise and concomitant illness may influence enzyme levels. Under optimal circumstances, CK testing will disclose 60% of female carriers. Bayesian probability calculations are often performed. Finally, in a comprehensive evaluation of a family, cDNA probes and DNA polymorphisms are used. In 50 to 70% of DMD males, gene deletions are identified to permit direct detection. Through a combination of predictive tests, risks may be substantially reduced in most families.

The tardive type of Becker is later in onset (twenties and thirties) and milder in course, permitting survival to more advanced ages.

In the tardive type of Dreifuss (also in gene locus Xp21.2), the onset may be as early as in the Duchenne type, but the progress is considerably slower, so that these patients may be gainfully employed. The shoulder-girdle musculature and the heart become involved, but there is no pseudohypertrophy. Flexion deformities of the elbows are characteristic.

Testicular Feminization Syndrome[2,4]

This syndrome offers an exception to the rule regarding chromosomal determination of phenotypic sex. Its biochemical basis is discussed in Chapter 11.

Patients with this syndrome are usually brought to medical attention as teenagers because of delay in menstruation, or the condition is discovered in early childhood because of "inguinal hernias" that are not hernias but testes in the inguinal canal. Further examination reveals a shortened vagina and the absence of uterus and adnexa. The buccal smear is negative, and the karyotype is that of a normal male: 46,XY. Hormonal assays are normal.

The familial transmission of the disorder fits the expectation for X-linked recessive inheritance. The locus is Xcen-q13.

Wiskott-Aldrich Syndrome[2,4]

This syndrome of eczema, thrombocytopenia, and frequent infections was described in three brothers by Wiskott in 1937. Aldrich defined the X-linked recessive mode of inheritance in 1954. Eczema and bloody diarrhea (with thrombocytopenia) are the usual manifestations early in infancy. Later in infancy, infections, particularly of the skin, middle ears, and lungs, become a more prominent problem. The immunologic deficiency is somewhat variable and may involve both cellular and humoral immunity. IgM and isohemagglutinins are usually diminished. Lymphopenia and thymic hypoplasia are often seen. Malignancies such as leukemia and lymphoma occur. Death is usual in infancy or early childhood. The locus is Xp11.

X-LINKED DOMINANT DISORDERS

Focal Dermal Hypoplasia (Goltz) Syndrome[1,2]

This syndrome appears to the X-linked dominant with lethality in the male. A diag-

nostic feature is atrophy of the skin that permits herniation of fat (Fig. 8–66). There may also be multiple papillomas of both skin and mucous membrane. Ocular anomalies include coloboma of the iris and choroid, strabismus, and microphthalmia. Digital anomalies, such as syndactyly, polydactyly, camptodactyly, and absence deformities, have been found. Cardiovascular anomalies in 5 to 10% of patients include aortic stenosis and atrial septal defect. The locus is Xp22.31.

Hypophosphatemic Rickets (Vitamin D-resistant Rickets)[3,4]

See Chapter 6 for more details. This X-linked dominant disorder is transmitted directly from an affected female to half of her sons and half of her daughters, and from an affected male to all of his daughters and to none of his sons. Affected females appear to have a somewhat milder form of the disease than males. The hypophosphatemia is secondary to diminished tubular resorption of phos-

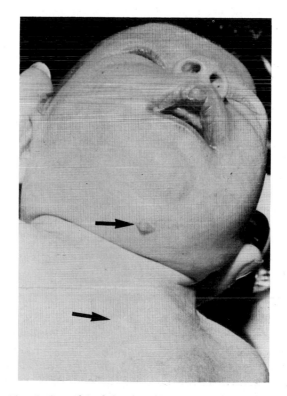

Fig. 8–66. Skin defects (arrows) in Goltz syndrome.

phorus and decreased gastrointestinal resorption of phosphorus and calcium. Growth in early infancy is normal until the serum phosphorus drops to a low level when the child is about 6 months of age. Clinical and radiographic evidence of rickets becomes gradually apparent (see Fig. 6–11). The lower limbs bow with weight bearing. Growth is slow, and ultimate height attainment is decreased. The gait may become waddling. Dolichocephaly, pseudofractures, and enamel hypoplasia are sometimes observed. Careful control of serum phosphorus levels may permit normal growth. The gene is assigned to Xp22.

Incontinentia Pigmenti[2,3]

This disorder, like OFD I, is thought to be X-linked dominant with lethality in the male. All patients are female, and there is a 2:1 ratio of liveborn females to males in affected families. The consistent feature is lesions of the skin, which may be vesicular, inflammatory, atrophic, or verrucous, but most characteristically are a "chocolate swirl ice cream" effect on the trunk and extremities (Fig. 8–67). Patchy alopecia, incomplete dentition with malformed teeth, strabismus, keratitis, cataracts, blue sclerae, syndactyly, hemivertebrae, microcephaly, and cardiac disease are frequent findings. Primary pulmonary hypertension leading to severe cor pulmonale may severely limit the life span. The skin lesions, which begin as inflammatory in appearance,

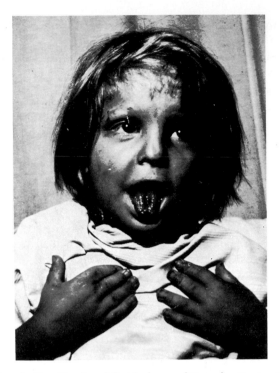

Fig. 8–68.   Hand and facial abnormalities of patient with orofaciodigital syndrome (OFD I).

progress through the "chocolate swirl" appearance, and are usually gone by 20 years of age. A serious problem for the affected individual is central nervous system involvement. About one third of the patients have varying degrees of mental retardation and spasticity; some have seizures. The counseling revolves around the specific clinical problems for the patient and the risks that may be anticipated for her future offspring: one-third affected females, one-third normal females, and one-third normal males. Gene localization is Xp11.

Orofaciodigital Syndrome (OFD I)[1,2]

This syndrome is found only in females. Pedigree analysis of their families has revealed an approximate 2:1 female to male ratio, suggesting that this disease is lethal in the male. The most reasonable explanation of the cause of the mode of inheritance is an X-linked dominant mutant gene. Because of lethality in the male, the genetic counseling risk is: two

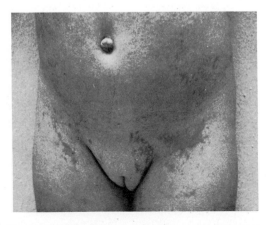

Fig. 8–67.   Skin lesions of incontinentia pigmenti.

thirds of the offspring of an affected mother will be female and one half of these females will be affected; the one third of the offspring who are live-born males will be normal.

Thus, the risks will be: one-third affected females, one-third normal females, and one-third males.

Diagnostic Features (Figs. 8–68, 8–69). *Oral.* Partial clefts in tongue, upper lip, alveolar ridge, palate. Irregularities of dentition (absence of teeth, supernumerary teeth). Webs between buccal mucosa and alveolar ridge. Hamartoma of tongue.

Facial. Laterally placed inner canthi, hypoplasia of alar cartilages, short philtrum, malar hypoplasia.

Digital. Asymmetric shortening of digits, some partial syndactyly, clinodactyly, and *unilateral* polydactyly.

Other. Moderate retardation, alopecia, and trembling.

Differential Diagnosis. *OFD II (Mohr syndrome).* This syndrome has many of the features of OFD I, but also has conductive hearing loss and bilateral polydactyly. OFD II is inherited as an autosomal recessive trait.

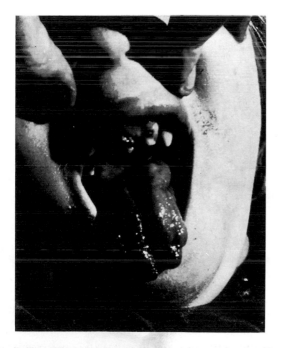

Fig. 8–69.   Close-up of cleft tongue and irregular dentition of patient with OFD I.

Contiguous Gene Syndromes

This term has been applied to a number of phenotypes caused by small deletions or duplications of chromosomes (e.g., Prader-Willi, Miller-Dieker, Langer-Giedion, retinoblastoma, Beckwith, Wilms, DiGeorge). Some of these syndromes are discussed in Chapter 3 (the deletions are illustrated) and some in Chapter 14.

Orphans

With each edition the chapter: Disorders and Syndromes of Undetermined Etiology has decreased in length as we have moved diseases from "undetermined" into established genetic and chromosomal categories. Because this is a textbook of genetics rather than a more general compendium of birth defects, those conditions from the previous editions that are still etiologic orphans will not be discussed.

REFERENCES

1. Birth Defects Encyclopedia. Ed.-in-Chief M.L. Buyse. New York, 1990.
2. McKusick, V.A.: Mendelian Inheritance in Man. 10th ed. Baltimore, Johns Hopkins University Press, 1992.
3. Nyhan, W.L. and Sakati, N.O.: Diagnostic Recognition of Genetic Disease. Philadelphia, Lea & Febiger, 1987.
4. Scriver, C.R. et al.: The Metabolic Basis of Inherited Disease, 6th ed. New York, McGraw-Hill, 1989.
5. Brook, J.D., et al.: Molecular basis of myotonic dystrophy: Expansion of a trinucleotide (CTG) repeat at the 3' end of a transcript encoding a protein kinase family member. Cell 68:799, 1992.
6. Fitch, N.: Classification and identification of inherited brachydactylies. J. Med. Genet. 16:36, 1979.
7. Huntington Disease Collaborative Research Group: A novel gene containing a trinucleotide repeat that is expanded and unstable on Huntington disease chromosomes. Cell 72:971, 1993.
8. Konigsmark, B.W. and Gorlin, R.J.: Genetic and Metabolic Deafness. Philadelphia, W.B. Saunders Co., 1976.
9. Nora, J.J., Berg, K. and Nora, A.H.: Cardiovascular Diseases: Genetics, Epidemiology, and Prevention. New York, Oxford University Press, 1991.
10. Rosenfeld, M.A., et al.: In vivo transfer of human cystic fibrosis transmembrane conductance regulator gene to the airway epithelium. Cell 68:143, 1992.
11. Spirio, L., et al.: A CA-repeat polymorphism close to the adenomatous polyposis coli (APC) gene offers improved diagnostic testing for familial APC. Am. J. Hum. Genet. 52:286, 1993.
12. Valle, D. and Gartner J.: Penetrating the peroxisome. Nature 361:682, 1993.

Chapter 9
Mapping the Human Genome

The process of finding the chromosomal locations of genes has come to be called *gene mapping*. Once the location of a gene on a chromosome is known approximately, its position can be determined precisely, in a process known as *positional cloning* (Chapter 7). Once a locus is found, the sequences of its usual and mutant alleles can be determined. Thus, mapping gene loci, and describing their DNA sequences, is in effect the description of the normal and morbid anatomy of the human genome.[17]

Interest in gene mapping dates from early in this century. Once Mendel's laws were rediscovered and chromosomes described, it rapidly became apparent that certain human traits, such as colorblindness, were transmitted on the X chromosome; that is, the traits exhibited *genetic linkage*. It came to be realized that it was possible in principle to identify persons carrying deleterious alleles from their genotypes at nearby polymorphic loci on the same chromosome. However, because only a few human polymorphisms were well characterized, it was not possible to make much use of genetic linkage in clinical and genetic counselling.

The efficiency of gene mapping has increased dramatically from approximately 1980 onwards, with the development of DNA technology (see Chap. 7). A gene can be mapped even when its product is not known (although knowledge of a gene's product may make gene mapping much easier), and then sequenced. Thus, it is possible to identify the product of a previously unidentified gene, and describe the fundamental defect in a previously unexplained single-gene disorder. Such information may lead to new, more rational therapies. In addition, gene mapping has the potential to identify loci influencing liability to common disorders. Thus, great interest and excitement surround gene mapping today. Figure 9–1 displays some of the disorders mapped to a single chromosome, in this case, chromosome 5. The morbid anatomy of all the human chromosomes is found in Appendix A.

OVERVIEW: THE USES OF GENE MAPPING

Diagnosis and Genetic Counseling

Chromosomal assortment during meiosis ordinarily ensures that a parent transmits half of their autosomal alleles, and those on one sex chromosome, to each offspring. This allows statements of genetic risk to be made, con-

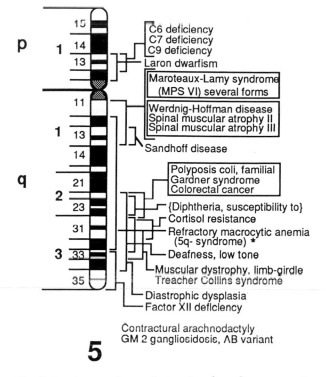

C6 deficiency
C7 deficiency
C9 deficiency
Laron dwarfism

Maroteaux-Lamy syndrome
(MPS VI) several forms

Werdnig-Hoffman disease
Spinal muscular atrophy II
Spinal muscular atrophy III

Sandhoff disease

Polyposis coli, familial
Gardner syndrome
Colorectal cancer

{Diphtheria, susceptibility to}
Cortisol resistance
Refractory macrocytic anemia
(5q- syndrome) *
Deafness, low tone
Muscular dystrophy, limb-girdle
Treacher Collins syndrome
Diastrophic dysplasia
Factor XII deficiency

Contractural arachnodactyly
GM 2 gangliosidosis, AB variant

Fig. 9–1. A map of gene loci assigned to chromosome 5.

sistent with Mendel's laws. For instance, on average half of the offspring of a heterozygote for an autosomal dominant disorder will inherit the mutant allele for the disorder.

Such a statement of risk may be less than satisfactory. In the case of an unborn child or of a gene causing an adult-onset disorder (see Chap. 28), it may be useful to know *definitely* whether a particular family member has inherited a deleterious allele.

For some single-gene conditions, prophylactic measures are available to avoid or delay the worst effects of the condition, which should not be applied to persons without the disease genotype. Familial adenomatous polyposis (FAP) provides an example. Persons at risk of this autosomal dominant condition can be screened endoscopically for adenomatous colonic polyps, and their colons can be removed before these become malignant. Endoscopy is an expensive and less-than-pleasant procedure. If applied to all persons at 50% risk, half are screened needlessly. Prophylactic colonectomy is clearly not appropriate for all persons at risk. Although the preclinical signs

of this condition (if detected) allow preventive measures to be started, if the disease genotypes of persons at risk of inheriting FAP were actually known, only those who actually had the disease allele would need to be screened. In fact, the chromosomal location of the FAP gene is known (it is on chromosome 5; see Fig. 9–1), from genetic linkage studies using DNA polymorphisms. It is possible to distinguish among persons at risk, between those with and those without the predisposing allele, and to restrict screening to the former.

The presymptomatic detection and management of some adult-onset single-gene conditions is less complex than that for FAP, and the prognosis less grim. However, for the majority, presymptomatic phenotypic diagnosis is not possible. Therefore the use of gene mapping techniques for presymptomatic diagnosis has a potentially wide application.

For many such disorders, therapy is not available, in which case some persons at risk may find presymptomatic diagnosis undesirable. It cannot prevent the effects, and the knowledge that they will develop the disorder may be unwelcome news. On the other hand, some persons who have inherited a disorder value an end to uncertainty about their risk, and persons who have not inherited a mutant allele may receive relief and reassurance from this information. Persons at risk, and their relatives, may desire presymptomatic diagnostic information to guide their reproductive decisions. Finally, depending on the nature of the condition, presymptomatic identification of persons with disease genotypes may be useful in developing and applying therapies to prevent or delay symptoms.

Dissecting Genetic Heterogeneity

Gene mapping may reveal that what has been taken to be a single clinical entity in fact results from mutations at different loci in different families. For example, the relatively uncommon form of autosomal dominant polycystic kidney disease (ADPKD) *not* caused by mutations at the PKD1 locus on chromosome 16 has a later onset and less rapid course than that due to PKD1 mutations. Such clinical variation is of immediate interest to affected persons and their families.[20] In addition, knowing that mutations at different loci can produce similar or identical structural or metabolic disorders is obviously relevant to understanding the pathogenesis of the disorder, and the normal function it disrupts.

Describing Loci and Mutations

If a gene can be located on a chromosome, its usual and mutant alleles can be sequenced, the function of its normal product determined, and the malfunction of mutant allele products ascertained. Such information may suggest therapies, or better therapies, for disorders caused by the mutant alleles.

When the gene product is known, the defective enzyme in inborn errors of metabolism for instance, it is possible to work backwards from the product, to find and describe the mutations that cause malfunction. However, for most single-gene disorders, the basic molecular defect is not known, and therefore gene mapping is, potentially, a source of valuable clinical insight. Examples of previously unknown genes causing common serious disorders, which have been found and characterized through gene mapping studies, include the CF locus, at which mutations cause cystic fibrosis,[22] and the DM locus, at which mutations cause myotonic dystrophy.[4]

When a locus is characterized in this way, it may become apparent that different mutations at the locus cause clinically distinct disorders. For instance, once the locus for Duchenne muscular dystrophy was sequenced, it was determined that the less severe Becker muscular dystrophy was allelic to Duchenne muscular dystrophy, being caused by mutations at the same locus.[29]

Once a locus is mapped and sequenced, it may be possible to construct diagnostic probes to detect common mutations at the locus, so that diagnosis by linkage analysis is no longer necessary.

Dissecting Multifactorial Liability to Disease

Sophisticated application of gene mapping techniques can reveal the genetic loci at which allelic variation influences liability to common disorders, for instance cardiovascular disease, psychoses, and diabetes. Such studies are just beginning, but will greatly increase our understanding of genetic variation in such liabilities, and, it is to be hoped, variation in response to treatment. These possibilities are further described later (see subsequent section entitled Genome anatomy and Dissecting Liability to Common Disorders), once methods of gene mapping have been set out.

METHODS OF GENE MAPPING

The positions of loci on chromosomes are determined in two basic ways. Genes can be mapped by analyzing coinheritance of phenotypes, information which reveals that the loci determining these phenotypes are near one another, on a chromosome. Such *genetic linkage analysis* is used to build up a *genetic linkage map*. Alternatively, various techniques can be used to determine the physical locations of specific genes and DNA sequences on chromosomes, and create a *physical map* of the genome. Physically mapping a gene requires knowledge of its product, or at least its DNA sequence. *Positional cloning* refers to the process of progressively refining information on the location of a gene, using linkage analysis and techniques of DNA manipulation, to find and sequence the locus (see also Chapter 7).

Genetic Linkage

Mendel's second law describes independent assortment: alleles at different loci should be inherited independently of one another. This is true for loci on different chromosomes. However, loci close together on the same chromosome tend to be inherited together, rather than independently, and are said to be *linked*. Therefore *alleles at linked loci tend to be inherited by offspring in the same combinations in which they occur in parents.* Linkage may be broken by *crossovers*, reciprocal exchanges of genetic material between homologous chromosomes, which occur during the formation of chiasmata during meiosis (Fig.

9–2). Chiasmata *recombine* the alleles at neighboring loci into nonparental combinations. The formation of chiasmata is a regular feature of meiosis, but if two loci are close together, a chiasma is unlikely to occur between them in any one meiosis, and the loci are said to be tightly linked. Loci farther apart on a chromosome are more loosely linked, because chiasmata are more likely to occur between them, and recombine the parental allele combinations. Loci may be *syntenic*, that is, located on the same chromosome but sufficiently far apart that they do not exhibit linkage.

An Example of Genetic Linkage

An example of the clinical application of genetic linkage information is useful at this point, to illustrate several basic principles.

Consider ADPKD, caused by mutations at the PKD1 locus. PKD1 is known to be on the short arm of chromosome 16. At the time of writing, PKD1 has not been sequenced, and PKD1 mutations cannot be detected directly. However, a region of hypervariable DNA (an HVR) has been identified 3′ to the α-globin gene cluster, and close enough to PKD1 to be used as a linked *genetic marker*, for following the inheritance of PKD1 alleles in families.[21] This 3′HVR, as its name suggests, has numerous alleles, which may be arbitrarily designated by letters. In the pedigree shown in Figure 9–3, marker allele A is coinherited with the PKD1 mutation that causes ADPKD in the family. A crossover between the two loci is not likely, so the fact that individual II.3 has inherited the A marker allele indicates that she has also inherited the ADPKD mutation. Although she is not yet affected, it must be expected that she will develop ADPKD if she lives long enough. Figure 9–3 includes diagrams of the allele combinations (often called **haplotypes**) on the chromosome 16 pairs of each pedigree member, to illustrate how marker and disease alleles are coinherited.

Note that:

1. It is possible to follow the inheritance of PKD1 alleles by observing the inheritance of the nearby 3′HVR marker al-

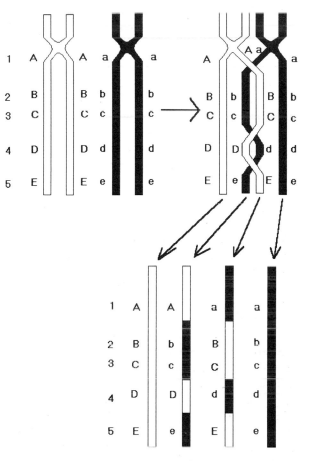

Fig. 9–2. When homologous chromosomes pair during meiosis, chiasmata may recombine parental allele combinations to produce recombinant as well as parental combinations in gametes. In this example, alleles at loci 2 and 3 have remained linked, whereas alleles at other loci exhibit recombination.

lele. The mutant PKD1 allele is inherited along with the A allele at the marker locus.

2. The marker is *informative*, i.e., useful in this process, because:
   A. it is polymorphic, so individuals are likely to be heterozygous for the marker, and
   B. the parent transmitting the PKD1 mutation is in fact heterozygous at the marker locus. If, for instance, I.1. were a BB homozygote, the 3′HVR marker would be *uninformative* because there would be no way of telling which of the identical B marker alleles was on the chromosome with the disease allele.

3. Family data are required to determine which marker allele is coinherited with the PKD1 mutation. The marker genotype of a single person does not reveal that person's disease genotype.

4. The marker allele is not the mutant allele, it is a marker for it, at a nearby locus. In different families, different marker alleles may be coinherited with the disease mutation. ADPKD could as easily be coinherited with B, for instance, or E.

5. For a polymorphic locus to be a useful marker, it must be close to the disease locus. Otherwise, crossovers may recombine marker and disease alleles and prevent accurate prediction. Recombination between PKD1 and the 3'HVR marker occurs in 5% of meioses; therefore this rate of prediction error is expected, using this marker.

Demonstrating Genetic Linkage

Now, the obvious question: How was it learned that the 3'HVR and PKD1 loci were linked?

Families in which ADPKD is being transmitted from generation to generation were typed for many polymorphic markers, and the data were then assessed to determine which, if any, marker alleles were co-inherited with ADPKD. Most markers were inherited independently of ADPKD, but it was observed that, in individual families, specific 3'HVR alleles tended strongly to be co-inherited with ADPKD phenotypes, and, by implication, normal and mutant PKD1 alleles. In short, genetic linkage is established by systematically analyzing the co-inheritance of alleles and the phenotypes they confer, in families.

Figure 9–4 illustrates the transmission of two markers and Huntington disease in a pedigree. One marker is linked to the disorder and the other not. (The figure also illustrates some of the predictive inferences about disease genotypes that can be drawn from linked marker genotypes, in a family.)

Units of Measurement. Because recombination between two loci becomes more likely

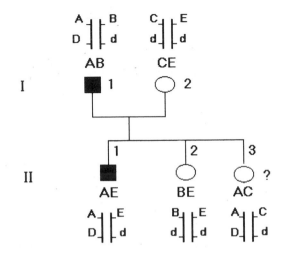

Fig. 9–3. Pedigree of family with polycystic kidney disease and marker alleles at the 3'HVR locus. See text.

the farther apart they are on a chromosome, the distance between loci on a genetic linkage map can be estimated from the rate of recombination between them. The rate of recombination, or *recombination fraction*, is symbolized θ. The unit of map distance is the centiMorgan (cM), which is equivalent to a recombination fraction of 1 in 100 meioses. For instance, between PKD1 and 3'HVR, $\theta = 0.05$; these loci are separated by 5 cM.

The total length of the human genome is estimated to be approximately 3300 cM. The total length of the haploid human genome is also estimated to be approximately 3 billion base pairs of DNA. Therefore one cM should be the equivalent of about 1 million bp. This is only approximate; in some regions of the genome recombination is relatively frequent (recombination "hot spots") and in others it is relatively infrequent. Also, in general, recombination is more frequent in female than male meioses, although this varies from chromosome to chromosome, and from region to region within individual chromosomes.[19]

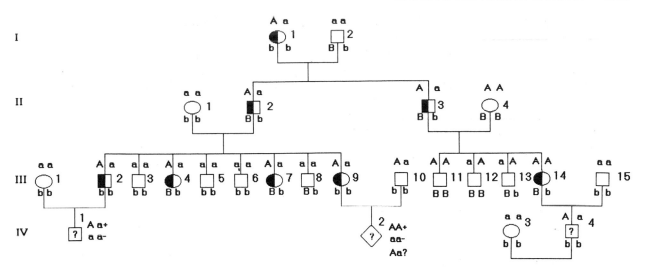

Fig. 9–4.   Pedigree of a family with Huntingdon disease showing the multiple tests and deductions often required to link markers and disease loci. Two polymorphisms have been typed, Aa and Bb. Is either linked to the Huntingdon disease locus? II.2 and II.3 inherited their affected mother's A allele and one of her b alleles, which suggests that the HD mutation was coinherited with A; b is uninformative. In the next generation, all six affected people have the A allele, and the six unaffected people have the a allele, which is strong evidence for linkage. The grandmother's b allele appears in both affected and unaffected individuals, so b is "exonerated." Once linkage has been established, it can be used for predictive testing. For example, one can now predict that only if IV.1 inherits A (and if no crossover occurs between A and HD) will he inherit the disease. The fetus IV.2 will almost certainly be affected if it is AA, and normal if it is aa. If it is Aa, it may or may not be affected: the A may have come from either parent. One would then have to find another, informative marker linked to HD, to predict the HD genotype. In some circumstances, one can make predictions about the offspring without knowing the status of the parent. In the case of IV.4, who is still young, we do not know whether he will be affected. If one of his future offspring were later found to be aa, however, we would know that it would be unaffected because it did not inherit an A allele from the grandmother.

Genetic Linkage Analysis

Determining that two loci are linked (except in very simple cases) requires complex calculations, which are ordinarily done using computer programs. Mapping the position of a locus on a chromosome requires much more extensive data organization and analysis. In addition, considerable effort is involved in data collection and marker genotyping. The standard reference on the topic, by Ott,[19] gives a very clear presentation of genetic linkage analysis. In a medical genetics textbook such as this one, it is only possible to set out the basic logic, in sufficient detail to serve as an aid to understanding references to genetic linkage in the medical literature.

The pedigree in Figure 9–5 shows the inheritance of a fully penetrant autosomal dominant condition and marker alleles at a polymorphic locus. This is the sort of pedigree that might be known to a primary care physician or specialist, collaborating in a study to map the locus for the disorder.

Note that the disease phenotype is coinherited with marker allele B. How do we decide whether the disease and marker loci are linked or not?

There are two possibilities to consider:

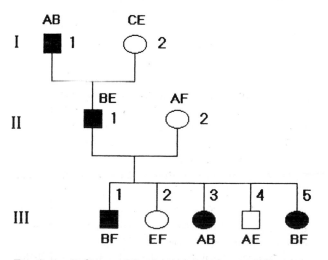

Fig. 9–5.   Pedigree of family with an autosomal dominant condition, and marker alleles at a polymorphic locus.

1. If the loci are linked, then the chromosome transmitted from I.1 to II.1 carries the disease allele and allele B at the marker locus.
2. The alternative to linkage is independent assortment. The two loci may not be linked, in which case the coinheritance of the disorder and B in this pedigree is a matter of chance.

Each of these alternatives could explain the observations. How do we rank their likelihoods, relative to one another?

The offspring of individual II.1 provide information to answer this question, because their genotypes reveal what has happened in five meioses, one for each offspring.

If marker and disease loci are linked, the coinheritance of disease with allele B and the nonaffected phenotype with allele E is exactly what is expected. Thus, *if the loci are linked,* the probability of this pedigree is 1.

If the loci are unlinked, each meiosis is an opportunity for recombination. The probability of recombination in a meiosis is 1/2. Therefore the probability that the disorder and allele B have been inherited together, and the usual allele and allele E have been inherited together, by chance, is $(1/2)^5$ or 1/32.

The probability of a set of observations, given some hypothesis, is called the *likelihood* of the observations.

For this pedigree, the ratio of the likelihoods of linkage *versus* independent assortment is:

$$1 : 1/32.$$

That is, on the evidence that this pedigree provides, marker and disease are 32 times more likely to be linked than assorting independently.

What if the pedigree were slightly different, as in Figure 9–6? On the hypothesis that marker allele B and the disease allele are linked, individual III.4 must represent a recombination event, the occurrence of a crossover between marker and disease loci in the meiosis between him and his father. One of the 5 meioses observed appears to be a recombinant, so the pedigree is most consistent with a recombination fraction of 0.2, or a dis-

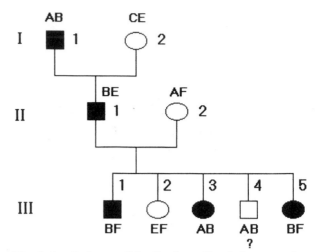

Fig. 9–6.   Pedigree of the family in Fig. 9–5, except that III-4 represents a crossover.

tance of 20 cM between loci. It can be calculated[19] that linkage at $\theta = 0.20$ is 2.6 times more likely than independent assortment, as an explanation for the pattern of inheritance of disease and marker alleles in the pedigree.

In the pedigrees in Figures 9–5 and 9–6, it can be specified which marker allele is on the chromosome carrying the disease allele, assuming that the two loci are linked, because the pedigrees extend over three generations, and we know the genotype and phenotype of I.1. This information about allele combinations on chromosomes is called the *phase* of linkage, and these are *phase-known* pedigrees.

It is usually difficult to obtain marker information on three generations of a family. However, the likelihoods of linkage and independent assortment can be calculated even though phase cannot be determined.

Consider the pedigree in Figure 9–7, which is simply the pedigree of Figure 9–6, without individuals I.1 and I.2. Lacking phase information, we must consider two possible ways in which the marker and disease alleles might be paired, shown in 5.a and 5.b. The disease allele could be on the same chromosome as marker allele B, in which case II.4 is a recombinant, or it could be on the same chromosome as marker allele E, in which case everyone in generation II *except* II.4 is a recombinant. In the absence of any other infor-

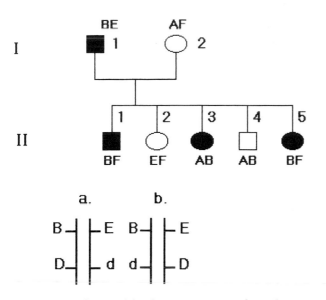

Fig. 9–7. Pedigree of family in Fig. 9–6, without the paternal grandparents.

mation, we must consider these two possibilities to be equally probable.

In the first case, recalling that θ symbolizes the recombination fraction, the probability of the pedigree is $\theta (1-\theta)$;[4] that is, the probability of one recombination times the probability of four nonrecombinants. In the second, it is $\theta^4 (1-\theta)$, the probability of four recombinants times the probability of one nonrecombinant. Because these possibilities are equally probable, their average value, the probability of linkage at distance θ in this pedigree is

$$1/2 \left[\theta (1-\theta)^4 + \theta^4 (1-\theta) \right],$$

Once again, this value may be compared with the probability of the pedigree, given independent assortment of marker and disease alleles. It can be calculated[19] that linkage at θ = 0.20 is 1.33 times as likely as independent assortment to explain the co-inheritance of disease and marker alleles in this pedigree. Note that this is consistent with a common-sense inspection of the data, which at least *suggests* that the disease genotype and allele B tend to be co-inherited.

By this point, it should begin to be apparent why linkage calculations are ordinarily done using computer programs, which can also take account of complications such as incomplete penetrance, variable age of onset (which makes the probability that an individual is a recombinant a function of his or her age), and unequal recombination frequencies in males and females.

Lod Scores. It is unlikely that any one pedigree will provide convincing evidence that two loci are linked, simply because it is usually not possible to assemble human pedigrees that include more than a few genotyped individuals in two or three generations. Therefore linkage between two loci is ordinarily demonstrated by combining information from a series of families.

For instance, data from 9 families were required to establish the PKD1 3'HVR linkage, and nearly 50 families were genotyped in detail, to position CF on chromosome 7.

The information from families is combined by calculating log odds, or *lod scores* (lods). A lod score is the $\log_{10}$ of the likelihood ratio: P (family | linkage) / P (family | independent assortment), that is, the probability of the family given linkage, divided by the probability of the family given independent assortment.

Lod scores can be added, allowing the information from different families to be combined.

Figure 9–8 shows a standard graphic presentation of linkage data. Lods are ordinarily calculated and plotted for a range of θ. The height of the curve above the abscissa gives the lod score for linkage, at various recombination fractions. Such curves can be plotted for individual families, and for the combined lods of linkage. Genetic heterogeneity is revealed when lod scores for one or more families are inconsistent with those of others.

What constitutes convincing evidence of linkage? By convention, a lod score of 3 (or greater) is accepted as demonstrating linkage. The literature almost invariably gives the impression that a lod score of 3 indicates a likelihood of linkage of 1000:1; this is not true, because tests for linkage, like any test based on probabilities, are expected to have some false-positive results. A lod score of 3 (or greater) has a probability of approximately 0.05

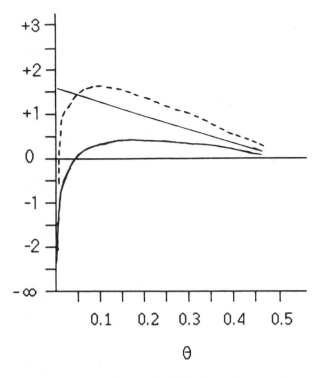

Fig. 9–8.   Curves showing lods for the pedigrees of Figures 9–5 (upper solid line) and 9–6 (lower solid line), and combined lods (dashed line) for values of θ from 0 to 0.5. Pedigree 9.5 is most consistent with θ = 0, and pedigree 9.6 with θ = 0.2.

(or less) of being due to chance.[9,19] This point is worth remembering, considering the large number of tests done in the process of mapping a disease locus, and the thousands of loci at which mutations can result in single-gene disorders. Conclusions of linkage based solely on a lod score of 3 will be in error far more often than one time in a thousand, and more convincing evidence of linkage is desirable.

If the cumulative lod score for two loci falls below −2, the loci are unlikely to be linked.

Ordering Loci

Genetic linkage data builds on itself, allowing the positions of loci to be mapped relative to one another. For instance, if θ = 0.05 for loci A and B, θ = 0.12 for loci B and C, and θ = 0.07 for loci A and C, this indicates that locus C is between A and B. This sort of logic is applied to order series of loci into linkage maps for chromosome regions, and, from these, to construct maps of entire chromosomes.

Reducing Error in Linkage Studies: Flanking Markers

Like any indirect prediction, predicting disease liability using linked markers is subject to error.

Obviously, if an individual possesses alleles at a marker locus, or at other loci, that cannot have come from his or her parents, either samples have been mixed up or parentage has been incorrectly attributed. Errors from such "technical" sources can be avoided without difficulty, by checking data before they are analyzed for linkage.

Recombination, however, is not preventable. Crossovers do occur, between marker and disease loci, at a rate that depends on the distance between them. Errors in prediction from this source can be avoided by genotyping *flanking markers*, lying on either side of the disease locus. This allows a crossover between the disease locus and one marker to be identified, so that the transmission of the disease allele can be followed despite the crossover. For a disease allele to become separated from both marker alleles, two crossovers must occur, one between the disease locus and each marker locus. This is highly unlikely, for reasonably close flanking markers.

Allelic Association

A mutation occurs on a specific chromosome. Therefore, for the first few generations after it occurs, copies of the mutation tend to be transmitted to offspring of the mutant individual in combination with whatever alleles were present at the other loci on that chromosome. As generations pass, crossovers will recombine the new allele and alleles at neighboring loci, and in time the probability that the mutant allele occurs in combination with any specific allele at a nearby locus should be a matter of chance.

For very closely linked loci, this process is slow, and *allelic association*, or *linkage disequilibrium*, is observed—the mutant allele occurs in combination with specific alleles at nearby loci more frequently than expected from the respective frequencies of the mutant and marker alleles.

Such allelic association can reveal the history of a mutation. From the frequencies of other alleles on the chromosome, in different populations in different parts of the world, it may be possible to infer where the mutation occurred. The strength of allelic association gives an indication of how long ago the mutation occurred.[2]

Allelic association can be put to practical use, since it allows disease genotypes to be predicted not from linkage analysis, but from the possession of a *specific* marker allele. It may be more convenient to test for the marker allele than for the mutant allele. Or, as is the case for prediction by genetic linkage analysis, the marker allele may identify loci at a gene that has not been characterized. For instance, the hemochromatosis allele is in linkage disequilibrium with the major histocompatibility (MHC) loci HLA-A3 and -B14, a fact that can be of use in identifying presymptomatic homozygotes.

Similarly, different 21-hydroxylase deficiency mutations are in linkage disequilibrium with alleles at MHC loci. MHC genotypes can be used to confirm diagnosis in atypical cases, including compound heterozygotes—persons possessing two different mutant alleles, among the collection responsible for this set of related conditions.

Linkage versus Mutation-Specific Probes

Once a gene and its disease-causing mutant alleles are sequenced, DNA probes can be synthesized that directly identify the mutant alleles. Compared to genetic linkage analysis, such probes might seem to provide a more efficient means of identifying persons with the mutant alleles. In practice, matters are not so straightforward.

For instance, over 200 CF-causing mutations have been described. In many European and North American populations, the most frequent of these, the ΔF508 mutation, accounts for about 70% of mutant alleles. Test-

ing couples for this mutation before they have children would detect only 49% of carrier couples. To detect 90% of mutations and 81% of carrier couples would require testing for several more mutations, and testing for dozens of mutations would be necessary, depending on their frequency in the population of interest, to detect directly 95% of mutations, and to directly identify 90% of carrier couples. Similarly, mutations causing Duchenne muscular dystrophy are numerous and varied, because the dystrophin gene is large, and therefore presents a big "target" for mutation. The same is true for hemophilia A and factor VIII mutations. These conditions have received particularly intense study precisely because they are relatively frequent. Among the thousands of single-gene disorders that are known, many others are likely to involve more than one mutation at the relevant locus, and it may be some time before mutations for rarer conditions are described. Therefore linkage analysis is likely to retain a prominent role in presymptomatic diagnosis of single-gene disorders.

DNA Marker Polymorphisms and a Complete Map of the Genome

The limiting factor in establishing the chromosomal positions of human genes is the availability of genetic markers. Linkage studies were originally undertaken using a few blood group and serum enzyme polymorphisms as markers, and were in a real sense "fishing expeditions", requiring considerable faith and perseverance.

Methods of manipulating and sequencing DNA have allowed an enormous increase in gene mapping activity by revealing extensive DNA sequence variation between individuals, and thus, in essence, providing thousands of marker loci. Also, DNA marker polymorphisms can be typed using standard techniques, rather than different techniques for each marker, making genetic linkage studies much more efficient. Most of the actual work of DNA typing can be done by automated machinery (see Chap. 7).

The chromosomal locations of over 2300 genes were known by late 1992,[7] and this number will continue to grow rapidly. However, considering that the human genome probably includes something like 100,000 loci, and that genes account for only perhaps 3% of its DNA, much gene mapping remains to be done.

A *complete map* of the genome of an organism is a set of DNA marker loci spaced fairly evenly along each chromosome, ideally only 1 or 2 cM apart. On such a map, the position of a locus can be sought systematically, allowing the task of mapping many thousands of loci to be approached efficiently.[3]

It is desirable that map marker loci have numerous alleles. This increases the proportion of the population that are heterozygotes, and thus the probability that recombination events can be detected in their offspring. The first DNA marker polymorphisms were restriction fragment length polymorphisms (RFLPs), which usually have only two alleles. Variable number tandem repeat polymorphisms (VNTRs) such as the 3'HVR mentioned above, are more useful, because they have numerous alleles. Particularly valuable are simple sequence repeats (SSR), which are highly polymorphic and seem to be widely and evenly scattered throughout the genome[27] (see Chap. 7).

The first comprehensive map of the human genome has appeared, with markers spaced, for the most part, at intervals of 15 cM or less.[18] It was rapidly followed by one with SSR markers spaced at, for the most part, 5 cM or less.[28] In view of the rapid technical advances being made in gene mapping, and the resources being devoted to this activity, a highly detailed map of the human genome can be expected within a few years.[23]

PHYSICAL MAPPING

Physical mapping is the process of determining the chromosomal positions of loci by physical means, as opposed to inference from pedigrees. This can be done in several ways.

Somatic Cell Genetics

It is possible to construct somatic cell hybrids, by fusing human and rodent cells. These hybrid cells can be maintained in cell culture, but, over time, gradually lose most of their human chromosomes. Panels of these hybrid cell lines can be assembled, each retaining a different human chromosome. If a particular human trait is expressed by one of these hybrid cell lines, it follows that the gene that determines this trait is on one of the human chromosomes in that cell line. This line of inference allowed many genes to be mapped in the 1970s and 80s. Such hybrid cells can be made from human cells containing translocations and chromosome fragments, allowing genes and marker polymorphisms to be localized to particular regions of chromosomes[24] (see Chap. 20).

In Situ Hybridization

DNA probes can be made radioactive, or fluorescent, and hybridized to the DNA of chromosomes. This allows the locations of the chromosome sequences complementary to the probe sequence to be observed microscopically, with high precision[10] (Fig. 9–9, see also Chap. 2).

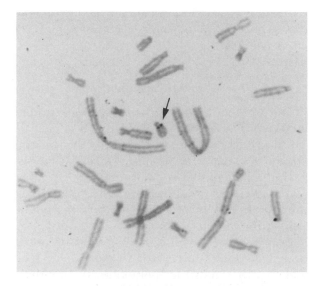

Fig. 9–9.   Arrow indicates site of hybridization. Probe is a 300 kb YAC containing NH 3053, mapping to q12.3.

Expressed Sequence Tags

A particularly efficient way of physically mapping genes begins by making cDNA from the mRNA of tissues such as brain, in which many genes are expressed. Automated machinery allows segments of this cDNA to be sequenced rapidly, and compared to sequences of known genes. A unique DNA sequence obtained from expressed DNA in this way serves in effect as a "tag" for the gene from which it is derived, an *expressed sequence tag* (EST). An EST can be used to construct a probe for in situ hybridization, to determine the chromosomal location of its gene. ESTs provide a rapid means of finding and characterizing previously undescribed genes, and therefore are potentially extremely useful for physical mapping. Because this approach focuses on genes rather than random DNA variation, it is likely to have a central role in gene mapping efforts.[1]

SEQUENCING THE HUMAN GENOME

Since 1986, great interest has been shown in obtaining the complete sequence of the human genome. This is an exciting idea, but is basically inefficient, considering that genes make up so little of the complete sequence of the genome. Interest has therefore shifted to techniques for finding and mapping genes more directly (see Expressed Sequence Tags, previous section).

It is possible to maintain sections of genomic DNA several hundred kilobases, or even several megabases in length, using yeast artificial chromosomes (YACs),[5] or related technologies. An ordered library of the genome, consisting of a few thousand YAC clones covering the entire genome, is a useful intermediate step between mapping individual loci and sequencing the genome from one end to the other. Such libraries will play a central role in the eventual sequencing the entire genome.[23] Until then, large-fragment libraries will allow genes of interest to be positioned quickly and sequenced along with neighboring DNA. Genes tend to occur in clusters or families that have evolved together, and gene

expression is often controlled by DNA sequences nearby, so it seems likely that much can be learned by sequencing outwards from loci of interest.

POSITIONAL CLONING: ACTUALLY FINDING GENES

(See also Chapter 7, Molecular Genetics)

"Finding" a "disease" gene, that is, determining the precise chromosomal position and usual sequence of a locus at which mutations cause a recognizable single-gene disorder, and then sequencing the mutant alleles that render its function aberrant, requires a combination of linkage analysis, DNA technology, cytogenetics and some luck.

Genetic linkage gives only a very approximate idea of a gene's location. Genes average a few thousand bases in length. In contrast, estimates of θ have confidence intervals of a few cM, that is, a few million bases.

As described previously (in Demonstrating Genetic Linkage), a locus at which mutations cause a single-gene disorder is positioned on the genetic linkage map by studying a collection of pedigrees in which the disorder is being transmitted. Once linkage to one marker is found, these pedigrees can be used to identify other nearby markers, including flanking markers. The aim is to find marker polymorphisms progressively nearer (more tightly linked) to the disease locus.

Closer markers are found by screening DNA libraries for clones that include the first marker as well as markers found subsequently. Eventually, it is possible to proceed by brute force, finding and sequencing overlapping DNA clones until the relevant gene is found and sequenced. This is tedious, because it implies proceeding along millions of bases in steps of a few thousand bases. Numerous techniques are available, using YACs for instance, to manipulate tens or hundreds of thousands of bases, and speed up progress from markers to the gene.

During this process of closing in on a gene, it is necessary to check for conserved DNA sequences of the sorts found near the start of genes, and coding sequences actually within genes. Not surprisingly, considering the expanses of DNA to be traversed, it is possible to stumble onto genes other than the one actually being sought, as well as much normal sequence variation. Therefore, as genes are found, sequences from individuals with and without the disease under investigation are compared, to determine whether a gene is indeed the one mutated in the disease. Once the relevant gene is found, the sequences of disease-causing mutant alleles can be described.

The preceding paragraphs give only a general outline of the process of positional cloning; strategies, tactics and details have differed, for the different human genes actually found to date.

As genes and their surrounding DNA sequences are explored, fascinating information is emerging about the nature of the DNA sequences that control gene function, and about previously unsuspected attributes of DNA. For instance, it has been observed that the mutation causing myotonic dystrophy not only occurs in the 3′ untranslated region of the gene, but is unstable. The mutation actually increases in length from generation to generation, with corresponding increasing severity of the disease phenotype.[4] This progressive increase in severity had been previously observed, and called *anticipation*. However, until its biologic basis was discovered, anticipation seemed best explained as an artifact, resulting from systematic biases in the ascertainment of families with disorders with variable age of onset, such as myotonic dystrophy. There was no evidence to suggest that a mutation could actually change over time. (The great majority of mutations are stable, and do not change over time, but unstable mutations do account for at least four other single-gene disorders, including the fragile-X syndrome and Huntington disease.)

GENOME ANATOMY AND DISSECTING LIABILITY TO COMMON DISORDERS

A complete map of the human genome makes it easier to search for loci that influence liability to common diseases and disorders, such as cardiovascular disease, mental and behavioral disorders, and common congenital malformations. As discussed (Chapter 12), liability to such conditions is familial, but they do not follow Mendelian patterns of inheritance. Numerous loci and environmental factors probably influence variation in liability for each condition. Identifying the alleles that confer liability might suggest therapies, or environmental exposures that could be avoided, to protect some or all persons at risk.

In effect, by knowing the anatomy of the genome, we can hope to "dissect" variation in liability to common disorders.

Common disorders can be divided into those for which the physiologic basis of liability is not well understood and those for which liability is better understood. The latter group includes some disorders for which liability may result from extreme values of some underlying quantitative attribute, and it is easiest to begin by considering such traits.

Quantitative Trait Loci

Extreme values of quantitative traits may be unhealthy. For instance, the genetic control of variation in blood pressure is of great practical interest, because hypertension is a frequent risk factor for cardiovascular disease. Can we identify the loci at which allelic variation influences variation in blood pressure, and risk of hypertension?

The genetics of hypertension has been studied in rats, taking advantage of the availability of a complete map of the rat genome. Rats from a hypertensive strain were crossed with rats from a normotensive strain, and then, in the offspring of these hybrids, the coinheritance of blood pressure and the marker alleles of the map was observed. Patterns of coinheritance of marker alleles and blood pressure indicated that a locus on rat chromosome 10 has a large role in determining blood pressure variation in these animals. There is extensive homology between rat chromosome 10, human chromosome 17, and rat, mouse, and human genes. This made it possible to demonstrate that the rat chromosome 10 locus with such a large effect on blood pressure differences between strains is the locus coding for angiotensin converting enzyme (ACE).[11,13]

The relevance of this finding to human hypertension is not yet clear. ACE-inhibiting drugs are effective in controlling hypertension, but in sarcoid (an inflammatory disorder), ACE levels are often much elevated, yet blood pressure is not. Needless to say, the relation between ACE polymorphism and circulating ACE levels in normotensive and hypertensive humans is under active investigation.[26]

Less Well-explained Conditions

For some common disorders psychiatric disorders are a particularly good example—the physiologic basis of liability is obscure. In such circumstances, the finding that a phenotype of disorder is coinherited with a genetic marker would provide strong evidence that allelic variation at a single locus influences liability.

Such studies have, to date, produced confusing results.[8] For both schizophrenia and bipolar affective disorder, familial aggregation of affected individuals is found, but is not consistent with single-gene inheritance. Nevertheless, it appears that, in some families, these might be single-gene disorders. For bipolar affective disorder, a linkage study of an extensive Amish pedigree at first gave evidence for a disease locus on the short arm of chromosome 11. However, when more family members were studied, the relevant lod scores fell from large positive values, approximately +5, to even larger negative values of −7 to −9.[14] Similarly, for schizophrenia a linkage study of seven families gave evidence of a liability locus on the long arm of chromosome 5, but subsequent studies have not confirmed this linkage.[6]

Several factors, alone or in combination, may explain such discordant results. It is likely that these common psychiatric conditions are etiologically heterogeneous, if for no other reason than that they occur frequently. Both conditions are difficult to diagnose, schizophrenia notoriously so. The genetic and environmental determinants of liability may be different in different populations. In particular, if there are indeed single-gene forms of schizophrenia or bipolar affective disorder susceptibility, these may be different in different populations.

Linkage analysis must incorporate some specific assumption about the mode of inheritance of the disorder being analyzed. In particular, linkage analysis is highly sensitive to any misdiagnosis of an individual as affected with a disorder versus not affected. After all, such a person represents a recombination! Undetected heterogeneity in liability for any reason—diagnostic error in either direction, or the presence of two genetic forms of a condition in a family—will confound linkage analysis.

In principle, genetic linkage strategies using a complete map allow genetic heterogeneity to be demonstrated.[10] Now that a reasonably complete map is available, such strategies are being applied to assess genetic variation in liability to psychoses and other common disorders.

Redefining Phenotypes: Dissecting Heterogeneity and Candidate Genes

Genetic studies of common disorders proceed in conjunction with other investigations aimed at clarifying liability.

For instance, if patients with a certain disorder respond to a particular drug, the metabolic basis of this response is relevant to liability to their condition. If some but not all patients respond, this difference may reflect allelic variation at a single locus (as many differences in drug response do; see Chap. 24, Pharmacogenetics). Genetic studies, including linkage studies, may provide clearer results if restricted to the families of individuals who show the drug response; the role of the gene in explaining at least a proportion of cases can be explored. In a similar way, if a disorder includes a range of signs, it may prove informative to restrict linkage studies to a proportion of cases showing particular signs. In effect, as pharmacologic or symptomatic differences are found, they can be used to identify etiologic heterogeneity. Genetic studies can then assess groups of families in which liability is similar.

For most common disorders, *candidate genes* can be identified, which may be suspected to influence liability. For instance, the ACE locus is an obvious candidate gene, in investigating variation in blood pressure. Genes coding for neurotransmitters and dopamine receptors are candidates in assessing liability to psychiatric disorders, and genes for growth factors in assessing liability to congenital malformations.

If it can reasonably be hypothesized that a particular gene is a candidate gene, allelic variation at which may influence liability to some condition, it may be possible to identify coding sequences in that gene, variation at which will influence the structure or expression of the protein produced by the gene. Probes for such sequences can be made: then, using PCR techniques, unrelated patients can be screened to determine whether the sequence variation is in fact associated with the occurrence of the condition. If an association is found, genetic linkage and epidemiologic studies can determine the extent to which variation at the locus influences liability variation in individuals, families, and the population as a whole. Such an approach is attractive, for instance, to determine whether allelic variation of the numerous dopamine receptor genes is associated with schizophrenia.[25]

If liability can be characterized closer to the level of gene action, previously indistinguishable disease phenotypes can be identified; in effect, genetic heterogeneity identifies new disease subclasses, and, it is to be hoped, points the way to more specific therapeutics.

ETHICAL ISSUES

Gene mapping is seen as having considerable commercial potential. As a result, genes are being mapped much more rapidly than therapies are being developed for the disorders that genomic information predicts.

The possibility of identifying individuals who are liable to develop disorders for which treatment is unsatisfactory or non-existent, before symptoms occur, is a cause for concern. As noted at the beginning of this chapter, for some single-gene disorders presymptomatic identification of persons at risk gives an opportunity to forestall the disorder. However, this is far from being the case for all single-gene disorders, including many that are extremely distressing. Persons at risk should not have to know their genotypes if they do not want to, nor should they be denied this information. Genotype information should be confidential. There is considerable risk that the availability of such genotypic information can result in genetic discrimination, including the denial of insurance or employment.[12]

The use of genotype information to predict liability to common disorders presents even more complex problems, because variation in liability is complex. Take risk of cardiovascular disease (see Chap. 23) as an example. Cardiovascular disease is the commonest cause of premature death in many populations. Most members of these populations (and their insurers and employers) will be interested in their liability profiles, and their genotypes at loci that influence variation in risk.

Single-gene conditions may greatly influence risk. The relatively small proportion of families in which LDL receptor defects are inherited, for instance, must be distinguished from others. For the rest of the population, it is important to recognize that while alleles follow Mendel's laws, these common disorders do not. Genes are not destiny. Specific alleles may influence risk, or even be necessary for disease to occur, but may not always produce disease. As is the case with some single-gene disorders, there may be straightforward ways of avoiding disease, regardless of genotype, by altering lifestyle. On the other hand, it is equally important to recognize that some individuals will be genetically unable to alter risk by environmental means, to lower their serum cholesterol levels by altering their diet, for instance.

Genetic variation in human populations, particularly variation that affects liability to common diseases, is not readily alterable, and is likely to be a consequence of natural selection (Chap. 10). The possibility of identifying individuals with high genetic liability to various disorders will create the danger of identifying a genetic "underclass." By way of illustration, a complete map of the dog genome is being constructed, with the goal of finding genes for such behavioral traits as aggressiveness, and presumably docility and loyalty. Positively nightmarish human scenarios are only too easy to construct. Efforts to map the human genome must be accompanied by extensive consideration of the implications, personal and societal, of the information that will be produced.[15]

SUMMARY

1. The approximate position of a gene on a chromosome can be mapped using genetic linkage analysis or physical mapping techniques. The gene can then be precisely located and its DNA sequence determined by positional cloning.
2. Genetic linkage analysis makes use of the fact that if loci are close together on a chromosome, the alleles at those loci tend to be transmitted to offspring in the same combinations in which they occur in parents. Alleles at loci close to another locus at which mutations cause a single-gene disorder, can be used as genetic markers to indicate which individuals at risk have actually inherited the mutant allele.
3. Physical mapping is the process of determining the chromosomal positions of loci by physical means. In situ hybridization involves using mRNA coding for a protein of interest to construct a labelled DNA probe, which can hybridize onto the complementary chromosomal DNA, revealing the location of the gene for the protein. A gene may also be localized to a chromosome by demonstrating its product in human-rodent hybrid cells containing only one human chromosome.
4. Positional cloning involves the combined application of genetic linkage analysis and physical mapping techniques to close in on and sequence a locus of interest. Once the locus is found, it can be determined whether specific mutations at the locus confer a specific phenotype, such as a single-gene disorder.
5. Work is in progress to clone the human genome into an ordered library of DNA segments, maintained in yeast artificial chromosomes (YACs). Such libraries will greatly facilitate mapping individual genes.
6. A comprehensive map of the human genome, that is, a set of relatively closely spaced markers covering each chromosome, has been constructed. A complete map, made up of more closely spaced markers, will greatly increase the efficiency of genetic linkage analysis by allowing a systematic search for markers linked to any locus of interest.
7. Using a complete map of the genome, it is possible to find loci at which allelic variation influences quantitative traits, for instance blood pressure, and to find loci which influence liability to disorders of complex inheritance, such as psychoses.
8. In investigating the physiologic basis of common familial disorders, it is often possible to identify candidate genes, at which allelic variation is suspected to influence liability to the disorder. By following the inheritance of candidate gene alleles and disease phenotypes in families, the influence of the alleles on liability can be measured, allowing mechanisms of disease to be better understood.
9. Genes influencing disease liability are being mapped much more rapidly than therapies can be developed for genetic disorders or common disorders with a genetic predisposition. Therefore the ethical implications of gene mapping require careful consideration.

REFERENCES

1. Adams, M.D., Kelley, J.M., Gocayne, J.D., et al.: Complementary DNA sequencing: Expressed sequence tags and Human Genome Project. Science 252:1651, 1991.
2. Arnason, A., Larsen, B., Marshall, W.H., et al.: Very close linkage between HLA-B and Bf inferred from allelic association. Nature 268:527, 1977.

3. Botstein, D., White, R.L., Skolnick, M., et al.: Construction of a genetic linkage map in man using restriction fragment length polymorphisms. Am. J. Hum. Genet. 32:314, 1980.

4. Brook, J.D., McCurrach, M.E., Harley, H.G., et al.: Molecular basis of myotonic dystrophy: expansion of a trinucleotide (CTG) repeat at the 3' end of a transcript encoding a protein kinase family member. Cell 68:799, 1992.

5. Burke, D.T., Carle, G.F. and Olson, M.V.: Cloning of large segments of exogenous DNA into yeast by means of artificial chromosome vectors. Science 236:806, 1987.

6. Byerley, W.F.: Schizophrenia: Genetic linkage revisited. Nature 340:340, 1989.

7. Chipperfield, M., Pearson, P., Gilna, P., et al.: Advances in human gene mapping. Science 258:87, 1992.

8. Ciaranello, R.D. and Ciaranello, A.L.: Genetics of major psychiatric disorders. Annu. Rev. Med. 42:151, 1991.

9. Edwards, J.H.: The linkage detection problem. Ann. Hum. Genet. 54:253, 1990.

10. Ferguson-Smith, M.A.: Invited editorial: Putting the genetics back into cytogenetics. Am. J. Hum. Genet. 48:179, 1991.

11. Hilbert, P., Lindpainter, K., Beckmann, J.S., et al.: Chromosomal mapping of two genetic loci associated with blood-pressure regulation in hereditary hypertensive rats. Nature 353:521, 1991.

12. Holtzman, N.A. and Rothstein, M.A.: Invited editorial: Eugenics and genetic discrimination. Am. J. Hum. Genet. 50:457, 1992.

13. Jacob, H.J., Lindpainter, K., Lincoln, S.E., et al.: Genetic mapping of a gene causing hypertension in the stroke-prone spontaneously hypertensive rat. Cell 67:213, 1991.

14. Kelsoe, J.R., Ginns, E.I., Egeland, J.A., et al.: Reevaluation of the linkage relationship between chromosome 11p loci and the gene for bipolar affective disorder in the Old Order Amish. Nature 342:238, 1989.

15. Kevles, D.J. and Hood, L.: The code of codes. Scientific and social issues in the Human Genome Project. Cambridge, MA, Harvard University Press, 1992.

16. Lander, E.S.: Splitting schizophrenia. Nature 336:105, 1988.

17. McKusick, V.A.: Mapping and sequencing the human genome. N. Engl. J. Med. 320:910, 1989.

18. NIH/CEPH Collaborative Mapping Group: A comprehensive genetic linkage map of the human genome. Science 258:67, 1992.

19. Ott, J.: Analysis of human genetic linkage. ed. 2. Baltimore, The Johns Hopkins University Press, 1991.

20. Parfrey, P.S., Bear, J.C., Morgan, J., et al: The diagnosis and prognosis of autosomal dominant polycystic kidney disease. N. Engl. J. Med. 323:1085, 1990.

21. Reeders, S.T., Breuning, M.H., Davies, K.E., et al.: A highly polymorphic DNA marker linked to adult polycystic kidney disease on chromosome 16. Nature 317:542, 1985.

22. Riordan, J.R., Rommens, J.M., Kerem, B-.S., et al.: Identification of the cystic fibrosis gene: Cloning and characterization of complementary DNA. Science 245:1066, 1989.

23. Roberts, L.: Two chromosomes down, 22 to go. Science 258:28, 1992.

24. Ruddle, F.H.: A new era in mammalian gene mapping: Somatic cell genetics and recombinant DNA methodologies. Nature 294:115, 1981.

25. Sobell, J.L., Heston, L.L. and Sommer, S.S.: Delineation of genetic predisposition to multifactorial disease: a general approach on the threshold of feasibility. Genomics 12:1, 1992.

26. Tiret, L., Rigat, B., Visvikis, S., et al.: Evidence, from combined segregation and linkage analysis, that a variant of the angiotensin I-converting enzyme (ACE) gene controls plasma ACE levels. Am. J. Hum. Genet. 51:197, 1992.

27. Weber, J.L. and May, P.E.: Abundant class of human DNA polymorphisms which can be typed using the polymerase chain reaction. Am. J. Hum. Genet. 44:388, 1989.

28. Weissenbach, J., Gyapay, G., Dib, C., et al.: A second-generation linkage map of the human genome. Nature 359:794, 1992.

29. Worton, R.G. and Thompson, M.W.: Genetics of Duchenne muscular dystrophy. Annu. Rev. Genet. 22:601, 1988.

Chapter *10*
Genetic Variation in Human Populations

THE LIVING AND THE DEAD, THINGS ANIMATE AND INANIMATE, WE DWELLERS IN THIS WORLD AND
THIS WORLD WHEREIN WE DWELL, ARE BOUND ALIKE BY PHYSICAL AND MATHEMATICAL LAW.

D'ARCY W. THOMPSON

Beyond the direct impact of genetic disorders on individuals and families, genetic variation in health has broad social and economic implications.

As has been stated (Chapter 1), the health care costs attributable to deleterious genes are considerable. In developing countries, genetic disorders emerge as a health care issue once morbidity and mortality from malnutrition and infectious disease are reduced.[23] In wealthy countries, the costs of health care and health insurance are disturbingly high. Therefore, it has seemed to many observers that the frequency of genetic disorders should be brought under control, even if this requires discouraging the reproduction of affected individuals.[14] We shall see that such ideas are misguided.

Moreover, the "burden" of genetic disease may seem to be worsening. Medical advances improve the chances that some persons with inherited disorders will survive and pass on their mutant alleles to their offspring (relaxed selection). Increasing exposure to environmental mutagens—radiation and toxic chem-

icals—can increase the frequency of deleterious mutations. How concerned should we be about such changes?

To address specific concerns about changes in the frequency of deleterious alleles, we must first consider, in a more general way, the influences that determine allele frequencies in populations.

HARDY-WEINBERG EQUILIBRIUM

Concern about a possible increase in the frequency of hereditary disease is not new. Indeed, it was probably stronger early in this century, when most hereditary disorders were untreatable, and the only option for avoiding their effects seemed to be preventing reproduction of affected individuals.

Shortly after Mendel's laws were rediscovered, G.H. Hardy, a prominent English mathematician, was presented with the seemingly reasonable proposition that brachydactyly (see Chap. 8) should in time come to affect three quarters of the population because of its autosomal dominant pattern of inheritance. Hardy recognized that this is not true, and published the correct relation between allele and genotype frequencies in populations. W. Weinberg, a German physician, had described this relation a short time earlier.

Hardy-Weinberg equilibrium, the fundamental theorem of population genetics, is a statement of the unsurprising fact that *in the absence of influences changing them, allele and genotype frequencies will remain constant from generation to generation.*

Consider a locus at which two alleles occur. Call them D and d, and assume that their frequencies in the population are p and q, respectively. For concreteness, let p = 0.99 and q = 0.01, and assume that dd homozygotes have an autosomal recessive disorder. The (haploid) gametes produced by the members of this population will be of two sorts, those carrying D and those carrying d, and must also occur with frequencies p and q. If these gametes combine at random to form zygotes, then the frequencies of the genotypes in the next generation are determined by the frequencies of D and d gametes. DD homozygotes occur in frequency p^2, and dd homozygotes in frequency q^2, whereas Dd heterozygotes occur in frequency 2pq, because a zygote can be heterozygous in two ways, by either combining a D sperm with a d ovum or vice versa.

This relation between allele and genotype frequencies is immediately useful in medical genetics. For instance in this example the disease frequency (the frequency of dd homozygotes), symbolized by q^2, will be

$$0.01 \times 0.01 = 0.0001,$$

or 1/10,000.

Conversely, if the disease frequency is known, the gene frequency can be calculated by taking its square root. The frequency of carriers or Dd heterozygotes is:

$$2pq$$
$$= 2\,(0.01)\,(0.99)$$
$$= 0.0198,$$

about 1/50, and nearly 200 times the frequency of affected individuals.

Such calculations guide the planning of carrier screening programs, when it must be known whether carriers are frequent enough to make screening an entire population worthwhile. Knowing population carrier frequencies is also important in advising families about recurrence risks for recessive disorders; an example is given in Chapter 5.

Figure 10–1 illustrates how allele and genotype frequencies are related in a random-mating population.

With a little algebra, it can be shown that a population consisting of individuals with DD, Dd, and dd genotypes in frequencies p^2, 2pq, and q^2 will produce D and d gametes in frequencies p and q, and that the allele and genotype frequencies will therefore remain con-

The relation between allele and genotype frequencies: examples.

If p = 0.5 and q = 0.5.

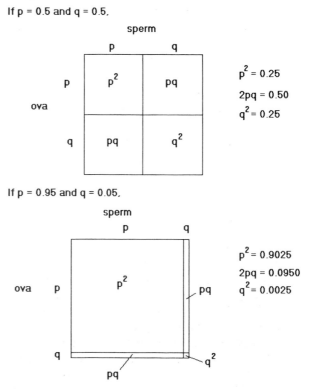

$$p^2 = 0.25$$
$$2pq = 0.50$$
$$q^2 = 0.25$$

If p = 0.95 and q = 0.05.

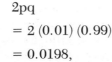

$$p^2 = 0.9025$$
$$2pq = 0.0950$$
$$q^2 = 0.0025$$

Fig. 10–1. Examples of the relation between allele and genotype frequencies. Allele frequencies determine genotype frequencies.

stant from generation to generation if not perturbed.

INFLUENCES THAT CAN ALTER ALLELE FREQUENCIES

Although allele frequencies do not change in the absence of influences changing them, such influences certainly operate.

Mutation can change the DNA sequence of a gene, transforming it into a new allele. *Selection* can act against certain phenotypes, so that individuals of different genotypes are not equally likely to survive and transmit their alleles to offspring. *Nonrandom mating* may change allele frequencies; that is, populations or groups of individuals can come to have different allele frequencies if their members mate preferentially with one another, and avoid mating with members of other groups. If a population is small, allele frequencies may fluctuate by *chance*, in the sample of gametes that is transmitted between generations. Finally, allele frequencies in a population can be altered by *in-migration* of individuals from a population with different allele frequencies, or differential *out-migration* of individuals whose genotypes are not representative.

Each of these influences can affect the prevalence of genetic disorders in human populations, and can contribute to population differences in the prevalence of a given single-gene disorder.

Mutation

A *mutation* is a permanent change in the genetic material. This may be an alteration of a single base in the DNA sequence, a more complicated change in DNA, such as an insertion or deletion of a base sequence, a gene duplication event that provides new material for evolution, or a change in chromosome structure or number. Here, we shall consider gene mutations in the DNA that alter messenger RNA, and thus the sequence, and potentially the function, of the polypeptide coded for by the mutated gene.

Most mutations are deleterious, and many mutations manifest as genetic disease. DNA sequence variations (single base changes) are about 9 times as common outside coding regions as within them, indicating that many mutations must be incompatible with survival to birth. This is hardly surprising; the genome represents instructions for the complex processes of cellular and organic growth and function. Random changes in such instructions are not likely to be helpful, in the same way that throwing a monkey wrench into a running motor would hardly ever improve its function. Highly developed cellular mechanisms of DNA repair exist, to maintain the genome without change; this is why, in the context of this chapter, we emphasize that "mutation" refers to a permanent change in DNA.

Mutations at any given locus are rare. The rate of mutations that produce a distinctive, autosomal dominant phenotype can be estimated by counting the numbers of persons with the phenotype born to unaffected parents. Each such individual arises from two gametes, only one of which has mutated to produce the phenotype. Therefore the mutation rate (m) can be estimated as twice the frequency of affected newborns with unaffected parents. For example, using this method the achondroplasia mutation rate has been estimated as 1.4×10^{-5}, from the observation of 7 new mutant cases among 242,257 births.

Mutations are the ultimate source of new alleles, and a mutation represents a change in allele frequencies.

Although mutation at any one locus is a rare event, the human genome is estimated to contain on the order of 100,000 loci, so there is ample opportunity for mutation to occur. There is extensive genetic variation in human populations, producing extensive phenotypic variation in, for instance, physical attributes such as size and skin color, and metabolic attributes such as immunologic responses and efficiency at utilizing nutrients. It is to the population's advantage to have a reservoir of genetic and consequently phenotypic variation among its members; such variation tends to ensure that at least some population members can adapt to changing environmental conditions.[8] In this way, genetic variation is allowing evolution to take place, so in a general sense mutation is beneficial to the species as a whole.

Selection and Biologic Fitness

In the context of health and disease, *selection* is the most obvious of the influences on allele frequencies.

Many mutant alleles manifest in patients—persons with an inherited disease, or deformity. These people may have less chance of passing on their genes than others, or perhaps no chance at all of reproducing. Their mutant alleles are therefore less likely to be transmitted to offspring than the alleles of unaffected persons. The *biologic fitness* of affected individuals is reduced, and *selection* is acting to reduce the frequency of the disease alleles in subsequent generations.

For instance, in one classic study it was found that the biologic fitness of individuals with achondroplasia was 0.196; that is, they had only about one fifth as many offspring as their unaffected sibs.

Biologic fitness can change dramatically if a therapy is found for a disorder, as, for instance, in the case of phenylketonuria (PKU) (Chapter 6). In a similar way, biologic fitness can change if social attitudes change: if, for instance, unusual physical appearance becomes less of an obstacle to mating. The biologic fitness of persons with achondroplasia has greatly increased in the course of this century.

Biologic fitness is an attribute of phenotypes, not of individual alleles. Clinically serious, even inevitably fatal conditions may cause little reduction in biologic fitness. For example, without treatment autosomal dominant polycystic kidney disease (ADPKD) will progress to cause death from renal failure. However, this rarely occurs before middle age, by which time most individuals with a mutant allele have completed their families and transmitted the ADPKD allele to half their chil-

dren, on average. The population frequency of ADPKD is unusually high for an autosomal dominant disorder, at least 1/2500, although the mutation rate is not,[9] presumably because ADPKD reduces biologic fitness only slightly.

Similarly, selection against the alleles for autosomal recessive disorders is small. Many autosomal recessive disorders are fatal in infancy or childhood, and the biologic fitness of affected homozygotes is therefore zero. This does not translate into strong selection against the disease allele because the great majority of mutant alleles are found in unaffected heterozygotes.

Mutation-selection Balance

If the frequency of a single-gene disorder is not changing, it must reflect a balance between the rate at which mutation generates alleles for the disorder and selection removes them. This suggests a simple way of estimating mutation rates.

For example, for an autosomal recessive condition that is *reproductively lethal*, causing infertility or death before reproductive age, the loss of affected homozygotes' mutant alleles should be balanced by new mutations. Thus, the mutation rate should equal the disease incidence. Many autosomal recessive disorders occur at frequencies consistent with such a *mutation-selection balance*, but there are interesting exceptions, which require us to reconsider our concepts of genetic disease.

Heterozygote Advantage

In some European populations, and North American populations of European descent, cystic fibrosis affects 1/3000 births or more. The biologic fitness of affected individuals was, until recently, close to 0, so in principle, a mutation rate of 1/3000 would be required to maintain the frequency of the disease. This value is improbably large, compared to direct estimates of mutation rates (see Mutation, above).

Hb S, the variant hemoglobin allele responsible for sickle cell disease, provides an even more striking example. Sickle cell disease is usually prereproductively lethal, yet rates of Hb S homozygosity reach 1% in West Africa, implying an equivalent mutation rate. Heterozygotes for the Hb S allele are relatively resistant to *falciparum* malaria infection, and hence more likely to transmit their genes to offspring than homozygotes for the normal, Hb A allele. This *heterozygote advantage* in fitness can explain the high frequency of the Hb S allele. Heterozygotes are about 20 times as frequent as homozygotes, and the increase in their fitness counterbalances the loss of alleles through the much-reduced fitness of homozygotes.

Heterozygote advantage may also explain the frequency of cystic fibrosis (CF) and other autosomal recessive disorders which are relatively common in Europeans, such as PKU. A 1.7% increase in fitness of CF heterozygotes, compared to homozygotes for the non-CF allele, would be sufficient to account for the frequency of the CF allele. In practice, such a small difference in fitness would not be measurable.

Further evidence for heterozygote advantage may come to light as DNA sequences of normal and mutant alleles, and nearby DNA variation, are documented. Studies of PKU, hemoglobinopathies, and CF show that a few mutation events have produced most of the mutant alleles responsible for these disorders. This is consistent with heterozygote advantage increasing the frequency of the mutant allele. If high mutant allele frequencies reflected extremely high mutation rates, many different mutations would be observed at the DNA level. If all mutant alleles were copies of a single mutation, this would suggest that the mutant allele had become frequent by chance at some point in prehistory when human populations were much smaller and chance fluctuations of allele frequencies were more probable (see next section).

From this discussion of heterozygote advantage, it should be apparent that the occurrence of single-gene disorders must be considered from the perspective of the overall fitness of the population, as well as the ill health of affected persons.

Population Genetic Isolation and Subdivision

Hardy-Weinberg equilibrium is really a statement of probabilities. If a population is large, and its members mate without reference to their genotypes, the laws of chance determine that gametes will combine to produce succeeding generations of offspring in which allele and genotype frequencies are unchanged. However, for most of its existence the human species has been divided into populations that were not "large." Tribes, settlements, and villages often numbered no more than a few dozen individuals, of whom only a portion were in their reproductive years and able to transmit alleles to offspring. Nor is the human species a single, random-mating population today. People tend strongly to choose mates from their own or nearby communities, even in densely populated industrialized countries where travel is not difficult. In all human societies, mating choices depend strongly on the geographic proximity of potential mates, which if nothing else determines whether they (or their families, in societies with arranged marriages) know of each other's existence.

Thus, the species is not one population, but is divided and subdivided into many populations, within which individuals tend to be related to one another, and between which some degree of *genetic isolation* occurs. Genetic isolation may increase with geographic distance between two populations, becoming progressively greater the farther apart the populations are. Bodies of water, mountain ranges, and other obstacles may act as barriers to population contacts and exchanges of mates. Some populations are *genetic isolates*, with little genetic exchange with other populations.[5]

Influences other than geography constrain mating choice. Where members of different races or ethnic groups live in the same area, people tend strongly to choose mates from within their own groups. Language differences are strong barriers to genetic exchange, as are social class, education, and religion. This general tendency to nonrandom mating gives human populations *genetic structure*.

Population genetic structure influences the geographic distribution of alleles, and causes populations to differ in allele and genotype frequencies. The influences on allele frequencies discussed earlier, mutation and selection, are direct: a mutation is a specific change at a locus, and selection occurs when there is a difference in fitness between genotypes. In contrast, nonrandom mating usually influences allele frequencies indirectly, because mating choices are usually determined by factors other than health and disease. However, the tendency to nonrandom mating affects all individuals and all loci, while mutation at any given locus is rare, and selective forces on most alleles are rather weak. Therefore it transpires that the indirect influences of population genetic structure account for much of the variation found among human groups in the frequencies of alleles and genetic diseases.

Genetic Drift and Founder Effect. Consider a locus at which two alleles, A and a, occur at equal frequencies. In a population with 1000 births per year, we would not expect the frequency of the two alleles to change from generation to generation, for the same reason that we would expect a coin tossed 2000 times to come up heads half the time and tails half the time.

However, in a population with only 10 births per year, allele frequencies might fluctuate from generation to generation by chance, in the same way that tossing a coin 20 times might well give something other than 10 heads and 10 tails. *Genetic drift* is the name given this random, or chance fluctuation of allele frequencies over time in a small population, because the "sample" of genes passed from one generation to the next is small.

Founder effect is a specific type of genetic drift. Some human populations are descended from a small number of founding individuals. An allele may occur in such a population at either an unusually high or low frequency because it was present in an unusually high or low frequency in these founders.

There are many examples of single-gene disorders occurring with unusual frequencies in human populations because of this founder effect. For instance, the Afrikaner population

of South Africa, which now numbers about 2.5 million, is largely descended from a few hundred persons who migrated there before 1700 from what is now Holland. Huntington disease, porphyria variegata, and lipoid proteinosis are all relatively frequent among Afrikaners. A well-documented instance of founder effect in a religious isolate is the high incidence of Ellis-Van Creveld syndrome among the Old-Order Amish of Lancaster County, Pennsylvania.

It is worth emphasizing that the founder effect may also produce an absence of single-gene disorders relatively common in other populations. Good examples come from Finland. A number of distinctively "Finnish" disorders, extremely rare or unknown in other parts of the world, have been described. On the other hand, disorders such as PKU and CF, which are relatively common elsewhere in Europe, are extremely rare in the Finnish population.

Genetic Isolation and Homozygosity. Genetic isolation is, in effect, a tendency for individuals to choose mates within their own population rather than outside. Because members of a genetic isolate tend to be consanguineous, one consequence of genetic isolation is increased homozygosity in population members. This has been termed random inbreeding, to distinguish it from the deliberate avoidance or choice of known biologic relatives as mates, which may be termed nonrandom inbreeding.

Random inbreeding acts to increase the incidence of recessive disorders in genetic isolates, and makes apparent the elevated frequencies of deleterious alleles in the population's "genetic heritage." For instance, the allele for tyrosinemia was introduced into the French Canadian population by a couple who migrated to New France around 1650. In this traditionally Roman Catholic population, closely consanguineous marriages were strongly avoided, and the parents of affected infants are found to be distantly rather than closely consanguineous. Indeed, the avoidance of consanguineous matings may act to delay the appearance of recessive traits in an isolate (see Autosomal recessive inheritance, pp 75ff).

Genetic Exchange Between Populations. When individuals mate with members of populations other than their own, alleles are transferred between populations. Such *genetic exchange* counteracts genetic isolation, and acts to reduce or eliminate population differences in allele frequencies.

The gradual flow of alleles between neighboring populations may produce a gradation in the frequency of an allele over distance, called a *cline*. A good example is the gradual increase in the frequency of the B allele of the ABO blood group system from west to east across Europe, attributable to the flow of B alleles from higher-frequency Asian populations. The wide distribution of variant globin alleles in the populations of Europe, Asia, Africa, and the Pacific has resulted from the gradual flow of advantageous alleles outwards from the locations where mutations first produced them.

OUR CHANGING ALLELE FREQUENCIES

Having considered the influences that determine the frequencies of alleles in populations, it is possible to assess how these frequencies may be changing, particularly the frequencies of alleles responsible for single-gene disorders.

Mutagenesis

In 1927, H. J. Muller showed for the first time that an environmental agent, x-rays, could cause mutations in Drosophila; in due course he received the Nobel Prize for this work. Since then, many physical and chemical agents have been found to be mutagenic. In industrialized societies, many human activities increase exposure to mutagenic agents—the use of x-rays and radioactive chemicals in medical diagnosis and industry, the use of nuclear energy to generate electricity, the testing of atomic weapons, and the widespread use of certain chemicals synthesized for a variety of purposes. Reasonably, concern arises that such activities may be increasing the mutation rate in germline cells, and consequently the prevalence of genetic disorders.

Demonstrating an effect of such human activities on the germline mutation rate, let alone any resulting change in the prevalence of genetic disorders, is extremely difficult if not impossible. The great majority of mutations are undoubtedly lost, unobserved, before birth or indeed before implantation occurs; therefore substantial changes in the mutation rate may go undetected. Also, a proportion of the background, or "spontaneous," mutation rate presumably results from radiation and chemical exposures that occur naturally, are not attributable to specific human activities, and are not readily avoidable.

Ionizing Radiation. The use of atomic bombs in World War II, and the prolonged period of nuclear-based national defense that followed, stimulated a great deal of research on the mutagenic effects of ionizing radiation in humans and other organisms.

Estimates of genetic radiation risk are expressed in terms of the *doubling dose*, the "amount of acute or chronic radiation that will produce the same mutational impact on a population as occurs spontaneously in each generation." All types of mutations are included, from point mutations to changes in chromosome number, so that the doubling dose estimate gives a comprehensible, socially relevant indication of expected total morbidity and mortality. Consideration is limited to a single generation because the effects of mutations that are not immediately lethal may occur over many generations.[18]

Long-term studies of the survivors of the atomic bomb attacks on Japan indicate that the doubling dose for humans is at least 1.69 sieverts* for acute exposure to radiation, and suggest that the doubling dose is at least 3.38 sieverts for chronic exposure. For comparison, it has been estimated that the average radiation exposure of US residents is 3.6 *milli*sieverts,[1] and that of UK residents 2.5 *mil*-

*The sievert is a unit of radiation dose equivalence used to measure exposures to mixtures of radiation of different types. One sievert equals the dose in grays multiplied by a quality factor which weights for the relative effectiveness of different types of radiation at damaging a biologic system. For example, for x-rays, 1 gray = 1 sievert; for fast neutrons, 1 gray = 10 sieverts. (One gray equals 100 rad.)

*li*sieverts.[13] Therefore it seems unlikely that exposure to the ionizing radiation that results from human activities is having an appreciable effect on the rate of genetic disease by increasing the mutation rate. Nevertheless, unnecessary radiation exposure must be avoided because it is known that radiation exposure increases the risk of cancer by increasing the mutation rate in somatic cells.

Chemical Mutagens. In tests on experimental organisms, tens of thousands of chemical compounds have been shown to be actually or potentially capable of causing germline mutations. These include compounds synthesized for a wide variety of purposes, and naturally occurring compounds including some found in common foods. In addition to causing chemical changes in DNA, mutagens may also increase the frequency of mutant genes by inhibiting DNA repair enzymes.

To assess fully the dangers of human exposure to such mutagens is impossible. As is the case for radiation exposure, it is not known how much of the "background" mutation rate is attributable to naturally occurring chemical mutagens. It cannot be assumed that inhabitants of industrialized nations are more exposed to mutagens than persons living in agricultural or hunter-gatherer societies, who may be exposed to relatively high levels of mutagens in their food. In industrialized populations, different individuals may experience different exposures to mutagenic chemicals during the course of their lives.

Chemical compounds may be screened for mutagenicity by assessing their ability to induce mutations in bacteria or cultured cells. Tests on living mammals are more directly relevant to assessing likely risks of exposure for living humans, but vastly more expensive. Such tests may focus on the ability of compounds to induce cancers, rather than germline mutations. Rats or mice are exposed to large doses of new compounds that might come to be widely used by the general public, or that are suspected of being potential mutagens by virtue of their chemical structure. There is considerable disagreement about how informative such testing is. Rodents metabolize some compounds differently from humans, and the doses administered are usually far larger than those to which humans might be exposed. For some compounds, these large doses may cause organ damage and cell proliferation, increasing the chances that the rodent will develop a cancer by means other than direct mutagenesis. Such doubts render extrapolations to germline mutation doubly difficult. Mutagenicity of chemical compounds varies widely, and ruling out the possibility that a particular compound may be a weak mutagen would require that it be tested on an impractically large number of organisms.[2,21]

Inhabitants of industrialized nations are exposed to large numbers of potentially mutagenic compounds, and it is clearly necessary to apply the most convincing mutagenicity tests possible to new compounds. Even a weak mutagen may present a serious public health risk if many people are exposed to it. And, as is the case for radiation exposure, cancer risks dictate that unnecessary exposures and high occupational exposures be avoided.

Population Surveillance. Because it is so difficult to demonstrate that specific human activities increase germline mutation rates, population registries have been established in several countries, to track the incidence at birth of chromosomal aberrations and mutations for certain single-gene conditions. An increase following a specific event may identify a mutation hazard. The Hungarian system, for instance, was in a position to evaluate the effects of the 1986 Chernobyl nuclear reactor incident; it found none.

Groups of industrial workers or other individuals potentially or actually exposed to high levels of a suspected mutagen can be closely monitored, to determine whether increased mutation rates result. Positive findings require that industrial exposures be reduced, and that exposures of the general population be controlled.

Another approach, increasingly practical as the necessary techniques become automated, is to screen large populations for mutations that cause changes in protein structure or DNA sequences.[19]

Conclusions. Usual human activities involving radiation and chemical mutagens seem less likely to be increasing our germline mutation rate than has been previously thought. Attention is better directed toward the health implications of existing genetic variation in human populations.[17]

Changing Selection

As has been explained (section entitled Selection and biologic fitness, above), the biologic fitness of individuals with a genetic condition can change as therapies or social attitudes change. In general, the biologic fitness of a phenotype depends on the environment in which individuals with that phenotype find themselves. Thus, a wide range of environmental changes may lead to changes in allele frequencies.

Changing Natural Selection. Certain alleles that were advantageous in the past may be less so now. A prime example is Hb S in populations of African origin who move to areas where malaria is not endemic. Frequencies of Hb S in such populations should gradually fall because selection no longer favors heterozygotes.

Another possible example is hemochromatosis. Approximately 10% of Europeans are heterozygotes for the allele that causes this autosomal recessive disorder, which results in iron overload. In the conditions of dietary scarcity that prevailed through most of human existence, it was undoubtedly advantageous to be able to retain dietary iron. What is now considered a deleterious allele may have conferred an advantage, accounting for its present high frequency.[7]

Yet another example is myopia, the inability of the eye to focus clear images of distant objects. The genetics of myopia is complex; being myopic is analogous to being of less-than-average height. There are various single-gene forms of extreme myopia; in most instances myopia is a consequence of the fact that ocular refraction is a quantitative trait, reflecting population genetic variation and, probably, variation in exposure to environmental influences on ocular development. About a quarter of the members of industrialized societies require corrective lenses for myopia, but myopia is rare or absent in hunter-gatherer societies, as is reduced visual acuity for any reason. This difference probably reflects the severe selective disadvantage conferred by poor vision in hunter-gatherer modes of life, which is not the case in agricultural and industrialized societies.[3]

Dysgenic Effects of the Treatment of Genetic Disease. When medical treatment ameliorates the effects of a hereditary disorder, and thereby increases the probability that affected persons will transmit alleles to future generations, selection against deleterious alleles is relaxed. Thus, in principle, medical treatment is *dysgenic*, and will increase the frequency of genetic disorders. What is the magnitude of this effect, and the appropriate level of concern?

Consider first an autosomal dominant disorder. Assuming that the frequencies of the disorder and of new mutations causing it are constant, the reduced biological fitness of affected persons results in a loss of mutant alleles from the population, which balances the gain resulting from fresh mutations. If the frequency of individuals with the disorder (heterozygotes for the mutant allele) is x, then

$$x(1 - f) = 2m,$$

where f represents the biologic fitness of affected individuals and m the mutation rate.

Complete relaxation of selection against an autosomal dominant, reproductively lethal mutation—a therapy or social change that changed the fitness of affected persons from 0 to 1—would cause the allele frequency to increase at a linear rate equal to the mutation rate. For instance, for a trait with a frequency of 0.0001 and a mutation rate of 5×10^{-5}, the trait frequency would double in one generation, rise to 0.0003 in the next generation, and so on. The proportion of familial to sporadic cases would increase. If selection against the mutation could be relaxed partially but not completely, a new mutation-selection balance would be established, with the frequency of the disease phenotype rising to

$$x - 2m/(1 - f).$$

If, in the example used here, fitness increased

from 0 to 0.5, the trait frequency would rise over several generations to a new equilibrium frequency of

$$x = \frac{2\,(0.00005)}{1-0.5}$$

$$= 0.0002$$

(see Figure 10–2).

Thus, assuming no countervailing measures are taken, the *potential* effects of relaxed selection for autosomal dominant traits are worrisome, particularly if treatment becomes available for several such disorders (but see below).

For an autosomal recessive lethal condition, a treatment that fully restored fertility would cause the frequency of the disease allele to increase by m mutations per generation. For example, for an initial allele frequency of 0.01 and a disease frequency of 0.0001, and assuming a (rather high) mutation rate of 10^{-4}, after 100 generations of complete selection relaxation the allele frequency would be 0.01 + (0.0001 × 100) = 0.02. This doubling of the allele frequency would cause a fourfold increase in the disease frequency, to 0.0004. The slow rate of increase is comforting, but again, the more disorders that can be ameliorated, the greater the total increase in recessive disease.

For X-linked recessive disorders it can be shown that, after four generations of com-

pletely relaxed selection, the allele frequency will double.

For conditions and disorders with a multifactorial etiology, it is impossible to predict the effects of improved treatment on the frequencies of any alleles relevant to liability. The numbers of genes involved, their modes of action, and their importance to the disease phenotypes are not known, nor, in many instances, are the environmental components of liability known.

Complete relaxation of selection against the alleles responsible for most single-gene disorders is certainly not immediately likely. For most disorders, effective treatments have not been found.[12] When affected individuals and carriers of genetic disorders have access to accurate information about the natural history of their disorder, many choose to avoid having affected offspring (see Chapter 28).

In general, concern about the dysgenic effects of medicine seems unnecessary, or even inappropriate. Advances in our understanding of genetic disorders have been rapid, compared to the rate at which medical interventions may be increasing the frequency of deleterious alleles, and this seems likely to continue. Therapeutic advances are really only an extension of other human efforts to achieve a less hostile environment by, for instance, controlling malaria, inventing glasses, and, during prehistory, developing agriculture and domesticating animals to achieve a relatively secure food supply.

Demographic Influences on the Frequency of Genetic Disease

Because much genetic variation within and between human populations is attributable to population genetic structure, it follows that demographic changes, particularly if these change human mating patterns, can alter the geographic distribution and frequency of genetic disease.

In many parts of the world, the change from an agricultural to an industrial economy, with increased population density and improved efficiency of transportation, has acted to break down the genetic isolation of populations and

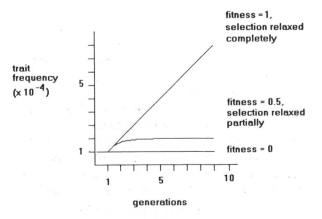

Fig. 10–2. Change in frequency of an autosomal dominant trait with relaxation of selection against the mutant allele.

increase the probability that individuals will choose mates from outside their populations of origin. In such circumstances, the frequency of recessive disease should decrease, because mates from different communities are less likely to be heterozygous for the same deleterious recessive alleles. Similarly, if the proportion of closely consanguineous matings changes, rates of recessive disease will change. As an example, over the last 50 years in Japan, first-cousin marriages became less frequent; decreases in the incidence of PKU and Wilson's disease are attributable to this change.[22] On a global scale, rates of population growth are relatively high in Asia and Africa, compared to rates elsewhere. Many African and Asian societies favor consanguineous matings, and as a result, the world frequency of recessive disease may increase.[4]

Migrant populations carry their alleles with them. Although thalassemia is a circum-Mediterranean disease, it is now also the most common genetic disorder at birth in some north European countries, reflecting the presence of migrant populations in these countries.[24]

The mutation rate is strongly related to parental age. A tendency for women to delay childbearing acts to increase the incidence of chromosomal anomalies, chiefly trisomy 21, and a tendency to earlier childbearing acts to reduce the incidence of these anomalies. Paternal age and single-gene mutation rates are associated in a similar manner; risk of new mutations to autosomal dominant conditions such as achondroplasia and Marfan syndrome is elevated four- or fivefold, in offspring of fathers older than 45 years. In the last decade or two, parental age at birth has been increasing in Europe and North America, but over the longer term, births to older parents have become less frequent in Europe. In consequence, it is likely that the incidence of genetic disease has fallen.[16]

THE PREVENTION OF GENETIC DISEASE

The occurrence of genetic disease reflects extensive genetic variation in human populations, variation that has been established by powerful, longstanding biologic and historical influences. Not surprisingly, it turns out to be extremely difficult to change human allele frequencies on purpose, and genetic disease cannot be "controlled" in any straightforward manner, as has proven possible for some infectious diseases. However, it is possible to organize successful programs to reduce the incidence of some common, severe genetic disorders.

Eugenics

Eugenics, or the directed control of the composition of the human gene pool, was formally proposed by Galton in 1865 and afterwards,[14] without a clear understanding of the nature of heredity. Galton was greatly interested in the inheritance of general ability and inability, or "hereditary genius," and this strain of thinking has persisted. Interest in eugenics peaked in the first third of the 20th century, following the rediscovery of Mendel's laws. Eugenics movements were organized in a number of developed countries, and encouraged such excesses as the sterilization of mental defectives and racial exclusion laws, aimed at preventing immigration of persons of "undesirable" ethnic origin. In Nazi Germany, eugenic arguments were used to justify the execution of individuals with hereditary and mental disorders, as well as mass extermination of Jews and members of other ethnic groups. Not surprisingly, eugenics fell into disrepute.[11,14]

More recently, in the US, there has been a recurrence of interest in eugenic policies, for example government-sponsored programs to discourage unintelligent individuals from reproducing.[14] The government of Singapore actively encourages its more intelligent citizens to marry and have children. Even setting aside the controversy that surrounds the definition of intelligence, it should be obvious that if the genetic basis of variation in a trait is not clearly understood, it is impossible to predict the effectiveness of programs to change population values for the trait, other than to acknowledge that they are likely to be small.

It is possible, however, to predict the effects of a hypothetic program to reduce the frequency of a specific deleterious allele.

It is difficult to envision lowering the frequency of an allele for an autosomal recessive disease. Only carrier couples who have had an affected offspring are readily identified. Humans have, on average, only a few offspring, and therefore many carriers will, by chance, have no affected offspring and remain undetected. Persuading parents of affected children to cease reproduction would reduce the disease frequency slightly, but would have little impact on the allele frequency. If all carriers could be identified, and prenatal diagnosis were universally available, carrier couples could avoid having affected offspring. However, this would actually tend to increase the allele frequency because these unaffected offspring would have a two-thirds chance of being heterozygotes.

In contrast, if every heterozygote for a mutant allele causing an autosomal dominant disorder could be persuaded not to reproduce, the frequency of the disorder would fall in one generation to twice the mutation rate. (This would be the opposite of relaxing selection against an autosomal dominant disorder, described above in the section entitled Dysgenic Effects of the Treatment of Genetic Disease.) Such a program would have little effect on the frequency of a disorder that markedly reduced biologic fitness. However, for common late-onset autosomal dominant disorders such as Huntington disease, the implications of being able to identify heterozygotes presymptomatically are considerable.

There is, one hopes, little possibility of drastically restricting personal reproductive behavior, as a eugenic program would require. Even if this could be done, enormous expense and effort would be required to achieve a reduction in the frequency of any one disorder, whereas, were such a regime instituted, many single-gene disorders would, logically, require eugenic control. Thus, a comprehensive program would require that most of the population limit its reproduction. It should be apparent that eugenic programs, although of historical and, unfortunately, continuing interest, are completely impractical.

Genetic Screening

Carrier Screening. In populations in which the frequency of a severe autosomal recessive disorder is sufficiently high, it may be practical to establish screening programs to detect heterozygote carriers. As examples, screening programs have been organized to identify Hb S carriers in populations of West African descent, thalassemia carriers in Mediterranean countries, and Tay-Sachs disease carriers in Ashkenazi Jewish populations.

The objective of such programs is to allow prospective parents to make informed choices about the health of their offspring. Some have been highly successful, for instance the thalassemia screening program in Cyprus, which requires couples to determine at the time of marriage whether they are carriers. This program has almost no effect on couples' decisions whether or not to marry. However, coupled with the availability of prenatal diagnosis, it has markedly reduced the frequency of affected births.[15]

Carrier screening programs must be carefully organized, and include a strong and culturally sensitive program of counseling and health education. Otherwise, great difficulties arise: carrier status is easily confused with disease status by the uninformed, and in ethnically mixed societies, screening and reproductive counseling are readily misrepresented as racist.

Prevention of Chromosomal Disorders. Even in wealthy countries, it is not possible (or desirable) to screen all pregnancies by amniocentesis, with the aim of decreasing the incidence of chromosome anomalies. This would be impossibly expensive. However, it is cost-beneficial to screen high-risk pregnancies, particularly those of older mothers. Such a screening program is substantially less costly than caring for the trisomic individuals that would otherwise be born to older mothers. Currently, maternal serum screening for alpha fetoprotein, unconjugated estriol, and human chorionic gonadotrophin (triple testing) is being evaluated, as a screening test for chromosome anomalies and neural tube defects, potentially applicable to all pregnancies (see Chap. 15).

Screening for Single-gene Disorders. Simple and inexpensive screening tests are available for several inborn errors of metabolism, and can be applied to all births in jurisdictions where disease incidences warrant. For instance, in the US, Canada and Europe all newborns are routinely screened for PKU, a relatively common and treatable condition (see Chap. 6).

It may prove practical to screen newborns for certain common single-gene disorders that are not currently treatable, such as Duchenne/Becker muscular dystrophy,[10] to alert families of affected individuals to the possible recurrence of the condition.

The Future. Genetic screening may become increasingly important in the coming years. Advances in DNA technology make it possible to identify presymptomatically not only carriers for recessive conditions, but also individuals who will develop adult-onset single-gene disorders and, less precisely, individuals at elevated risk of common multifactorial disorders.

Significant ethical concerns exist about the appropriate use and abuse of genetic screening (see also Chap. 9). Should populations be screened for a genetic disorder for which treatment is far from satisfactory, or nonexistent? Should persons be told they will develop adult-onset disorders? Could such persons be refused health insurance?[20] Where health insurance is provided as an employee benefit, should companies be able to refuse to hire individuals at risk of genetic disorders? Such questions are being debated against a backdrop of increasing public and political awareness of the cost, and value of public health. In answering them, we will have to acknowledge that genetic disorders, in families and in individuals, are a consequence of genetic variation in the population.

SUMMARY

1. Genetic variation in human populations, including variation in the frequency of genetic disease, is a manifestation of population history and natural selection.

2. Allele frequencies remain constant from generation to generation, in the absence of influences changing them. This allows carrier frequencies to be estimated in calculating recurrence risks for families and in planning carrier screening programs.

3. Genetic variation, including alleles responsible for single-gene disorders, originates through mutation. Selection, or the reduced biologic fitness of persons with genetic disorders, acts to remove deleterious alleles from the population. However, selection against alleles causing recessive and adult-onset disorders is slight. The relatively high frequency of alleles for some common autosomal recessive disorders may result from slightly increased biologic fitness of heterozygotes (heterozygote advantage).

4. Nonrandom mating subdivides the human species into many populations, and produces genetic variation between these groups, including extensive variation in the frequency of genetic diseases.

5. It is extremely difficult, if not impossible, to observe changes in mutation rates in human populations. An appreciable increase in the prevalence of genetic disorders attributable to human-mediated radiation exposure can be ruled out. An increase attributable to increasing exposure chemical mutagens has not been demonstrated.

6. Technologic, therapeutic, and social developments may increase the biologic fitness of individuals with genetic disorders. Any resulting change in the frequency of genetic disease will be slow, compared to the rate of improvement in treatment.

7. Demographic changes may influence the frequency of genetic disease by changing the frequency of consanguineous matings or the distribution of parental age.

8. The prevalence of deleterious alleles in populations is not readily alterable. However, genetic screening programs can help prospective parents to make informed decisions about the health of their offspring.

REFERENCES

1. Ionizing radiation exposure of the population of the United States. Report No. 93. Washington, DC, NRCP, 1987.
2. Ames, B.N. and Gold, L.S.: Carcinogens and human health: Part 2. Science 251:12, 1991.
3. Bear, J.C.: Epidemiology and genetics of refractive anomalies. *In* Refractive Anomalies. Research and Clinical Applications, edited by T. Grosvenor and M.C. Flom. Boston, Butterworth-Heinemann, 1991, pp. 57–80.
4. Bittles, A.H., Mason, W.M., Greene, J., et al.: Reproductive behavior and health in consanguineous marriages. Science 252:789, 1991.
5. Bodmer, W.F. and Cavalli-Sforza, L.L.: Genetics, evolution, and man. San Francisco, W. H. Freeman and Company, 1976.
6. Cooper, D.N., Smith, B.A., Cooke, H.J., et al.: An estimate of unique DNA sequence heterogeneity in the human genome. Hum. Genet. 69:201, 1985.
7. Cox, T.M.: Prevalence of the hemochromatosis gene. N. Engl. J. Med. 302:695, 1980.
8. Crow, J.F.: Basic concepts in population, quantitative and evolutionary genetics. New York, W. H. Freeman and Company, 1986.
9. Davies, F., Coles, G.A., Harper, P.S., et al.: Polycystic kidney disease re-evaluated: a population-based study. Q. J. Med. 79(NS):477, 1991.
10. Greenberg, C.R., Jacobs, H.K., Halliday, W., et al.: Three years' experience with neonatal screening for Duchenne/Becker muscular dystrophy: gene analysis, gene expression, and phenotype prediction. Am. J. Med. Genet. 39:68, 1991.
11. Harper, P.S.: Huntington disease and the abuse of genetics. Am. J. Hum. Genet. 50:460, 1992.
12. Hayes, A., Costa, T., Scriver, C.R., et al.: The effect of mendelian disease on human health. II. Response to treatment. Am. J. Med. Genet. 21:243, 1985.
13. Hughes, J.S., Shaw, K.B., and O'Riordan, M.C. The radiation exposure of the UK population 1988 review. Chilton, NRPB, 1988.
14. Kevles, J.D.: In the Name of Eugenics. New York, Knopf, 1985.
15. Modell, B.: The ethics of prenatal diagnosis and genetic counselling. World Health Forum 11:179, 1990.
16. Modell, B. and Kuliev, A.M.: Impact of public health on human genetics. Clin. Genet. 36:286, 1989.
17. Neel, J.V.: Priorities in the application of genetic principles to the human condition: A dissident view. Perspect. Biol. Med. 35:49, 1991.
18. Neel, J.V. and Lewis, S.E.: The comparative radiation genetics of humans and mice. Annu. Rev. Genet. 24:327, 1990.
19. Neel, J.V., Schull, W.J., Awa, A.A., et al.: The children of parents exposed to atomic bombs: Estimates of the genetic doubling dose of radiation for humans. Am. J. Hum. Genet. 46:1053, 1990.
20. Ostrer, H., et al.: Insurance and genetic testing: Where are we now? Am. J. Hum. Genet. 52:565, 1993.
21. Rall, D.P.: Carcinogens and human health: Part 2. Science 251:10, 1991.
22. Saito, T.: An expected decrease in the incidence of autosomal recessive disease due to decreasing consanguineous marriages. Genet. Epidemiol. 5:421, 1988.
23. World Health Organization: Community Approaches to the Control of Hereditary Diseases. Geneva, Hereditary Diseases Programme, WHO, 1985.
24. World Health Organization: The Haemoglobinopathies in Europe: Combined Report on two WHO Meetings. Copenhagen, World Health Organization Regional Office for Europe, 1988.

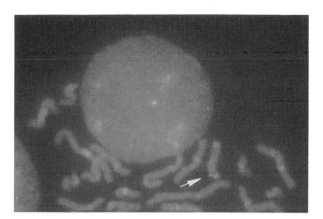

Plate 1

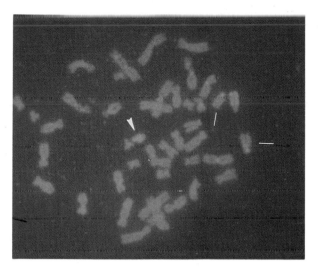

Plate 2

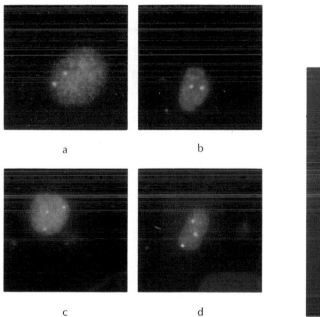

a

b

c

d

Plate 3

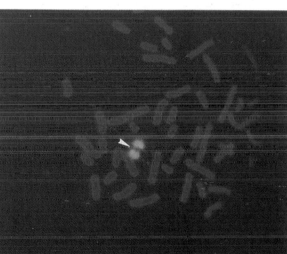

Plate 4

Plate 1.   Partial metaphase after in situ hybridization with two probes located in the distal bands of chromosome 13q. The probe closest to the centromere is labeled with a red fluorochrome, and the more distal probe is labeled with a green fluorochrome. Chromosomes are counterstained with DAPI. Plate 2.   Metaphase containing an extra small "marker" chromosome whose origin was not distinguishable by G-banding. In situ hybridization was performed using chromosome 15 "paint" labeled with a red fluorochrome. Both normal chromosomes 15 and the small unknown chromosome (arrow) light up with this probe, indicating the derivation of the marker from chromosome 15. Chromosomes are counterstained with DAPI. Courtesy of M-T Yu. Plate 3.   Use of chromsome-specific probes for indentification of aneuploidy in interphase nuclei. The top two nuclei show two sites of hybridization with a chromosome 21-specific probe: the bottom two nuclei show three sites, indicating trisomy 21. Courtesy of S. Gersen, Integrated Genetics. Plate 4.   Metaphase from male with dicentric iso-Y chromosome, after in situ hybridization with probe DYZ1, which is specific for repetitive sequences in the heterochromatin of the Y long arm. Arrow indicates the labeled regions at both ends of the dicentric Y.

Chapter 11

The Genetics of Development and Maldevelopment

JUST AS THE TWIG IS BENT THE TREE'S INCLINED.

ALEXANDER POPE

Because the human embryo is largely hidden from the investigator, little is known of human developmental genetics, and much must be extrapolated from lower organisms. Nevertheless, rapid advances are being made in understanding the complex sequence of interactions that occur as a functional organism elaborates itself from the fertilized egg. There is a wealth of relevant animal models,[8,16] but, because of space limitations, we will confine this discussion mainly to examples in man.

Thanks to the recent development of extremely sensitive biochemical techniques for identifying, characterizing, and tracing macromolecules, combined with electron and light microscopy, rapid progress is being made in understanding how cells function, communicate with one another, migrate, and form themselves into tissues that interact with other tissues to shape themselves into organs.

CELLULAR ULTRASTRUCTURE

A generation ago, the cell was represented as a more or less uniform jelly, with the nucleus and a few organelles floating in it. Now it is known to be a highly organized structure. A convoluted membrane, the *endoplasmic reticulum*, forms canals that limit the diffusion of solutes and channel them to different areas of the cell. Some enzymes are bound to membranes; others are packaged in lysosomes. The *mitochondria*, in constant movement, carry their own DNA sequences, as well as the enzymes of oxidative phosphorylation that provide the cell with energy. Clusters of ribosomes (*polyribosomes*) reel off newly synthesized strands of polypeptides from the messenger RNA. *Microtubules* provide a skeleton for the cell that enables it to adopt forms other than spherical or cuboidal. Contractile *microfilaments* provide motility and another means to alter cell shape.

The bilayered nuclear *membrane* has pores through which molecules pass in and out. Membranes themselves have a complex structure, consisting of a fluid double layer of phospholipids transfixed by glycoproteins that act as surface receptors for other molecules, such as hormones and antigens, and as transport vehicles. These proteins are mobile in the plane of the membrane, and on the inside they

245

can interact with the microfilaments and microtubules, to allow events within the cell to modify the properties of the surface, such as the ability to recognize other cells. They may also allow events on the outside to initiate changes on the inside, such as mitosis or morphogenetic movements. Cells may be linked to other cells by specialized junctions that hold tissues together, set up impermeable barriers (tight junctions) at strategic points, or provide channels (gap junctions) connecting the inner surfaces of adjacent cells.[1]

The processes by which the egg develops into an organism include *differentiation*, in which cells become structurally and functionally different from one another, *induction*, whereby a signal from one organ or tissue causes another tissue to begin following another developmental pathway, and *morphogenesis*, the emergence of formed structures and the synchronized integration of various tissues into structured organs.

Maldevelopment can arise at any of these levels, and as a result of point mutations, chromosome aberrations, environmental insults, or interactions of genes and environment. This chapter will deal mainly with errors in development resulting from single mutant genes. Those resulting from the interaction of polygenic systems and environmental factors (multifactorial disorders) will appear in Chapter Twelve, and other examples of gene-environment interactions appear in Chapter Sixteen (Teratology) and Twenty-four (Pharmacogenetics).

DIFFERENTIATION

As the fertilized egg becomes multicellular by a series of mitotic cell divisions, each cell receives a replica of the original complement of genes. Yet many hundreds of different cell types appear in the adult organism.

One model assumes that the same genotype will respond differently to cytoplasm of different compositions, that the cytoplasm of the original egg is not homogeneous, and that there are regional differences in the distribution of various components. The first few cell divisions will result in cells with cytoplasms that differ in their composition. If identical nuclei respond differently to these differences in cytoplasm, they will create new cytoplasmic differences between cells, which will bring about further variations in nuclear response, and the cells will become more and more different by a series of progressively more specialized nucleocytoplasmic reactions. This process requires a system of cytoplasmic signals to which certain genes respond and others do not, i.e., selective gene regulation.

Regulation of Gene Activity

Central to the problem of differentiation is the idea of differential gene activity. For example, a reticulocyte (an immature red blood cell) makes mostly globin molecules, and a pancreatic islet cell makes mostly insulin. This activity implies a differential activity of the globin and the insulin genes in the respective cell types.

Rapid progress has been made in understanding the mechanisms by which genes are regulated in microorganisms. Progress in understanding gene regulation in mammals suggests that higher organisms have evolved more complex means of controlling gene activity.

Regulation can occur at the level of chromatin structure, transcription initiation, RNA processing, and translation. Chromosomal proteins become rearranged to expose the DNA to the transcribing enzymes. The promoter appears to be suppressed by methylation of cytosine, and loss of methylation is correlated with onset of transcription (DNA methylation is also involved in X-chromosome inactivation).

DNA sequences have been identified that are involved in the regulation of transcription. **Promoters** immediately upstream from the start site of transcription are responsible for the initiation of transcription by the RNA polymerase. **Enhancers**, which increase the rate of transcription, can be farther away and even downstream from the gene. One model suggests that regulation acts through proteins that bind with the enhancer and promoter, with looping out of the intervening DNA for transcription. Other factors can affect regulation by interacting with these proteins—these, of course, will be trans-acting, as in the case of steroid receptors that allow certain genes to be "turned on" in response to steroids.

While still in the nucleus, the "silent" regions of the hnRNA within the region that codes for the polypeptide are excised by splicer "snurps"[22] enzymes, as are some regions beyond the sequence to be translated. The 5′ end of the remaining mRNA, where translation starts, is "capped" by a methylated guanosine very early in transcription. This capping and methylation are vital to the initiation of *translation*. About 150 untranslated nucleotides remain, mostly at the 3′ end, which is modified by the addition of a stretch of adenylic acid residues (poly A). The poly (A) appears to protect the mRNA from enzymatic breakdown in the cytoplasm. It is also useful to the biochemist, who can purify mRNA by fishing it out of solution on a column lined with poly U (to which poly A binds), but presumably that is not why it is there.

It has recently been recognized that the same messenger RNA can be cut and spliced differently under different conditions—alternative splicing. This may be a clue to how cells with the same genome can become different (*differentiation*) and to how a mutation in a single gene can affect different tissues or organs (*pleiotropy*).

In the cytoplasm, the process of polypeptide synthesis begins. Attachment to the ribosome, initiation of translation, elongation of the growing polypeptide chain, and termination of translation involve a number of additional factors, and the complexity of the process becomes more obvious as our knowledge increases. Gene activity, or the process of transferring the information at one gene locus from DNA to protein structure, involves some 200 or more other loci, encoding, for example, aminoacyl synthetases, ribosomal proteins, translation factors, tRNAs, and the enzymes involved in RNA modification. Thus there are many opportunities to bring about the regulation of gene activity, so necessary for the process of development. Most of the control, however, seems to operate at the level of transcription.

SELECTIVE GENE REGULATION

Development involves a progressive and prescribed limitation of gene activity. In some organisms, if the two daughter cells resulting from the first cleavage division are separated, each will develop into a complete organism. After a few divisions, however, the individual cells lose this ability and will not, if separated, continue development beyond a certain stage. In older embryos, experiments in which tissues are transplanted from one region to another show that the developmental options open to cells become progressively limited, until there is finally commitment to only one type. This is referred to as *determination*, which is followed by differentiation.

That this progressive restriction is accompanied by differential gene regulation is shown by identifying the various species of messenger RNA in different tissues. In the sea urchin, there are about 20,000 different mRNAs in the blastula, and about half of these are present in the gastrula, along with many new species. Each stage of differentiation involves the activation of new sets of structural genes and the production of new protein species in the differentiating cell population. Differentiated cells all have a certain number of mRNAs in common, presumably those coding for the "housekeeping" enzymes necessary for cell function in general, but each makes large amounts of a few particular mRNAs, those coding for the proteins specific to that particular cell type. For example, a reticulocyte spends most of its synthetic efforts on hemoglobin. The globin genes may make over 140,000 copies of globin mRNA, whereas a liver cell makes only a few, even though they both have the same number of globin genes.

Nuclear-Cytoplasmic Interactions

What determines the selectivity of gene activation? Cytoplasmic factors are certainly involved. When enucleated frog eggs are injected with nuclei from differentiated cells, a small proportion will develop into tadpoles, indicating that something in the egg cytoplasm is able to reactivate the appropriate genes in the injected nucleus. This is the classic "cloning" experiment of Briggs and King that made it possible to produce a large number of genetically identical tadpoles, causing some to worry about the implications for man. However, no one has succeeded in transplanting a nucleus from the cell of an adult organism into an enucleated egg that then developed to adulthood.[5]

Nuclei from frog kidney cells injected into enucleated newt eggs become active in RNA synthesis and produce several proteins that are normally present in frog oocytes, but not those that are specific for frog kidney cells. Clearly, then, the oocyte cytoplasm must contain factors, presumably specific molecules, that can activate certain genes and suppress others.

There is good evidence from many species of lower organisms that the egg cytoplasm does contain macromolecules that are distributed differently to the four cells resulting from the first two cleavage divisions. In the snail, for example, there is unequal distribution of certain macromolecules, possibly maternal mRNAs, which results in different patterns of protein synthesis in descendants of these cells well before they become morphologically different. In mammals, the early embryo's cells seem able to regulate their organization after being rearranged, so that any unequal partitioning of regulatory macromolecules must occur later than in snails and frogs.

Chromosomal Differentiation

Recent studies of chromosome ultrastructure (see Chap. 2) are revealing something of the mechanisms by which selective transcription of the DNA is achieved.[5,19]

To recapitulate a current view, the nuclear genetic material consists of strands of DNA associated with histone and nonhistone proteins. The DNA is, at intervals, wrapped around histone octamers in a precise manner, forming nu bodies. When acetylated, these histones unfold, and the associated DNA sequences are extended into a form that exposes them to the RNA polymerase and initiates transcription of that particular gene.

Selective Gene Activation

This provides a model for gene activation but is nonspecific—we still do not know why certain regions of the DNA are activated in certain cells and others are not. Further insight comes from study of systems in which the activity of specific genes varies greatly in response to *hormones*. The hormone binds to a specific cytoplasmic receptor in the target tissue to form a complex that is translocated into the nucleus, binds to specific acceptor sites on the chromatin, and activates transcription.

Steroid receptors provide a fascinating example. Proteins that bind to glucocorticoids and progesterone, respectively, have a "finger" region that binds to the DNA of genes that are activated by that hormone. Genetic engineering techniques made it possible to replace the DNA-binding region of the progesterone receptor with that of the glucocorticoid receptor. The resulting "hybrid" molecule bound to the DNA where the genes normally activated by glucocorticoids are, but these genes now responded to progesterone!

One of the best known examples of selective changes in gene activation during development is the switch from production of hemoglobin F in the fetus to hemoglobin A in the adult (see Chapter 6), but almost nothing is known of how this happens. The switch begins at 32 to 36 weeks of gestation. Before this, most red cells contain 90 to 95% hemoglobin F ($\alpha_2\gamma_2$) and 5 to 10% A ($\alpha_2\beta_2$). Tissues forming blood cells are continually producing new generations of red blood cells, and at about 34 weeks of gestation some cells containing mostly hemoglobin A appear. At term, the red cell population contains about 2 to 5% of these cells, and about 50% of the cells have large amounts (>20%) of both F and A. The proportion of hemoglobin-F-containing cells ("F cells") produced decreases to about 5% in adults, but remains higher in the heterogeneous types of hereditary persistent fetal hemoglobinemia (HPFH) and the β-thalassemias, and can increase again in normal adults in response to certain types of anemia.

Cultured erythroid stem cells form clones which, in embryos before 32 weeks of gestation, all produce large amounts of hemoglobin F. In cultures from newborn infants, each clone may produce either large amounts of F, large amounts of A, or intermediate amounts of both A and F. In cultures from adults, most clones produce cells that form mainly A. Thus the switch from the embryonic to the adult state is not accomplished by a gradual increase in β-chain synthesis and decrease in γ-globin gene activity. Rather, the commitment occurs at the stem cell stage. As the differentiation of the stem cell tissue proceeds, a progressively greater proportion of clones is committed to hemoglobin A production. But the differentiated tissue still contains a small proportion of undifferentiated cells that can form clones of F cells. Discovery of a locus control region (LCR) just upstream of the ε gene gives a clue to the nature of the switch. The evidence suggests that the β and γ genes compete with each other for interaction with the LCR, with the outcome depending on the availability of trans-acting factors that alter the ability of the globin genes to interact with the LCR, but the mechanism is far from clear.[21]

Learning to regulate the switch has some exciting implications for therapy. Saudi Arabs have unusually high levels of hemoglobin F, and those who have sickle cell disease have it in a much less severe form than do Africans. Similarly, patients with beta thalassemia are less severely affected if they also have the HPFH gene (see Chap. 6) or some other form of elevated F production. Because hemoglobin F is an adequate substitute for A, if one could learn to prevent the switch from F to A production at term in patients with sickle cell disease, the harmful effects could be prevented.

There are now a number of human examples in which new enzymes appear and others disappear at specific stages of development and in different tissues. One is the enzyme lactic dehydrogenase (LDH), a tetramer that exists in five electrophoretically different forms known as isozymes. The five isozymes represent varying combinations of two chains—four alpha; three alpha, and one beta; two alpha and two beta; one alpha and three beta; or four beta chains. Since there are two chains, two gene loci must code for them. The proportions of the five isozymes are different in different tissues, and in the same tissue at different stages, indicating that the relative activities of the two genes vary from time to time and place to place. The isozymes vary somewhat in their properties, such as degree of inhibition by lactate, and their varying proportions in different cells presumably have some functional significance. For instance, in striated muscle, lactate resulting from strenuous exercise inhibits the "muscle" type LDH, which weakens the muscles; this weakening may be why sprinters sometimes collapse at the end of a dash. This would be perilous for heart muscle which, conveniently, has more of the isozyme that is not inhibited by lactate.

Epigenetic Control

Brief mention should be made of regulation beyond the level of translation, the so-called epigenetic level. Enzyme activity can be regulated, for instance, by controlling the rate of degradation of the enzyme rather than its synthesis or by the way the molecule is folded in different cytoplasmic states. Polymerization and addition or deletion of part of a peptide chain are other ways of achieving epigenetic control.

Diseases Caused by Defective Differentiation

Many genetic defects can be attributed to errors of differentiation, in which a specific cell type does not appear or takes some abnormal form. For instance, in the pituitary dwarf mouse, the eosinophils fail to differentiate, resulting in a specific growth hormone deficiency, and various hereditary chondrodystrophies result from failure of specific aspects of cartilage differentiation.

MORPHOGENESIS

Morphogenesis, or the emergence of form in the developing organism, is much more complicated than the activation or inactivation of genes. To account for the migration of cells, their aggregation into tissues, the synchronized spreading, bending, and thickening of tissues, the transfer of development instructions from one tissue to another (induction), and, in short, the whole complexly integrated series of interactions that eventually result in the adult organism seems a superhuman task. Yet a beginning has been made.

We cannot cover the whole subject of morphogenesis and its genetic control in this chapter, but will refer briefly to a number of representative examples.

There is no doubt that morphogenetic processes are influenced by genes, since there are large numbers of mutant genes that alter the shapes of organs. Many of these are well described in structural terms, but little is known of their precise modes of action. Mutant genes can be useful in revealing the normal, and there are a large number of mutant genes in the mouse and in other animals that produce phenotypes resembling human diseases and malformation.[8,16] How genes influence morphogenesis is beginning to become clear with the recent advances in molecular genetics referred to at the end of this chapter.

INDUCTION

Induction, to the embryologist, is the process by which a signal from one tissue initiates a change in the developmental fate of another. For instance, according to the classical view, the optic cup, growing out from the brain, induces the ectoderm that lies over it to form a lens, and the two structures integrate with one another to form the eye. Recently, the use of mutant genes has shown that induction is under genetic control but that inductive relations are more complicated than previously suspected. For example, the very early chick limb consists of an ectodermal jacket surrounding an apparently undifferentiated mesoderm. Inductive interactions have been analyzed by the use of mutant genes causing such things as extra digits or winglessness. By combining mutant ectoderm with normal mesoderm, and vice versa, and seeing how the resulting limb develops, it has been shown that the overlying ectoderm induces the mesoderm to form digits. But the *number* of digits

depends on an inductive stimulus to the ectoderm from the mesoderm. Thus morphogenesis of the hand depends on a series of genetically controlled reciprocal inductive interactions between ectoderm and mesoderm. Retinoic acid may be the morphogen. It is likely that some of the malformations of hands and feet seen in human babies result from disturbances in inductive relationships.

According to a recent comprehensive review,[12] induction is far more complex than the classical view had suggested. At least in amphibia (which are more amenable to experimental analysis), the patterned distribution of different organs begins with the establishment of the animal and vegetal regions of the early embryo, which differ in developmental potency (the range of tissues into which the region can differentiate). Inductive interactions across the boundaries of regions of different potency establish morphogenetic fields that reflect developmental potency rather than developmental fate—that is, they are larger than the area fated to give rise to a particular organ, and become progressively restricted. For example, the series of inductions that result in formation of a lens begins in gastrulation, long before there is even an optic cup. Several tissues are early inductors of the lens; their effects are cumulative and synergistic. The ability of non-neural ectoderm to respond to lens induction becomes restricted to head ectoderm (which is also being induced to form nose and ear) and finally to the cells that actually form the lens.

The chick limb also provides interesting examples of selective gene regulation through environmental modification in development.[3] The early limb bud mesenchyme contains cells whose progenitors will form either cartilage or muscle. In culture, the cells form muscle if there is a high level of nicotinamide in the medium and, consequently, of NAD in the cell. Low levels of nicotinamide and of NAD will result in differentiation to cartilage. In the limb bud, at this stage, the developing vascular system has already resulted in heavily capillarized, nutrient-rich, and avascular nutrient-poor zones. The nutrient-rich zone, which presumably has lots of nicotinamide, is the area that will form muscle, and the nutrient-poor zone, low in nicotinamide, is the area that will form cartilage. Thus differentiation of the mesenchymal limb cells depends on an environmental difference brought about by a previous morphogenetic event, vascularization.

In some cases, abnormal development of an organ results from *failure of induction due to asynchrony* rather than an abnormal inductive mechanism. There is a gene that causes absent or small kidneys in the mouse, for example. Embryologic studies show that the migration of the ureter is delayed so that it is late in reaching the kidney-precursor tissue. This finding suggested that the kidney tissue required an inductive stimulus from the ureter bud to initiate its differentiation and that the abnormal kidney resulted from a diminished or absent stimulus. In culture, when mutant ureter and mutant kidney precursor were put together, kidney differentiation occurred. Thus the ureter could induce, and the kidney precursor could respond; abnormality resulted from failure to bring the two together at the right time.

These examples show how a mutant gene may reveal normal developmental mechanisms, as well as how they go wrong. Such studies can contribute to the understanding of human malformations.

SHAPE AND PATTERN

The most complex developmental problem of all is the means by which genes control the shape of organs and the patterns seen in such profusion and with such beauty wherever one looks in nature.

The influence of genes on pattern is beginning to be analyzed in higher organisms. The mouse mutant gene "reeler," for example, deranges the form of the cerebellum and cerebrum. The various organized layers are unrecognizable, the various cell types being intermixed instead of sorted out into their normal orientation. Experiments have shown that dissociated isocortical cells from mutant day 18 embryos will form aggregates normally but do not organize themselves into an external mo-

lecular layer and an internal nerve-fiber zone as do aggregates of normal cells of this age (but not a day earlier or later). Thus the mutant produces a defect in self-organization of the mutant brain cells at a particular stage of development, showing that this property is under genetic control.[5]

In another example, a morphogenetic change caused by a mutant gene has been traced to a property of the cell membrane. The mutant gene talpid in the chick causes midline facial defects, fusion of mesenchymal precartilage condensations, and polydactyly. Cell aggregation experiments demonstrate that these result from increased adhesiveness and decreased motility of the mesenchymal cells.[8]

The immotile cilia syndrome is an interesting example of abnormal morphogenesis in humans.[6] In this condition, there appears to be a genetically determined defect in the ultrastructure of cilia, resulting in immobility. In the respiratory tract, this results in obstruction, as secretions are not cleared by the cilia, with repeated infections. Male patients are sterile, because the sperm are immobile. About half the patients have their internal organs on the "wrong" side, possibly because embryonic cilia are involved in determining lateral asymmetry in organogenesis, but are inactive in affected embryos, so the determination of laterality becomes random. About one eighth of the sibs also have situs inversus, suggesting autosomal recessive inheritance.

Much new information has been provided by a technique that makes use of the remarkable regulatory powers of the early mouse egg. If the membrane (zona pellucida) surrounding the cells of the early mouse embryo (blastocyst) is removed and two such eggs are placed together, they will merge, forming a larger blastocyst that is a mixture of the cells from the two eggs. If one egg is genetically albino and the other black, the resulting embryo will grow into a normal-sized black and white striped mouse. The pattern of such *allophenic* mice demonstrates that the cells forming each stripe come from one ancestral cell that migrates from the neural crest into the appropriate area and then multiplies to give rise to all the pigment cells that populate that stripe.

THE MODES OF ACTION OF MUTANT GENES

Theoretically, for every process involved in normal development, one might expect malformations resulting from mutations of each gene affecting that process. Thus one might have malformations resulting from a mutant *structural protein* (defective hair and teeth in hydrotic ectodermal dysplasia); absent or abnormal *enzymes* (dislocation of the lens in homocystinuria); defective properties of *cell adhesiveness* (the "talpid" chick); defective capacity of cells to *migrate* or orient themselves (the "reeler" mouse); failure of cells to *die* at the proper time (syndactyly); excessive cell death (the rumpless chicken); failure to *respond to signals* from other tissues either by contact (anophthalmia resulting from failure of the ectoderm to respond to induction by the optic cup) or a humoral inducer (testicular feminization); *asynchronies* in growth resulting in inductive failure (anophthalmia resulting from delayed growth of the optic cup; the kidneys of the Danforth short mouse); and no doubt many other causes. The wealth of mutant genes in the mouse and in other mammals provides a fruitful field for research into the developmental links between mutant gene and phenotype, with the possibility of extrapolation to analogous human syndromes. See also the discussion of homeobox genes at the end of this chapter.

Gene-Environment Interactions

Environmental teratogens may also strike at various points in the developmental network or may interact with mutant genes affecting the same developmental processes. A particularly instructive example is the interaction of 5-fluorouracil (FUDR) and the mutant gene "luxoid" (lu) in the mouse. A low dose of the teratogen, or the mutant gene in the heterozygous condition, produces only a minor defect, polydactyly of the hind foot. The homozygous mutant, or a high dose of the teratogen, produces polydactyly and tibial absence. The combination of a low dose of teratogen and the heterozygous gene will produce polydac-

tyly and tibial defect even though neither would individually. One wonders whether an analogous situation may exist in man. Why, for instance, does a synthetic progestin produce a masculinization of the genitalia in only a minority of babies exposed to it at the appropriate gestational age? Could these babies be heterozygous for a recessive gene that causes the adrenogenital syndrome in the homozygote?

Another example shows that *malformations can be prevented by prenatal measures*. The mutant gene "pallid" in the mouse causes ataxia, resulting from failure of the otoliths of the inner ear to form. Maternal manganese deficiency causes a similar condition in the rat. The genetically determined ataxia in pallid mice was corrected by giving their mothers large doses of manganese during pregnancy.[7]

A mutant in the rabbit provides another example of the prenatal prevention of hereditary malformations. The recessive mutant gene causes amputations of the limbs of variable severity. The trouble appears after the limb has formed and results from hemorrhages, followed by death of the distal tissues. The hemorrhages are associated with the presence of large nucleated red blood cells (macrocytes) in the blood stream. These seem to obstruct the small vessels in the limbs, causing the hemorrhage and tissue death. Treatment of the pregnant mother with oxygen or with vitamin B_{12} and folic acid prevented the appearance of the macrocytes and, consequently, of the malformations.[17]

Finally, we must mention the numerous examples of gene-environment interactions involving multifactorial threshold characters (Chapter 12). An embryo's genes may place a particular developmental variable near a threshold of abnormality, so that a relatively small additional environmental influence may place that organ beyond the threshold, and a malformation results. In another embryo, not near the threshold, the same environmental insult will have no effect. An example described in detail in Chapter 12 is cleft of the secondary palate, in which the variable is the time at which the embryonic palatal shelves reach the horizontal, so they may fuse, and the threshold is the latest stage of development when they can reach each other when they do become horizontal.

The Developmental Basis of Pleiotropy, Penetrance, and Expressivity

Pleiotropy. Pleiotropy refers to the fact that a single mutant gene may have several end effects, as in numerous inherited syndromes. The multiple effects of single genes can be explained in several ways.

First, the several end effects may be secondary, tertiary, or even more removed results of the initial defect, forming a "pedigree of causes" (Fig. 11–1). Thus, in sickle cell disease, the basic molecular defect leads to *destruction of red cells*, which leads to anemia, pallor, and fatigability; to *intravascular sickling*, which causes leg ulcers, infarcts of various organs, and splenic rupture; and to *marrow enlargement*, which causes bone pain and the "tower skull." In phenylketonuria, the mental defect, growth retardation, hypopigmentation, skin rash, and seizures are all, no doubt, results of the basic enzyme defect, but some of the steps are not yet clear.

In many syndromes, the developmental connections are entirely obscure. What biochemical defect, for instance, is common to the degeneration of the retina and extra fingers of the Laurence-Moon-Biedl syndrome? As mentioned previously, alternative splicing could be an explanation. If alternative splicing led to an mRNA involved in finger development, and another involved in retinal development, a mutation in the LMB gene could result in anomalies of both finger and retina development.

Pleiotropy could also occur if the same polypeptide were common to more than one protein. A mutant polypeptide would then result in more than one mutant protein, and more than one end effect. A great challenge for students of developmental mammalian genetics will be to trace the developmental connections revealed by pleiotropic mutant genes.

Penetrance and Expressivity. Little is known about the developmental basis of penetrance and expressivity. A convenient, if oversimplified, model is based on the developmental variable/threshold concept (see Chapter 12). If a group of individuals (such as a particular strain of mice) has a genotype and environment that place it near the threshold, the effect of a major mutant gene may be to throw all the individuals beyond the threshold, and one would say that the gene had full penetrance (Fig. 11–2). In another group, who are far from the threshold, the effect of a mutant gene may place only a few individuals beyond the threshold, and the gene would be said to have low penetrance. Similarly, if individuals near the threshold were mildly affected and those far beyond the threshold were severely affected, it is clear that there would be a correlation between penetrance and expressivity, as there often seems to be in experimental animals, in which this can be adequately tested.

Phenocopies

Phenocopies are individuals with a mutant phenotype but a nonmutant genotype—that is, some environmental factor has simulated the effects of a mutant gene. Much has been deduced about the mode and time of action of mutant genes by analysis of their phenocopies, but this approach is only just beginning to be applied in man. An interesting example is given by Lenz,[13] who showed that, depending on the stage of exposure, the teratogenic effects of thalidomide on the limb could resemble those of three different mutant genes causing absence of the radius.

The Genetics of Human Male Sexual Development

An example illustrating many of the preceding concepts is provided by recent studies on the various types of male pseudohermaphrodite.

Male differentiation proceeds in a stepwise fashion.[18] The gonad in the early embryo is an undifferentiated primordium, into which germ cells migrate from the yolk sac. If the germ cells contain a Y chromosome, the gonad differentiates into a testis. Otherwise it forms

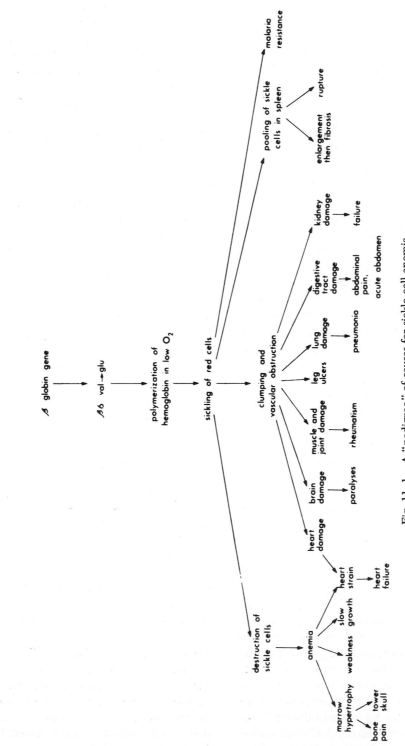

Fig. 11–1. A "pedigree" of causes for sickle cell anemia.

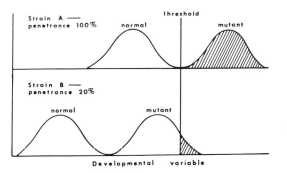

Fig. 11–2. Hypothetical model showing penetrance of gene on two different genetic backgrounds. Note that the same model accounts for strain differences in response to a teratogen—for instance, cleft palate caused by cortisone in the A/J and C57BL inbred mouse lines (see Chapter 12).

an ovary. The stimulus to testis differentiation is provided by a gene, SRY, on the short arm of the Y chromosome[9] which codes for a cell membrane antigen, the H-Y antigen (H stands for histocompatibility, because in mice it causes male skin grafts to be rejected by females). This antigenic component is the inductive stimulus that switches the gonad into the male developmental pathway.

Some time after the gonad differentiates, the embryo lays down two sets of ducts: In females, the müllerian ducts are the precursors of the fallopian tubes, uterus, and upper part of the vagina; in male embryos, the wolffian ducts will form the vas deferens, seminal vesicles, and epididymis, the ducts leading from the testis to the penis. Development of these ducts depends on a stimulus provided by the male hormone, testosterone, produced by the embryonic testis (induction). The testis also produces a hormone (the müllerian inhibitory substance) that inhibits further differentiation of the adjacent müllerian ducts.

In the absence of a testis (i.e., in the normal female or castrated male embryo), the müllerian ducts continue to differentiate and the wolffian ducts regress. Later on, the external genitalia form. In the presence of the male hormone 5α-dihydrotestosterone, the genital folds and tubercle form a penis; in its absence, they form the labia and clitoris (morphogenesis). Finally, it has been discovered in rodents that various target organs are "imprinted" by male hormone at various period

of development so that at puberty they will respond in a male pattern (determination). These include the secretion of gonadotrophic hormone by the hypothalamus, the way the liver metabolizes steroid hormones, the maturation of the prostate gland and seminal vesicles at puberty, and various behavioral characteristics.

What starts this cascade of male-determining events? The SRY gene on the short arm of the Y produces the mRNA for a testis-determining factor (TDF) which signals the Sertoli cells (which surround and nurture the germ cells) to produce the müllerian duct inhibitor. The Sertoli cells probably control the differentiation of other testicular cell types, such as the Leydig cells that secrete androgens which initiate differentiation of the wolffian ducts and various other aspects of male differentiation.

The sex-reversal gene in the mouse, which converts females into males, and the rare human XX males and XY females, result from translocation of the SRY gene from the Y to the X chromosome.

Mutant genes can interrupt or divert the process of male sexual development at various points, leading to various kinds of male pseudohermaphroditism, as follows.

Failure of Testis Differentiation

Differentiation of the primordial gonad into a testis requires a Y chromosome carrying the locus of the testis determining factor, but this is not enough. There is a mutant gene, probably on the X chromosome, which prevents the formation of testes in an XY individual, who is therefore anatomically female, because no testosterone or müllerian inhibiting substance will be produced. Presumably the normal allele at this locus interacts with the SRY gene to promote testis differentiation. The condition is known as *familial XY gonadal dysgenesis*. The gonads are not ovaries, but "streak gonads" like those of XO Turner syndrome, suggesting that there is also a locus on the X chromosome which must be present in duplicate to maintain normal ovarian development.

In some families, some affected individuals do manage to achieve some degree of testis differentiation, so that although the internal anatomy is female, there are varying degrees of masculinization of the external genitalia (variable expressivity). These may represent what the microbial geneticists would call "leaky" mutants.

Absence of Müllerian Duct Inhibition

In the rare *uterine hernia syndrome*, the affected males are normal except that they have müllerian ducts and an infantile uterus that may present in an inguinal hernia. The inheritance is probably autosomal recessive. Presumably, the mutant gene either prevents the production of the müllerian inhibitory substance by the testis or renders the müllerian duct anlage unresponsive to the hormone.

Defects in Testosterone Synthesis

There are several recessively inherited forms of male pseudohermaphroditism in which the mutant gene causes a deficiency of one of the enzymes involved in testosterone synthesis. Most of them also involve synthesis of steroids by the adrenal cortex (pleiotropy) and are referred to as the adrenogenital syndromes. In males, there are varying degrees of undermasculinization of the external genitalia, which may extend to a fully female anatomy, and varying degrees of breast enlargement (gynecomastia) at puberty. It is not clear why the wolffian ducts manage to differentiate successfully. Perhaps the defect in testosterone synthesis appears after wolffian duct differentiation has been induced, or the defect is incomplete, and the wolffian duct needs less of a stimulus than the genital tubercles in order to proceed with development in the male pathway. The gynecomastia may result from a failure of "imprinting" of the breast tissue at a critical period that normally prevents the pubertal male breast from responding to estrogenic hormones from the adrenal cortex.

Failure of Target Tissue Response to Androgen

Perhaps the most interesting type of male pseudohermaphroditism is testicular feminization (TF). X-linked forms exist in the rat and mouse, and the human type fits this familial pattern too. The affected individuals have an XY karyotype, testes, no uterus or fallopian tubes, and female external genitalia. At puberty, feminization occurs. The basic defect is in the response of the target organs. The testis in TF males produces testosterone. Because there is müllerian duct inhibition, the testis must also produce the inhibitory hormone. The biochemical defect is now becoming clear.

In the normal male, testosterone enters the target cell and is enzymatically reduced to 5α-dihydrotestosterone (DHT). The DHT binds to a cytosol receptor protein and the complex enters the nucleus, where it attaches to the chromatin and in some way promotes the transcription of messenger RNA for whatever protein the target cell is to produce in response to the hormonal stimulus. Because most cases of testicular feminization are deficient in the cytosol receptor protein, the target tissues are unresponsive to the hormone. Thus the failure of the external genitalia to masculinize and the lack of secondary sex characteristics.[18]

Mutations in the androgen receptor gene can lead to various defects ranging from the full-blown TF syndrome to otherwise asymptomatic azoospermia.

Another form of androgen insensitivity results from a deficiency of testosterone 5α-reductase, the enzyme that converts testosterone to DHT. The patients have normal wolffian duct derivatives, but their external genitalia are feminine. At puberty there is marked virilization, with male muscularity and enlargement of the external genitalia. There is little or no beard growth, suggesting that growth of the external genitalia is testosterone-dependent, but that beard growth depends on DHT.

This catalogue of gene-determined classes of male pseudohermaphroditism is far from complete, but it serves to demonstrate that mutant genes may interfere with male sex differentiation at many points and to show how study of their effects is contributing to our understanding of the normal process.

NEW INSIGHTS FROM DNA TECHNOLOGY

The extraordinary recent advances in DNA technology are bringing genetics and embryology together as never before. Thanks to PCR, it is now possible to identify specific messenger RNAs and specify where and when they appear in the embryo, thus revealing where and when particular genes begin to act. Genes can be transfected into embryos to study their developmental effects; for example, transfection of the Sry gene for male sex development into XX embryos caused them to become males, thus proving the sex-determining function of the gene.[9] Sometimes transfected genes inserted at random into the genome disrupted a normal gene and caused a mutation, as in the case of the mouse ld (limb deformity) gene. The mutant gene causes defects of kidneys, as well as limbs. mRNA from the mouse gene was used to isolate the human homologue from a genomic DNA library. The human gene was mapped by in situ hybridization, and shown to be homologous to the human limb-deformity (ld) gene; it is expressed in both kidney and limb buds.

It is now possible to mutate genes more precisely by homologous recombination, and this approach has been used to create animal models to study the pathogenesis of morphogenetic syndromes. This "knockout" technique is a conceptual breakthrough that is already helping to unravel the puzzles of immunology, development biology, and the pathogenesis of genetic disorders such as cystic fibrosis, the hemoglobinopathies, and Gaucher's disease,[23] and it is beginning to make inroads into behavioral genetics. For example, knocking out the gene for a particular kinase enzyme results in specific and profound effects on learning and memory.[20]

The field is moving so rapidly that we cannot provide an extensive discussion here, but have selected a few illustrative examples for a brief presentation.

The example that is giving the most profound insights into how genes control development is the discovery of the homeobox genes. Homeotic mutants have been known in Drosophila for decades; they alter the organization of whole body segments, changing the aristae on the head into legs, for instance, or making wings grow out of the abdomen. They were hailed as evidence that genes control the topography of the developmental landscape, not just the details. In particular, homeotic mutants seemed to determine the anterior-posterior gradient. More recently these genes, now called homeobox genes, were cloned and found to be highly conserved in evolution, being found in organisms ranging from hydra to humans. They occur in groups, in the same order in the mouse as in Drosophila, and this order corresponds to the order in which they are expressed along the anterior-posterior axis. Some may be involved in formation of the blastopore lip (at least in Xenopus) and may perhaps produce the "organizer" that induces the dorsal mesoderm, as Spemann demonstrated by his classical transplantation experiments more than 70 years ago.[2]

A mutant form of one of these genes, produced by homologous recombination, was put into mouse inner-cell-mass blastomeres and the resulting mosaic mice were interbred to produce heterozygous mutant mice. Homozygotes derived from these had a lethal syndrome resembling (unexpectedly) the di George syndrome, with absence of parathyroids and thyroids, and heart malformations.[9] Another group of segmentation genes, pax, is involved in the early spatial organization of the mouse central nervous system. Several known mouse mutants have been mapped to the Pax region, including Splotch, a mutant that affects neural crest cells, located on the proximal part of chromosome I. It was known that this region is homologous with a region on human chromosome 2 that contains the gene for Waardenburg syndrome, and, sure enough, in several families segregating for Waardenburg syndrome, patients have a mutation at this locus. Conversely, a candidate cDNA for human aniridia was cloned, and several aniridia patients had deletions in it, confirming that it did indeed represent the aniridia gene. This gene is the human homologue of *Pax-6* and a mutant Pax-6 gene (small eye, Sey) causes deficiencies of the eyes and nose.[10]

Another approach that is bringing genetics and embryology closer together is the use of antisense oligodeoxynucleotides (a-ODNs). An oligonucleotide for a specific gene sequence is added to a cell or organ culture, where it will bind to the complementary DNA sequence and inhibit transcription, or to the complementary RNA sequence, where it will inhibit processing or translation of that gene product. In effect, it copies the effect of mutating a gene without altering the gene—a sort of molecular phenocopy. This is making it possible to demonstrate developmental effects that might be difficult to analyze otherwise, for example if the mutant gene had such serious effects that it killed the early embryo. Thus, when an a-ODN for the nerve growth factor was added to cultures of early kidney anlagen, it inhibited nephron formation and subsequent ureter bud branching.[9]

Thus the tools of molecular biology are bringing genetics and embryology together in new and illuminating ways, and the prospects of untangling some of the complexities of how genes regulate development are bright.

SUMMARY

Development from a single cell to an organism containing many cells and organ systems of diverse function is a complex process that cannot be studied in the human at many critical stages. Cells containing the same genetic information, through the process of differentiation (resulting largely from differential gene activity), become specialized to develop along different lines, to form different structures, and to perform different functions.

Differential gene activity is regulated at various levels, including organization of the chromosome, transcription, processing of the messenger RNA, translation, and beyond at levels of epigenetic control.

Morphogenesis (the emergence of form in the developing organism) is even more complicated than gene regulation. Cell migration and aggregation and inductive interactions (under genetic influence) participate in the morphogenetic process leading to the development of shape and pattern. The use of DNA technology is clarifying the role of genes in morphogenesis.

Maldevelopment may result from failures at the genetic level or chromosomal level, from potent environmental pathogens, and from interactions between polygenic diatheses and less potent environmental triggers.

REFERENCES

1. Bennett, M.V.L. and Spray, D.L., Editors: Gap junctions. Cold Spring Harbor Laboratory, Cold Spring Harbor, NY, 1985.
2. Blumberg, B., Wright, C.V.E., De Robertis, E.M. and Cho, K.W.Y. Organizer—specific homeobox genes in *Xenopus laevis* embryos. Science 253:194, 1991.
3. Caplan, A.I. and Ordahl, C.P.: Irreversible gene repression model for control of development. Science 201:120, 1978.
4. Dagg, C.P.: Combined action of fluorouracil and two mutant genes on limb development in the mouse. J. Exp. Zool. 164:479, 1967.
5. DiBerardino, M.A., et al.: Activation of dormant genes in specialized cells. Science 224:946, 1984.
6. Eliasson, R., et al.: The immotile-cilia syndrome. N. Engl. J. Med. 297:1, 1977.
7. Erway, L.C., Fraser, A.S. and Hurley, L.C.: Prevention of congenital otolith defect in pallid mutant mice by manganese supplementation. Genetics 67:97, 1971.
8. Fraser, F.C.: Relation of animal studies to the problem in man. *In* Handbook of Teratology, vol. 1, edited by J.G. Wilson and F.C. Fraser. New York, Plenum Press, 1977, pp. 75–96.
9. Gilbert, S.F. Synthesizing embryology and human genetics: Paradigms regained. Am. J. Hum. Genet. 51:211, 1992.
10. Gruss, P. and Walther, C.: Pax in Development. Cell 69:719, 1992.
11. Holliday, R.: The inheritance of epigenetic defects. Science 238:163, 1987.
12. Jacobsen, A.G. and Sater, A.: Features of embryonic induction. Development 104:341, 1988.
13. Lenz, W.: Genetic diagnosis: Molecular diseases and others. *In* Human Genetics, edited by J. de Grouchy, F.J.G. Ebling, and I.W. Henderson. Amsterdam, Excerpta Medica, 1972.
14. McLaren, A.: Mammalian Chimaeras. Cambridge, Cambridge University Press, 1976.
15. Maniatis, T., et al.: Regulation of inducible and tissue-specific gene expression. Science 236:1237, 1987.
16. Patterson, D.F., et al.: Models of human genetic disease in domestic animals. *In* Advances in Human Genetics, vol. 12, edited by H. Harris and K. Hirschhorn. New York, Plenum Press, 1982.
17. Petter, C., et al.: Simultaneous prevention of blood abnormalities and hereditary congenital amputations in a brachydactylous rabbit stock. Teratology 15:149, 1977.
18. Pinsky, L. and Kaufman, M.: Genetics of steroid receptors and their disorders. *In* Advances in Hu-

man Genetics, vol. 16, edited by H. Harris and K. Hirschhorn. New York, Plenum Press, 1987, pp. 299–472.

19. Pritchard, D.J.: Foundations of developmental genetics. London, Taylor and Francis, 1986.
20. Silva, A.J., Paylor, R., Wehner, J.M., and Tonegawa, S.: Impaired spatial learning in α-calcium-calmodulin kinase II mutant mice. Science 257:206, 1992.
21. Stamatoyannopoulos, G.: Human hemoglobin switching. Science 252:383, 1991.
22. Steitz, J.A.: "Snurps." Sci. Am. 258:56, 1988.
23. Travis, J. Scoring a technical knockout in mice. Science 256:1392, 1992.

Chapter 12
Multifactorial Inheritance

WOODEN LEGS ARE NOT INHERITED, BUT WOODEN HEADS ARE.

A. E. WIGGINS, A NEW DECALOGUE OF SCIENCE

METRICAL TRAITS

Everyone knows that close relatives tend to resemble each other with respect to a number of quantitative, or metrical, characters such as height, weight, size of nose, "intelligence test scores," and so on. The question of how closely relatives resemble each other and how much of the familial tendency is due to genes shared in common is one that has received a good deal of attention from mathematical geneticists, and there is an extensive literature on the subject.[16] We will review only a few basic principles here.

For any particular metrical character, a first approach to the question of the genetic basis is to see whether the frequency distribution of the trait has a single mode, or peak, or more than one mode. Two or three peaks strongly suggest that a major genetic difference is segregating in the population, as in the case of isoniazid degradation (Fig. 12–1). A symmetrical curve with one peak (as in the case of blood pressure or intelligence) suggests that no single factor is making a major contribution to the variation in the trait.

Heritability

Many quantitative traits have a frequency distribution that fits the familiar bell-shaped curve known as the normal curve. A normal curve will result when the trait in question is determined by a large number of factors either genetic, environmental, or both, each making a small contribution to the final effect. If genetic factors are involved, they will not be common ones with a major effect on the trait (or the distribution would not be unimodal). A simple model would be that the magnitude of the trait is determined by a number of genes, each adding a small amount to the value of the trait or subtracting a small amount from it, and each acting independently of the others (i.e., acting additively, with no dominance or epistasis). This is known as *polygenic* inheritance. There are many individuals in the middle of the distribution, and few at the extremes because it is unlikely for an individual to inherit a large number of factors all acting in the same direction.

To take an obviously simplistic example, if height were determined by one gene locus with three alleles, one adding 2 inches to the height (h^+), one subtracting 2 inches (h^-), and one neutral (h), and if h were twice as frequent as the other two alleles, the expected distribution of heights could be found by calculating the frequencies of pairs of gametes from the available pool, as in Table 12–1 and

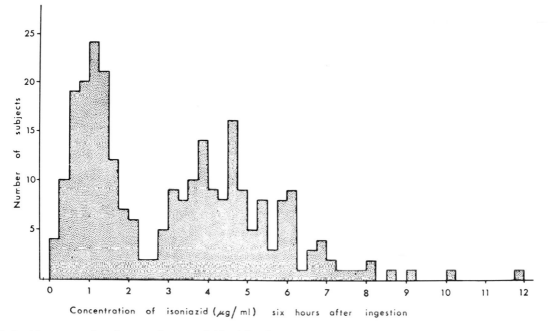

Fig. 12–1. Frequency distribution of isoniazid blood levels 6 hours after a standard dose. The distribution is bimodal, illustrating the presence of two phenotypes—fast and slow inactivators (see Chap. 24).

Figure 12–2. Thus, if the mean height was 68 inches, $1/16$ of the population would be h^-h^- and 64 inches tall, $1/16$ would be h^+h^+ and 72 inches tall, $4/16$ would be hh and 68 inches tall, $2/16$ would be h^+h^- and also 68 inches tall, and so on.

If we add another locus, also with three alleles in the same proportions, the distribution of heights begins to look like the normal curve (Fig. 12–3). Thus a relatively small amount of genetic variation can produce a distribution that is fairly normal. In this case, only 1/256 individuals would inherit all four minus or plus alleles and be at the extremes of the distribution. On the other hand, a number of environmental factors, each adding or subtract-

Table 12–1. Frequencies of Genotypes for Height if Determined by Three Alleles at a Single Locus*

		Sperm		
		1 h⁺	2 h	1 h⁻
Eggs	1 h⁺	h⁺h⁺ 1 72"	h h⁺ 2 70"	h⁺h⁻ 1 68"
	2 h	h⁺h 2 70"	h h 4 68"	h h⁻ 2 66"
	1 h⁻	h⁺h⁻ 1 68"	h h⁻ 2 66"	h⁻h⁻ 1 64"

h = average   h⁻ = minus 2 inches   h⁺ = plus 2 inches
*After Carter, C.O.: Human Heredity. Baltimore, Penguin Books, 1970.

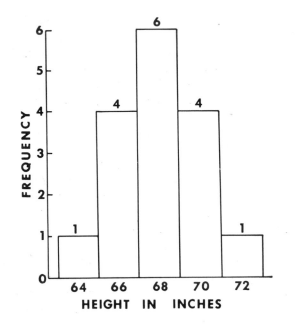

Fig. 12–2. Frequency distribution of heights from Table 12–1.

ing a small amount to the final result, will also result in a normal distribution, even without genetic variation. In most cases, the variation in the population results from a number of genes and environmental factors acting together to determine the final quantity. This can be termed *multifactorial* inheritance. The proportion of the total variation in the trait that results from additive genetic variation is the *heritability* of the trait.

The problem then is to determine how much of the variation in the multifactorial trait is due to genes and how much to environmental factors. One can reason as follows: If all the variation were caused by environmental factors (which did not themselves show a familial tendency), there would be no tendency for relatives to resemble one another—i.e., the correlation between relatives would be 0. What would it be if the inheritance is polygenic, with no environmental variation? Consider, for instance, the correlation between father and son. We will assume, for the purpose of this argument, that the heights of the mothers are representative of the general population. Because the son gets half of his father's genes, if the father's genes for the trait in question are such that he deviates from the mean by

a certain amount, the son should, on the average, deviate by half as much. For a series of such pairs, this would lead to a father-son correlation (and regression of son on father) of 0.5. A similar situation would exist for pairs of brothers, who have half of their father's genes in common (Fig. 12–4).

This relationship was first formulated by Sir Francis Galton as the *law of filial regression*. The regression line in Figure 12–4 represents the mean value of the sons' heights for any father's height. The regression line shows that for any father's value, the mean value of the sons would be halfway between the father's and the mean of the population. In other words, the mean of the sons "regressed" from the mean of the fathers toward the mean of the population. Obviously, the more environmental, nonfamilial variation there is, the lower the correlation will be. Conversely, the less important environmental factors are (i.e., the higher the heritability), the closer to 0.5 will be the correlation between first-degree relatives. Thus it is possible to estimate the proportion of the total variation caused by genetic variation (heritability) from the correlation between various groups of relatives. For first-degree relatives, if all the variation were genetic (a heritability of 1), the correlation would be 0.5. If there was no genetic variation (heritability 0), the correlation would be 0. The closer the correlation is to 0.5, the closer the heritability is to 1. Twins provide a useful extension to this approach, since monozygotic

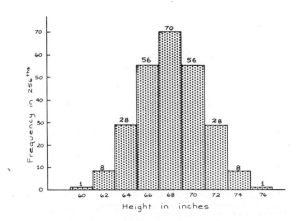

Fig. 12–3. Frequency distribution of heights assuming two loci each with three alleles.

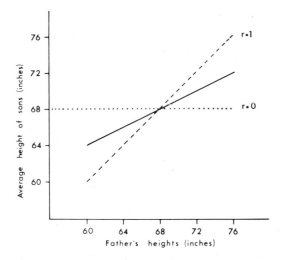

Fig. 12–4. Regression toward the mean of sons' on father's phenotype for a polygenic character. For any father's value, the mean value for sons is halfway between father's value and the mean of the population (assuming no assortative mating).

twins are genetically identical and should therefore have a correlation of 1 if the variation in the trait is entirely genetic, whereas dizygotic twins are genetically no more similar than sibs. Conversely, the variation between pairs of monozygotic twins provides an estimate of the environmental variation.

Remember that this assumes (idealistically) that there are no major genetic factors contributing to the variation, no dominance or epistasis, no assortative mating, and no environmental factors that tend to cluster within families.

In fact, familial environmental factors also increase the correlation between relatives. Some attempt to measure these can be made by comparing, for instance, similarities between half-sibs, to estimate the common environment, or between pairs of unrelated children raised in institutions and raised in foster homes, respectively, but the practical difficulties are great. Furthermore, it has been postulated that the genes act additively; nonadditive interactions, such as dominance or epistasis, would modify the correlations in a complicated way. They will, for instance, lead to parent-child correlations being lower than sib-sib correlations. Assortative mating increases the genetic variation, by increasing homozygosity.

Finally, it should be emphasized that heritability estimates have nothing to do with the degree to which genes determine that trait, but refer only to *genetic variation* in a particular population. They are made on specific populations in a specific range of environments and should not be extrapolated uncritically to other populations and environments. An estimate of heritability of skin color, for instance, based on a Swedish population would be much lower than that for the population of the United States, even though the genetic determination of skin color is the same. The difference is in the amount of *variation* due to genetic differences.

A variety of statistical techniques have been developed to estimate the various components of the variation in a trait, for instance, comparisons between monozygotic and dizygotic twin pairs, twins reared together and reared apart, and correlation between child and biologic parents and between child and foster parents.[16] Estimates of heritability have been made for many quantitative human traits, but they should in most cases be regarded as no more than indications of whether the role of genes in determining the trait is relatively large or small.[16] Chapter 15 provides further discussion.

THRESHOLD CHARACTERS

Many relatively common defects and diseases that are clearly familial cannot be made to fit all the expectations for mendelian inheritance, in spite of enthusiastic attempts to do so, sometimes by statistical methods more vigorous than rigorous. It was first recognized by the great American population geneticist, Sewall Wright, in 1934, that the inheritance of a discontinuous character (polydactyly in the guinea pig) could be accounted for by multifactorial inheritance of a continuously distributed variable, with a *developmental threshold* separating the continuous distribution into two discontinuous segments—polydactylous and not-polydactylous.[17] Gruneberg showed that many discontinuous but seemingly nonmendelian traits in mice fitted this model and called them "quasicontinuous variants."[10]

Developmental Thresholds

A well-documented example of a developmental threshold is cleft of the secondary palate. To close, the palatal shelves must reorient themselves from a vertical position, on either side of the tongue, to a horizontal plane above the tongue, where their medial edges meet and fuse. During the time of reorientation, the head continues to grow, carrying the base of the shelves farther apart. If the shelves become horizontal late enough, they may have lost the ability to fuse, or the head will be so wide that they will be unable to meet, and a cleft palate will result. The latest point in development when the shelves can reach the horizontal and still fuse can be considered a *threshold*. All embryos in which the shelves become horizontal later than this will have cleft palates. Other thresholds may involve other developmental asynchronies, such as neural tube closure; physiologic characteristics, such as renal tubular reabsorption; a mechanical relationship—e.g., the degree of occlusion of the coronary artery that cuts down the blood supply to the heart muscle to the point where a heart attack ensues.

To return to the palate, the important point is that a continuous, multifactorial variable—stage at which shelf movement to the horizontal occurs—is separated into discontinuous parts—normal and cleft palate—by a threshold. If the continuous variable involves a post-

natal process, e.g., blood pressure, it is possible to place any given individual on the distribution, but for a prenatal process, it is possible to tell only whether or not the individual fell beyond the threshold.

However, it is possible to make some deductions about how such a trait will be distributed in the population and in the relatives of affected persons. Furthermore, for traits that fit the predictions, one can then estimate the heritability of the underlying variable from the observed frequencies in families, as we will see.

Models of Quasicontinuous Inheritance

Several mathematical models have been proposed from which estimates of heritability of liability to the disease can be calculated.[8]

A Scots quantitative geneticist, Falconer, proposed the term *liability* to represent the sum total of genetic and environmental influences that make an individual more or less likely to develop a disease or defect.[6] The liabilities of individuals in a population form a continuous, normally distributed variable. A person develops overt disease if his liability reaches a certain threshold.

In the case of cleft palate, many things influence the stage at which the shelves move to the horizontal—the force within the shelves that promotes their movement to the horizontal, the size of the resisting tongue, changes in the growing head and jaw that provide more space for the shelves to move into, and so on. Each of these is influenced by genetic and environmental factors. This, then, is a multifactorial model.[7,8] The stage at which the shelves reach the horizontal would represent the liability to cleft palate—the later, the more liable—and the latest stage at which they can still bridge the gap will be the threshold. Note that genes and environmental factors can also influence the threshold—in this case by altering the size of the gap through changes in shelf width and head width. Figure 12–5 represents palate closure as a multifactorial threshold character.

Figure 12–6 illustrates a population in which liability for a given disease is normally distributed (solid curve), and all individuals be-

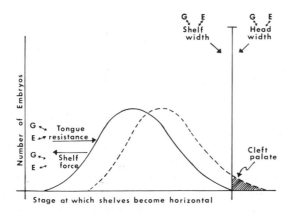

Fig. 12–5. Diagram of factors influencing palate closure, illustrating its multifactorial threshold nature. The dotted line represents a population exposed to some factor that delays closure, e.g., cortisone.

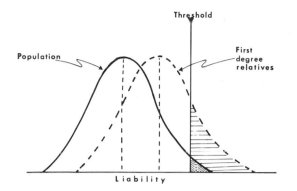

Fig. 12–6. Hypothetical frequency distribution for a threshold character, showing the distribution of the population (solid line) and that of first-degree relatives (broken line).

yond a certain threshold (T) actually have the disease (diagonal hatching). Thus the affected individuals have a mean liability near the right-hand tail of the distribution. The usual family study ascertains a series of such individuals, as probands, and measures the frequency of affected individuals in the near relatives. What will the frequency be in the proband's sibs and children?

The broken line in Figure 12–6 illustrates the distribution of liabilities for first-degree relatives, assuming that all the variation is genetic (a heritability of 1). By the law of filial regression, it will have a mean halfway between the mean of the probands and the mean of the population, and the frequency of the disease will be higher than that of the general population (horizontal hatching). How much higher?

If liability is normally distributed, an estimate can be deduced from a property of the normal curve, which is that there is a fixed relationship between the distance from the mean (measured in standard deviations) and the number of individuals that lie under the curve beyond that distance. For instance, by consulting a normal curve area table, we can see that if a threshold were set two standard deviations from the mean, 2.27% of individuals would lie beyond the threshold and be affected, and at three standard deviations from the mean, 0.13% would be affected.

Thus we can estimate, from the frequency in the population, how far the threshold is from

the mean. For a frequency of 1 per 1000, for instance, the table tells us that the threshold is 3.1 standard deviations from the mean. If all the variation is genetic, the mean of the distribution of liabilities for first-degree relatives should be intermediate between that of the affected probands (say 3.3 standard deviations) and that of the general population, or about 1.65 standard deviations. If so, we would expect (from the normal curve) that about 5% of the first-degree relatives would be affected. If the heritability is less than 1, the observed frequency in the relatives would be correspondingly lower, so it is possible to estimate the heritability by the difference between the observed figure and that expected if the heritability were 1. Mathematical details and appropriate tables can be found elsewhere.[5,15,16]

Note that traits with a high heritability can have a relatively low recurrence rate. For example, for cleft lip and palate, in which the frequency in sibs of probands is 3 to 5%, heritability is estimated as 70 to 90%.

Family Features of Multifactorial Threshold Diseases

The family distributions of certain common congenital malformations show certain features that are neatly explained by the multifactorial threshold model, as first pointed out by the English medical geneticist, Cedric Carter, for pyloric stenosis.[2] Some of the features are explained equally well by other models, but some are not.

Relation of Recurrence Risk to Population Frequency. With the aid of a number of reasonable mathematical approximations, it has been shown that for a threshold character with high heritability, the frequency of occurrence of the trait in first-degree relatives of affected individuals is approximately the square root of the frequency in the population. This relationship holds (approximately) for a number of common congenital malformations and not for diseases known to show mendelian inheritance or diseases with a known major environmental component, which suggests that the former are, indeed, multifactorially determined threshold characters.

It also follows that the recurrence risk for a given defect will be higher in a population with a high frequency than in one with a low frequency, though not proportionately. This has been shown for neural tube defects, for example; in Northern Ireland the population frequency is close to 1% and the risk for sibs is 10%, a 10-fold increase, whereas in London the corresponding figures are 0.29 and 4.4%, a 15-fold increase.

If the recurrence risk in sibs of affected individuals is not known, it can be predicted from this relationship. However, this is not a very sensitive approach; e.g., population frequencies of 1/10,000 and 1/1000 would predict risks in sibs of 1 and 3%, respectively.

Nonlinear Decrease in Frequency with Decreasing Relationship. We have already seen that the distribution of the underlying variable in first-degree relatives of affected individuals will have a mean halfway between the mean of the affected relatives and the mean of the population. For second-degree relatives, the mean will be between the mean for the first-degree relatives and that of the population, and so on. Thus, if the distance between the curve for the first-degree relatives and the curve for the population is 1, the distance for the second-degree relatives will be $^{1}/_{2}$, and for the third-degree relatives $^{1}/_{4}$, and so on. However, the proportion of affected relatives will be represented not by these ratios but by the *area under the curve* beyond the threshold for the respective distributions (Fig. 12–7). Because the tail of the curve becomes progressively flatter, the drop in frequency should be greater between first- and second-degree relatives (on the steep part of the curve) than between second- and third-degree relatives (on the flatter part of the curve). This has been shown for several common congenital malformations, including pyloric stenosis, dislocation of the hip, clubfoot, and cleft lip with or without cleft palate.[2]

In the case of cleft lip, for instance, the frequency of the defect is about 40 per 1000 for the first-degree relatives, 7 for second-degree relatives, and only 3 for third-degree relatives.

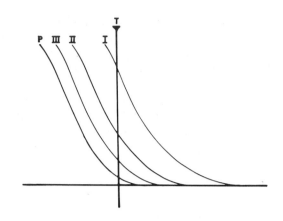

Fig. 12–7.   Relation of the tail of the frequency distribution to the threshold for the population (P) and the first (I), second (II), and third (III) degree relatives of affected individuals.

Increased Risk of Recurrence after Two Affected Children. As we have said, with threshold characters one cannot tell where, on the distribution of liability, a given individual is. However, parents who have an affected child must have contributed a relatively large number of genes for liability to the child and are therefore likely to be carrying more than the average number of such genes themselves. That is, they tend to lie between the population mean and the threshold (see Fig. 12–6). Their future children will thus have a greater than average risk of being affected. If they do have a second affected child, they can be assumed to carry still more predisposing genes, so they will lie still closer to the threshold, and the recurrence risk will be even greater than for parents after one affected child. This has been shown to be true for cleft lip and palate, pyloric stenosis,[2] and spina bifida aperta, where the recurrence risk after one affected child is about 4% and after two affected children about 10% (see Chap. 13).

Increased Recurrence Risk with Increased Severity of Defect. It is reasonable to suppose that, for a threshold character, a person with a severe form of the defect would be nearer the tail of the distribution of liability than a person with a mild one. If so, the risk of recurrence should be higher in patients with the more severe defects. In the case of cleft lip, for instance, the recurrence risk is about 2.5% for probands with unilateral cleft lip and 5.6% for bilateral cleft lip and palate.[7]

Recurrence Risk and Sex of Proband. In defects that occur more frequently in one sex than the other, it must be assumed that the threshold is nearer the tail of the distribution in the sex less often affected. If, for instance, the defect appears less often in females than males, females must have more genes for liability in order to fall beyond the threshold and be affected. If so, the recurrence risk should be higher for the relatives of female patients. This was first shown for congenital hypertrophic pyloric stenosis. This is a condition in which the muscle at the exit to the stomach enlarges, and closes off the canal, so that the baby vomits its feedings. It affects about five times as many males as females. For instance, the risk is about 20% for sons of affected females as compared to 5% for sons of affected males (Table 12–2). Similar, though less striking, differences occur in the case of cleft lip and, in the opposite direction, for cleft palate, when there is an excess of females.[7] In each case, *the recurrence risk is higher when the proband is of the less frequently affected sex.*

IMPLICATIONS

These features suggest that a number of relatively common familial diseases and defects fit the multifactorial threshold model. It should be pointed out, however, that other models will predict these features too. For example, if a major gene difference were causing bimodality or trimodality in the left-hand side of the distribution, the criteria would still fit as long as one of the more resistant populations extended beyond the threshold. The problem is that one cannot determine the shape of the distribution by observing only the tail that falls beyond the threshold. Thus a variety of models can be constructed that will fit the empirical data just about as well (or as badly) as the one above. These include a major gene combined with polygenic and environmental variation,[12] a single locus with two alleles acting additively (i.e., trimodal) and environmental variation;[15] a mixture of cases determined by a major locus with incomplete dominance and reduced penetrance or by environmental factors or variations of these.[6,9] *Cultural inheritance*, the familial transmission of cultural patterns, can also be incorporated.[3]

Discussions of the relative merits of the multifactorial versus the major gene models, both with a threshold, have generated more heat than light,[7,9] and the truth probably lies somewhere in between for many common, familial, disorders. The polygenic model is unrealistic—Nature does not deal in large numbers of genes with small, equal and additive effects. But so is the major gene model—a process as complex as palate closure, for instance, can be interfered with in many ways; surely there is more than one place where a major gene might interfere. And clearly any such "major" gene(s) must have greatly reduced penetrance, thus approaching the multifactorial model.

The major gene model promises the prospect of identifying the major genes and thus improving understanding, prognosis, and prospects for prevention or treatment. The rapid expansion in the capabilities of molecular genetics may help to search out some of the genes contributing to susceptibility in multifactorial disorders. The following chapter provides some examples—e.g., diabetes mellitus, peptic ulcer. The multifactorial model encourages us to look at the epigenetic aspects of liability distributions and thresholds, as illustrated by the work on facial clefts.[8,11] Both have their value.

Table 12–2. Frequency (%) of Pyloric Stenosis in Children and Sibs of Male and Female Probands*

Proband	Sons	Daughters	Brothers	Sisters
Male	5.5 (11 ×)	2.4 (24 ×)	3.8 (8 ×)	2.7 (27 ×)
Female	18.9 (38 ×)	7.0 (70 ×)	9.2 (18 ×)	3.8 (38 ×)

*The numbers in brackets represent the increase over the population frequency.

In any case, one should resist the temptation to invoke the concept, as some have done, for familial conditions that have not been tested by the above criteria. Neither should multifactorial be used to refer to etiologic heterogeneity—that is, when different cases of the disease have different causes.

In counseling, we find it useful to develop with the parents of an affected child the idea that susceptibility is the result of the adding up of "a lot of little things," none of which is in itself abnormal, so that they should not feel guilty about having "bad genes" or having unknowingly exposed the baby to a prenatal insult.

What can be done to reduce the frequency of such conditions? One approach is to try to identify the individual components contributing to susceptibility—for instance, familial joint laxity with congenital hip dislocation, differences in face shape with cleft lip, or blood group O secretor status with duodenal ulcer. The more components identified, the better the identification of susceptible individuals. DNA technology can identify markers of susceptibility in an increasing number of multifactorial disorders.[1] Another approach recognizes that multifactorial threshold characters often vary in frequency with season of birth, socioeconomic class, geographic region, and other environmental differences. This shows that extrinsic factors may shift the relationship of underlying distribution and threshold; we must now learn to identify these factors. The preventive approach would then be to protect genetically susceptible individuals from precipitating factors or find ways of shifting the distribution away from the threshold. The reduced recurrence risk for neural tube defects following periconceptional vitamin supplementation may be an example (see Chap. 13).

SUMMARY

Many quantitative or metrical traits such as height and intelligence fit a unimodal curve with a normal distribution, suggesting that no major genetic factor is segregating but rather that the trait is determined by many genes, each contributing a small amount to the final result (polygenic inheritance). In most cases the trait (or variation) is produced by an interaction of polygenic and environmental factors. This system of genetic-environmental interaction is termed *multifactorial inheritance*. For a given population, the proportion of the variation in the trait that results from the genetic variation is the heritability of the trait.

Certain discontinuous characters may be produced by the imposition of a developmental threshold on a continuously distributed variable (quasicontinuous variation). Several models of quasicontinuous inheritance have been proposed. For common traits, it may be difficult, if not impossible, to distinguish the multifactorial threshold model from one that is based on a major gene with reduced penetrance in some cases and on many genes, each with a small effect, in the majority of cases, or from other similar models.

Several features characterize multifactorial threshold diseases, including the relation of recurrence in first-degree relatives to the population frequency, nonlinear decrease in frequency with decreasing relationship to the proband, increased risk after two affected first-degree relatives, increased risk with increased severity of the defect, and a higher recurrence risk when the proband is of the less frequently affected sex. These variations in recurrence risk are usually not large enough to make much difference to genetic counseling.

REFERENCES

1. Bock, G. and Collins, G.M. (Editors): Molecular approaches to human polygenic disease. Ciba Foundation Symposium 130, Chichester, UK, John Wiley & Sons, Ltd., 1987.
2. Carter, C.O.: Genetics of common single malformations. Br. Med. Bull. 25:52, 1969.
3. Cloninger, C.R., et al.: Multifactorial inheritance with cultural transmission and assortative mating. II. A general model of combined polygenic and cultural inheritance. Am. J. Hum. Genet. 31:176, 1979.
4. Elston, R.C. and Yelverton, K.C.: General models for segregation analysis. Am. J. Hum. Genet. 27:31, 1975.
5. Falconer, D.S.: The inheritance of liability to diseases with variable age of onset, with particular reference to diabetes mellitus. Ann. Hum. Genet. 31:1, 1967.
6. Farrell, M., and Holder, S.: Familial recurrence—pattern analysis of cleft lip with or without cleft palate. Am. J. Hum. Genet. 50:270, 1992.

7. Fraser, F.C.: The multifactorial/threshold concept—uses and misuses. Teratology 14:267, 1976.

8. Fraser, F.C.: Evolution of a palatable multifactorial threshold model. Am. J. Hum. Genet. 32:796, 1980.

9. Fraser, F.C.: Mapping the cleft-lip genes. The first fix? Am. J. Hum. Genet. 45:345, 1989.

10. Gruneberg, H.: Genetic studies on the skeleton of the mouse. IV. Quasicontinuous variations. J. Genet. 51:95, 1952.

11. Mendell, N.R. and Spence, M.A.: Empiric recurrence risks and models of inheritance. Part I. Birth Defects Original Article Series XV(5C):39, 1979.

12. Morton, N.E., and MacLean, C.J.: Analysis of family resemblance. III. Complex segregation of quantitative traits. Am. J. Hum. Genet. 26:489, 1974.

13. Murphy, E.A.: The genetic dynamics of disease. Am. J. Med. Genet. 8:35, 1981.

14. Rotter, J.I.: Genetic approaches to ulcer heterogeneity. *In* The Genetics and Heterogeneity of Common Gastrointestinal Disorders, edited by J.J. Rotter, I.M. Samloff and D.L. Rimoin. New York, Academic Press, 1980, pp. 111–128.

15. Smith, C.: Discriminating between modes of inheritance in genetic disease. Clin. Genet. 2:303, 1971.

16. Vogel, F., and Motulsky, A.G.: Human Genetics. Problems and Approaches. Berlin, Springer-Verlag, 2nd edition, 1986.

17. Wright, S.: An analysis of variability in number of digits in an inbred strain of guinea pigs. Genetics 19:506, 1934.

Chapter 13

Some Malformations and Diseases Determined by Multifactorial Inheritance

ALL INTEREST IN DISEASE AND DEATH IS ONLY ANOTHER EXPRESSION OF INTEREST IN LIFE.

THOMAS MANN

Multifactorial diseases are, in general, common, and diseases caused by major mutant genes are uncommon. "Common" is generally taken to mean of the order of 1 per 1000. For an increasing number of disease entities, there are data consistent with multifactorial inheritance; a selection of these will be presented in this chapter.

The genetic counseling of families having diseases determined by multifactorial inheritance may be more difficult than for those having single mutant gene disorders because the risks given are usually average risks rather than precise probabilities. Empiric recurrence risks are becoming increasingly available, but are often incomplete for a given disease even if the multifactorial etiology is reasonably well established. For example, although recurrence risks after one affected first-degree relative may be known, the recurrence risk after two or three affected first-degree relatives may not be established. Under these circumstances, it is reasonable to apply generalizations from experience with multifactorial diseases in which such empiric risks have been established to multifactorial diseases for which there are no established risks. Several theoretical models for calculating such risks (Table 13–1) are available.[6,13,24]

From the theoretical model and from experience with cleft lip and palate, spina bifida-anencephaly, and some congenital heart lesions, the recurrence following the birth of two affected first-degree relatives would be two to three times greater than that after one. For more than two affected first-degree relatives there are few data for any diseases, but the theory and experience with some congenital heart lesions suggest that the risk becomes quite high (Table 13–1).

ANENCEPHALY-SPINA BIFIDA

The neural tube defects are among the most fascinating of the common birth defects, pre-

Table 13–1.   Recurrences Risks (%) for Multifactorial Diseases According to Number of Affected First-Degree Relatives and Heritability

Affected Parents		0			1			2		
Population Frequency (%)	Heritability (%)		Affected Sibs			Affected Sibs			Affected Sibs	
		0	1	2	0	1	2	0	1	2
1.0%	100	0.7	7	14	11	24	34	63	65	67
	80	0.8	6	14	8	18	28	41	47	52
	50	0.9	4	8	4	9	15	15	21	26
0.1	100	0.1	4	11	5	16	26	62	63	64
	80	0.1	3	8	3	10	18	32	37	42
	50	0.1	1	3	1	3	7	7	11	15

This table, adapted from Smith,[23] provides theoretic recurrence risks for a multifactorial threshold character. It can be used as a guide when no empiric figures are available. For instance, to estimate the risk for the next child of schizophrenic parents who have a schizophrenic child, the frequency is close to 1%, heritability is, say, 80%, so the risk would be about 47%. For a parent with cleft lip and palate who has two affected children, the frequency is about 0.1, the heritability is 80%, and the risk would be about 18%. The risk decreases with each unaffected child, but not very much, e.g., in the last example, if there were also 2 unaffected children, the risk for the next would be 15 instead of 18.

senting many puzzles, and some tantalizing hints of solutions. Anencephaly and spina bifida appear to be etiologically related because they often occur together, and the frequency of each is increased in sibs of children with the other. It is not necessary to discuss the anatomic defects in detail. Spina bifida is a failure of fusion of the bony spinal arch. In *spina bifida occulta,* the defect is limited to the bony arch and is covered by skin. In *spina bifida cystica,* the covering of the spinal cord, the meninges, protrudes through the opening in the spine (meningocele) and perhaps the cord as well (meningomyelocele). Hydrocephalus (water on the brain) may also occur. This has led to some confusion in family studies, reported in the literature, that have combined data from cases of isolated hydrocephalus and of hydrocephalus with spina bifida. Hydrocephalus with spina bifida should be considered secondary to the spinal defect; hydrocephalus without spina bifida should be considered separately. *Anencephaly* is an absence of skin, skull, overlying membranes, forebrain, and midbrain, which produces still-birth or death shortly after birth. Embryologically and genetically, spina bifida cystica and anencephaly may be variations of the same basic defect, a failure of the embryonic neural tube to close.

The usual findings in patients with spina bifida with meningomyelocele are paralysis of the lower extremities and urinary and fecal incontinence. Progressive hydrocephalus may be arrested by neurosurgical intervention, but the course has usually been one of progressive deterioration with an infection often being the terminal event. Advancements in surgical management are improving the outlook. Paradoxically, improved surgical procedures may lead to an increase in the number of living but crippled children because these procedures may save the lives of children who would otherwise have died, but leave many of them with varying degrees of handicap.

A recurrence rate of 2 to 6% in first-degree relatives has been derived from a number of European and North American studies.[8] As expected with multifactorial threshold conditions, the higher the population frequency the higher the recurrence rate. In Belfast, for example, it is almost 10%. Whether the proband has anencephaly or spina bifida aperta, the sibs are at risk for either one or the other or both. The recurrence risk after two affected first-degree relatives is about 10% (Table 13–2).

In this group of lesions there is an excess of females. There is also a small excess of first-born infants and infants in which the maternal

Table 13–2.   Rates (%) of Recurrence of the Same Defect in a Child of Given Relationship to an Affected Person*

Defect	f/1000	Sex Ratio	Relative(s) Affected ♂	Parent	♀	Brother	Sister	Sib	2 Sibs	Parent + Sib	2nd Degree	3rd Degree
Heart malformation												
VSD	2.5		2.0		6.0			3.0				
PDA	1.2		2.5		3.5–4.0			2.5				
Tetralogy	1.1		1.5		6–10			2.4				
ASD	1.1		1.5		4–4.5			2.5				
PS	0.8		2.0		4–6.5			2.0				
AS	0.4		3.0		13–18			2.0				
Coarctation	0.6		2.0		4.0			2.0				
Transposition	0.5							2.0				
Endocardial cushion	0.4		1.0		14.0			3.0				
Legg-Perthes[†]	0.7	5.2				3.6	4.3	3.8				
Anencephaly[†]	3.0	0.6				3.2	6.5	5.4	10			0.3–1.3
Spina bifida[‡]	3.0	0.8		3.0		3.8	3.1	3.4				
Pyloric stenosis	3.0	5.0	♂ 5.5		18.9	3.8	9.2	6.0				
			♀ 2.4		7.0	2.7	3.8					
Scoliosis, idiopathic (adolescent onset)	1.8	0.15						5.0			3.7	1.5
Talipes equinovarus	1.2	2.0				2.0	6.0	2.9			0.5	0.2
Dislocated hip[§]	5.0	0.3	♂	6.0				♂ 1.8		36	1.5	0.3
			♀	17.0				♀ 11.4				
Cleft lip ± palate	1.0	1.6		4.0		3.9	5.0	4.3	9	15?	0.7	0.4
Cleft palate	0.45	0.7		5.8		6.3	2.3	2.9		15?	0.4	0.3
Hirschsprung disease	0.2	3.7	N.R.		Rare	2.6	7.2	5.0				
Schizophrenia	8.0	1.0			15.0			10–15			2.0	1.5
Manic depressive (bipolar)	6.0	0.8			14.0			14.0				

*To find the probability of occurrence for a child whose mother has pyloric stenosis, look up pyloric stenosis, parent, ♀. The probability is 18.9% for a male and 7% for a female child. If the mother has VSD, the recurrence risk for a child of either sex is 6.0; if the father has VSD, the recurrence risk is 2.0.

[†]Attack rate to age 15.

[‡]Rates given are for anencephaly and/or spina bifida.

[§]Neonatal diagnosis.

N.R. = not reported

age exceeds 40 years. Multiple vertebral defects, with or without spina bifida occulta, also fit into the group of neural tube closure defects, with similar risks of sibs having spina bifida cystica or anencephaly.[5]

The neural tube defects show the most striking epidemiologic variations of any of the common malformations, suggesting that the environmental contribution to liability is comparatively large.[8] The range of frequencies extends from less than one to more than 10 per thousand births. The frequency is higher in Western than Eastern Britain and in Eastern than Western North America, high in the Irish, Welsh, and Sikhs, and low in Mongolians and Blacks, and higher in the less well-off socioeconomic groups. In some regions, it occurs more often in babies conceived in the late winter or early spring, and in many parts of the world a slow decline is occurring, since a high in the 1930s. Correlations have been suggested with a variety of environmental factors including soft water, zinc deficiency, consumption of cured meat and of tea, and prevalence of potato blight.

What specific factors are responsible for these curious correlations is a tantalizing question, so far unanswered. Some factors suggest poor nutrition, and support for this idea comes from some studies suggesting that nutritional supplementation of at-risk mothers may reduce the recurrence rate of neural tube defects. This exciting advance was confirmed by a randomized collaborative trial organized by the British Medical Research Council, which showed that the active ingredient is folic acid.[15] The effect has been shown only for mothers known to be at high risk, but it is reasonable to suppose that it would also apply to the population at large. The role of alpha-fetoprotein screening in prenatal diagnosis is discussed in Chapter 15.

CARDIOVASCULAR DISEASE

A genetic-environmental interaction appears to be the underlying cause of the majority of familial manifestations of cardiovascular disease, including congenital heart disease, coronary heart disease, hypertension, and rheumatic fever.[17] This topic is covered in detail in Chapter 23.

CLEFT LIP AND CLEFT PALATE (FIG. 13–1)

The evidence that congenital clefts of the primary and secondary palate are multifactorially determined threshold characters has been discussed in Chapter 12. The secondary palate closes later in development than the primary palate, which forms the gum and lip, and the genetic and environmental factors that influence its closure are likely to differ from those that influence closure of the primary palate.

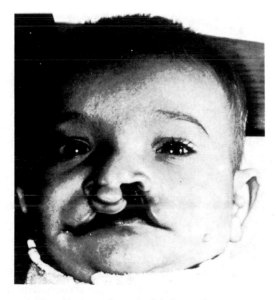

Fig. 13–1. Bilateral cleft lip and palate.

On the other hand, abnormal development of the primary palate, leading to a cleft lip, may interfere with secondary palate closure, leading to cleft palate with the cleft lip. Thus, on both embryologic and genetic grounds, congenital cleft lip (CL) and cleft lip with cleft palate (CLP) appear to be etiologically related,[10] and in data combining the two they may be designated CL(P). Isolated cleft of the secondary palate (CP) is an etiologically independent entity. Nevertheless, some mutant genes cause CL(P) in some individuals and CP in others—the cleft lip with lip-pit syndrome, for example.

In a large number of syndromes CL(P) or CP may be one of the features. A few are associated with recognizable chromosomal aberrations, about a third are caused by major mutant genes, and for most the cause is not known. A survey lists 142 syndromes involving orofacial clefts, of which 103 were monogenic.[7] Each of these syndromes is rare, and together they may account for perhaps 5% of all cases, most of the rest being multifactorially determined. For counseling, it is important to distinguish cases associated with syndromes from the multifactorial type, because the recurrence risks are different. Inclusion of unrecognized cases of syndromes in family studies may account for the fact that the recurrence risk for sibs of patients with CL(P) is reduced from 4% to 2% if the proband has an additional malformation.

Cleft Lip with or without Cleft Palate— CL(P). Most cases of CL(P) or CP without associated malformations appear to fit the multifactorial model,[10] though we reiterate that, on the basis of present evidence, there is little to distinguish models in which the genetic component is polygenic from those involving a major gene with reduced penetrance plus polygenic variation and some phenocopies.[13] An association of CL(P) with the transforming growth factor alpha has been found, but no linkage. Even after known syndromes have been eliminated from the data, there is likely to be considerable heterogeneity. For counseling, one must rely on average recurrence risks, which for most families will be similar for the various models.

More males than females are affected with CL(P). There are striking differences in frequency between races: Orientals have relatively high frequencies (1.7/1000 births), Caucasians are intermediate (1/1000), and Africans tend to have low frequencies (0.4/1000). These differences persist in different geographic regions, suggesting that they do not result from environmental factors, and it is tempting to think that they may be associated with differences in face shape.[11]

As expected for multifactorial traits, the risk for relatives of affected persons drops off sharply from first- to second-degree relatives. Thus it is about 4% for sibs and children, 0.7% for uncles, aunts, nephews, and nieces, and 0.4% for first cousins. Occasionally these figures are useful for counseling; for instance, the sib of a person with CL(P) can be advised that the chance of having an affected child is about 0.7% or 1 in 140 (Table 13–2).

The recurrence risk is somewhat higher in the sibs of female probands than of male probands, in the sibs of patients with a severe defect than in those with a mild form, and after two affected sibs than after one (Table 13–2). There are few data on the risk for sibs of an affected child with an affected parent. The available figures suggest a figure of about 15%, but the numbers are small.

In spite of many attempts to demonstrate environmental factors associated with CL(P), no association has been convincingly demonstrated between CL(P) incidence and such things as seasonal trend, geographic location (except when there are differences in racial groups), social class, maternal age or parity, or paternal age. Several prenatal factors have been tentatively implicated, such as pernicious vomiting of pregnancy, antiemetics, maternal bleeding, toxemia of pregnancy, and toxoplasma, but their significance is not clear. Some anti-epileptic drugs, particularly diphenylhydantoin, may increase the frequency of cleft lip (and other defects) in exposed embryos. The risk is about 2%, suggesting that exposure to the drug shifts the distribution of liability somewhat less than being a first-degree relative of a person with cleft lip.

Cleft Palate (CP). Isolated cleft palate is rarer than CL(P), with an average frequency in Caucasians of about 0.45 per 1000 births. More females than males are affected. There is little racial variation. The frequency appears somewhat higher than average in older mothers of high parity.

The recurrence risks for CP are similar to those for CL(P)[10] except that the risk is higher for sibs of male probands (6.3%) than for sibs of female probands (2.3%), as expected for a multifactorial threshold character (Table 13–2). The rather low concordance rate in MZ co-twins (23% vs. 10% in DZ co-twins) suggests that the environmental contribution to causation is larger than it is for CL(P) and there is more evidence for an admixture of families segregating for a major gene.

CONGENITAL DISLOCATION OF THE HIP (CDH)

It is difficult to establish reliable figures for the prevalence of this defect either in populations or families because of variations in diagnostic efficiency. Subluxation and dislocation of the hip may be demonstrated by appropriate examination in the first few days of life (the **neonatal diagnosis group**). An unknown fraction of these cases, if untreated, would go on to frank dislocation at the time of weight-bearing, and the rest would correct themselves spontaneously. Those diagnosed only after the first few weeks are referred to as the **late diagnosis group**. The more effectively patients are diagnosed in the neonatal period, the fewer cases will appear in the late diagnosis group. Effective neonatal screening has been introduced only recently, and family data will include varying proportions of the two types, depending on the age group involved. The following discussion presents figures for the neonatal diagnosis group, which will overestimate the number that would go on to frank dislocation, but because early detection should lead to immediate treatment, these are the appropriate figures to indicate that a subsequent child will require treatment.

For probands with early diagnosis CDH and normal parents, the risk is about 2% for brothers and 11% for sisters, or a risk for all sibs of 6%—a strong indication for careful screening at birth. No data are available for offspring in this group. For children of CDH patients, the risk is about 6% (−) for sons and 17% for daughters, or an overall risk of 12% for all children.[27]

The data are consistent with a multifactorial etiology. Susceptibility varies with the degree of acetabular dysplasia, which appears to be polygenically inherited, and with the degree of laxity of the joint capsule. Thus a dominantly inherited joint laxity is frequently found in the families of patients with CDH, particularly in the neonatal diagnosis group. Associations with environmental factors have also been identified. There is an excess of first-born children and of breech births. CDH occurs more often in babies born in the winter than in summer months (perhaps because tight swaddling may elicit frank disease in a predisposed baby) and also (at least in Edinburgh) in the upper socioeconomic groups.

Closed reduction and immobilization in a hip spica cast is recommended, but the success of treatment depends on early diagnosis and prompt therapy.

DIABETES MELLITUS

Diabetes mellitus, a group of diseases involving abnormal glucose metabolism and resulting in "too much sugar in the blood," has been referred to as a "geneticist's nightmare." Every possible mode of inheritance has been postulated for its undoubtedly familial nature, and there is still no agreement. Part of the problem is genetic heterogeneity. The existence of two major groups, of early and late onset, was recognized early in the game, but the situation is much more complicated than that, and the more one looks, the more heterogeneity one finds.

To begin with, there are more than 40 rare genetic syndromes, of which diabetes is a feature showing (as one would expect with something as complex as the control of glucose metabolism) many ways to produce the diabetic phenotype.[2] The more common forms of diabetes mellitus separate into two major groups, the insulin-dependent (IDDM) and the non-insulin dependent (NIDDM). Much (but by no means all) of the confusion in early genetic studies resulted from not treating the two types separately.

Insulin-dependent diabetes mellitus (IDDM) tends to have an onset in childhood, and was therefore referred to as "juvenile onset" DM. It has a frequency of 1 to 3 per 1000 by age 17. Patients are thin, prone to diabetic coma because the metabolic upset results in ketosis, and require insulin. At least one subgroup manifests antibodies against the pancreatic islet (insulin making) cells, which are thereby destroyed, so that this type can be thought of as an auto-immune disease.

No simple mendelian pattern is found.[2] Concordance in MZ twins is less than 50%. Recurrence rates for sibs vary from 5 to 10% and for offspring around 2% during the first decade of life. A striking advance has been the discovery of a strong association with certain haplotypes at the HLA locus (see Chapter 18). One model suggests that susceptibility depends on a locus within the HLA complex— one allele predisposes to the autoimmune DR3 associated, form of IDDM, a second predisposes to a form with anti-insulin antibodies and associated with DR4, which generally has an onset earlier in childhood than the DR3 type. The DR3/DR4 heterozygote has the highest risk of all for early onset IDDM (relative risk 14.3). HLA-DR types are being examined to see if it is possible to further partition these specificities into diabetes-prone and diabetes-resistant alleles using DQA or DQB typing.[1a,16]

Non-insulin-dependent diabetes mellitus is much more common, affecting 5% or more of the adult population. It tends to occur in obese individuals, usually after age 40, and can often be controlled by diet or drugs. It is more prevalent in populations that suffer from "overnutrition." Concordance in MZ twins approaches 100% suggesting that the necessary environmental factors are usually present. Estimates of risks for first-degree relatives range from 5 to 10% for clinical diabetes (NIDDM) and 15 to 20% for an abnormal glucose-tolerance test. An interesting subgroup of NIDDM is a type with early onset of diabetes mellitus with the adult onset phenotype, and is discussed in the following paragraph.

Maturity-onset diabetes of the young (MODY) is a mild juvenile diabetes mellitus without the severe complications of typical juvenile diabetes. There is evidence that this phenotype is inherited as an autosomal dominant in some families.

With cloning of the HLA region and insulin gene, and recognition of RFLPs, the molecular basis for the various types of diabetes is rapidly being clarified.

THE EPILEPSIES[14]

The familial nature of epileptic seizures has been recognized at least since the time of Hippocrates. There has been some progress in our understanding since then, particularly in our appreciation of the complexity of the subject, but there are still many gaps in our knowledge.

To begin with, epilepsy is not a disease, but a symptom of a great variety of derangements of neuronal function, which is why the title of this section is in the plural. McKusick's catalogue lists over 100 mendelian conditions of which epileptic seizures may be one manifestation. Most chromosomal syndromes have an increased risk of seizures. Brain damage may result in focal epilepsy. Convulsions may accompany high fevers. If there is no overt cause, as is the case in about 85% of epileptics, the familial patterns seem to fit the multifactorial category. This group has been referred to as "idiopathic," "cryptogenic," or "centrencephalic" and more recently as "primary generalized" epilepsy.

Studies of monozygotic (MZ) and dizygotic (DZ) twins leave no doubt that genetic factors are important in determining the patterns of the electroencephalogram, both normal and epileptiform, as well as the occurrence of seizures, for which concordance rates are as high as 90% for MZ and 15% for DZ pairs. However, no simple mode of inheritance appears. For genetic counseling, one must rely on empiric estimates of recurrence risks.

Primary generalized epilepsy is characterized by a 3/sec spike-wave EEG pattern. This pattern appears in about 40% of the sibs of affected children, the highest frequency occurring between 5 and 15 years of age. About one fourth of these sibs have seizures, whereas few of the sibs with normal EEGs have seizures. This finding suggests that the genotype determining the 3/sec spike-wave EEG trait increases liability to seizures. For counseling, the following figures provide guidelines. A child who has a parent or a sib with 3/sec spike-wave epilepsy has about a 15% chance of having at least one seizure and about an 8% chance of having recurrent seizures, as compared to a population frequency of about 2%. If the child has both a parent and a sib affected, the chance of being epileptic is about 15%. The risk decreases the longer the child remains free of seizures and if the EEG is still normal after 5 years of age.

Sibs of a person with focal epilepsy have about a 3% chance of having seizures, somewhat higher than the rate for the general population. Sibs of a child with febrile seizures have an increased risk for febrile seizures (about 10%) and also increased risk of nonfebrile seizures (about 5%). Furthermore, if febrile seizures develop between 14 and 35 months of age, the probability of recurrence in the child is much higher if a near relative also had febrile seizures than if there is no such family history.

In summary, it seems reasonable to suppose that liability to seizures is determined by a multifactorial system that determines not only the probability that an individual will have primary generalized epilepsy, but the probability that a major brain-damaging factor, be it mutant gene, aberrant chromosome, or trauma, .will be accompanied by seizures. The importance of the family history in the evaluation of a child with seizures is evident.

HIRSCHSPRUNG DISEASE (CONGENITAL AGANGLIONIC MEGACOLON)

This disorder, with a population frequency of about 1 in 5000 and an M:F sex ratio of about 3.7 to 1, recurs in approximately 5% of sibs. If the proband is male, the recurrence risk is 2.6%; if the proband is female, the recurrence risk is 7.2%.[21] The hereditary predisposition is consistent with multifactorial inheritance, although a mixed model has also been proposed. Very few cases of parent-to-child transmission have been reported, and these have been maternal in origin. The clinical picture varies from severe constipation to acute obstruction of the bowel. Roentgenographic study reveals a dilated and hypertrophied colon proximal to a narrowed segment that lacks normal ganglion cells in Auerbach's plexus.

LEGG-PERTHES DISEASE

This disease, aseptic necrosis of the capital femoral epiphysis, fits the expectation for a multifactorial threshold disease.[12] It occurs five times as often in males as in females. The annual incidence in children under 15 years of age is at least 3.1 per 100,000, with an attack rate of 1:1400. As expected for a multifactorial threshold character with a high sex ratio, the recurrence rate is higher for sibs of female probands than for sibs of male probands, although the difference is not significant and not as striking as in pyloric stenosis. The frequency is 1:26 for siblings, 1:340 in second-degree relatives, and 1:350 for third-degree relatives. Finally, the square root of the population frequency is 2.6%, close to the sib frequency of 3.8%.

MENTAL RETARDATION

"Intelligence" in the general population is more or less normally distributed as one would expect for a character with a polygenic hereditary component influenced by a number of subtle environmental factors. Thus, if one arbitrarily decides that anyone with an IQ of less than 70 is retarded, some individuals will be retarded simply because they received an assortment of genetic and environmental factors, each detracting a small amount from the level of intelligence, that placed them in the lower tail of the normal distribution without any one of these factors being in itself abnormal. Some may be retarded because of a major insult to the brain, which may result from a chromosomal anomaly, a major gene, or an environmental cause such as birth trauma, prenatal viral damage, or postnatal meningitis. These cases, which are relatively rare, form a small hump near the lower tail of the distribution of intelligence; i.e., the curve is "skewed to the left."

Thus, the causes of mental retardation fall into the same four categories as do other common, familial disorders: those caused by major mutant genes, chromosomal aberrations, major environmental insults, and a multifactorial etiology. As one might expect, children with specific causes of mental retardation, as in the first three groups, tend to be more severely retarded than those in the multifactorial group, because the damage in the former groups results from an insult that is likely to be major. Also consistent with this concept is the following seemingly paradoxical fact: The intelligence of the near relatives of children with specific and therefore severe types of retardation (excluding those similarly affected) is like that of the general population, whereas the intelligence of near relatives of children with nonspecific and therefore milder mental retardation tends to be lower than average. The first group are either similarly affected or unaffected, and therefore normal. The second group are in the multifactorial category and therefore show regression toward the mean.

When dealing with a case of mental retardation, the genetic counselor first tries to place the child in one of the four etiologic categories by a thorough family prenatal and perinatal history, physical examination, and appropriate chromosomal and biochemical screening. If a specific cause is found, counseling is given accordingly. If the condition does not fall into one of the first three categories, it is assumed, by exclusion, to fall in the multifactorial group. On the average, then, the intelligence of the sibs will be midway between that of the two parents. The empiric risks presented in Table 13–3, taken from the large study of Reed and Reed,[19] serve as a rough guide in the appropriate family situation.

The evidence for X-linked nonspecific types of mental retardation, some of which have the

Table 13–3. Risk of Mental Retardation in Children and Sibs of Retardates*

Number of Retarded: Parents	Children	Risk for	Risk (%)
0	—	child	1
1	—	child	11
2	—	child	40
0	1	sib	6
1	1	sib	20
2	1	sib	42

*IQ less than 70.

fragile X chromosome, carry a higher risk if the proband is a boy, particularly if the family history suggests an X-linked recessive pattern or the karyotype reveals a "fragile X."[25]

PYLORIC STENOSIS

This, the first of the multifactorial threshold characters, is a disorder in which projectile vomiting, undernutrition, dehydration, and electrolyte imbalance result from a muscular hypertrophy of the pylorus. Incising the hypertrophied pyloric muscle permanently relieves the condition. The frequency in North American and European populations is about 3 per 1000.

The M:F sex ratio is 5:1. Carter's observation that the recurrence risks are much higher to the first-degree relatives of affected females than to the first-degree relatives of affected males was the clue to its multifactorial threshold nature.[4] As discussed in Chapter 12, if a disease is found more frequently in one sex (in this case males), individuals of the other sex (females) require a greater genetic predisposition for the disease to develop because they are, on the average, farther from the mean. If a greater number of "liability genes" are required for the disease to become manifest in the female, it follows that her first-degree relatives would also have greater genetic liability and a higher frequency of the disorder than the first-degree relatives of a male patient, with less genetic predisposition.

Although the overall recurrence risk to first-degree relatives of patients with pyloric stenosis is about 6%, it is preferable to use the more specific risks as shown in Table 13–2, which take into account the greater genetic liability of affected females. Empiric risk figures after two affected first-degree relatives are not available, but one would predict a two- to threefold increase in risk.

TALIPES EQUINOVARUS (CLUBFOOT)[26]

There is more than one type of "clubfoot," but the most common type is talipes equinovarus, in which there is plantar flexion and adduction at the midtarsal joint, the forefoot is supinated, and the heel is inverted. There may be associated malformations such as generalized joint laxity (10%), inguinal hernia (7% of affected boys), and minor deformities of the extremities (4 to 5%). About 1 to 2 infants per 1000 live births have this anomaly, and twice as many males as females are affected. If postural talipes equinovarus, talipes calcaneovalgus, and metatarsus varus are included, the prevalence increases to 4 per 1000 live births.

The recurrence risk is 2.9% in first-degree relatives or 24 times the frequency in the general population. As expected for a multifactorial threshold character, the recurrence risk for talipes calcaneovarus appears higher for the sibs of female probands (6%) than for the sibs of male probands (2%). There is an additional risk for sibs of about 1% for having metatarsus varus, suggesting a common factor in the etiology of these conditions. (Similarly, for the sibs of patients with metatarsus varus, there is about a 4% risk of metatarsus varus and an additional 2.5% risk for talipes equinovarus.) Patients with talipes equinovarus and talipes calcaneovarus have a somewhat increased frequency of congenital dislocation of the hip, possibly because familial joint laxity predisposes to all three conditions.

ULCER, PEPTIC[20]

The familial nature of peptic ulcers has been recognized for a long time and has often been referred to as multifactorial, or even polygenic; only recently has there been progress in sorting out the genetic factors. Recognition of genetic heterogeneity is the key to understanding. Duodenal and gastric ulcer are both familial, independently. Group O nonsecretors are at increased risk, but the association is weak and its basis is not clear. Much clearer is the relationship of duodenal ulcer to serum pepsinogen. Human pepsinogens consist of two immunochemically distinct groups, I and II. PG I is produced by the chief cells in the fundus of the stomach. About half of the patients with duodenal ulcer have an increased serum level of PG I, and the elevated *serum PG I trait shows autosomal dominant inheritance.* Because an increase in chief cell mass is usually accompanied by an increase in parietal (acid-producing) cell mass, this dominant gene presumably causes an increase in both pepsin and acid secretion and thus an increase in liability to ulcer. The relative risk for gene carriers is not yet established, but is likely to be significant. This group of ulcer patients is further separable on the basis of the gastrin response to a protein meal. Ulcer families in which there is no increase in serum PG I can be separated into those with and without rapid gastric emptying.

Thus, the genetics of peptic ulcer still remain multifactorial, but is certainly not polygenic in the strict sense. Recognition of genetic heterogeneity allows better understanding of the pathophysiologic mechanisms and development of more rational modes of therapy or prevention, individualized for the particular family.

REFERENCES

1. Badner, J.A., et al.: A genetic study of Hirschsprung disease. Am. J. Hum. Genet. 46:568, 1990.
1a. Baisch, J.M., et al.: Analysis of HLA-DQ genotypes and susceptibility in insulin-dependent diabetes mellitus. N. Engl. J. Med. 322:1836, 1990.
2. Bell, G.I., et al.: The molecular genetics of diabetes mellitus. Ciba Foundation Symposium on Molecular Approaches to Human Polygenic Disease. Chichester, U.K., John Wiley and Sons, 1987, p. 169.
3. Bear, J.C.: Liability to cleft lip and palate: interpreting the human data. Issues and Reviews in Teratology, edited by H. Kalter. New York, Plenum Press. 1988, vol. 4, p. 163.
4. Carter, C.O.: Genetics of common single malformations. Br. Med. Bull. 32:21, 1976.
5. Carter, C.O., Evans, K.A., and Till, K.: Spinal dysraphism: genetic relation to neural tube malformations. J. Med. Genet. 13:343, 1976.
6. Cloninger, C.R., Rice, J.R., and Reich, T.: Multifactorial inheritance with cultural transmission and assortative mating. Amer. J. Hum. Genet. 31:176, 1979.
7. Cohen, M.M., Fraser, F.C., and Gorlin, R.J.: Craniofacial disorders. *In* Principles and Practice of Medical Genetics, edited by A.E. Emer and D.L. Rimoin, Edinburgh, Churchill Livingstone, 2nd Ed., 1990, Vol. I, p. 749.
8. Elwood, J.H., and Elwood, J.M.: Epidemiology of Anencephalus and Spina Bifida. Oxford, Oxford University Press, 1980.
9. Elwood, J.H., and Elwood, J.M.: Investigation of area differences in the prevalence at birth of anencephalus in Belfast. Int. J. Epidem. 13:45, 1984.
10. Fraser, F.C.: The genetics of cleft lip and cleft palate: yet another look. *In* Current Research Trends in Prenatal Craniofacial Development, edited by R.M. Pratt and R.L. Christiansen. New York, Elsevier North Holland, Inc., 1980, p. 357.
11. Fraser, F.C., and Pashayan, H.: Relation of face shape to susceptibility to congenital cleft lip. A preliminary report. J. Med. Genet. 7:112, 1970.
12. Gray, I.M., Lowry, R.B., and Renwick, D.H.G.: Incidence and genetics of Legg-Perthes disease (osteochondritis deformans) in British Columbia: Evidence of polygenic determination. J. Med. Genet. 9:197, 1972.
13. Kidd, K.K.: Empiric recurrence risks and models of inheritance Part II. Birth Defects Original Article Series XV (5C):51, 1979.
14. Metrakos, J.D., and Metrakos, K.: Genetic studies in clinical epilepsy. *In* Basic Mechanisms of the Epilepsies, Chapter 24. Boston, Little, Brown and Company, 1970, p. 700.
15. MRC Vitamin Study Research Group: Prevention of neural tube defects. Results of the Medical Research Council vitamin study. Lancet 338:131, 1991.
16. Nepom, G.T.: A unified hypothesis for the complex genetics of HLA associations with IDDM. Diabetes 39:1153, 1990.
17. Nora, J.J., Berg, K., and Nora, A.H.: Cardiovascular Diseases: Genetics, Epidemiology and Prevention. New York, Oxford University Press, 1991.
18. Rice, J., et al.: Multifactorial inheritance with cultural transmission and assortative mating. Am. J. Hum. Genet. 30:618, 1978.
19. Reed, R.W., and Reed, S.C.: Mental Retardation: A Family Study. Philadelphia, W.B. Saunders Co., 1965.
20. Rotter, J.I.: The genetics of peptic ulcer: more than one gene, more than one disease. Prog. Med. Genet. 4:1, 1980.
21. Passarge, E.: Genetics of Hirschsprung's Disease. Clin. Gastroenterol. 2:507, 1973.
22. Rotwein, P.R., et al.: Polymorphism in the 5'-flanking region of the human insulin gene and its possible relation to type 2 diabetes. Science 213:1117, 1981.
23. Smith, C.: Recurrence risks for multifactorial inheritance. Am. J. Hum. Genet. 23:578, 1971.
24. Spence, M.A., et al.: Estimation of polygenic recurrence risk for cleft lip and palate. Human Hered. 26:327, 1976.
25. Weaver, D. and Sherman, S.: A counselling guide to the Martin-Bell syndrome. Amer. J. Med. Gen. 26:39, 1987.
26. Wynne-Davies, R.: Family studies and aetiology of club foot. J. Med. Genet. 2:227, 1965.
27. Wynne-Davies, R.: A family study of neonatal and late-diagnosis congenital dislocation of the hip. J. Med. Genet. 7:315, 1970.

Chapter 14

Nontraditional Inheritance

NO SOONER HAD CHROMOSOMAL HEREDITY, WITH ITS MENDELIAN LAWS BEEN DEFINED . . . THAN EXCEPTIONS WERE DESCRIBED. AS FAR BACK AS 1909 . . .

J.L. JINKS

For many years, it has been obvious that certain familial diseases in some families did not fit comfortably into mendelian patterns. Multifactorial inheritance has been invoked to explain a great many nonmendelian conditions, but it turns out that there are familial diseases that fail to conform to either mendelian or multifactorial expectations, for example, mitochondrial inheritance and genomic imprinting. There are also genetic disorders that involve chromosomes, but are not caused by nuclear chromosomal trisomies, translocations, or other abnormalities that one sees described in the usual discussions of chromosomal anomalies. These include uniparental disomy and segmental aneusomy.

We have crowded under nontraditional inheritance certain modes that were scattered throughout various chapters in the last edition and have designated nontraditional inheritance as a category (however heterogeneous) that would benefit from separate treatment. To illustrate the intensity of interest in these forms of inheritance, at the Eighth International Congress of Human Genetics in October 1991, one subject in this category attracted so many geneticists to the lecture

hall that the city fire marshal had to threaten to shut down the entire Congress until the overflow of people dispersed to two satellite halls to listen to the proceedings over loud speakers.

It is not always easy to distinguish these nontraditional forms of inheritance within families. Mitochondrial inheritance is fairly straightforward if one ignores the possibility that galtonian as well as mendelian inheritance may exist in this mode. However, there is overlap between the family patterns in diseases resulting from genomic imprinting, segmental aneusomy, uniparental disomy, and germline mosaicism. The existence of nontraditional modes of inheritance is of more than academic interest. It has a direct bearing on genetic counseling. We must now exercise caution in making statements such as, "This appears to be a fresh mutation of an autosomal dominant disorder, so the recurrence risk in this sibship is negligible, only the population frequency of, say, 1 in 5000." If germline mosaicism is a possible mechanism, the recurrence risk could be appreciably higher, and it is now incumbent on the geneticist to take this into account in the evaluation. There is, at present, no unanimity of opinion as to how best to share this sort of information in the counseling of a specific family.

GERMLINE MOSAICISM

Mosaicism means two or more cell lines differing in genotype or karyotype derived from a single zygote. In this presentation, we shall define *germline mosaicism* as the production of a substantial proportion of gametes with the same mutation, which is consistent with the use of the term in *Drosophila* and mice, as well as in humans. It results when a mutation occurs after fertilization in a cell that gives rise to germ cells. As a rule, this term applies to gonads from which more than 1% of the end cells or stem cells carry the same mutation.[4] If mosaicism involves both germline and somatic cells, the term used is *gonosomal mosaicism*. Mosaicism that is confined only to somatic cells may be manifested as patchy or segmental abnormalities, but is not transmitted to subsequent generations. X-linked disorders have provided opportunities to study somatic, gonosomal, and germline mosaicism.

It is estimated that in the human female there are about 23 to 30 mitotic cell divisions before meiosis and that there are 8 million oocytes present at birth culminating in the eventual release of about 300 to 400 mature ova. In the male, at least 100 mitotic divisions take place, leading to the eventual release of $>10^{12}$ sperm cells.

In theory, germline mosaicism in the human subject may be recognized by examining germ cells. In the female parent of an affected child, such studies would be meddlesome at best. However, detection at the molecular level is the specific method of diagnosis. Without resorting to molecular studies, what clues would lead one to believe that germline mosaicism is the mechanism operating in a given family? A disease that is generally considered to be dominant, but which occurs in two offspring of parents, neither of whom have any evidence of the disease, may be accounted for by germline mosaicism. The majority of cases of osteogenesis imperfecta (OI Type II) result from new dominant mutations. Byers and coworkers[2] have reported families with recurrent perinatal lethal OI Type II in which germline mosaicism was evident on the basis of an unaffected parent having affected offspring by two different spouses (Fig. 14–1). If a condition, the inheritance of which is uncertain, appears in two or more offspring of unaffected parents, it is usually first assumed to be recessive. But if one or more of the affected children of normal parents later has an affected child, germline mosaicism may be suspected. An example in the literature is pseudoachondroplasia.[5] The difficult counseling situation is: what do you tell the family that presents with only one child with a disorder that is established as being autosomal dominant? In the past, the counselor would say that the child represents a fresh mutation and that the recurrence risk in the sibship would be very small—i.e., on the order of twice the mutation rate for that condition. It may be prudent now to touch lightly on the possibility of germline mosaicism in counseling, if this can be done without arousing undue confusion and anxiety.

UNIPARENTAL DISOMY

If both homologues of the same chromosome derive from one parent in the absence

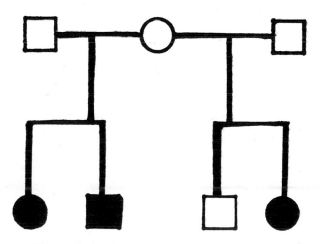

Fig. 14–1. An apparently unaffected parent who has affected children by two different unaffected spouses is one reason to suspect the mechanism of germline mosaicism.

of a homolog from the other parent, *uniparental disomy* is said to exist. In 1988, Spence and co-workers[13] reported the first case of uniparental disomy in a female with cystic fibrosis (CF), short stature, and an apparently normal diploid complement, who was demonstrated to have inherited much or all of both copies of her chromosome 7 from her mother and no marker alleles from her father. This would account for the child being homozygous for the CF gene when only the mother was a carrier, but it does not explain the shortness of stature. One possibility that has been suggested for the child's short stature was genomic imprinting (see below). The following year, another patient with both CF and shortness of stature attributed to uniparental disomy was reported, as was a case of father-to-son transmission of hemophilia A. These cases suggested that uniparental disomy may not be as rare as first believed and that it involves sex chromosomes as well as autosomes. In the patient with hemophilia A, both sex chromosomes were inherited from the father and none from the mother. In the discussions of uniparental disomy, the following definitions are sometimes used: if two different homologues derive directly from one parent, the term used is *heterodisomy;* if both homologues are identical and derive from one parent, *isodisomy* is used.

Several models may be proposed for how uniparental disomy can occur. Gamete complementation (Fig. 14–2a) in which one gamete carries the diploid number of a specific chromosome and the second gamete lacks that chromosome entirely. One can visualize this mechanism for chromosome 7—or perhaps, more easily, for the father of the son with hemophilia A supplying both the X and Y chromosomes in the absence of a sex chromosome contribution from the mother. This requires a nondisjunctional event preceding formation of both the sperm and the egg.

Figure 14–2b and c illustrate possible mechanisms of monosomy and trisomy leading to uniparental disomy. In monosomy, a normal and a nullisomic gamete produce a monosomic zygote, which through duplication yields an isodisomic cell. In trisomy, a normal gamete and a gamete carrying the diploid number of given chromosome produce a trisomic zygote, which can yield through nondisjunction a cell with uniparental disomy. This may be the most common mechanism. A postfertilization error, as shown in Fig. 14–2d, may through nondisjunction lead to isodisomy.

Uniparental disomy should be considered in families in which there is a recessive disorder when only one parent is shown to be a carrier; and in X-linked recessive disorders transmitted from father to son or present in the homozygous form in females. More precise diagnosis of this mode of inheritance may be obtained through the use of DNA markers such as alpha-satellite probes.

GENOMIC IMPRINTING[6]

According to mendelian principles, an autosomal gene is transmitted from a parent of either sex to an offspring of either sex, and

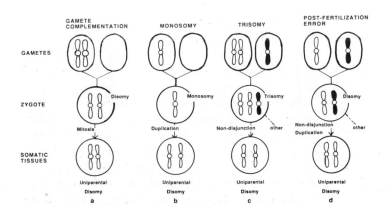

Fig. 14–2. Proposed mechanisms for uniparental disomy. See text for discussion.

the parental source should not influence the expression of the gene. Unfortunately, many traits and conditions clearly do not follow neat segregation ratios. The challenge is how to explain the exceptions—particularly those in which the sex of the transmitting parent seems to affect the expression of genes. *Genomic imprinting* is used to describe "the differential expression of genetic material, at either a chromosomal or allelic level, depending on whether the genetic material has come from the male or female parent."[6] This epigenetic allele-inactivation process must involve some sort of modification of nuclear DNA of somatic cells in order to cause recognizable differences in phenotype. What must be visualized at the outset is that an "imprintable" allele is inherited in a mendelian manner, but the expression of the allele is determined by the sex of the transmitting parent.

Figure 14–3A and B shows what maternal and paternal imprinting might look like. The action of genomic imprinting is to *suppress* the imprintable allele, whether it is normal or abnormal. It is not yet established if it is single genes or segments of chromosomes or both that are responsible for imprinting. In the case of X-chromosome inactivation, the most clear-cut example of imprinting, it is clearly a large segment of the chromosome that is inactivated. Apparently the imprinting of DNA occurs during gametogenesis and is reversible in the next generation. Note that in the pedigree of maternal imprinting there is no phenotypic expression of the imprintable allele when transmitted from the mother. There are nonmanifesting carriers, and the trait or disease is allowed to "skip a generation" before reappearing in the offspring of *carrier males*. So, if we are dealing with a trait in which *maternal imprinting* is a factor, it appears only in the offspring of males and if the trait is expressed in a female, she can only transmit it in the carrier state. The trait may then reappear in the next generation or be transmitted in the carrier depending on the sex of the transmitting parent. The mother can transmit the carrier state, but not the disease. In *paternal imprinting*, the opposite occurs: only mothers transmit the trait and affected fathers transmit only the carrier state.

All of this convoluted discussion is necessitated by the fact that we are describing two separate modalities of inheritance. The mode we are accustomed to working with is the transmission of a normal or abnormal allele. The simultaneously occurring second mode, imprinting, turns expectation on its head, because the transmission of imprinting (through single genes or segments of chromosomes) is the transmission of the *suppression* of an imprintable allele. For the process to be recognizable, the suppressed or silenced allele should be of large effect. It is thought that imprinting represents a form of regulation in the control and expression of the mammalian genome. Nuclear transplantation experiments in mice show that it plays a fundamental role in the development of the early embryo and its membranes.

Uniparental disomies were described in the previous section and the suggestion was made that imprinting might account for the intrauterine and postnatal growth retardation found in two children who inherited the CF gene in duplicate from their mothers (and were thus homozygotes having the disease cystic fibro-

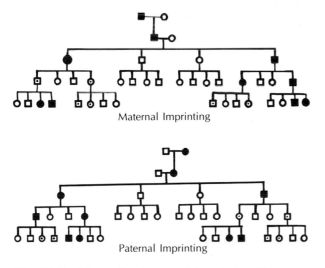

Fig. 14–3. Maternal and paternal imprinting. The action of imprinting is to *suppress* the imprintable allele so that, in maternal imprinting, the allele is not expressed when transmitted by the mother, but is expressed (is not suppressed) when transmitted by the father. The converse is found in paternal imprinting—expression of the allele when transmitted by the mother, but not by the father.

Table 14–1. Features of Prader-Willi and Angelman Syndromes

Prader-Willi syndrome:
   Infancy
      Hypotonia, hyporeflexia
      Cryptorchism
      Poor feeding caused by difficulty in sucking
         and swallowing
   Later childhood
      Enormous appetite, obesity
      Small hands and feet
      Short stature
      Hypogonadism
      Facies: dolichocephaly; almond-shaped
         eyes; small, down-turned mouth
      Behavioral problems
      Mild to moderate mental retardation

Angelman (happy puppet) syndrome:
   Jerky puppet-like movements
   Paroxysmal laughter
   Hyperactivity
   Ataxia
   Epilepsy
   Abnormal EEG
   Absence of speech
   Facies: jolly, happy-puppet appearance,
      open mouth, protruding tongue, widely-
      spaced teeth, prominent mandible,
      microcephaly
   Ocular hypopigmentation

sis). The possibility has been put forward that growth retardation not related to CF might result from the presence of uniparental disomy for chromosome 7 (and consequent absence of the homologous genetic material from the other parent). The idea is that the two homologues are imprinted in the parental gonads in such a way that the absence of either of them interferes with normal development. This idea is based not only on these cases in humans, but on studies in mice that show that a major differential growth defect occurs if certain segments of chromosomes represent uniparental disomy of maternal or paternal origin.

Deficiencies of chromosomes or even small parts of chromosomes are poorly tolerated in humans. One such deficiency that has attracted great interest in the literature of genomic imprinting is the chromosomal deletion 15q11-13. This deletion occurs in as many as half of the patients with Prader-Willi syndrome, which is discussed and illustrated in

Chapter 3, Autosomal Chromosomal Anomalies. Curiously, the same deletion is also seen in a distinctly different condition, Angelman syndrome. The classic clinical picture of Prader-Willi (see Chap. 3) evolves from infancy through later childhood. Angelman (happy puppet) syndrome has a distinctly different phenotype. The features of the two syndromes may be compared in Table 14–1.

What is most interesting is that, if the chromosome 15 with the deletion is inherited from the father, the result is Prader-Willi syndrome, but if the chromosome with the 15q11-13 deletion is of maternal origin, Angelman syndrome occurs. It has not been established at this time that the deletions in chromosome 15 in Prader-Willi and Angelman syndromes encompass precisely the same area, but DNA studies are compatible with a common segment. The same genetic markers have been used to evaluate Angelman and Prader-Willi syndromes occurring in first cousins in the same family with a translocation.[12] Angelman, like Prader-Willi syndrome, also occurs in the absence of a deletion in about half the cases.

(In the literature one often finds Prader-Willi and Angelman syndromes referred to as *segmental aneusomy* or *contiguous gene* syndromes. Other conditions frequently discussed in this category include Miller-Dieker, DiGeorge, WAGR, and Xp22.3 deletions. Segmental aneusomy may encompass uniparental disomy, microdeletions or segmental monosomy, and microduplications or segmental trisomy.)

The next step in evaluating the 15q11-13 region was to study cases of Prader-Willi and Angelman syndromes in which no deletion of DNA could be found. Nicholls and coworkers[10] found that both chromosomes 15 with no deletions in patients with Prader-Willi had been *inherited from the mother*. This would appear to mean that the lack of the 15q11-13 region on a paternally imprinted chromosome (or, in these cases, the lack of the entire paternal chromosome 15) is responsible for the Prader-Willi phenotype. Cases of Angelman syndrome have been found in which no deletion was detected and the *uniparental disomy was of paternal origin*.[3] This may sound paradoxic, but it can be clarified by looking back at the two idealized pedigrees depicted in Figure 14–3. Imprinting produces suppression not expression of a trait.

Cancers represent another class of chromosome deficiencies in which the parental origin of the chromosome plays a role in the expression (or suppression) of tumors such as Wilms tumor, familial glomus tumors, and retinoblastoma (see Chapter 21, Genetics and Cancer).

Several human disorders, often affecting growth, behavior, and intrauterine survival, are recognized in which the severity appears to depend on the sex of the parent transmitting the disease and may thus be suspected of being influenced by imprinting.[7] A more severe, earlier-onset form of Huntington disease occurs if the gene is transmitted through the father. When the myotonic dystrophy gene is inherited from the mother, a more severe form of the disease results. The severity of neurofibromatosis I and II, spinocerebellar ataxia, cerebellar ataxia, Wiedemann-Beckwith, and fragile-X syndromes may depend on whether the gene is transmitted by the father or the mother. Many cases of the phenomenon of "skipped generations" in human disease may be explained by imprinting.

The biology of imprinting has been investigated in some detail in the mouse, and areas of homology between mouse and human chromosomes are candidates for study of genomic imprinting. In transgenic mice, the differential expression of the transgene is related to methylation-modification of DNA, which may determine when a particular allele is inactivated. The function of methylation appears to represent a secondary level of gene regulation. Again, think of imprinting as suppression of a gene.

The concept of imprinting requires us to return to our data bases and re-evaluate pedigrees for this possibility.

MITOCHONDRIAL INHERITANCE[1]

In the sense that the X and Y chromosomes may be considered to be chromosomes 23 and 24, the hereditary material of the mitochondria may be termed chromosome 25, although

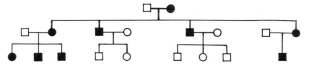

Fig. 14–4. Idealized pedigree of mitochondrial inheritance. Transmission of the gene is only through the female, and it affects all offspring, male and female.

it is non-nuclear and does not behave in the same way as nuclear chromosomes. For several decades, it has been recognized that transmission of hereditary influences was not confined to the nucleus, but could be attributed to factors in the cytoplasm, particularly the mitochondria. Because cytoplasmic constituents are present in the ova but not the sperm, a clue to this mode of inheritance has been that transmission is entirely maternal (matrilineal), and thus a characteristic of cytoplasmic inheritance is that all or almost all offspring of an affected mother are affected (Fig. 14–4). Some diseases known to be associated with a mitochondrial mutation (such as Leber optic atrophy)[8] show the striking matrilineal transmission illustrated in Figure 14–4, although not all offspring of affected females are affected.[14] By contrast, another disease in which there has been documentation of a mitochondrial DNA deletion (Kearns-Sayre syndrome or progressive external ophthalmoplegia) is often sporadic and may be genetically heterogeneous.

Although other constituents of the cytoplasm could be implicated in maternal inheritance, the mitochondrion attracts major scrutiny. It is an organelle that multiplies by division like microorganisms, and plays an important biochemical role in energy functions (e.g., aerobic oxidation, the citric acid cycle). The mitochondrion itself (Fig. 14–5A) may be visualized as a sack of enzymes with an external membrane and an internal membrane "crinkled" into folds (cristae and tubuli). The genome or chromosome of the mitochondrion consists of 16,569 base pairs structured in a circular manner in two strands, one heavy and one light (Fig. 14–5B). Both strands of *mitochondrial DNA (mtDNA)* are *transcribed and translated* in contrast to what occurs with nu-

A

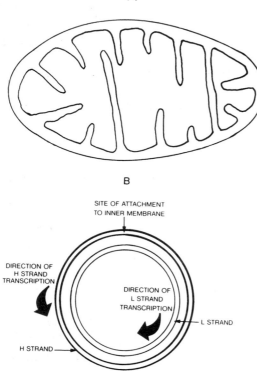

B

SITE OF ATTACHMENT
TO INNER MEMBRANE

DIRECTION OF
H STRAND
TRANSCRIPTION

DIRECTION OF
L STRAND
TRANSCRIPTION

L STRAND

H STRAND

Fig. 14–5. A. Diagram of internal structure of a mitochondrion as revealed by electron microscopic study of cell section. B. Diagram of mitochondrial chromosome showing the heavy (H) and light (L) strands with opposite directions of transcription.

clear DNA, and the genetic code differs in some cases from the universal genetic code (e.g., AUA codes for methionine, not isoleucine). Each mitochondrion contains several copies of circular chromosomes and each cell (with many mitochondria) contains thousands of copies of the mitochondrial chromosome, as opposed to only two copies of each nuclear chromosome being present per cell. This multiplicity of mitochondrial chromosomes in each cell provides a basis for mosaicism between normal and mutant mtDNA.

The mitochondrial genome is transcribed as a single messenger RNA (mRNA) that is ultimately cleaved into the various components, which participate in a number of functions, the most important being the synthesis of ATP (adenosine triphosphate) by the process of oxidative phosphorylation, which involves five multi-polypeptide enzyme complexes (four of

these five complexes are under the combined control of nuclear DNA and mtDNA). Of the 69 separate polypeptides known to be required for oxidative phosphorylation, 13 are coded by mitochondrial DNA.

The high rate of gene mutation of mtDNA (on the order of 10 times the rate in nuclear DNA) and the variable allotment of mutant mitochondrial genomes in each cell leads to a wide range of bioenergetic capacities. Normal and mutant mtDNA co-exist within cells and tissues, perhaps as a protective mechanism to prevent the threat to survival that could occur if mitochondrial mutants took complete control. It is possible to visualize that mutations in mtDNA could have variable and perhaps profound effects on the bioenergetics of development and maldevelopment. However, to this time, only a small number of clinical entities have been attributed to mitochondrial inheritance, including Leber optic atrophy, Kearns-Sayre syndrome, myoclonic epilepsy with ragged red fibers, and infantile bilateral striated necrosis. Neuromuscular diseases, including cardiomyopathies and cardiac rhythm disturbances, appear to be prominent candidates for consideration for mitochondrial inheritance.

More common categories of developmental abnormalities may also justify investigation. For example, could the preferential inheritance of congenital heart disease (and some other common anomalies) through the maternal line[11] mean that in some families mitochondrial mutations are operating? If one is dealing with two populations of mitochondria within cells and tissues, both influencing the bioenergetics of development, it is possible to visualize that an all-or-none phenotypic result may not occur in maldevelopment that is not due to a single mutation of large effect. Perhaps the presence in congenital heart disease of "matrilineal inheritance," without all offspring being affected, reflects this possibility. The gradual accumulation of mitochondrial mutations during a lifetime has been suggested as an important contributor to aging.[9] Dietary or pharmacologic replacement of redox substances (such as ascorbic acid) has been suggested as a way of increasing bioenergetic capacity in the presence of accumulating mitochondrial mutations with aging.[5] In the presence of mitochondrial mutations underlying congenital and/or genetically transmitted diseases, could pharmacologic or dietary supplementation also prevent or modify adverse outcomes? Clearly, the study of the mitochondrial genome may result in some substantial changes in our thinking about genetic processes.

FUTURE PROSPECTS

It is too early to propose a major role in human disease for the types of nontraditional inheritance discussed here. In writing on this subject and allowing a free flow of imagination, the author of this chapter is inclined to believe that a study of nontraditional inheritance will not only fill in some large gaps in our knowledge, but will require us to re-examine many of our established positions.

SUMMARY

Several forms of inheritance that do not fit traditional modes have commanded increasing attention.

Germline mosaicism may be suspected in families in which unaffected parents have two or more offspring with a disease generally considered to be dominant—and especially if one or more of the affected children later has an affected child.

Uniparental disomy may be considered in families in which there is an autosomal recessive disorder, but only one parent demonstrated to be a carrier; and in X-linked disorders transmitted from father to son or present in the homozygous form in the female.

Genomic imprinting should be thought of as suppression of a gene. There are nonmanifesting carriers and skipped generations. In maternal imprinting, expression of the imprintable allele is suppressed when the mutant gene comes from the mother, and the phenotype is expressed only when the mutant gene comes from the father. In paternal imprinting, the reverse is the case.

Mitochondrial inheritance comes through the mitochondrial genome (or chromosome) and is recognized when there is transmission through females and not males.

REFERENCES

1. Anderson, S., et al.: Science and organization of human mitochondrial genome. Nature 290:457, 1981.
2. Byers, P.II. et al.: Perinatal lethal osteogenesis imperfecta (OI Type II): A biochemically heterogeneous disorder usually due to new mutations in the gene for Type 1 collagen. Am. J. Hum. Genet. 42:237, 1988.
3. Cassidy, S.B., et al.: Trisomy 15 with loss of the paternal 15 as a cause of Prader-Willi syndrome due to maternal disomy. Am. J. Hum. Genet. 51:701, 1992.
4. Edwards, J.H.: Familiarity, recessivity and germline mosaicism. Ann. Hum. Genet. 53.33, 1989.
5. Hall, J.G., et al.: Gonadal mosaicism in pseudoachondroplasia. Am. J. Med. Genet. 28:143, 1987.
6. Hall, J.G.: Genomic imprinting: Review and relevance to human diseases. Am. J. Hum. Genet. 46:857, 1990.
7. Hall, J.G.: Genomic imprinting and its clinical implications. N. Engl. J. Med. 326:827, 1992.
8. Howell, N., et al.: Leber hereditary optic neuropathy: Identification of the same mitochondrial ND1 mutation in six pedigrees. Am. J. Hum. Genet. 49:939, 1991.
9. Linnane, A.W., et al.: Mitochondrial DNA mutations as an important contributor to ageing and degenerative diseases. Lancet i: 642, 1989.
10. Nicholls, R.D. et al.: Genetic imprinting suggested by maternal heterodisomy in nondeletion Prader-Willi syndrome. Nature 342.281, 1989.
11. Nora, J.J., and Nora, A.H.: Maternal transmission of congenital heart diseases: New recurrence risk figures and the questions of cytoplasmic inheritance and vulnerability to teratogens. Am. J. Cardiol. 59:459, 1987.
12. Smeets, D.F.C.M., et al.: Prader-Willi syndrome and Angelman syndrome in cousins from a family with a translocation between chromosomes 6 and 15. N. Engl. J. Med. 326:807, 1992.
13. Spence, J.E., et al.: Uniparental disomy as a mechanism for human disease. Am. J. Hum. Genet. 42:217, 1988.
14. Sweeney, M.G., et al.: Evidence against an X-linked locus close to DXS7 determining visual loss susceptibility in British and Italian families with Leber hereditary optic neuropathy. Am. J. Hum. Genet. 51:741, 1992.

Section II

Special Topics

Chapter *15*

Prenatal Diagnosis of Genetic Diseases

DISEASES DESPERATE GROWN BY DESPERATE APPLIANCE ARE RELIEVED OR NOT AT ALL.

SHAKESPEARE

One of the most exciting chapters in the history of genetics as applied to medicine is the development of techniques for the diagnosis of congenital disease before birth. Before this, genetic counseling could provide only probabilities of recurrence, based on the mendelian laws or empirical data, and couples at risk for such diseases could never have a child without taking the chance that it might be affected. Now it is possible, for certain diseases, to provide a definite answer—yes or no. If the fetus is affected, the parents have the choice of terminating the pregnancy and beginning again.

Techniques for the prenatal detection of disease are broadly summarized in Table 15–1 and amplified in the sections that follow.

INDICATIONS FOR PRENATAL DIAGNOSIS

Birth defects can be divided into those in which the probability of occurrence, or of recurrence in subsequent children of the same parents, is high enough to justify the procedure and those in which it is not. Just where the cut-off point should be is a matter of judg-

Table 15–1. Methods Used in Prenatal Diagnosis of Genetic Disease

Amniocentesis
  Study of fetal cells: cytogenetic and biochemical
  Study of amniotic fluid: alpha fetoprotein (AFP) and
    acetylcholinesterase (ACHE)
Chorionic Villus Sampling (CVS)
  Study of cells: cytogenetic and biochemical
Maternal Blood
  Maternal serum AFP, human chorionic gonadotrophin
    (HCG), estriol, and fetal cells
Visualization and Manipulation of the Fetus
  Ultrasound, radiography, fetoscopy, biopsy, and sampling

ment, and there are no hard-and-fast rules. For the individual case, the most important factor is the parents' view of the risks and benefits; for society, questions of cost and the distribution of resources complicate the picture.[20]

AMNIOCENTESIS

Amniocentesis is the removal of fluid from the amniotic sac. It has been used diagnostically since the mid-1930s for detecting fetal distress and, more recently, for following the

291

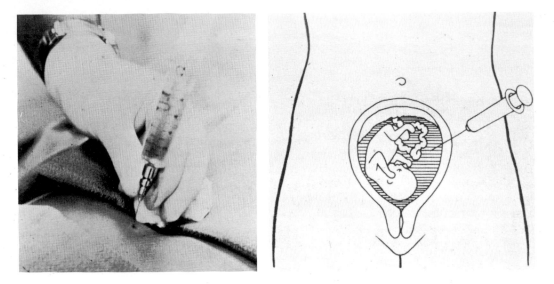

Fig. 15–1.   Technique of withdrawing amniotic fluid.

progress of Rh hemolytic disease. In the mid-1950s, it was found that fetal cells in the amniotic fluid could be used to determine fetal sex (by observing the sex chromatin) and blood type. In the late 1960s, techniques were developed for obtaining karyotypes[7] and enzymatic assays[23] from fetal cells, and prenatal diagnosis began to revolutionize genetic counseling.

The Procedure

Amniocentesis should be done by a physician skilled in the technique, after the patient has had appropriate counseling and has given her informed consent. A needle is inserted through the anterior abdominal and uterine walls into the amniotic cavity (Fig. 15–1) with ultrasonic visualization (Fig. 15–2), and about 10 to 20 mL of fluid are withdrawn. The optimal time for the procedure is about 16 weeks after the beginning of the last menstrual period; before this the amount of fluid is small (there is about 125 mL at 15 weeks), and the cells do not grow well. The longer one waits after this, the less time there is to grow the cells, make the appropriate tests, and obtain a diagnosis while there is still time to perform an abortion. Because cultures occasionally fail, requiring another tap, and for some biochem-

ical tests it takes 3 to 6 weeks before the results are known, the schedule may be tight.

The amniotic fluid is primarily fetal urine and contains cells sloughed off from the skin, respiratory tract, and urinary tract. Diagnostic determinations, both cytologic and enzymatic, on cells from the amniotic fluid are highly reliable, with error rates well under 1%. Duplicate cultures are advisable, in case of contamination and to help in distinguishing between fetal mosaicism and aberrations arising in culture.

After removal of the cells, the supernatant fluid can be examined for biochemical abnormalities of enzymes, hormones, and other constituents, alpha-fetoprotein in particular.

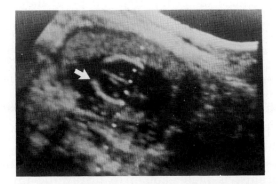

Fig. 15–2.   Intrauterine cavity as scanned by ultrasound. Arrow points to the skull of the developing fetus.

Hazards of Amniocentesis

Several large collaborative studies have evaluated the hazards of the procedure.[2,6] The British study (but not the U.S. or Canadian ones) found that the procedure adds about 1% to the risk of spontaneous abortion and that there may be an additional 1% risk for neonatal problems, such as respiratory difficulties, and postural deformities, such as clubfoot. There was also a small increase in late complications of pregnancy such as premature separation of placenta or rupture of the membranes, and postpartum hemorrhage. Although there are some minor disagreements in the figures between the various collaborative studies, there is no doubt that the hazards are small. Nevertheless, they should be made known to the patient and taken into consideration when deciding whether the procedure is indicated in a particular case.

Patients should also be made aware of the possible technical problems and difficulties in interpretation.[23] There is a small possibility that no fluid is obtained (2 to 5%) or that the culture fails to grow well (5 to 10%), requiring a second amniocentesis. Puncture of the placenta may result in a bloody sample, poor growth of cultured cells, and increased alphafetoprotein levels. Mosaicism or polyploidy in the cultures will complicate the interpretation. There may be difficulties in deciding whether minor variations in chromosome morphology are significant abnormalities or normal variants; these may be resolved by study of the parental karyotypes. Clerical and technical errors should not, but do, occur, albeit rarely. The presence of twins should be detected by ultrasound and will complicate the situation. In Rh negative women, there is a risk of maternal immunization by fetal red cells, and the administration of Anti-D immunoglobulin (RhoGAM) is recommended, although it is not yet possible to evaluate its effectiveness.

CHORIONIC VILLUS SAMPLING

A technique has been developed which allows earlier diagnosis. This is chorionic villus sampling. As early as 8 weeks after the last menstrual period, a needle is inserted (under ultrasound guidance) through the vagina and the cervix of the uterus, and bits of the chorionic membrane (which is fetal tissue) are aspirated, for culture or direct chromosome preparations.[24] Earlier diagnosis has several advantages. The procedure can be done while the pregnancy is still "private" and, if an abnormality is found, abortion is simpler, less stressful, and less dangerous than it is at 20 weeks. On the other hand, the new technique raises more ethical problems, such as pressure to do the test for increasingly trivial reasons and, in particular, for the determination of sex for social, rather than medical reasons.[6,10] No doubt lots of interesting debates are in store. In the meantime, collaborative studies are under way to collect data on reliability and risks of the procedure. In collaborating study centers, the risks do not appear to exceed substantially the risk of amniocentesis.[3] There is general agreement that cultured cells are necessary in addition to direct preparation to maximize accuracy of diagnosis.

CYTOGENETIC ANALYSIS

Increased risk of chromosomal aberrations is the most common reason for diagnostic amniocentesis and chorionic villus sampling. Because significant chromosomal imbalance is present in about 1/200 live-born babies, it has been argued that prenatal diagnosis should be done for all pregnancies, but the logistics, as well as our ignorance of the long-term effects, make such a proposal unacceptable at present.[7]

Maternal Age. The most common indication is maternal age. The age at which the risk becomes high enough to be an indication for amniocentesis is a question of policy that varies from center to center. In the USA, it is standard practice to recommend prenatal diagnosis to all women who will deliver at age 35 or older. Table 15-2 summarizes the risk of having a chromosomally abnormal infant at different maternal ages. In the United States, testing all births to mothers over 35 would involve about 6% of all births and detect 30% of babies with trisomy 21. There is some sug-

Table 15–2.   Risk of Chromosomal Abnormalities in Liveborns Related to Maternal Age*

Maternal Age	Risks per 1000
33	2.9–3.5
35	4.7–5.2
37	7.6–7.9
39	12.3–12.1
41	20.1–19.0
43	32.6–30.2
45	53.0–48.2
47	86.2–77.5
49	140.1–125.3

*Modified from Hook[12a]

gestion of an increase associated with paternal age of 55 or over, but if there really is one, it is small and does not constitute an indication for amniocentesis.

Aneuploidy. A previous aneuploid child is the second most common indication, the risk of recurrence being 1 or 2%, irrespective of maternal age.

The question of whether recurrent abortion should be included in this category raises a complex issue, still not resolved. Because 50% or more of early spontaneous abortions have unbalanced chromosome complements, a previous abortion of unknown karyotype is quite likely to have been trisomic. If an abortus is trisomic, the probability of a second abortion is not increased, but if there is one, it is likely (85%) to be aneuploid.[13] Some have argued that this justifies amniocentesis for a woman who has had an aneuploid abortus or one who has had two spontaneous abortions if (as is usually the case) neither abortus had been karyotyped. It would also be an argument for routine karyotyping of abortuses. However, until we know the probability of a *live-born* aneuploid baby in such cases, it seems premature to accept recurrent abortion as an indication for amniocentesis. On the other hand, recurrent abortion may be an indication for karyotyping the parents, as a significant number of these (perhaps 5%)[18] will have a balanced chromosomal rearrangement, which *is* an indication.

Balanced Chromosomal Rearrangement. A balanced chromosomal rearrangement in one parent is a less common but important indication for amniocentesis. The risk of having a viable child with an unbalanced complement depends on the size and location of the rearrangement (Chapter 3) and may be very low for many translocations,[13] but it would be wise to offer amniocentesis nonetheless.

Determination of Sex. This may be offered to a woman at risk for being a carrier of an X-linked gene causing a disorder that cannot yet be diagnosed prenatally. The parents then have the option of abortion if the fetus is male and therefore at risk. Abortion of a male who has a 50:50 chance of being normal is a harder decision for parents to make than if the fetus is known to be affected, or if the decision to have an abortion is made early in pregnancy on the basis of high risk without knowledge of the sex. Earlier diagnosis, by chorionic villi biopsy, may make the decision easier.

BIOCHEMICAL DISORDERS DETECTED IN AMNIOTIC FLUID CELLS

Any disease in which a biochemical defect is demonstrable in fibroblasts is potentially detectable in cells cultured from the amniotic fluid. The relevant enzyme must be demonstrated in fetal cells at the time the test is to be done, and the defect in mutant cells must be great enough to permit their discrimination from those of heterozygous and normal fetuses. There are hundreds of eligible conditions, many of which have actually been diagnosed prenatally. Because the diseases involved are often rare, and the assays complex, appropriate facilities may exist in only a few laboratories, and arranging for an assay at the right time may present logistical problems. Early consultation is therefore important.

Molecular Techniques for Diseases of Known Molecular Basis

The techniques of molecular genetics have greatly increased the scope of prenatal diagnosis by making it possible to detect mutant genes at the level of the DNA, so that diagnosis no longer necessarily depends on demonstrating the relevant protein (or lack of it) in the amniotic fluid cells or fetal blood. Probes have been used to diagnose Duchenne muscular dystrophy, hemophilia, alpha- and beta-thalassemia, and sickle cell anemia.

Restriction Fragment Length Polymorphisms (RFLPs) for Diagnosis When the Molecular Basis is Unknown

This class of genetic markers has had practical applications in prenatal diagnosis and is discussed in Chapter 7. RFLPs have proven useful not only for prenatal diagnosis, but as a class of genetic markers that have greatly accelerated the progress of mapping the human genome. Of course, the RFLP must be heterozygous and the cis/trans relationship known, so not all families are informative for predicting whether an offspring has inherited the gene.

Linkages with other markers can also be useful for prenatal diagnosis of dominant disorders, few of which are detectable biochemically in fibroblasts. This depends on the gene in question being closely linked to a marker that is detectable in amniotic fluid cells and the mating being informative—i.e., the marker is heterozygous and, in the parent carrying the mutant gene, it is possible to determine from family studies whether the genes are in the cis or trans configuration. The presence of the gene for myotonic dystrophy was predicted prenatally in the fetus through its close linkage to the secretor locus, and congenital adrenal hyperplasia has been diagnosed by use of its linkage to the HLA locus. As more markers are mapped, and RFLPs in particular, more such opportunities will become available. The molecular basis for the gene for myotonic dystrophy has been shown to involve a CTG triplet repeat.[1]

The list of disorders eligible for prenatal diagnosis continues to grow. Because the list is continually expanding, call the nearest medical genetics center when in doubt. The significance of cells not normally present in amniotic fluid will be considered in the discussion of neural tube defects.

PREIMPLANTATION DIAGNOSIS

It has become possible to diagnose disorders detectable by DNA analysis in very early embryos, before they implant, i.e., in the first week after conception.[12,25] The ability to do this depends on: (1) the ability to recover eggs or early embryos by the techniques of assisted human reproduction—in vitro fertilization (IVF) and related methods, such as uterine lavage; (2) the demonstration that mammalian (including human) early embryos will reorganize themselves and continue development normally after removal of one or a few cells (embryo biopsy) for diagnosis; (3) the advent of PCR and related techniques that amplify the DNA from one or a few cells to quantities adequate for diagnostic tests.

Techniques of early embryo biopsy include removal of the first polar body, aspiration of one or more cells from the embryo at the 4- to 16-cell stage, excising a few cells at the blastocyst stage (when the embryo is a hollow sphere) or, later still, removing cells from the trophoblast, the tissue that will form the membranes around the embryo.

Diagnostic techniques must be applicable to minute amounts of tissue, ideally to single cells. Measurement of some *enzymes* is now at this level of resolution, but there are problems with the products of maternal ribosomes, still present in the early embryo, and the fact that some of the enzymes of interest are not yet present at this early stage.

Aneuploidy of chromosomes leading to viable offspring (21, 18, 13, X and Y) can be detected in single cells by fluorescent in situ hybridization (FISH), which is useful for rapid screening of fetal cells obtained by CVS or amniocentesis (see Chapter 2). Their use for preimplantation diagnosis is limited to diagnosis of sex when there is a risk of a severe X-linked disorder (to back up the results of DNA analysis) or in the rare case where the mother has a translocation involving one of these chromosomes. It is not practical to *screen* preimplantation embryos, because of the high cost of obtaining them. Neither would the technique be suitable for polar body analysis because there are false negatives, so several cells must be examined.

PCR in theory allows preimplantation diagnosis of any disorder detectable by *DNA analysis,* and progress is being made. Early trials have involved mostly determination of sex, but other conditions are under study, particularly cystic fibrosis, hemophilia A, and the fragile X syndrome. But there are problems: amplification is successful in only about 80% of cells, and the technique is so sensitive that there is a risk of contamination by foreign DNA. So far, sensitivity of the technique is less than 100%, and pregnancies following preimplantation diagnosis will have to be monitored by traditional methods for some time to come.

Polar body analysis also presents problems. The rationale is that if the polar body from an egg of a woman heterozygous for a deleterious gene carries the mutant gene, the egg must have the normal allele and vice versa. But PCR amplification is not always successful, and there may be crossing over between the gene and the centromere, making the interpretation ambiguous.

Because of the difficulties in obtaining eggs or early embryos by the inefficient techniques of assisted reproduction, the high cost, and the less than satisfactory diagnostic precision, preimplantation diagnosis is not likely to become a major contender in the prenatal diagnosis field. Nevertheless, it has the promise of giving a small number of women at risk of having children with a genetic disorder, and who find the prospect of abortion intolerable, a means to have offspring free of that disorder.

DISORDERS DETECTABLE BY EXAMINATION OF AMNIOTIC FLUID

Abnormalities of the amniotic fluid may be diagnostically useful in cases in which the fetal secretions contain abnormal concentrations of enzymes or metabolites.

Alpha-fetoprotein. There is one amniotic fluid component that has become an important diagnostic indicator, and that is α-fetoprotein (AFP). This protein is synthesized by the yolk sac, and later by the fetal liver. The fetal serum concentration rises from about the sixth week of gestation to a peak between 12 and 14 weeks of gestation and then gradually falls. Little appears in the fetal urine or the amniotic fluid, the serum-amniotic fluid ratio being about 200:1. It may be the fetal equivalent of albumin. Both elevated and reduced levels of serum alpha-fetoprotein have diagnostic implications.[15]

When the fetus has an open neural tube, as in anencephaly or open spina bifida, α-fetoprotein appears in increased concentration in the amniotic fluid, probably by leakage of fetal cerebrospinal fluid. Contamination of amniotic fluid with fetal blood will lead to misleadingly high values. The sensitivity and specificity of the test are very high. Other conditions in which elevated amniotic fluid AFP concentrations have been reported in the second trimester are, for the most part, serious. These include intrauterine death, Rh isoimmunization, exomphalos (some), congenital nephrosis, duodenal atresia, esophageal atresia, and some types of congenital cystic kidney disease. AFP may also be high in twin pregnancies, but these are identified by ultrasound.

About 90 to 95% of neural tube defects are open, i.e., not covered by a full-thickness layer of skin. This represents all the anencephalics (which can be diagnosed by ultrasound) and roughly 80 to 90% of the other neural tube defects. Thus any woman who has, or has had, a baby with a neural tube defect, and therefore has about a 5% risk for each subsequent child (Chapter 13), is a candidate for amniocentesis and AFP determination. Also eligible is any couple in which either has an affected sib or parent, because the second-degree relatives of an affected child have a risk of about 2% of being affected. Furthermore, multiple vertebral anomalies, or spinal dysraphism, appear to fit into the category of neural tube defect, so a family history of these anomalies has the same implications for prenatal diagnosis as does that of anencephaly or spina bifida cystica (Chapter 13).

Acetylcholinesterase (ACHE) is a useful adjunct to AFP determination that is being used in more and more centers to increase specificity. This test is not gestational age-dependent as is alpha-fetoprotein; however, ACHE is detected in ventral wall defects and gastroschisis, but apparently not omphalocele.[22]

MATERNAL BLOOD

Amniocentesis for mothers ascertained retrospectively, by having already had a child with a neural tube defect, would detect only about 10% of all affected fetuses. An opportunity for more effective screening was provided by the discovery that AFP can be measured in maternal serum, using a sensitive radioimmune assay, and that when it is elevated in the amniotic fluid, it may also be increased in the mother's serum. This has raised the possibility of screening all pregnancies routinely. Such a prospective approach would allow a much higher detection rate, but also introduces some difficult problems.[8]

The optimal time for serum screening is around the sixteenth week of pregnancy. The specificity of the test is lower than that for amniotic fluid AFP measurements—that is, there are more false positives. If the upper limit of normal is set at the 97th percentile, 3% of screened pregnancies will be initially registered as abnormal. These will include some that simply represent the upper limit of normal variation, and some in which the AFP is elevated for causes other than a neural tube defect. These include underestimation of the gestational period, multiple pregnancy, and intrauterine death. The sensitivity of the test is not as high as that for amniotic fluid AFP (there are more false negatives), being about 90% for anencephaly, 80% for open spina bifida, and 5% for closed spina bifida, for an overall sensitivity of 64%.

The sensitivity for detecting low levels of serum alpha-fetoprotein is even less than for high levels. Low serum AFP levels are associated with trisomies 21, 18, and 13—and possibly other chromosomal anomalies. Such screening is being utilized in many centers. The false-positive rates are still excessive, leading to many otherwise normal pregnancies going to amniocentesis. The other side of the argument is that the great majority of patients delivering babies with trisomies are now not in the age 35 and older group, and

there is a body of opinion that suggests that amniocentesis is being underutilized in the younger age groups. An obvious compromise is being sought through improving the specificity and sensitivity of serum AFP screening for chromosomal anomalies.[5] Human chorionic gonadotrophin (HCG), free gonadotrophin, and unconjugated estriol have been used to supplement AFP, particularly in the diagnosis of Down syndrome.

Uncertainties make it difficult to determine whether a routine screening program is advisable. Clearly, no such program should begin without adequate laboratory facilities and counseling services and a good public education program. There is considerable concern, for example, about kits on the market that allow the obstetrician to measure serum alpha-fetoprotein in the office, without developing adequate norms and without the necessary back-up resources to handle the increased need for genetic counseling and amniocentesis. Although policy statements have been distributed by the American Society of Human Genetics to define quality maternal serum AFP programs in an effort to encourage state regulation, to date the response has been poor.[4]

Monetary cost-benefit calculations must take into consideration the population frequency of the defect, the nature of the health care services, anticipated inflation and interest rates, and many other variables. And who can estimate the intangible costs of emotional stress resulting from the screening program on the one hand and from having an affected child on the other? How does one measure the trauma imposed on a couple who, *without having sought testing*, find themselves having to decide whether to abort a fetus who might be only minimally handicapped, or die in infancy, or survive with varying degrees of physical and mental handicap? Will parents be more likely to reject an affected infant when they have been falsely reassured by a negative screening test? Will a false positive serum test impair the developing parent-child relationship?

One thoughtful analysis of the potential benefits and costs of a screening program for neural tube defects in Great Britain concludes that in 100,000 births, a screening program would avert 187 cases, but of these only 36 would have resulted in handicapped survivors, the rest being stillborn or dying in the neonatal period.[2] On the debit side, there would be 10 cases of fetal loss and 9 cases in which the infant had problems as a result of the procedure. In the words of the author: "Inevitably, different individuals will reach different conclusions about the human benefits and costs. Some will judge that advancing the deaths of severely affected fetuses, who would die irrespective of the screening program, is a substantial benefit; others will be influenced only by the ability of screening to reduce the number of handicapped survivors. Similarly, some will regard the accidental loss of unaffected pregnancies and damage to otherwise normal infants as indefensible, whereas others will argue that lost pregnancies are easily replaceable, and that the accidental damage to normal infants is less than the morbidity of spina bifida. Perhaps firmer evidence on both benefits and costs is needed, together with wide discussion of the ethical issues, to enable society as a whole to decide whether or not a national screening program should be implemented."[2]

DIAGNOSIS BY FETAL METABOLITES OR CELLS IN MATERNAL BLOOD

Because fetal blood cells and diffusible metabolites cross the placenta, they provide another approach to prenatal diagnosis, which has already been exploited in the case of alpha-fetoprotein and neural tube defects. Few other examples exist, however. In the case of methylmalonic aciduria, the accumulating methylmalonic acid spills over into the mother's blood and appears in her urine. This allows prenatal diagnosis without amniocentesis, and, in the case of the B_{12}-dependent type (Chap. 6), the opportunity for prenatal treatment. Efforts are now being made to test fetal cells in the maternal circulation, utilizing flow cytometry and amplification of fetal DNA by polymerase chain reaction (PCR). Monoclonal antibodies, fluorescent in situ hybridization (FISH), and chromosome-specific DNA

probes are also under investigation.[6] These procedures may eventually greatly reduce the need for more invasive procedures.

VISUALIZATION OF THE FETUS

Major anatomic defects do not have a recognized biochemical basis and can be recognized only by some means of visualizing the fetus. These include ultrasound, radiography, and fetoscopy.

Ultrasound (Sonar). This technique, first developed in 1917 for the detection of enemy submarines, makes use of high-frequency, low-intensity, pulsed ultrasonic waves, from which the reflections are displayed on a cathode-ray oscilloscope, much as radar uses radio waves. It has become a remarkably sensitive, noninvasive technique that is becoming routine in obstetric care to estimate fetal age and detect twins, and in prenatal diagnosis to locate the placenta, guide the fetoscope (see Fetoscopy) and demonstrate anatomic abnormalities[21] such as anencephaly; many cases of spina bifida (in combination with alpha-fetoprotein measurements); some types of short-limbed dwarfism, major skeletal defects and other conditions resulting in anatomic abnormality. As techniques continue to improve, certain heart malformations, polycystic kidneys, and other deformities are being added to the list (Figs. 15–3 through 15–6).

For the many inherited deformities in which the expressivity is variable, this technique (as well as radiography and fetoscopy) can be used on the understanding that a positive finding is good evidence that the fetus has the condition, but that absence of a positive finding does not rule it out. This makes a less satisfying option than if there were a clear-cut answer, but one that some couples may nonetheless find helpful.

Radiography. X-ray examination of the fetus applies only in conditions involving parts of the skeleton that are mineralized early enough to be useful. Skeletal ossification is sufficiently well advanced by 16 weeks to allow visualization of the tubular bones but not of parts of the pelvis, spine, and skull.[14] Conditions that have been diagnosed in the sec-

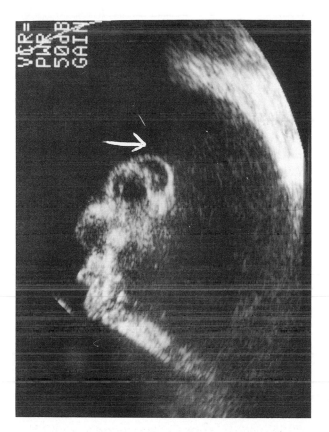

Fig. 15–3. Anencephaly. Sagittal image at 19 weeks' gestation showing absence of the calvarium superior to the orbit. Courtesy of Wayne Persutte, University Hospital, University of Colorado.

ond trimester by radiography, usually in conjunction with ultrasound, include absence of the radius and limb reduction in certain types of short-limbed dwarfism. Conditions in which second-trimester radiography has not been successful include heterozygous achondroplasia, dominant osteogenesis imperfecta, and recessive osteopetrosis.[14]

Amniography, in which radiopaque dyes are injected into the amnion, provides beautiful visualization of the fetal outlines when the dye is picked up by the vernix caseosa, the fatty layer that covers the fetal skin. Unfortunately, the technique does not seem to be reliable in the second trimester, perhaps because the vernix is not sufficiently developed by then.

Fetoscopy. This technique involves direct viewing of the fetus by a fiberoptics system, passed into the amnion through a needle, and video augmentation. A placenta covering the

anterior surface of the uterus may preclude this approach, and the hazards to the fetus are still formidable (about 5% in experienced hands), but may diminish as techniques improve. The technique is most valuable in conditions in which there is no biochemical or other disorder detectable in fibroblasts, but diagnoses can be made from external examination of the fetus or by sampling the fetal blood or skin. These conditions include certain hemoglobinopathies, hemophilia, deformities of the limb, and other disorders associated with structural anomalies or skin diseases that can be diagnosed by biopsy.[23] If the safety of the technique improves enough, it could be used for chromosomal or biochemical analysis of fetal cells when gestation is already approaching the maximum at which termination

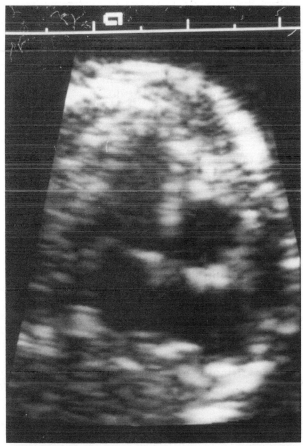

Fig. 15–4. Right ventricular hypoplasia. Four-chamber view of the fetal heart at 24 weeks gestation. Courtesy of Wayne Persutte.

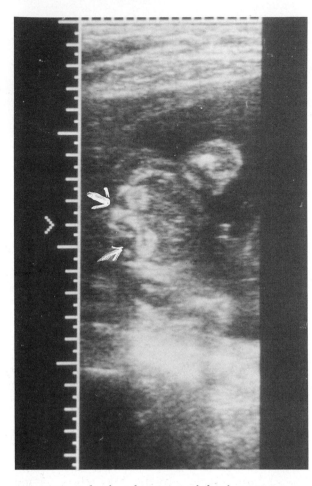

Fig. 15–5.   Infantile polycystic renal dysplasia. Transverse view of the fetal abdomen at approximately 22 weeks. Courtesy of Wayne Persutte.

can still be done because karyotyping and other enzyme determinations can be done much more rapidly on fetal blood cells than on cultured amniotic fluid cells.

FETAL THERAPY

One advantage of prenatal diagnosis is the possibility of treating the disorder in question before birth, but progress so far has not been encouraging.

One success story in this area is the treatment, or prevention, of hemolytic disease of the newborn caused by maternal Rh immunization (Chapter 19). One type of *fetal thrombocytopenia* is also caused by maternal immunization, in this case by fetal platelets.

It can be treated by transfusion of platelets into the fetus.

A small group of *inborn errors of metabolism* can be treated by supplying a missing product in utero, much as they are treated after birth. They are so rare that reports of prenatal treatment are anecdotal. They include treatment of vitamin B_{12}-responsive *methylmalonic acidemia* with large doses of vitamin B_{12} (no evidence that results are any better than those of postnatal treatment); treatment of multiple carboxylase deficiency with biotin; maternal treatment with dexamethasone to prevent masculinization of female external genitalia in congenital adrenal hyperplasia (variable results); and (theoreti-

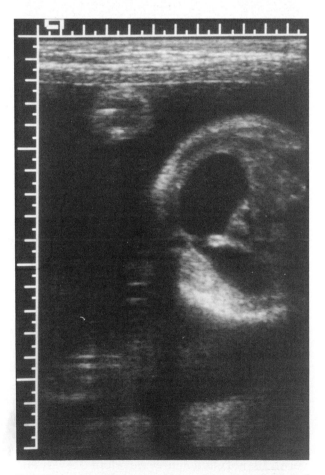

Fig. 15–6.   Duodenal atresia. Transverse view of the fetal abdomen at 27 weeks gestation in patient with Down syndrome showing dilated fetal stomach, constricted pylorus, and dilated proximal duodenum—the typical "double bubble." Courtesy of Wayne Persutte.

cally) treatment of *galactosemia* by maternal dietary galactose restriction.[9a]

Injection of genetically normal fetal stem cells into the affected fetus is a promising approach. These primitive cells from bone marrow or liver are not rejected immunologically by the fetus as adult stem cells would be, and may colonize the marrow or liver, where they may produce the missing product. Theoretically, this approach should apply to any of the disorders now treated by postnatal marrow or liver stem cell transplants. Trials with thalassemia are in progress.

Methods of treatment are being developed for many *anatomic disorders*, mostly nongenetic, that can cause fetal damage, e.g., by blocking circulation of fluids or pressing on developing organs. These include hydrocephalus, hydronephrosis, diaphragmatic hernia, pleural effusions, and cardiac arrhythmias. Results have been disappointing so far. Risks are high and the potential for harm is great. Much more work is needed in defining risks for mother and fetus, refining techniques, and learning how to select cases that will benefit.[22]

ROLE IN GENETIC COUNSELING

The advent of prenatal diagnosis is producing profound changes in the practice of genetic counseling. It is a great boon to many families at risk for certain genetic diseases, for whom it provides an opportunity to have healthy children rather than having to remain childless or to take the chance of having a child with a serious disorder and bear the emotional and financial cost of caring for such a child. In most centers, the results are normal in 96% or more of the cases tested, avoiding many months of anxiety for these families.

On the other hand, the fact that electing prenatal diagnosis implies a possible induced abortion raises some difficult ethical and moral questions.[16,20] In the following paragraphs, we summarize some general considerations, both practical and philosophic, relating to the role of prenatal diagnosis in genetic counseling.

Prenatal diagnosis is clearly a team effort, requiring a physician skilled in amniocentesis and preferably in ultrasonography, a genetic counselor, and a laboratory with good quality control, which is equipped to do the appropriate tests and has developed its own norms. If possible, therefore, prenatal diagnosis should be done in a center geared to deal with numbers of cases and using tests with the highest possible specificity and sensitivity.

The couple should be referred early, at or before 14 weeks after the last menstrual period. This allows adequate time to interview the couple, take a family history to determine whether the indications for prenatal diagnosis are valid and what tests should be done, and to make the necessary preparations if other than routine assays are required. It also gives the couple a chance to get used to the idea and prepare themselves to make an informed decision when the time comes.

Sometimes couples referred for prenatal diagnosis arrive at the center with the idea that they are more or less obligated to go through with it. Genetic counseling should ensure that they understand the risks that the fetus will be abnormal, the consequences of having a baby with the disorder in question, the hazards to mother and fetus of the procedure, and the options open to them. They should feel free to make an uninfluenced choice to decline amniocentesis and take their chances, and may very well do this if they find that the risks are in the less than 5% range, particularly if they object to abortion on moral or emotional grounds. Or they may accept amniocentesis and abortion if the diagnosis is positive. Or, if they object to abortion, they may accept amniocentesis with the intention of continuing the pregnancy even if the diagnosis is positive. They may want the chance to prepare themselves for care of a defective child either at home or in a foster home or institution. In some cases, treatment may be available, or knowing of the condition may allow referral to a high-risk obstetric center for "special delivery," as in the case of spina bifida before birth. Finally, parents who elect one option at the time of amniocentesis may change their minds in the face of a positive diagnosis and should be free to do so.

They should understand that the test relates only to the specific condition for which they are being tested and does not guarantee normality. The baby may have an anomaly that is not detectable by the methods used.

Conversely, the counselor should discuss the possibility of unexpected findings, such as a neural tube defect when the indication is maternal age or an XYY fetus when the indication is a parental translocation. The XYY fetus, in particular, is a difficult problem for parents to handle, because there are so many false ideas and areas of ignorance about the prognosis for this condition. The possibility of not telling the parents of such findings may come up, but most counselors feel that the parents should be fully informed unless they have specifically requested (in writing) that they should not be told of such findings.

Mosaicism in the cultured amniotic fluid cells presents a counseling quandary. If the aneuploid cell line is found in more than one culture flask, it probably did not result from nondisjunction after the amniocentesis. Therefore the mosaicism is likely to involve the fetus, the placenta, or both. If it does involve the fetus, the significance with respect to future development is unclear. Mosaicism for some trisomics—8, 9, and 10, for example—may (or may not) lead to viable defective offspring, even though a fully trisomic fetus is usually nonviable. On the other hand, several cases of mosaicism for trisomy 20 have been reported in which the baby was normal at birth and no longer had any signs of the aneuploid cell line, which may have been at a selective disadvantage and disappeared without doing any harm. Information on which to base decisions in such cases will accumulate slowly. In the meantime, whether to abort the fetus is a decision that will depend mainly on the parents' perception of ambiguous and ill-specified risks. Some centers have adopted a multiple-cultures method using coverslips. We strive to obtain 20 separate colonies by coverslip technique to reduce the chance of misdiagnosing mosaicism.

It is useful to decide ahead of time whether to reveal the sex of the fetus. Parents have the right to know this, but some find that knowing the sex takes some of the excitement and mystery away from the anticipation of birth, and this should be considered.

Parents should also be advised of the possibility that the culture may fail, so that there may be a need for a second tap or at least an unexpected delay in the results. One mother related that she and her husband were managing the stress of waiting nicely until told they would have to wait another 2 weeks, during which time they "didn't even speak to each other, the tension was so bad." Forewarned is forearmed.

If the diagnostic tests do reveal a problem in the fetus, another counseling session will ensue; parents may find the real situation very different from the anticipation.

A subject that causes much soul-searching among geneticists, ethicists, and others is the question of how severe a defect should be to justify prenatal diagnosis.[20] As techniques improve, increasingly subtle disorders will become detectable. Some diseases, such as Tay-Sachs or Krabbe disease, are so terrible that there would be a general agreement that the procedure is justified. But what about albinism, cleft lip, thalassemia minor, simple polydactyly?

The current practice is to balance the probability of occurrence of the defect against the probability of damage from the procedure. That is, if the probability of occurrence of a diagnosable birth defect is less than the 1 or 2% probability of damage from the procedure, the procedure is not justified. Though convenient, this rule-of-thumb ignores the question of severity. A couple may feel that the burden of having a child with, say, Down syndrome far outweighs the burden of an abortion or other hazard of the procedure. Thus, the two risks are not equatable because the stakes are different. How the burden can be taken into account in deciding who is eligible for prenatal diagnosis is still unresolved. Each family will have its own perception of the cost of having an affected child, and the couple, fully informed of the risks, costs, and benefits of the various options, is in the best position to make the decision. Society, on the other hand, should play a role in determining the distribution of resources, which are never plentiful enough to meet the demands. The physician must strive to meet the needs of the former within the limitations of the latter.

Diagnosis of fetal sex for simply social reasons is perhaps the extreme example of a trivial "anomaly" and one that causes the most argument.[9] To most families, the sex of the baby is unimportant, compared to the possibility of a deformity, but to the occasional family it is not trivial; for various social and cultural reasons it may be very important to have a baby of a particular sex. Some geneticists are reluctant to make the resources of prenatal diagnosis available when the aim is to abort a perfectly healthy fetus who just happens to be of the unwanted sex. Others remain true to the philosophy that parents have the right to make the decision. We feel that both should act according to their consciences. No legal restrictions should be placed on the use of amniocentesis, and counselors who object on the grounds of morals, ethics, or personal distaste can refer such couples elsewhere. The expense and hazards of amniocentesis and the unpleasantness of a second-trimester abortion should ensure that the demand for sex ascertainment for social reasons will remain small. If, on the other hand, it becomes possible to determine the embryonic sex by some simple test early in pregnancy (as seems likely), there will be major social repercussions, and society will have to have a say in how to use this two-edged tool.

The development of prenatal diagnosis has involved the convergence of many disciplines, ranging from molecular genetics to biomedical instrumentation, on the common goal of reducing human suffering. It has also stimulated a great deal of interaction among scientists, physicians, ethicists, and lay people. Few other advances in medicine have created so much concern about the moral, ethical, and social implications.[16,20] With wisdom, respect, objectivity, and good will, we must continue to work toward minimizing the costs and maximizing the benefits of this medical achievement.

SUMMARY

The detection of genetic disease in the fetus has added a new dimension to genetic counseling. Techniques beyond screening procedures include cytogenetic or biochemical analysis of fetal cells obtained from the amniotic fluid, analysis of the fluid itself, and visualization of the fetus by ultrasound, radiography, or fetoscopy. The indications, roughly in descending order of frequency are:

1. Maternal age. Risk of a chromosomal problem increases with maternal age. Amniocentesis for examination of chromosomes is offered at most centers in the USA to mothers who will be 35 or older at the time of delivery.

2. Abnormalities detected by screening of maternal blood: serum AFP, HCG, free beta-HCG, and unconjugated estriol.

3. Anencephaly or spina bifida (other than simple occulta type) and related types of vertebral anomalies in a previous child (5% risk), or second degree relative (e.g., the patient's sib or her husband's sib, 2% risk). Ultrasound and increased α-fetoprotein in the amniotic fluid are used as indicators. Increased maternal serum α-fetoprotein provides an opportunity for mass screening for neural tube defects (and decreased serum AFP for some chromosomal anomalies).

4. Previous chromosomal problem in the family, such as (a) a previous child with trisomy or (b) a previous child with an unbalanced chromosomal rearrangement, if one parent has the balanced rearrangement.

5. A significant family history for one of a large number of autosomal recessively inherited and a few X-linked or autosomal dominant inborn errors of metabolism. The list is continually growing. Consult your nearest genetic counselor.

6. X-linked diseases that cannot be diagnosed specifically but for which parents can be offered amniocentesis for sex determination and the option of termination if it is a boy and therefore at high risk.

7. Other familial conditions in which there is a detectable biochemical difference in the amniotic fluid.

8. Various familial conditions involving gross skeletal or visceral malformations—anencephaly, certain short-limbed dwarf-

isms, missing limbs, renal agenesis, poly-cystic kidneys (though not all cases by 20 weeks). Fetoscopy is still in the developmental stage, but is in use for conditions diagnosable by blood examination (e.g., sickle cell disease, thalassemia, hemophilia) and structural anomalies (e.g., dwarfism associated with extra digits).

To make maximum use of this means of reducing the frequency of birth defects *the physician must be alert to these indications as revealed in the family or personal history.*

To evaluate the hazards, costs, and benefits of prenatal diagnosis to society is a complex task. It is certainly a boon to certain families.

REFERENCES

1. Brook, J.D., et al.: Molecular basis of myotonic dystrophy: Expansion of a trinucleotide (CTG) repeat at the 3' end of a transcript encoding a protein kinase family member. Cell 68:799, 1992.
2. Chamberlain, J.: Human benefits and costs of a national screening programme for neural tube defects. Lancet 2:1293, 1978.
3. Crane, J.P., Beaver, H.A., and Cheung, S.W.: First trimester chorionic villus sampling versus mid-trimester genetic amniocentesis—preliminary report of a continuing prospective trial. Prenatal Diag. 8:355, 1988.
4. Cunningham, G.C., and Kizer, K.W.: Maternal serum alpha-fetoprotein activities of state health agencies: A survey. Am. J. Hum. Genet. 47:899, 1990.
5. DiMaio, M.S., et al.: Screening for fetal Down's syndrome in pregnancy by measuring maternal serum alpha-fetoprotein levels. N. Engl. J. Med. 317:342, 1987.
6. Elias, S., et al.: Prenatal diagnosis of aneuploidy using fetal cells from maternal blood (Abst.). Am. J. Hum. Genet. 51:A4 (Suppl.), 1992.
7. Ferguson-Smith, A.A.: Prenatal chromosome analysis and its impact on the birth incidence of chromosome disorders. Br. Med. Bull. 39:355, 1983.
8. Ferguson-Smith, M.A.: The reduction of anencephalic and spina bifida births by maternal serum alpha feto-protein screening. Br. Med. Bull. 396:365, 1983.
9. Fraser, F.C., and Pressor, C.: Attitudes of counselors in relation to prenatal sex determination simply for choice of sex. *In* Genetic Counseling, edited by H.A. Lubs and F. de la Cruz. New York, Raven Press, 1977.
9a. Goldberg, J.D., and Golbus, M.S.: In utero therapy for genetic diseases. *In* Treatment of Genetic Diseases. Edited by R. Desnick. New York, Churchill Livingstone, 1991.
10. Gosden, J.R., et al.: Rapid sex determination in first trimester prenatal diagnosis by dot hybridation of DNA probes. Lancet 1:540, 1984.
11. Gusella, J.F., et al.: A polymorphic DNA marker genetically linked to Huntington's disease. Nature 306:234, 1983.
12. Handyside, A.H., et al.: Birth of a normal girl after in vitro fertilization and preimplantation diagnostic testing for cystic fibrosis. N. Engl. J. Med. 327:905, 1992.
12a. Hook, E.B.: Rates of chromosome abnormalities at different maternal ages. Obstet. Gynecol. 58:282, 1981.
13. Jackson, L.: First trimester diagnosis of fetal genetic disorders. Hosp. Practice 20:801, 1985.
14. Lachman, R., and Hall, J.G.: The radiographic prenatal diagnosis of the generalized bone dysplasias and other skeletal abnormalities. Birth Defects 15(5A):3, 1979.
15. Merkatz, I.R., et al.: An association between low maternal serum alpha-fetoprotein and fetal chromosomal abnormalities. Am. J. Obstet. Gynecol. 148:886, 1984.
16. Milunsky, A., and Annas, G.J. (Eds.): Genetics and the Law. New York, Plenum Press, vol. III, 1985.
17. Modell, S.: Prevention of the haemoglobinopathies. Br. Med. Bull. 39:386, 1983.
18. Pantzar, T.P., et al.: Cytogenetic findings in 318 couples with repeated spontaneous abortion. Am. J. Med. Gen. 17:615, 1984.
19. Pearson, J.F.: Fetal surgery. Arch. Dis. Child. 58:324, 1983.
20. Powledge, T., and Fletcher, J.: Guidelines for the ethical, social and legal issues in prenatal diagnosis. N. Engl. J. Med. 300(4):168, 1979.
21. Roberts, C.J., et al.: Diagnostic effectiveness of ultrasound in detection of neural tube defect. Lancet 2:1068, 1983.
22. Rodick, C.H., and Fisk, N.M.: Intrauterine therapy. *In* Antenatal Diagnosis of Fetal Abnormalities. Edited by J.A. Drife and D. Donnai. New York, Springer-Verlag, 1991.
22a. Saleh, A.A., et al.: Amniotic fluid acetylcholinesterase (ACHE) is found in gastroschisis but not omphalocele (Abst.). Am. J. Obstet. Gynecol. 166:349, 1992.
23. Scrimgeour, J.B. (Ed.): Towards the Prevention of Fetal Malformation. Edinburgh, Edinburgh University Press, 1978.
24. Simoni, G., et al.: Efficient direct chromosome analyses and enzyme determinations from chorionic villi samples in the first trimester of pregnancy. Hum. Genet. 63:349, 1983.
25. Verlinsky, Y., and Kuliev, A. (Eds.): Preimplantation Genetics. New York, Plenum Press, 1991.

Chapter *16*
Human Teratology

A SUBSTANTIAL COLLECTION OF THE MONSTROSITIES OF NATURE, WELL EXAMINED AND DESCRIBED . . .

FRANCIS BACON: ADVANCEMENT OF LEARNING

Fifty years ago, it was generally held that the uterus was an almost impregnable barrier protecting the embryo from environmental insult. Congenital malformations were, by exclusion, considered genetic in origin. ("Congenital" simply means "present at birth" without implying a cause.)

One of the first challenges to this view was made by an Australian ophthalmologist, Gregg, in 1941, who noted an unusual number of cataracts in children he was seeing in his practice and a history of maternal infection with rubella (German measles) during the pregnancy. Deafness and heart malformations were soon recognized as additional teratogenic effects of maternal rubella.[31] At about the same time, Josef Warkany, a Viennese Cincinnati pediatrician, began a classical series of studies that laid the foundation of experimental mammalian teratology.[31] He showed that a maternal dietary deficiency of the vitamin riboflavin could cause malformations in the offspring of the deficient rat mothers. A different pattern of malformations was produced by a deficiency of vitamin A. It was clear that environmental agents could harm the embryo, after all.

In the early 50s, it was shown that another environmental agent, maternal hypoxia, could cause malformations in the offspring of exposed rat or mouse mothers, and the pendulum of opinion began to swing to the view that birth defects were, by and large, caused by environmental insults.

The first drug shown to be teratogenic in experimental animals was cortisone,[8] and the McGill group brought genetics back into the malformation picture by showing that the frequency of cortisone-induced cleft palate in mice depended on the genotype.

Many other substances, including drugs such as aspirin and antihistamines were found to be teratogenic in experimental animals, but only at what were referred to as "sledge-hammer" doses,[8] well out of the range likely to occur in people, and there was little concern about the possibility of drugs being teratogenic—until thalidomide. This sleeping pill, which was also good for nausea of pregnancy, was not good for embryos. Even one pill, at the right (wrong) stage, could cause severe deformities of limbs, heart and intestines. Experimental teratology suddenly became important to physicians, drug manufacturers and regulatory agencies. By then, teratogens had been recognized as valuable tools for the study of development and its errors, and a set of principles had emerged.[33]

PRINCIPLES OF TERATOLOGY

Malformations can be caused by agents that change the genetic material of the germ cells—*mutagens*—or by agents that damage the somatic tissues of the embryo—*teratogens*. Most mutagens are also teratogens, but not necessarily vice versa. Whether a given agent is teratogenic depends on its chemical and physical nature, the developmental stage of exposure, the dose, the genotype of mother and embryo, and possible interactions with other environmental factors.

Periods of Vulnerability. Certain periods of organogenesis are particularly vulnerable to teratogens. Viable malformations are not produced prior to implantation (second week in the human). After that, each organ has its own periods of vulnerability, or *critical* periods. These differ for different organs, and for different teratogens. In general, they occur some time before the actual developmental event. Presumably, they represent periods when something vital to subsequent organogenesis is happening, that is attacked by the teratogen.

In the case of thalidomide and the human heart, for example, the period of exposure that interferes with closure of the ventricular septum is in the fifth week, two weeks before the septum closes. This is what is treacherous about teratogenic insults: many organ systems, such as the heart, are vulnerable at a time when the mother is just becoming convinced she is truly pregnant and not "just a week or two late." She then decides to stop drinking alcohol or taking retinoic acid for her acne, but this may already be too late.

Which Agents are Teratogenic? Although relatively few agents have been identified that are potent teratogens capable of causing malformations in an appreciable proportion of individuals exposed at a vulnerable period of embryogenesis, possibly hundreds of agents are teratogenic within a given set of circumstances, such as hereditary predisposition to a

malformation and hereditary sensitivity to a drug or virus, or some interacting environmental factor such as nutritional deficiency.

Relationship to Dose. In experimental animals the teratogenic dose range usually overlaps the dose that will kill some of the embryos. There are exceptions, however. Conversely, teratogenic effects may occur at doses well below the embryo-lethal dose and even more so the maternal toxic dose. Thalidomide is an outstanding human example.

Hereditary Predisposition to a Given Teratogen. There are species and individual differences in response to the teratogenic effects of an agent. The genotype of the embryo and mother are highly critical.

One of the first examples of genetic differences was that of cleft palate induced by cortisone in the mouse. The same dose produced a frequency of 100% in the A/J inbred strain and only 20% in the C57BL/6 strain.

When F1 embryos were treated in an A strain mother, the frequency of cleft palate induced by cortisone was much higher than when the genetically identical F1 was treated in a C57BL/6 mother. That meant that not only the fetal, but the maternal genotype was important in determining teratogenic susceptibility. Furthermore, susceptibility of the embryonic palate to cortisone correlated well with the stage at which the palate normally closes. Palates that normally closed later were more susceptible. Thus a *normal, genetically determined difference in developmental pattern* influenced the susceptibility of the embryo to an environmental insult.

As another example, about 1% of C57BL/6 mice "spontaneously" have a ventricular septal defect, but none has atrial septal defect. Exposure of the pregnant female at day 8 of gestation to a single large dose of dextroamphetamine produces ventricular septal defects in 11% of offspring. The A/J strain has a low spontaneous frequency of atrial septal defect but not ventricular septal defect. Treatment of A/J females with dextroamphetamine produces atrial septal defects in 13%. Thus, the C57 appears to have a hereditary predisposition to ventricular septal defect, and the A/J to atrial septal defect. The same teratogens caused different lesions in the two strains of mice. The predisposition to a rather specific type of heart defect is seen in human studies, in which affected members of a family tend to have the same anomaly—ventricular septal defect in one family; atrial septal defect in another.

Genetic differences in susceptibility became particularly important when it was discovered that thalidomide was teratogenic in man. The malformations so readily produced by thalidomide in the human could not be reproduced in a number of traditional animal models. And not all pregnant women who ingested thalidomide during vulnerable periods of embryogenesis produced malformed infants. The ample experimental evidence of genetic differences in response to a teratogen makes it impossible to predict with confidence, from animal studies, whether a new drug or other agent will be teratogenic in man. It is also still not possible to predict in the human which individual will be predisposed to react adversely to a drug and which may be relatively safe from its teratogenic effects.

Of particular interest is the Ah locus studied by Nebert and his group in several inbred strains of mice, which has potentially great relevance to human mechanisms. When an exogenous chemical enters a cell, the Ah locus is activated, leading to an increase in enzymes which detoxify the chemical to a harmless substance. "Responsiveness" at the Ah locus to handle exposure to hydrocarbons through synthesizing cytosolic receptors is genetically determined both in laboratory mammals and humans (see Chap. 24).

Interaction of Teratogens and Other Agents. Experimental studies show that drugs taken in combination with other drugs may produce malformations even though either drug taken singly would not. It is too often the case that a pregnant woman is treated for a disorder with not one but several drugs. Furthermore, a given drug may be teratogenic only through interaction with another environmental factor, such as a virus or nutritional deficiency. From the clinical point of view, this is another pitfall in the path of safe drug administration, and, from the research point of view, it is a further

obstacle to defining specific human teratogens.

Specificity of Teratogens. Finally, certain drugs and viruses cause malformations and patterns of malformation that are characteristic (e.g., phocomelia from thalidomide and patent ductus arteriosus, deafness, and cataracts from rubella virus). These patterns must be related to special properties of the teratogens: In the case of drugs, there are specific metabolic effects; in the case of rubella virus continued proliferation interferes with the host's normal processes of growth and development.

Hereditary Predisposition to the Malformation. The *three components of a typical teratogenic exposure* leading to a malformation are: (1) genetic predisposition to a malformation; (2) genetic predisposition to the effects of a given teratogen; and (3) administration at a vulnerable period of embryogenesis.

From experience with human beings and experimental animals, it would seem likely that in most instances of maldevelopment produced by a teratogen there is a genetic predisposition to the specific malformation that results. The defect occurs when an exposure occurs at a vulnerable period of embryogenesis. There are probably few teratogens like thalidomide and rubella virus that produce such a high frequency of malformations following maternal exposures in the first trimester. Even in some of these cases, there is evidence of genetic predisposition to the malformation, as will be discussed in the section on the rubella syndrome.

ROLE OF TERATOGENS IN HUMAN MALFORMATIONS

The question of teratogens in human malformations may be looked at from two perspectives: that of the patient and his family and that of the research investigator.

It is relatively easy to identify an agent as teratogenic if it produces a high frequency of an uncommon anomaly. The goal becomes even easier to reach if the agent has just been introduced or is not in widespread use. Thalidomide and lithium are examples. However, it is extremely difficult—some may say impossible—to identify a teratogen that is widely used and causes a small increase in common anomalies. Yet, as hazards to public health, agents in the latter category can be much the more important.

Problems in Implicating Teratogens

Human teratogenicity of drugs (or other potential teratogens) can be evaluated by two approaches. In *prospective* studies, women who take the drug during pregnancy are registered, and fetal outcomes are compared with those of comparable women who did not take the drug. These are relatively unbiased, but expensive because they require large numbers unless the frequency of malformations following exposure is high.

In *retrospective* studies, mothers of offspring with malformations are compared with comparable mothers of offspring without malformations (or with different malformations) with respect to exposure during pregnancy. These are more subject to bias, and require some intelligent guesswork as to what malformations to study.

Even with thalidomide (50 to 80% malformation rate), it took 4 years from the time the drug came on the market until a sufficiently compelling data base was produced to encourage its withdrawal. How much greater is the challenge to discover low-level teratogens! But what if a drug causes malformations in only 1 or 2% of those exposed, does it really matter all that much? It matters most tragically to those who must live with the burden of disability and death, particularly if the use of the drug was not absolutely essential. From the point of view of society it also matters. If a drug is commonly used in pregnancy, then the potential exposure rate is high, and even if the malformation rate following exposure is only 1 or 2%, this could mean thousands of babies born every year in North America alone with birth defects that could have been prevented.

A critical error that flaws many epidemiologic studies is the failure to associate the time of exposure to the teratogen with the vulnerable period of embryogenesis for the defect in question. To illustrate this point, many studies have looked at transposition of the great arteries (TGA). Truncoconal septation is completed by about day 34. Any teratogenic influence on this structural development must take place before day 34. Therefore, a drug given after day 34 cannot be considered responsible for transposition of the great arteries, nor can a case where teratogenic exposure after day 34 that failed to produce transposition be tallied as showing no effect.

The magnitude of the problem of using the first 3 months as the vulnerable period for TEA rather than the first month (a 67% mismodeling bias) is illustrated by the following calculations. If one builds into a study a 67% error through mismodeling, the number of cases needed to show no association of a teratogen with birth defects at a fourfold increase in risk balloons from only 140 cases to 2299 cases needed in a retrospective study or to 12,122 cases (rather than 1663) in a prospective study. What if the increase in risk is only twofold (as in increasing congenital heart defects from 1 to 2% in exposed groups)? Then *60,231* cases would be required to show "no effect" in a prospective study.

No study could tolerate a 67% mismodeling bias. Precision in design greatly reduces the number of cases needed to reach confident conclusions. Financial resources will no longer permit the profligacy of enormous but imprecise studies. Small, elegant, well-designed studies will achieve the answers with greater economy and accuracy.

Malformation registries are beginning to provide the data for case-control and cohort studies large enough to elucidate teratogenic factors not detectable by sample sizes available to a single center.

SYNDROMES PRODUCED BY TERATOGENS

Table 16–1 is a selected list of the known or suspected human teratogens, arbitrarily divided according to the strength of the evidence into class 1—no doubt, 2—very likely, and 3—possible. Because it is so difficult to impli-

Table 16–1.   Selected Teratogens in Humans Implicated with Varying Degrees of Confidence

Teratogens	Confidence Class	Approximate Frequency of Maldevelopment
Infections		
Rubella	1	90% (see text)
Cytomegalovirus[24]	1	1/1000
Herpes simplex virus (HSV) as teratogen	3	?
HSV (type 2) as neonatal infection	1	—
Syphilis[10]	1	very high
Toxoplasmosis	1	≈15%
Parvovirus	1	?
Maternal Conditions		
Diabetes[2]	2	5%
Fever	2	?
Lupus erythematosus[34]	1	very high
Phenylketonuria—untreated	1	very high
Drugs, Chemicals, and Radiation		
Alcohol (chronic alcoholism)	1	30%
Amphetamines[11]	2	?≈5%
Anticoagulants (warfarin)	2	5–10%
Anticonvulsants		
Hydantoin (Phenytoin)	2	5–10%
Phenobarbital	3	?
Trimethadione	1	?≈20%
Valproic acid	1	≈5%
Chemotherapeutic agents	1	high
Cocaine[30]	1	≈15%
Hypoglycemics	3	?
Lithium[22]	1	10%
Mercury, organic	1	high
Minor tranquilizers		
Diazepam	2	? (very low)
Meprobamate	3	? (very low)
Penicillamine	2	moderate
Radiation[4]	1	dose dependent
Retinoic acid, etretinate	1	10–15%
Sex Hormones	1	
Male	1	? low
Female	2	?5%
Stilbestrol	1	?
Thalidomide	1	50–80%

cate an environmental agent as a teratogen, for reasons referred to above, we must admit the possibility that there may be dozens, or hundreds of agents that cause malformations in special circumstances of genetic and environmental susceptibility, that would not be detected by our present surveillance systems. If the agent is widespread, even if it causes malformations in only a small fraction of exposed individuals, the total amount of damage may be large. With constant vigilance, and improved surveillance systems, the number of identified teratogens continues to grow. We will mention some of the more significant ones. More extensive reviews are available.

Rubella Syndrome

The original triad of defects (cataracts, deafness, and patent ductus arteriosus) resulting from maternal infection with rubella was expanded, after the epidemic of 1964–65, to include several other kinds of damage, including large liver and spleen, hepatitis, bone lesions, anemia and psychomotor retardation.

The virus appears to infect the various organs and produce its teratogenic effects by direct tissue damage.

It was also realized, after several pregnant nurses caring for infants with the rubella syndrome themselves produced affected children, that the virus could persist in these children for months, or sometimes years after birth.

The risk that a child would be affected if the mother had the disease seems higher than originally thought. In cases with serologic confirmation of maternal infection, the risk of some defect attributable to rubella is 85% if infection occurs within the first 12 weeks of pregnancy, falling to 65% (almost all deafness) for infection in the 15th to 16th week. There is an increase in deafness in the relatives of deaf children with the rubella syndrome, suggesting that the genotype influences the response of the ear to the environmental insult.

Fortunately, a vaccine is now available and the congenital rubella syndrome is a preventable disease.

The Thalidomide Syndrome

In late 1960, a sudden increase in babies with reduction deformities (missing bones) of the limbs (Fig. 16–1) was noted in West Germany. In some cases, the whole limb was missing, with the hand or foot attached directly to the body—referred to as phocomelia (seal limb). There was a frantic search for the cause. Heredity and viruses were quickly ruled out. Then a pediatrician-geneticist, Widukind Lenz, noticed that several mothers reported having taken a sleeping pill containing a new drug, thalidomide. When he asked the mothers specifically about thalidomide, many more remembered they had taken it, and he became convinced that thalidomide was the cause of the deformities. At the same time, an outbreak of phocomelia occurred in Australia, and an obstetrician, William McBride, also noticed the association with thalidomide, which was there being used to treat nausea of pregnancy. The first reports of Lenz and McBride were received with some skepticism, but further evidence came pouring in and the drug

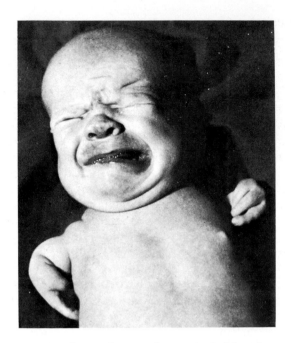

Fig. 16–1.   Phocomelia in infant with thalidomide syndrome.

was soon taken off the market. In the United States, the drug was never put on the market because Dr. Frances Kelsey of the Food and Drug Administration was worried about reports of neuritis in some cases of chronic use, so the U.S. was spared the tragedy experienced by countries where it was used, including Germany, Great Britain, Australia, Canada, and Japan. There is a characteristic pattern of defects, affecting virtually all organ systems.[28]

Thalidomide illustrates two principles of teratology. There was no effect if the pill was taken earlier than 20 days after conception or later than 36 days. The critical period was 25 to 30 days for the arms, 28 to 34 days for the legs and 27 to 29 days for major heart defects.[17] Secondly, there are marked species differences. Human embryos are exquisitely sensitive, whereas most strains of mouse and rat are very resistant.

It is humbling to think that, in spite of the tragic harm done by this, the most potent human teratogen, and the enormous amount of research on it, the mechanism by which it disrupts development remains a mystery.

Alcohol

Alcohol is a teratogen that has been around much longer than any other drug, but it was only in the late 60s that the damage it does to the fetus was first recognized.[5] In spite of a voluminous literature since then, not all the answers are in. The frequency of the full-blown fetal alcohol syndrome is 1 or 2 per thousand, and 1 in 300 babies may show some detrimental effects. As more subtle effects are recognized, and more prospective studies are completed, the estimates of damage will rise. A touching story of the tragic effects on children and their families is told by an adoptive father.[7]

Growth deficiency, mild to moderate psychomotor retardation, with tremulousness, hyperactivity, distractibility, mild to moderate microcephaly, short palpebral fissures, short nose, and a thin, smooth upper lip are the main characteristics (Fig. 16–2).

The risk of damage to the fetus is as high as 50% for children of severe chronic alcoholics. Effects on IQ, learning, and other neurobehavioral measures can be found in the children of moderate drinkers,[29] and there is some evidence that even the occasional binge may be harmful.[5] Even 10 grams of alcohol a day (one drink) may produce a detectable reduction in birth weight.[29] Thus maternal alcohol consumption is one of the four largest contributors to human mental retardation (with Down syndrome, spina bifida, and fragile X) and the only one of these that is preventable. It is important to note that alcohol exposure damages the brain even after the period of organogenesis, so that to give up drinking even in the second or third trimester is of some benefit to the offspring.

The existence of animal models leaves no doubt that ethyl alcohol, and not some concomitant of the alcoholic environment does the damage. An elegant mouse model suggests that the facial characteristics result from damage to mesodermal cells inducing the forebrain.[5]

Anticonvulsants

Women have been on antiepileptic drugs for many years, but it was not until 1968 that an alert British physician, Meadows, noticed that there was an increase in malformations in infants of mothers on one of these, diphenylhydantoin (DPH, Dilantin). In spite of initial scepticism, particularly from neurologists, a number of studies have confirmed the existence of a fetal hydantoin syndrome.

Wide-spaced eyes, epicanthal folds, broad depressed nose bridge, short nose and bowed upper lip, and characteristic hypoplasia of finger tips and nails are some of the characteristics (Fig. 16–3). It is difficult to predict the probability that an exposed offspring will have the syndrome or a major malformation (cleft lip or heart malformation in particular) because it varies with whether other anticonvulsant drugs are used as well, the dosage, the stage of pregnancy, and probably the genotype. Estimates range around 10% for the full syndrome (higher for partial forms), with about a 5% risk of a major malformation. Mothers who have had an affected child are at much higher risk (9/10). A suggestion that fetuses with the "slow" form of epoxide hydrolase activity are most likely to be affected provides a possible means of prenatal diagnosis, but needs further testing. Other anticonvulsants such as barbiturates, tridione, and carbamazine are also teratogenic to some degree.[6]

The latest to join the list is valproic acid; exposed babies have about a 5% risk of neural tube defect or heart malformation. This has the distinction of being the only drug so far whose teratogenicity was first recognized in a surveillance system.[16]

Claims that the epileptic genotypes themselves have a teratogenic potential, as manifested by an increase in malformations in children of epileptic fathers, are not well substantiated. If there is an increase, it must be small. Management of the epileptic woman who wants children is difficult. It is not wise to take her off medication—provided she is on for a good reason. The best approach is to be sure she knows about the teratogenic risk before she gets pregnant and, if she does conceive, to keep her on the lowest possible dose, preferably of just one drug, with monitoring

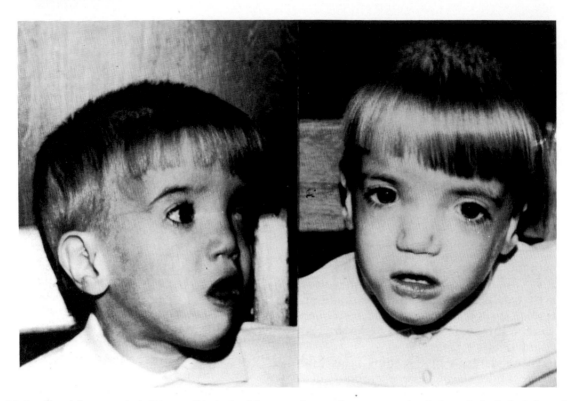

Fig. 16–2. Facial features, including small palpebral fissures, frequently seen in individuals with fetal alcohol syndrome. From Nora, J.J., and Nora, A.H.: Genetics and Counseling in Cardiovascular Diseases. Springfield, Charles C Thomas, 1978.

of blood levels. Prenatal diagnosis can be offered, particularly for neural tube defects if valproic acid is the drug of choice.

Cocaine

Because of its increasingly widespread use, cocaine must receive more than just a notation in Table 16–1. Volpe has reviewed the problem.[30] From 10 to 45% of women in urban teaching hospitals and 6% in private suburban hospitals have had exposure to cocaine during pregnancy. The major consequences are to the central nervous system (cerebral infarction and intracranial hemorrhage), microcephaly, low birth weight, prematurity, seizures, sudden infant death syndrome, and *possibly* long-term neurologic, cognitive, and behavioral problems.

Radiation

Data on the teratogenic effects of X-irradiation (as distinct from the mutagenic and carcin-

ogenic effects) are scanty.[4] There are reports of malformed babies (mostly microcephalic) born to mothers following therapeutic irradiation for cancer, and an increase in microcephaly was shown in children of mothers exposed to, but not killed by, the atomic bomb in Japan. Studies in rats and mice have shown that teratogenic doses of x rays are well above those used in the usual diagnostic procedures, so we counsel reassurance when consulted by women who had, for example, a gallbladder series or a tubal insufflation and then found out that they were pregnant at the time.[4]

Retinoic Acid, Etretinate, and Related Products

Additions to the list of human teratogens include retinoic acid, a precursor of vitamin A.[25] The 13-cis form, isotretinoin (Acutane), is good for the treatment of cystic acne, a seriously disfiguring condition for some patients. Because of its teratogenicity in animals, it was approved for human use only with the warn-

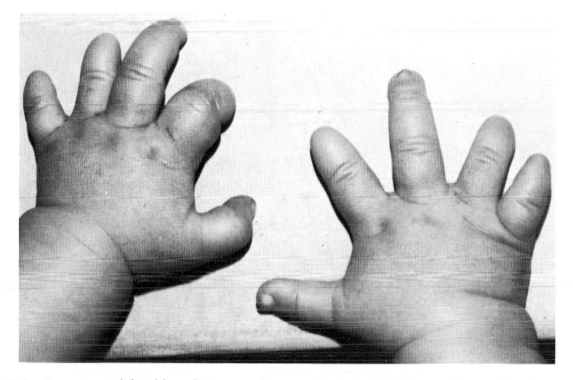

Fig. 16–3. Severe terminal digital hypoplasia commonly associated with the fetal hydantoin (phenytoin) syndrome. From Nora, J.J., and Nora, A.H.: Genetics and Counseling in Cardiovascular Diseases. Springfield, Charles C Thomas, 1978.

ing that it should not be used by women in the reproductive age range. Nevertheless, a significant number of reports are now appearing of malformations occurring in babies exposed before their mothers knew they were pregnant. Malformations of the ear, brain and heart are described; in a prospective study,[11] of 57 exposed offspring had malformations. Use during pregnancy is contraindicated except for severe cystic acne, and then only with rigorous monitoring.[25] Etretinate, used for treating psoriasis, has recently been implicated in birth defects. Whether large doses of vitamin A may be teratogenic is still an open question, but it would be prudent to avoid megadoses of vitamin A during pregnancy.

MATERNAL TERATOGENIC CONDITIONS

Besides the various hazards from the mother's environment to which the embryo is exposed, there are several maternal conditions that can increase the probability of malformations.

Diabetes Mellitus

The frequency of malformations is increased in the offspring of maternal diabetics with a risk of about 18% for major malformations.[2] Apart from the rare "caudal dysplasia" or sacral agenesis, the malformations do not occur in a characteristic pattern. Heart malformations and neural tube defects are among the more common, being frequent enough to justify prenatal diagnosis. The risk of malformation appears to fall as control of the diabetes improves.

Phenylketonuria

Sometimes medical advances have unexpected price-tags and this is true of the successful dietary treatment of children with phenylketonuria. When the first cohort of treated girls with PKU reached the age of reproduction, a high frequency of microcephaly, mental retardation, and malformations, particularly of the heart, was noted in their babies. Here it is not the fetal genotype but the excess phenylalanine to which the fetus is exposed by virtue of its mother's genotype that does the damage (Fig. 16–4). Women with other forms of hyperphenylalaninemia (see Chap. 6) may also be at risk. Dietary control of the mother's phenylalanine levels appears to reduce or perhaps prevent the damage but it must begin early in pregnancy, preferably before conception.[18]

Maternal Fever (Hyperthermia)

Evidence is accumulating for the teratogenicity of maternal fever (high fever over some days), either infectious or induced in saunas or hot baths.[32] The degree of risk is not known. Microphthalmia and neural tube defects are among the most characteristic defects. Animal models suggest that mitotic inhibition is the mechanism.[32]

ATTEMPTED ABORTION, TERATOGENS, AND MALFORMATIONS

It is not uncommon that a newborn with multiple congenital anomalies is the firstborn child of a very young mother, often unwed or wed after conception. A careful history based on good rapport between the mother and the genetic counselor frequently reveals an attempted abortion with various drugs taken in large doses. Two important requirements for teratogenesis are met under these circumstances: the drugs are taken at the most vulnerable period of organogenesis (just when the mother first realizes she is pregnant), and the dose of the drug is very large, not large enough to kill mother or embryo, but large enough to

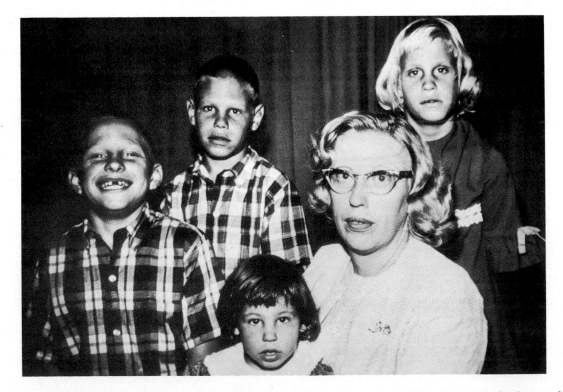

Fig. 16–4.   This mother with elevated serum levels of phenylalanine (maternal phenylketonuria) gave birth to 4 children with microcephaly. Photograph courtesy of Dr. William Frankenburg.

malform. In the case of aminopterin there is a documented relation between attempted abortion and malformations.

SUMMARY

Teratogens act by causing damage to the cells, tissues, or interactions between tissues of developing embryos, in contrast to mutagens, which produce changes in the genetic material.

The three components of a typical teratogenic exposure are (1) hereditary predisposition to a malformation; (2) hereditary predisposition to the effects of a given teratogen; and (3) administration of the teratogen at a vulnerable period of embryogenesis. A number of human teratogens and their effects are reviewed.

The teratogenic hazards to which the human fetus is exposed are numerous and complex. Presumably the known environmental teratogens represent the tip of the iceberg; it is extremely difficult to detect an agent that has a low risk of producing a common malformation; yet if exposure to the agent was common it could cause many malformations. We know enough to appreciate the complexities of interactions between teratogens, other environmental factors, and genes in experimental animals, but our knowledge in the human being is still very limited.

REFERENCES

1. Anderson, H., Bengt Barr, E.E., and Wedenberg, D.: Genetic disposition—A prerequisite for maternal rubella deafness. Arch. Otolaryngol. 91:141, 1970.
2. Becerra, J.E., Khoury, M.J., et al.: Diabetes mellitus during pregnancy and the risks for specific birth defects: A population-based case-control study. Pediatrics 85:1, 1990.
3. Begelow, S.W., and Nebert, D.W.: The murine aromatic hydrocarbon responsiveness locus: A comparison of receptor levels and several inducible enzyme activities among recombinant inbred lines. J. Biochem. Toxicol. 1:1, 1986.
4. Brent, R.L.: Radiation teratogenesis. Teratology 21:281, 1980.
5. Ciba Foundation Symposium 105. Mechanisms of Alcohol Damage in Utero. Edited by R. Porter et al. London, Pitman, 1983.
6. Dansky, L.V., and Finnell, R.H.: Parental epilepsy, anticonvulsant drugs, and reproductive outcomes. Epidemiologic and experimental findings spanning three decades: (2)Human studies. Reprod. Toxicol. 5:301, 1991.
7. Dorris, M.: The broken cord. New York, Harper and Row, 1989.
8. Fraser, F.C.: The use of teratogens in the analysis of abnormal developmental mechanisms. In First International Conference on Congenital Malformations. Philadelphia, J.B. Lippincott Co., 1961.
9. Fraser, F.C.: Interactions and multiple causes. In Handbook of Teratology, vol. 1. Edited by J.G. Wilson and F.C. Fraser. New York, Plenum Press, 1977, pp. 445–463.
10. Grossman, J.: Congenital syphilis. Teratology 16:217, 1977.
11. Hall, J.: Warfarin and fetal abnormality. Lancet 1:1127, 1976.
12. Hanson, J.W., et al.: Teratogen update: Fetal hydantoin effects. Teratology 33:349, 1986.
13. Heinonen, O.P., et al.: Birth defects and drugs in pregnancy. Littleton, Mass., Publishing Sciences Group, Inc. 1977.
14. Kallen, B.: Search for teratogenic risks with the aid of malformation registries. Teratology 35:47, 1987.
15. Kelley-Buchanan, C.: Peace of mind during pregnancy. New York, Facts on File Publications, 1988.
16. Lammer, E.J., Sever, L.S. and Oakley, G.P.: Teratogen update: Valproic acid. Teratology 35:465, 1987.
17. Lenz, W.: Chemicals and malformations in man. In Second International Conference on Congenital Malformations, New York, International Medical Congress Ltd., 1964, p. 263.
18. Levy, H., et al.: Comparison of treated and untreated pregnancies in a mother with phenylketonuria. J. Pediat. 100:876, 1982.
19. McBride, W.G.: Thalidomide and congenital abnormalities. Lancet 2:1358, 1961.
20. Munro, N.D. et al.: Temporal relations between maternal rubella and congenital defects. Lancet II:201, 1987.
21. Nora, J.J. et al.: Homologies for congenital heart diseases: Murine models influenced by dextroamphetamine. Teratology 1:413, 1968.
22. Nora, J.J., Nora, A.H., and Toews, W.H.: Lithium, Ebstein's anomaly and other congenital heart defects. Lancet 2:594, 1974.
23. Nora, J.J., Nora, A.H., and Blu, J., et al.: Exogenous progestogen and estrogen implicated in birth defects. JAMA 240:837, 1978.
24. Peckham, C.S., et al.: Cytomegalovirus infection in pregnancy: Preliminary findings from a prospective study. Lancet 1:1352, 1983.
25. Public Affairs Committee, Teratology Society. Recommendations for isotretinoin use in women of childbearing age. Teratology 44:1, 1991.
26. Schardein, J.L.: Chemically induced birth defects. New York, Marcel Dekker, Inc., 1985.
27. Shepard, T.H.: Human Teratogenicity. Adv. Pediat. 33:225, 1986.
28. Smithells, R.W., and Newman, C.G.H.: Recognition of thalidomide defects. J. Med. Genet. 29:716, 1992.
29. Streisguth, A.P., Barr, H.M. and Sampson, P.K.: Moderate prenatal alcohol exposure: effects on child's IQ and learning problems at age 7 1/2 years. Alcohol. Clin. Exp. Res. 14:622, 1990.
30. Volpe, J.J.: Mechanisms of disease: Effect of cocaine use on the fetus. N. Engl. J. Med. 327:399, 1992.
31. Warkany, J.: Congenital Malformations. Chicago, Year Book Medical Publishers, 1971.
32. Warkany, J.: Teratogen Update: Hyperthermia. Teratology 33:365, 1986.
33. Wilson, J.G.: Embryotoxicity of drugs in man. In Handbook of Teratology, vol. 1. Edited by J.C. Wilson and F.C. Fraser. New York, Plenum Press, 1977, pp. 309–355.
34. Winkler, R.B., Nora, A.H., and Nora, J.J.: Familial congenital complete heart block and maternal systemic lupus erythematosus. Circulation 56:1103, 1977.

Chapter *17*
Dermatoglyphics

TRANSMIT THE PRELUDES THROUGH HIS HAIR AND FINGER-TIPS.

T.S. ELIOT, PORTRAIT OF A LADY

Dermatoglyphics are the dermal ridge configurations on the digits, palms, and soles. They begin to develop about the thirteenth week of prenatal life as the fetal mounds on the digit tips, interdigital, thenar, and hypothenar areas of the hand and the corresponding areas of the foot begin to regress.[3,5] The pattern formation is complete by the nineteenth week.

Certain syndromes include unusual combinations of dermatoglyphic patterns. These can help to establish a probability index for a particular diagnosis, as first demonstrated by Walker in the case of Down syndrome.[11] This approach has been extended to a number of other syndromes,[4] but there are now so many invalid claims for associations of dermatoglyphic patterns with syndromes and diseases that the literature must be approached with caution.[7] Nevertheless, dermatoglyphic analysis is still a useful, but underappreciated, screening procedure, especially for Down syndrome (see page 320). Even when a specific syndrome cannot be identified abnormal dermatoglyphics are a sign of prenatal growth disturbance that may have some diagnostic value—for example in cases of mental retardation when there is some question of whether the cause was perinatal or prenatal.

TERMINOLOGY

Finger Patterns. The patterns on the finger tips are of three main types, classified by the number of triradii present. A triradius is a three-way "fork" resulting from the confluence of three ridge systems (Fig. 17–1). A simple arch (A) has no triradius; a tented arch has a central triradius. The loop has a single triradius and is called ulnar (U) or radial (R), depending on the side to which it opens. The whorl (W) has two or more triradii and may be a double loop or, more commonly, a circular type of pattern.

The *ridge count* is a quantitative way of measuring finger patterns. The number of ridges is counted between the center of the pattern and the farthest triradius. Thus arches have a count of 0, and whorls tend to have the highest values. The total ridge count is obtained by summing the counts for the 10 fingers.

The frequency of these patterns for Caucasians is shown in Table 17–1. Conventionally the digits are numbered from thumb to little finger. Arches and radial loops have the lowest overall frequency; when present, they occur most often on digit 2, especially in the

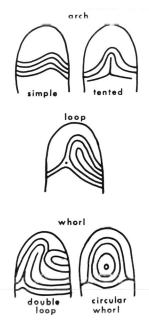

Fig. 17–1. Three basic finger patterns. The arch has no triradius or central triradius. The loop has a single triradius and opens to one side. The whorl has two or more triradii.

case of radial loops. Whorls occur most often on digits 4, 1, and 2. Ulnar loops are the most common pattern. A common distribution is shown in Figure 17–2.

The pattern frequencies vary somewhat with side and with sex, females having slightly more arches and fewer whorls than males. There are also racial differences in pattern frequencies. Orientals, for example, have a higher frequency of whorls than European-Americans.[1]

Palmar Patterns. The palm can be divided into the hypothenar, thenar, and four interdigital areas I_1, I_2, I_3, and I_4 (Fig. 17–2). The normal palm has a triradius at the base of the palm between the thenar and hypothenar areas. This is the axial triradius (t). A variety of patterns (loops and whorls) found in the hypothenar area are classified by the location and number of triradii. A pattern in either I_3 or I_4 is common, and a pattern in the thenar/I_1 and the I_2 area is less common. The main line from the a triradius usually exits in the hypothenar area, that from b in I_4, that from c in I_3 and that from d in I_2. The axial triradius t is usually proximal, but may be displaced distally. The amount of distal displacement is

Table 17–1. Frequency (%) of Pattern Types on the Fingers*

	Digit					
Pattern	1	2	3	4	5	Total
A	3	10	8	2	1	5
U	65	36	72	58	86	63
R	0	23	4	1	0	6
W	32	31	16	39	13	26

*The values for left and right and male and female do not differ appreciably and have been combined for simplicity. Adapted from Holt, S.B.: The Genetics of Dermal Ridges. Springfield, Charles C Thomas, 1968.

measured as a percentage of the height from the distal wrist crease to the proximal crease at the base of the third digit; the normal state, t, is defined as a height of 0 to 14%, t' as 15 to 39% and t" as greater than 40% of the total height. This method of classification is less age-dependent than the alternative method, measuring the atd angle. As both methods are used in the literature, Dr. M. Preus has established values from her data for converting the angle measurements to t, t', or t". She defines t as less than 46 degrees and t" as greater than 63 degrees.

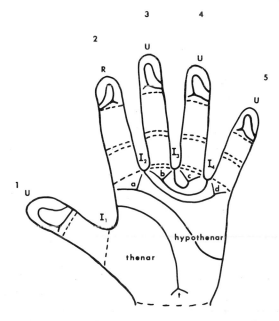

Fig. 17–2. One of the more common finger and palm patterns.

Soles. Because of the difficulties in printing the foot, observations are limited largely to the hallucal area, although other areas can also give valuable information. The patterns in the hallucal area are shown in Figure 17–3. The most frequent patterns in normal individuals are the whorl and the large distal loop (>21 ridges).

Flexion Creases. Strictly speaking, the flexion creases are not dermatoglyphic patterns but have come to be included in dermatoglyphic analysis. They represent places of attachment of the skin to underlying structures and are formed between the seventh and fourteenth week of development.[5]

The palmar creases generally consist of a distal and proximal transverse crease and a thenar crease (Fig. 17–4). About 6% of normal individuals have at least one **simian crease**—a single crease extending across the entire palm—or a **transitional** simian crease—two transverse creases joined by an equally deep, short crease (type 1, bridged) or a single crease with a branch above and below the main crease (type 2). Considerable variations in reported frequencies depend on whether transitional forms are counted as simian creases. About 11% of normal individuals have a **Sydney line**, in which the proximal transverse crease extends across the entire palm, rather than stopping short of the ulnar border.

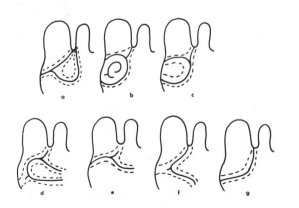

Fig. 17–3. Hallucal patterns in order of frequency: (a) distal loop; (b) whorl; (c) tibial loop; (d) fibular loop; (e) proximal arch; (f) fibular arch; (g) tibial arch (no triradius).

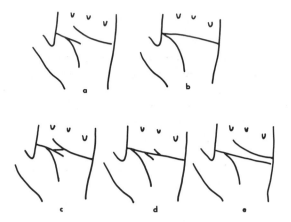

Fig. 17–4. Palmar creases: (a) normal; (b) simian; (c) transitional type 1; (d) transitional type 2; (e) Sydney.

METHODS OF OBSERVATION AND PRINTING

If the dermal ridges are too small or poorly developed to observe directly, as with the newborn subject or presbyopic observer, an ordinary otoscope provides a satisfactory light and magnification for observation. The position of the hand or foot is adjusted to get the best interplay of available and direct light. Depending on the interests of the observer and the nature of the patient's defect, the patterns may be recorded directly or printed for a permanent record.

Several techniques for printing are available.[10] For infants, Hollister* ink pads and paper are useful. The area to be printed should be clean, dry, and warm; after being "inked" with the pad, the hand is placed lightly on the paper. Too much pressure will blur the print. For ages over 4 years the Faurot[†] inkless methods works well. Placing the paper over a sponge rubber pad helps one to get a complete print when the hand is too large to manipulate easily. Care must be taken not to use too much ink or pressure. Cellulose tape applied after dusting the hand with charcoal, or rubbing with pencil carbon paper provides clear prints and is particularly useful for small and uncooperative patients.[3]

*Hollister, Inc., 833 New Orleans St., Chicago, Ill.
†Faurot Inc., 299 Broadway, New York, N.Y.

USES AND LIMITATIONS OF DERMATOGLYPHIC ANALYSIS

The strong resemblance of dermatoglyphic patterns in pairs of monozygotic twins suggests that their determination has a major genetic component. This is substantiated by the correlation for ridge count between pairs of individuals of various degrees of relationship, which correspond closely to the expectation for a trait determined by multiple additive genes, with a heritability of 1 (Table 17–2). One would therefore expect that when a large number of genes are missing or present in excess the dermatoglyphics will be altered. This appears to be so. In several chromosomal syndromes these alterations are consistent enough to be of diagnostic value.

Intuitively, one might expect that the dermal ridge patterns reflect the conformation of the fetal hand at the time of ridge development, as first suggested by Cummins (1926). If so, we would expect the dermal ridges to be altered when the limbs are deformed, and they are.[4] We would therefore not expect the dermatoglyphic patterns to be diagnostically useful if the patient has gross malformations of the limbs; the patterns reflect the obvious anatomic defect. They may be useful, however, as a reflection of more subtle morphologic changes in the embryo. Webbing between the digits (cutaneous syndactyly), for instance, is a feature of a number of syndromes, but it is sometimes difficult to decide on gross examination whether it is present in a minor degree. Fusion of the triradii at the base of the digits is good evidence that the developmental disturbance resulting in syndactyly was present when the ridges formed, even if the syndactyly is not obvious at birth.

Examination of dermatoglyphics may help to decide whether a causative agent acted early or late. For example, the unusual longitudinal main line configurations in a number of patients with one form of joint contractures suggest that the defect was present in these patients at least as early as the 13th to 19th week.

ZYGOSITY DIAGNOSIS IN TWINS

If dermatoglyphic patterns are in large part genetically determined, then the hands of monozygotic twins should resemble one another as closely as do the two hands of a single individual, which are also genetically identical. This appears to be true, and the argument can be used in reverse to develop an aid to the diagnosis of zygosity. That is, the more closely the hands of twins resemble one another, the more likely it is that the twins are monozygotic. Several methods have been developed to estimate the probability of monozygosity.[1,2]

BIASES AND PITFALLS

It is often assumed that a pattern on one finger has no relation to the patterns on other fingers of the same individual, but in fact there is a tendency for them to be alike more often than expected if they were independent of one another. This has been shown in both normal individuals and those with Down syndrome. Chi square tests on differences in pattern frequency between groups assume independence of observations and are therefore unreliable indicators of statistical significance. Furthermore, dermal patterns are largely inherited, and inclusion of several members of a single sibship will bias the sample. Neglect of these points, use of too small a sample, failure to match control populations for race and sex, and inappropriate use (or nonuse) of statistical tests can lead to much confusion, as has been pointed out for the dermatoglyphics of pa-

Table 17–2. Correlations between Various Pairs of Relatives for Total Finger Ridge-Count

Relationship	Observed	Expected
MZ twins	0.95	1.0
DZ twins	0.49	0.5
Sibs	0.50	0.5
Father-child	0.49	0.5
Mother-child	0.48	0.5
Mother-father	0.05	0.0
Midparent-child	0.66	0.7

tients with congenital heart disease,[7] leuke-mia, and schizophrenia, for example.

Another bias in establishing the dermato-glyphic features of a syndrome may arise if the etiology is unknown. Because syndromes are identified by a characteristic association of fea-tures, each of which may sometimes be ab-sent, cases with relatively few features or lacking the supposedly "cardinal" features may not be accepted as "true" cases of the syn-drome. This creates a bias in assessing the frequency of the various features of the syn-drome. If a dermatoglyphic pattern is a fea-ture of the syndrome or related to it, it is subject to this bias.

DERMATOGLYPHIC FEATURES OF SYNDROMES

Chromosomal Syndromes

Trisomy 21 (Down) Syndrome. The der-matoglyphic features of Down syndrome are summarized in Table 17–3. The most useful is the hallucal tibial arch, which is so rare in normal individuals that its presence in a child suspected of having Down syndrome is strong evidence in favor of the diagnosis.

Long before the chromosomal basis of Down syndrome was established, Cummins demon-strated characteristic differences in dermal configurations between affected and normal children. In 1957, the Canadian geneticist Norma Ford Walker used these differences to estimate the probability that a child has Down syndrome by the dermatoglyphics alone.[11] In

Table 17–3. Dermatoglyphic Features of Trisomy 21 (Down) Syndrome

	Down Syndrome %	Control %	Ratio %
Hallucal tibial arch	72	ca 0.5	144.0
Small distal loop (<21 ridges)	32	11.0	2.0
Single crease on digit 5	17	0.5	34.0
Bilateral t″	82	3.0	27.3
Bilateral simian crease	31	2.0	15.5
10 ulnar loops on fingers	31	7.0	4.6
Radial loop on digit 4 or 5	13	4.0	3.3
Bilateral I_3 pattern	46	26.0	1.8
Thenar pattern	4	11.0	0.4

the log ratio method, which she used, each dermatoglyphic character in the index is as-signed a ratio according to its frequency in patients with Down syndrome as compared to that in normal individuals. By multiplying the individual ratios the probability of Down syn-drome vs. normality is derived. The ratios are expressed as a $\log_{10}$ so that scores for each character may be added. Characters that are more frequent in patients with Down syn-drome will have a positive score and those that are less frequent will have a negative score. The total scores for a group of Down syn-drome subjects and a group of controls will form two frequency distributions that ideally would not overlap, but in practice do so. The distributions may be divided into a non-Down zone, a zone of doubt, and a Down zone. (See Fig. 17–5B.) Individuals not falling into the zone of doubt can be diagnosed as having or not having Down syndrome with a high de-gree of confidence. Figure 17–5 illustrates a simple and effective method, developed by Preus, that allows such identification in over 80% of suspects.[6] A simpler version, using both dermatoglyphic and clinical traits, provides even better discrimination.[9] Such an index can be useful in the stressful intervals between the time the suspicion of Down syndrome arises and the time the karyotype can be read, par-ticularly if there is a question of surgical in-tervention. It may also help in deciding whether a karyotype should be requested when the index of suspicion is low. Other indices are reviewed in Preus' paper.[6]

Other chromosomal syndromes have der-matoglyphic abnormalities, some of which are diagnostically useful. For example, the high frequency of digital arches in trisomy 18 is so characteristic that less than 6 arches, or the presence of 2 or more whorls, is strong evi-dence against the diagnosis.

It is not appropriate to discuss the details here. They are covered in reviews.[10,12]

WHEN ARE THE DERMATOGLYPHICS ABNORMAL?

In practice, when evaluating a patient sus-pected of having a prenatal developmental

I Digital patterns

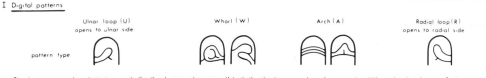

pattern type — Ulnar loop (U) opens to ulnar side · Whorl (W) · Arch (A) · Radial loop (R) opens to radial side

The digits are numbered starting with the thumb as number one. If both thumbs have an ulnar loop, circle UU under digit 1, etc. Circle one score in each of the five digit groups.

Digit 1		Digit 2		Digit 3		Digit 4		Digit 5	
AA,AU,AR,AW	+.19	UU	+.61	UU	+.12	RR,UR	+.89	RR,RU,RW,RA	+1.42
UU	+.12	UW,UA,WA	-.29	WW,WA,WR	-.17	RA	+.65	WW,WA	+.14
UW	-.10	WW	-.73	UW	-.29	RW	+.30	UU,UA	-.02
WW	-.30	AA	-.80	UA,UR	-.61	AU,AW	+.23	UW	-.10
RR,RU,RW	-.48	RU	-.84	AA,RR,AR	-.89	UU	+.07	AA	-.37
		RR,RA,RW	-1.54			UW	-.17		
						WW,AA	-.24		

TOTAL SCORE I =

II Palms and soles   Circle one score in each of the four groups

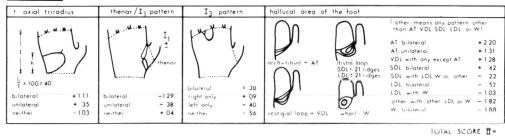

t axial triradius	thenar/I₁ pattern	I₃ pattern	hallucal area of the foot
bilateral +1.11	bilateral -1.29	bilateral +.30	AT bilateral +2.20
unilateral +.35	unilateral -.38	right only +.09	AT unilateral +1.31
neither -1.03	neither +.04	left only -.40	VDL with any except AT +1.28
		neither -.56	SDL bilateral +.42
			SDL with LDL,W or other -.22
			LDL bilateral -.52
			LDL with W -1.03
			other with other,LDL or W -1.82
			W bilateral -1.88

arch–tibial – AT   distal loop SDL < 21 ridges   LDL ≥ 21 ridges
vestigial loop – VDL   whorl – W
(other means any pattern other than AT,VDL,SDL,LDL or W)

$\frac{l_i}{l} \times 100 \pm 40$

TOTAL SCORE II =

III Stigmata   Circle one score in each of the three groups

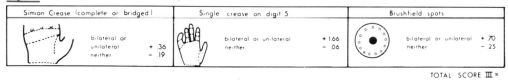

Simian Crease (complete or bridged)	Single crease on digit 5	Brushfield spots
bilateral or unilateral +.36	bilateral or unilateral +1.66	bilateral or unilateral +.70
neither -.19	neither -.06	neither -.25

TOTAL SCORE III =

A   TOTAL LOG INDEX SCORE = I + II + III =

Probability of Down syndrome

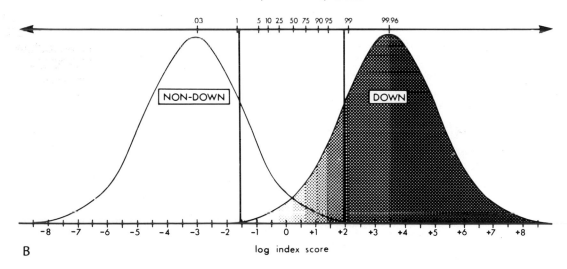

B   log index score

Fig. 17–5. A simple dermatoglyphic screening test for Down syndrome. A, Log index score. B, Probability of Down syndrome. For each area determine the pattern in the patients, and circle the appropriate score in A. For example, if the patient has radial loops on the fourth fingers, or a radial loop and an ulnar loop, circle + .89. Sum the circled scores for a total score, and read off the probability of the patient having Down syndrome from B. From Preus, M.: A diagnostic index for Down syndrome. Clin. Genet. 12:47, 1977.

Table 17–4. A Scoring Method for Quantifying the Degree of Abnormality in Dermatoglyphic Patterns

Area	Pattern	Score*	Area	Pattern	Score*
Digits	8–10W	1	Palm	t″ bilateral	2
	7–10A	6		t″ unilateral	1
	4–6A	2		Thenar 1₁, bi- or unilateral	2
	RL on I (score once only)	25		I₂ Pattern bi- or unilateral	6
	RL on III (score once only)	2		Thenar exit to A-line, bilateral	5
	RL on IV or V (score once only)	3		Thenar exit to A-line, unilateral	2
	10 U	1		Absent, fused, misplaced triradius a, b, or d	6
Hallucal	Tibial A or vestigial distal L	17		Absent triradius	1
	A other than tibial	1		Simian crease, bilateral	6
	Tibial L	1		Simian crease, unilateral	3
	Fibular L	4		Sydney line, bilateral	5
	Distal L with fibular L under it	10		Sydney line, unilateral	2

*The score is the reciprocal of the percentage frequency of the trait in the general population × 10.

disturbance, one may wish to judge how abnormal the dermatoglyphics are, without having any particular syndrome in mind. As a rough guide, developed by Preus, each feature is assigned a score, and the reciprocal of its percentage frequency in the general population is multiplied by 10 to convert it to a whole number. Thus a feature with a population frequency of 5% has a score of 2 (Table 17–4). For a particular patient, the degree of deviation from normality can be estimated from Table 17–5, which is based on 188 normal controls, with a mean score of 2. For example, a score of 8 is higher than those of about 95% of the controls. Thus the score is a rough guide as to how abnormal the dermatoglyphics are.

In a series of children karyotyped because of suspected abnormality, only 25% of those with normal karyotypes had a score of >5, versus 65% of those with abnormal karyotypes.

Table 17–5. Cumulative Distribution of Dermatoglyphic Scores for Normal Controls

Score	% of Controls	% of Controls with This or Lower Score
<1	20	20
1–2	44	64
3–4	14	78
5–6	10	88
7–8	6	94
9–10	3	97
11–	3	100

SUMMARY

Dermatoglyphic patterns are laid down fairly early in embryogeny, and determined largely by the genotype. Abnormal patterns are evidence of developmental disturbance. These can be diagnostically useful, particularly in Down syndrome.

REFERENCES

1. Holt, S.B.: The Genetics of Dermal Ridges. Springfield, Charles C Thomas, 1968.
2. Maynard-Smith, S., and Penrose, L.S.: Monozygotic and dizygotic twin diagnosis. Ann. Hum. Genet. 14:273, 1955.
3. O'Leary, E. et al.: A simple technique for recording and counting sweat pores on the dermal ridges. Clin. Genet. 29:122, 1986.
4. Penrose, L.S., and Loesch, D.: Diagnosis with dermatoglyphic discriminants. J. Ment. Defic. Res. 15:185, 1971.
5. Popich, G.A., and Smith, D.W.: The genesis and significance of digital and palmar hand creases: Preliminary report. J. Pediatr. 77:1017, 1970.
6. Preus, M.: A diagnostic index for Down syndrome. Clin. Genet. 12:47, 1977.
7. Preus, M., Fraser, F.C., and Levy, E.P.: Dermatoglyphics in congenital heart malformations. Hum. Hered. 20:388, 1970.
8. Preus, M., and Fraser, F.C.: Dermatoglyphics and syndromes. Am. J. Dis. Child. 124:933, 1972.
9. Rex, A., and Preus, M.: A diagnostic index for Down syndrome. J. Pediat. 100:903, 1982.
10. Schuman, B., and Alter, M.: Dermatoglyphics in Medical Disorders. New York, Springer Verlag, 1976.
11. Walker, N.F.: The use of dermal configurations in the diagnosis of mongolism. J. Pediatr. 50:19, 1957.
12. Wertelecki, W., and Plato, C., Editors: Dermatoglyphics—fifty years later. Birth Defects: Original Article Series XV(6), New York, Alan R. Liss, 1979.

Chapter *18*

Immunogenetics

A LITTLE INCOMPATIBILITY IS THE SPICE OF LIFE

OGDEN NASH. I DO, I WILL, I HAVE

The following pages may contain more than the average reader cares to know about antibodies and antigens, and less than some special readers need. We hope that the one will be able to grasp the concepts and the other will find adequate references to the literature.[7,10]

DEVELOPMENT OF IMMUNITY

The basis of immunity is the capacity within each individual to recognize what is "self" and what is "nonself."[2] This capacity is vital to survival. When bacteria, or viruses, or cancer cells, appear, the body can recognize the invaders as being "nonself" and try to destroy them before being destroyed by the invading cells. The appearance of lymphoid tissue (in the human at about 12 weeks in utero) coincides with and is directly related to the beginning of immune defense capability.

There is innate immunity (which will not be discussed in any detail here) and there are two major immune systems—the bursa system and the thymus system—which originate and differentiate from the same stem cells. The term bursa is maintained from its historical context reflecting early immunologic research in the chicken and continued in the term B cell, now meaning bone-marrow cell, rather than bursal cell. The term T cell is for thymus-derived cell. There is extensive cooperation between T cells and B cells and with MHC class I and class II molecules (which will be discussed later).

Bursa System. The so-called bursa system is responsible for humoral immunity carried by circulating *antibodies*, small globulin molecules that arise in response to stimulation from an antigen. An *antigen*, then, is a substance (a protein or related material) that stimulates the formation of an antibody. The antibody is able to recognize the antigen and combine specifically with it. The result depends on the nature of the antigen and antibody, but may be, for instance, the destruction of the cell, agglutination of red blood cells, or the release of histamine, with its symptoms so well known to hay-fever sufferers.

To illustrate how the bursa system works in the development of immunity, let us hypothesize that the body is invaded by bacteria, in this example, beta-hemolytic streptococci, group A, type 3. The first cells to try to halt this invasion are white blood cells, macrophages, which engulf the bacteria by a non-immunological process (innate immunity). Following this initial contact, a series of transformations takes place in which antigens (mostly intact proteins) processed by the macrophage are taken up by small lymphocytes that become transformed to lymphoblasts and then to plasma cells. The lymphocytes that become transformed to plasma cells are bone marrow-derived B cells. It is in the plasma cells that the immunoglobulins, which constitute the antibodies, are manufactured.

Each lymphocyte of a subset of B cells is programmed to make one antibody. The complexity of this programming will be discussed in subsequent paragraphs. The antibody is bound on the surface of the cell where it acts as a receptor. When an antigen enters the body, it selects and is selected for by an antibody receptor that fits, and there follows a transformation of the cell that results in clonal proliferation and the production of soluble circulating antibody. For thymus-dependent antigens, T-helper cells are required to produce an immune response.

There are five classes of immunoglobulins designated: IgG, IgM, IgA, IgD, and IgE, separable on the basis of their physicochemical properties. Each is called upon for certain functions. Soluble immunoglobulins are released into the circulation as antibodies, capable of combining specifically with the corresponding antigens. In the case of the invasion of bacteria, the antibodies inactivate the antigens in collaboration with other constituents of the blood, such as complement and polymorphonuclear cells. In the example of the beta-hemolytic streptococcus, group A, several antigens stimulate antibody production, including erythrogenic toxin, streptolysin O, and M substance, a protein fraction of the cell.

How can the body produce antibodies with the wide variety of specificities needed to match the large number of antigens it must respond to? Current thinking is that the genes that specify each antibody are not present in the early embryo, but are formed from component pieces by a shuffling process as the B lymphocytes differentiate and mature. This shuffling, or somatic rearrangement, allows production of an enormous number of cell lines in each of which a unique gene is assembled that in turn leads to a unique antibody.[6] A similar shuffling process takes place for the T-cell receptors to produce the great diversity required for a multitude of immune responses.

Some of the functions of the specific classes of immunoglobulins have been defined. IgG takes part in reactions against a variety of bacteria, viruses, and toxins. In this illustration, it plays the central role in fighting the streptococcal invasion. IgA has the remarkable property of being secreted locally into saliva, intestinal juice, colostrum, and respiratory secretions (where it protects mucous membranes). IgM is prominent in early immune responses to most antigens. It may be adapted to deal with particular antigens such as bacterial cells, activate complement, and provoke immune lysis as in the case of skin graft rejection. IgM and IgG antibodies are the immunoglobulins that participate in the classic activities of antibodies, such as agglutination, hemolysis, precipitation, and complement fixation.

IgE is involved in allergic diseases, and IgD appears to interact with IgM as the predominating immunoglobulins on the surface of the B cell involved in lymphocyte activation and suppression.

Because our clinical example presents a first exposure to a certain type of streptococcus, the patient will become clinically ill while developing antibodies to fight the infection. The response to the streptolysin O antigen is a rising antistreptolysin O (ASO) titer, which assists in the diagnosis of the streptococcal infection. The development of antibodies against the M substance confers a permanent immunity against the specific type-3, group-A, beta-hemolytic streptococcus.

Now what would happen should the patient be exposed to another invasion of type-3 group-A streptococci? The body would recognize this group of foreign proteins as a previous invader, and there would be a prompt and vigorous response that would eradicate the invader without allowing it a sufficient foothold to produce clinical illness. The patient is said to be "immune," and this is a manifestation

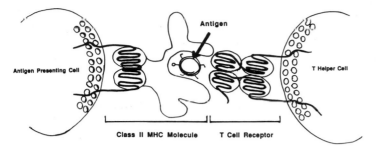

Fig. 18–1. The trimolecular complex of MHC molecule, antigen, and T-cell receptor involved in the induction of a normal or autoimmune response. Modified and redrawn from Sinha, A. A., Lopez, M. T., and McDevitt, H. O.: Autoimmune diseases: The failure of self-tolerance. Science 248:1380, 1990.

of "immunological memory." A small lymphocyte originating from the marrow (a B cell) serves as the "memory cell." On antigenic stimulation, "memory" is rapidly translated into the activity of antibody production. The memory cell immediately recognizes the M substance of the type 3 organism.

The defense mounted against the invasion of streptococci, in our example, may not always result in an unqualified victory. The immune response may turn against some patients and produce damage. Such is the case with rheumatic fever and glomerulonephritis, two examples of autoimmune disease.

Thymus System. The second system of immunity, the thymus system, is mediated by entire cells, lymphocytes. It is important in organ transplantation and is a necessary defense against intracellular invaders—a major factor in the body's natural defense against cancer, as well as against many viral, bacterial, fungal, and protozoal diseases. The sequence of events following the introduction of foreign cells such as a kidney allograft is similar to that found in the invasion of bacteria discussed earlier. The antigens present in the cells of the kidney allograft are detected as being "nonself" by small thymus-dependent lymphocytes, probably after the antigens have been processed by the macrophages. These lymphocytes are now sensitized. They are transformed to lymphoblasts, which divide into many new lymphocytes, each one sensitized to the grafted kidney and the foreign kidney cells. Unlike humoral antibodies, which may circulate freely in the blood, the functional activity in cellular immunity remains fixed to lymphocytes as a T-cell receptor (TCR), which is analogous to the membrane-bound antibody

on the surface of the B cell. The T cell recognizes foreign antigens only when they are complexed with MHC molecules as shown in Figure 18–1. What happens next is not precisely understood, but the sensitized lymphocytes return to the kidney allograft, which has been recognized as "nonself," and initiate a rejection of the graft, which includes enlisting the aid of macrophages. A second graft would result in a much more rapid and strenuous rejection—that is, there is immunologic memory. The memory cells are small lymphocytes, derived from the thymus (T cells), that may live in the circulation for 10 years.

Antigen Processing. How cells break up viruses and other intracellular invaders into fragments suitable for presentation to the immune system has been commanding a lot of recent attention.[5] The primary method is for the cell to reduce the viral protein into peptide fragments utilizing enzymes from the complex called the low molecular mass polypeptide. The peptides are carried by means of specialized transporter proteins into the endoplasmic reticulum (ER) of the cell, where they bind to MHC class I proteins and are then conveyed to the cell surface, where this complex of MHC and polypeptide is inserted into the cell membrane in such a way that it may be recognized by receptors on immune cells. A second pathway has been proposed that does not require transporter proteins for the peptide to enter the ER and is associated with the MHC class I molecule HLA.A21.[4]

STRUCTURE AND FUNCTION OF IMMUNOGLOBULINS

One of the great mysteries that is now yielding to the techniques of molecular biology is how the genes of the antibody-producing cells manage to achieve the enormous diversity necessary for them to produce a specific antibody for any antigen they may meet. The details are voluminous and complex and their elucidation led to the award of the 1987 Nobel Prize to Tonegawa.[14] We hope that the following guide will provide the basic concepts.[6,8,9]

The basic structure of the antibody (immunoglobulin) molecule is shown in Figure 18–2. It consists essentially of two heavy chains, in a "Y" formation, with two light chains bound to the arms of the Y. The stem of the Y and the proximal part of the two arms have a constant (C) structure. The outer halves of the four chains in the two arms of the Y are variable (V), and form a sort of basket, with the inside surface of the basket having a surface that conforms to the shape of a particular antigen. This is the antigen-binding site, and the variability in the four variable regions provides the vast number of possible surfaces that ensures that there will be at least one cell that makes an antibody that fits a particular antigen.

How is the variability of the variable region achieved? A current concept is that in the embryonic cell the genetic material for the variable region exists in several pieces and that a process of shuffling and splicing (somatic rearrangement) brings them together as an active gene. For the light chains, there are perhaps 150 copies of the gene for the variable

region, all slightly different, separated by a long stretch of noncoding DNA from J regions (corresponding to the part of the globulin connecting the V and C regions), each of which is linked by an intervening sequence, to a C gene. Recombination, and deletion of the extra V, J, and noncoding sequences, brings one V region, one J region, and a C gene together to form an active gene for a light chain. Transcription and splicing out of the intervening sequences leaves a messenger RNA ready for translation into the light chain, which will then be incorporated into an immunoglobulin molecule. Possible combination of one out of 150 V regions and one of 6 J regions allows for 900 possible different genes for the variable region. Variability in the V-J joining sites increases the number of V/J combinations another tenfold.

The heavy chain adds further variability. There are as many as 80 heavy-chain V genes, 6 J genes, and a D region between the V and C segments with about 50 members, giving about 24,000 possible combinations, So a total of perhaps 300 separate genetic segments in the embryonic DNA can generate billions of possible antibody specificities.

When an antigen (of bacterial origin, for example) is first presented to the body, it binds to the prelymphocyte that carries on its surface the antibody that has the site that fits that antigen, and that cell is stimulated to proliferate and form a clone of antibody-producing B lymphocytes, as predicted in the Burnet-Jerne *clonal selection* hypothesis. The body is now immunized.

What type of immunoglobulin will be produced is dictated by the heavy-chain constant region. Downstream from the V, D, and J sequences are the genes for the various heavy chains—mu for IgM, gamma for IgG and so on. By a similar recombination process, the assembled variable chain gene is joined to a delta, mu, gamma, epsilon or alpha sequence, and the corresponding D, M, G, E, or A immunoglobulin will be produced and remain on the cell surface. If the sequence is gamma, IgG will be produced and released into the circulation. An epsilon sequence will result in IgE, which will bind to a mast cell and react

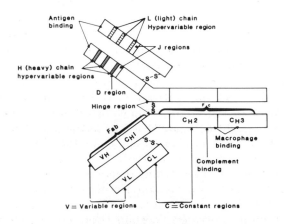

Fig. 18–2.   Antibody molecule. See text.

with its specific antigen there to trigger the release of histamine from the mast cell—and so on.

Immunoglobulins as Genetic Markers. Some of what we know about the genetic control of immunoglobulins comes from studies of markers inherited as antigenic determinants on the immunoglobulin molecules. Four sets of antigenic markers are presently recognized. Three of these, the Gm, Am and Mm systems, are closely linked; and one, the Km (formerly Inv), is independently inherited. The Gm marker is on the heavy chain of IgG, the Mm on IgM, and Am on IgA. Km is a marker on kappa-type light chains. Subclass specificities are further designated as G1m(1), G3m(14), Km(1) and so on. Gm haplotypes have been studied extensively in populations and have proved useful in the investigation of genetic drift and migration.

HLA and MHC[1]

HLA (human leukocyte antigen) is the international designation for the region constituting the major histocompatibility complex (MHC) in a man. The region is located on the short arm of chromosome 6 and consists of an increasing number of recognized loci that play a role in immunologic response. These loci are generally grouped into three classes: classes I and II contain the highly polymorphic HLA genes (Fig. 18–3). Class I and class II molecules are membrane-bound heterodimers and their genes are structurally related to immunoglobulin and the T-cell receptor genes.

The loci in class I are responsible for the expression of antigens on T cells (thymus-dependent lymphocytes) and the loci in class II are expressed predominantly on B cells. Class III loci code for certain components of complement, tumor necrosis factor (TNF), and some immunologically unrelated genes, such as 21-OH (21 hydroxylase—see adrenogenital syndrome). The important T-cell loci are called HLA-A, HLA-B, and HLA-C, and the B-cell loci of major interest are HLA-DR, HLA-DQ, and HLA-DP, which have been subdivided from the original D locus (now called Dw and tested for by mixed leukocyte culture rather than by the standard serologic method). Various analyses have shown more complexity of the D loci (DZ, DO, DX) than we shall discuss. The terminology is constantly changing, to the frustration of students and teachers who are not immunogeneticists. For this volume, we shall make no effort to tabulate the HLA antigens because this information was outdated even before the print was dry on several past editions. As we mentioned earlier, the T lymphocytes and their subsets (helper, cytotoxic, and suppressor) are primarily involved in cellular immunity, and the B lymphocytes in the production of circulating antibody (after they differentiate into plasma cells). The HLA-A, B, and C antigens are not present just on the surfaces of T lymphocytes, but on essentially all nucleated cells, whereas the antigens specified by the D loci are mainly confined to B cells and macrophages.

The term *haplotype* is used to refer to the genes on *one* chromosome. Thus a haplotype of the major histocompatibility complex would have an antigen or determinant from each of the loci in Figure 18–3. An example of a haplotype detectable by the usual serologic method would be A1, B8, Cw1, DR3. A specificity that has a "w" (for workshop) in it is still somewhat provisional, and the serologic diagnosis is less firm. The loci are so polymorphic that most people have eight specificities (four on each haplotype). If there is only one specificity detected at a locus, it is either homozygous, or carries an antigen that is not detectable by present methods. Another practical point is that in attempting to define the phenotype of a given patient, it is still not uncommon to have strong reactions for A and B specificities, but weaker findings for antigens at the C and DR loci. Cross reactions are common between certain defined antigen groups.

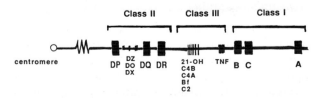

Fig. 18–3.   Relationship of MHC loci on chromosome 6.

The HLA loci show linkage disequilibrium (Chapter 5), both between themselves and with other loci. For example, if the frequency of the A allele is 0.17 and of B8 is 0.11, at equilibrium the frequency of A1B8 should be 0.17 × 0.11 = 1.9%. In fact, the frequency varies from 13 to 40% in various populations. That is, the two alleles show association. Possibly the B8 mutation originated in such a relation to A2 that equilibrium has not been reached, or this particular combination carries some selective advantage. This interpretation is supported by the fact that both the individual loci and associations of loci vary widely among different populations.

HISTOCOMPATIBILITY—THE GENETIC BASIS OF TRANSPLANTATION[2,6]

That every human being differs genetically from every other human being (except for monozygotic twins) does not require elaboration. The fact that "nonself" is open to immunologic attack whether it is a virus, bacterium, cancer cell, or transplanted organ would appear to present a formidable barrier to transplantation. How, then, can one even consider transplanting an organ, which cannot avoid being genetically dissimilar from its recipient? Fortunately, of all the genetic differences between the donor and recipient, only certain of them play significant roles in whether a transplanted organ will be accepted as "self" or rejected as "nonself." The histocompatibility antigens, as discussed in the previous section, and the ABO blood groups are of major importance.

Great progress has been made in elucidating the genetic basis of the histocompatibility (HLA) antigens. The situation is complicated because of the large number of histocompatibility antigens. There are several thousand possible phenotypes, which is why it is unlikely that one will find an unrelated donor who is entirely histocompatible with a would-be recipient.

Mixed Leukocyte Culture

Mixed leukocyte culture (MLC) or mixed lymphocyte reaction (MLR) is the original test for histocompatibility at the HLA-D locus. Before the 1975 workshop it was called the MLC locus. The test consists of culturing leukocytes from donor and recipient together. If stimulation occurs, the cells are antigenically different. The basis of the test is that lymphocytes exposed to materials that are antigenically incompatible (including other lymphocytes) undergo a lymphoblastic transformation, which can be observed under the microscope. This test may be used whenever there is a living donor and at least one week available to complete the study, but cannot be applied to cadaver donors for heart and liver transplants because there are only a few hours to prepare for the procedure. This MLC test is also obviously reserved for situations in which there is a paired organ, specifically kidney. An ideal living donor would be an identical twin, but few candidates for transplantation are lucky enough to have one available. The next best alternative would be a sib, in which the chance of being histocompatible is 1 in 4. (This is straightforward mendelian genetics. Think of parental haplotypes and the probability that two sibs would receive identical haplotypes from their parents.)

Perhaps the clearest way to illustrate the features of histocompatibility in the human is to begin with a clinical situation. A patient has irreparable brain injury and is about to die in the emergency room of a hospital that has an active transplantation service. The relatives are approached about possible donation of the patient's organs to the transplantation service at his death. They agree. What steps now follow to prepare for organ transplantations and reduce the risk of incompatibility and rejection? They include lymphocyte crossmatch, histocompatibility antigen matching, and ABO incompatibility testing.

ABO Incompatibility

ABO incompatibility is a strong barrier to transplantation, so the donor's blood group must be compared with the blood groups of potential recipients in the same way that blood groups are matched for transfusion (see Chapter 19). If the donor is type A, the only suit-

Table 18–1. Terminology of Tissue Transplantation

Terminology	Adjective	Definition	Result
Autograft	Autologous	Graft in which donor and recipient are the same individual	Acceptance
Isograft	Isogeneic	Graft between individuals with identical histocompatibility antigens (e.g., MZ twins)	Acceptance
Allograft	Allogeneic	Graft between genetically dissimilar members of same species (e.g., man to man)	Rejection
Xenograft	Xenogeneic	Graft between species (e.g., ape to man)	Rejection

able recipients would be type A or AB. However, if the donor is type O, he may be considered a universal donor—that is, he would be compatible in this first step of matching with recipients of groups O, A, B, and AB.

Lymphocyte Cross-match

The lymphocytes of the donor are presumed to reflect the antigen content of the donor organs. These donor lymphocytes are cross-matched with the blood serum of the recipient in an effort to detect in the recipient the presence of antibodies already formed against the donor antigens. Such preformed antibodies could be responsible for hyperacute rejection of the donor organ. This second step in deciding whether to proceed with transplantation cannot, of course, be taken until some potential recipients are selected for cross-matching on the basis of the information obtained in step 1.

Histocompatibility Antigen Matching

The specific antigens possessed by the donor are identified by serologic means, using the lymphocytes as the source of antigen. Although potent antirejection drugs are now available, survival of cadaveric renal allografts is still best in those having the closest HLA match between donor and recipient[12]—particularly at the DR locus. In the case of cadaveric donors, HLA matching makes sense clinically as an index of genetic similarity. If one is dealing with a living donor of a paired organ and there is a favorable MLC reaction, but an HLA antigen difference with the recipient, the MLC finding would take precedence.

ORGAN TRANSPLANTATION

The central problem in transplantation is how to violate a basic biological law—the rejection of "nonself"—and get away with it. As we pointed out in the previous section, grafts between identical twins and grafts between other individuals completely compatible in ABO and histocompatibility specificities are not recognized as "nonself." However, in the clinical setting, most candidates for transplantation do not have an identical twin available, or even a compatible sib (a 1 in 4 chance), and the limitations in present techniques of histocompatibility matching and donor availability do not permit ideal matching.

A brief historic review can mention only that transplantation was described in Greek mythology and early Christian legends. Tagliacozzi, in the 16th century, gained a reputation for being able to reconstruct noses (lost in duels and to syphilis). He appreciated (empirically?) that one could not transplant the nose from one person to another and thus devised the operation, used to this day, of utilizing a flap from the patient's own upper arm (autograft). The terminology of transplantation is provided in Table 18–1.

Several workers have been responsible for the accelerated advancement in knowledge in transplantation in our own century, among them Jensen, Carrel, Murphy, and Medawar. The series of classic experiments by Medawar in the 1940s provided the basis for contemporary transplantation research. Certain principles have emerged from the work of Medawar and other investigators:

1. Allograft immunity is cell-mediated (although humoral mechanisms play a role).
2. Grafts between genetically dissimilar individuals may first appear to be ac-

cepted, but are then rejected within a period of about 10 days, depending on the strength of the genetic difference (first-set rejection). If another transplant from the same donor (or donor of the same genotype) is attempted, rejection is accelerated (second-set rejection). The process may require only 3 to 6 days. The recipient has been sensitized (has immunologic memory) and quickly attacks the graft.

3. The foreign cells may be accepted as "self," especially in the immunologically immature (or deficient) individual, rather than rejected as "nonself." Methods, such as induction of tolerance, that take advantage of this weakness in the immunologic armor may provide the answer to long-term survival of allografts without resorting to drastic immunosuppression.

Rejection

The mechanism of rejection has been described in the section on development of immunity. Certainly, the cell-mediated immunity of the thymus system plays the major role. Small lymphocytes are transformed to lymphoblasts after detecting the foreign antigen, and they return to the graft as "sensitized" cells capable of participating in the graft rejection. Figure 18–4 illustrates rejection of a skin allograft between genetically dissimilar strains of mice, acceptance of an isograft between mice of the same genetic constitution, and temporary acceptance (overriding of rejection) of an allograft between genetically dissimilar mice under the influence of immunosuppressive medications.

This points up the problem faced by the physician managing a patient with an organ transplant. Because the patient is at risk from rejection, his immunologic mechanisms against "nonself" must be suppressed. But immunosuppression is not yet sufficiently specific, and thus the patient's immune system is suppressed not only with respect to the transplant, but also with respect to bacterial and

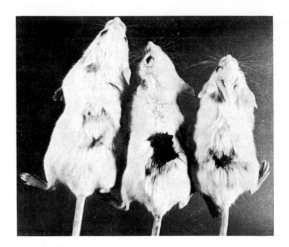

Fig. 18–4 From left to right: A/J mouse receiving transplant of A/J skin without rejection; A/J mouse receiving C57 skin without early rejection because of cyclophosphamide immunosuppression; A/J mouse without immunosuppression showing active rejection of C57 skin.

viral infections and cancer. He walks a tightrope between rejection and infection.

It has already been pointed out that, if there were complete histocompatibility, as in identical twins, immunosuppressants would be unnecessary. Because this situation rarely occurs, the need is for techniques that will define more accurately the histocompatibility of donor and recipient. Serologic tests are the most popular and are becoming more definitive. Mixed lymphocyte cultures are too time-consuming (1 week) to be applicable to cadaver donors when only hours are available—until there is an important advance in long-term organ preservation.

A recent advance that has added substantially to survival of grafts is the anti-rejection drug, cyclosporine. But what is needed to make organ transplantation an unqualified therapeutic success is an authentic breakthrough in immunology. The need is for immunologic specificity. The recipient should not have his ability to fight infection and cancer disastrously compromised. The ideal would be to leave the recipient with only one immunologic blind spot, that is, the inability to recognize the transplanted organ as being "nonself." It is true that 5-year survivors of kidney transplants are common. However, kidney recipients have advantages over heart recipients in that there is more time to get a good tissue match (including the opportunity to use relatives as donors) and the recipient is initially immunosuppressed by his uremic condition. Although 1-year survival in heart transplantation is now approaching 80%, if heart transplantation is ever to become a genuine therapeutic alternative able to meet the needs of the great excess of potential recipients, ways to utilize poor histocompatibility matches, specifically xenografts, would be necessary.

Graft verses Host (GVH)

Not only does the recipient recognize the transplant as being "nonself," but if the donor tissue is immunologically competent, e.g., lymphoid tissue, the transplant may recognize the recipient as being "nonself" and attempt to attack it. This is the problem in using incompatible bone marrow transplants to treat patients with immune deficiencies or leukemia. If a transplant of blood-forming tissue is introduced into a subject following total-body irradiation and destruction of host immunity, the transplanted incompatible immune-competent cells raise antibodies against the host leading to wasting and death. Similarly, a rapidly fatal graft-versus-host reaction may follow a blood transfusion that contains incompatible immune-competent lymphocytes in patients, such as those with Swiss-type agammaglobulinemia, who have no immunologic defense. This can be avoided by irradiating the blood first, to kill the lymphocytes.

SELECTED DISEASES IMPORTANT IN IMMUNOGENETICS

Infectious disease is the classic métier for immunology. Later came the so-called autoimmune and immune deficiency diseases. We began the chapter with an example of a streptococcal infection and developed the problem to the point where the body, in defending itself against the bacterial invasion, could also, in a minority of cases, begin to attack itself with the weapons being used on the streptococcus—thus producing rheumatic fever. It is also possible that there is an immune basis

for other cardiovascular diseases, and certainly the growing awareness of the importance of immunity in cancer has opened an enormously productive area for investigation. This is why the present section is titled "Selected Diseases . . ."

Diseases of Immune Deficiency

Table 18–2 lists a selection of diseases which may be categorized as immune deficiencies. The terminology is according to a proposal by a committee of the World Health Organization. The classification highlights the possible types of deficiency: antibody (B cell); cellular (T cell); combined (B and T cells); phagocytic dysfunction; and complement abnormalities. Most of these disorders are of genetic interest and some will be discussed in other chapters.

Agammaglobulinemia (Bruton Disease, Hypogammaglobulinemia)

Agammaglobulinemia, the commonest of the immune deficiency diseases, involves a defect in immunoglobulin synthesis or in B-lymphocyte differentiation.

Diagnostic Features and Clinical Course. A history of frequently recurring severe bacterial infections, such as pneumonia and sepsis in a male child, usually between 3 to 6 months of age, is the initial basis for entertaining the diagnosis. A family history of other males dying of overwhelming infection may

Table 18–2. Diseases of Immune Deficiency

Disease	Deficiency	Inheritance
Congenital hypogammaglobulinemia (Bruton Disease)[4]	B cell	X-R
Immunodeficiency with hyper IgM	B cell	X-R
DiGeorge syndrome	T cell	?
Agammaglobulinemia	B and T cells	X-R
Agammaglobulinemia, Swiss	B and T cells	R
Ataxia-telangiectasia	B and T cells	R
Wiskott-Aldrich syndrome	B and T cells	X-R
Granulomatous disease	Phagocytes	X-R and R
Chediak-Higashi syndrome	Phagocytes	R
Job syndrome	Phagocytes	R
C1r and C1s	Complement	R
C2 deficiency	Complement	R
C5 dysfunction	Complement	?

also be obtained. Immunoelectrophoresis and quantitative immunoglobulin determinations reveal absence or virtual absence of IgG and IgM and absence of IgA. Plasma cells are rarely found, but lymphocytes are present in low titer. Tonsils are unusually small, and adenoids are not visible by lateral pharyngeal radiographs. Patients have adequate cellular immunity and ability to reject allografts. There is no excessive vulnerability to viral and fungal infections. Patients recognized early and treated promptly with gamma globulin and chemotherapy may do well during childhood. Complications of adolescence and early life include a dermatomyositis-like syndrome of arthritis, contractures, and brawny edema that ends fatally. The gene locus is Xq21.3-q22.

Treatment. Gamma globulin is administered regularly in monthly maintenance therapy after the initial loading dose to raise the IgG level to about 200 mg/mL. Vigorous specific antimicrobial therapy is given for individual bacterial infections.

Progressive sinopulmonary disease remains a problem, but with good medical attention the prognosis is fair, and survivors are now reaching adulthood.

Agammaglobulinemia, Swiss Type

The Swiss type of severe combined agammaglobulinemia is genetically heterogeneous. A more common X-linked type and at least one autosomal recessive form exist. There is no large difference in their clinical courses.

Diagnostic Features and Clinical Course. In agammaglobulinemia, both humoral and cellular immunity are deficient. Patients do not have tonsils or adenoids and have a vestigial or dysplastic thymus. Viral and fungal infections, as well as the bacterial infections encountered in Bruton disease, threaten the life of the patient. The capacity to reject allografts is lost. Patients are also at risk from fatal graft-versus-host reactions (GVH) from blood transfusions that include lymphocytes. A smallpox vaccination may result in a fatal progressive vaccinia. Laboratory studies reveal an absence or marked decrease in IgG,

IgM, and IgA. There is a gross deficiency in lymphocytes and plasma cells.

This disease has been invariably fatal. Death usually occurs before a child is 1 year of age in the autosomal recessive form, and within the first 2 years in the X-linked recessive patients. Persistent infections of the lungs, chronic diarrhea, wasting, and runting precede a fatal infection.

Treatment. Bone marrow transplantation from carefully matched, histocompatible, related donors has been therapeutically effective in providing the patient with immune competence without producing a fatal GVH reaction.

Differential Diagnosis. The differentiating features of this disorder from some of the other immunologic deficiency states are presented in Table 18–2.

Complement and Complement Deficiency

The participation of complement in antigen-antibody reactions has been recognized for a long time, but the complexity of its role and the existence of diseases resulting from its deficiency have been recognized only recently.

The complement system comprises 20 proteins present in an inactive form in body fluids that serve as effectors of immunologically induced inflammation. Its complexity precludes detailed description here. In summary, the binding of C1 to antibody triggers an enzyme cascade culminating in the cleavage and fixation of C3 on the receptors of phagocytic cells, erythrocytes, platelets and lymphocytes. The activated proteins participate in a series of proteolytic reactions leading to the changes in vascular permeability, attraction of leukocytes, enhancement of phagocytosis, and damage to cell membranes that occur in the inflammatory process.

There are over 25 inherited disorders of components of the complement system, some leading to immunologic defects, some to autoimmune disorders, and one to hereditary angioneurotic edema. This is a dominant disease in which patients, who are deficient in C1 inhibitor, have episodes of edematous swelling in various parts of the body. If it involves the larynx, it may be fatal.

Genetic polymorphisms exist at many complement loci, and have greatly aided mapping. Three components map within the class III region of the MHC (see Fig. 18–3).

The HLA System and Disease

The HLA system is by far our most polymorphic set of loci, and this makes it particularly suitable for linkage studies, since virtually everyone is heterozygous for at least some alleles in this region. Perhaps this is why so many genetic conditions have shown linkage or some relationship to HLA. Most, but not all, of these diseases have an immune component (see below). There is an apparent increase in risk of recurrent spontaneous abortion to offspring if both parents share more than one HLA antigen. This problem was first considered to be immunologic, but was later attributed to a genetic mechanism.[3]

Table 18–3 displays only a partial list of diseases in which a high relative risk for susceptibility has been shown to be associated with particular antigens or haplotypes. The list grows with almost every new issue of *The New England Journal of Medicine*.

A comprehensive review of this subject cannot be accommodated in a general genetics textbook of manageable size, but references are provided for those who wish to pursue the subject further.[1,7]

Table 18–3. HLA and Selected Disease Associations

Disease	HLA Type
Ankylosing spondylitis	B27
Reiter disease	B27
Juvenile rheumatoid arthritis	B27
Graves disease (hyperthyroidism)	DR3
	B8
Multiple sclerosis	DR2
Juvenile diabetes (susceptibility)	DR3
	DR4
Juvenile diabetes (protection)	DR2
Celiac disease	DR3
Systemic lupus erythematosus	DR2
	DR3

Autoimmune Diseases

The concept of what constitutes an autoimmune problem has expanded considerably during the past decade from diseases of connective tissue to encompass a wide variety of disorders involving almost every organ or system, even extending to the biologic process of aging. Approximately 40 such diseases are now in this category, and they afflict about 6% of the population.

We started the chapter with a discussion of a bacterial invasion of streptococci, and it seems appropriate to end with the possible results of such an invasion. Most patients who have untreated streptococcal infections eventually raise successful immune responses and recover without sequelae. However, a small proportion of those who recover experience distressing to devastating complications, such as glomerulonephritis (an inflammatory kidney disease) and rheumatic fever.

To continue with rheumatic fever as our model, there has been some evidence that the group A beta-hemolytic streptococcus shares a common antigen (cross-reactive antigen) with human heart muscle. The blood of patients with acute rheumatic fever can be demonstrated to contain antibodies to this cross-reactive antigen. One can thus speculate that in raising antibodies to fight a streptococcal infection, the patient may also raise antibodies capable of attacking the heart. There are objections to this model, which will not be enumerated here, but whatever the mechanism, there is likely to be a combination of susceptible HLA and non-HLA genes underlying the autoimmune reaction.

Autoimmunity has been visualized as a failure to discriminate between "self" and "nonself" antigens—a failure to tolerate "self." Consider the trimolecular complex (Fig. 18–1) formed by MHC molecules, antigen, and T-cell receptors as the basis for both a normal and an autoimmune response.[11] A specialized cell with an MHC molecule presents an antigen to a T cell for recognition as "self" or "nonself." Viruses appear to play an important role in the pathogenesis of autoimmunity. Chronic infections, especially with "slow virus," show features of autoimmunity. Juvenile diabetes frequently follows a viral infection. "Virogenes," in which certain viruses become integrated into the genome, may produce antigens that call forth an antibody response with deposition of immune complexes in blood vessels and along glomerular basement membranes. And, of course, antibodies can be raised against hybrid molecules, in which a hapten that is not itself immunogenic can become conjugated with protein to elicit an immune response. The possibilities in this area of research seem to be almost endless.

Monoclonal Antibodies[13]

Our discussion of immunogenetics would be incomplete without mention of monoclonal antibodies, a technologic breakthrough that has dramatically advanced knowledge of antibody structure and function, provided sensitive probes for use in many areas of research, and enhanced the production of diagnostic and therapeutic weapons.

Antibodies have been used for diagnosis, treatment and prevention of diseases for a long time and, more recently, to label molecules for tracing in biologic research. One problem has been making antibodies with unique specificity in sufficient quantities. This is the need that monoclonal antibodies have fulfilled.

The key was the myeloma, a tumor of the antibody-producing white cells that produces antibody in large quantities. Each tumor seems to originate from a single cell; it makes only one antibody. How can it be persuaded to make a particular antibody of choice? Cells from a mouse myeloma are fused to normal mouse spleen cells to form a hybridoma. The spleen-donor mouse has previously been immunized against the antigen for which an antibody is required. Some of the spleen cells will make the antibody of choice, but spleen cells will not persist indefinitely in culture. Fusion with a myeloma cell confers immortality on the spleen cell, and some of the resulting hybridomas will make the required, and only the required, antibody. These can be selected and implanted in mice, where they grow and produce monoclonal antibody in large quantities.

Such antibodies have been of great use, for example, to dissect the structure of the immunoglobulins themselves and the recombination process that provides their diversity, to improve the specificity of serologic agents for diagnosis and immunization, to label molecules for tracing in biologic experiments, and to bring radioactive or cytotoxic agents to the tumors they are to attack.

SUMMARY

Immunity develops from a basic stem cell through two systems: (1) the so-called bursa system ("B cells"), which is bone-marrow derived and is responsible for the production of circulating antibodies (immunoglobulins) to combat bacterial and viral infections, toxins and some particulate antigens; (2) the thymus system ("T cells"), which is responsible for cellular immunity, plays a major role in transplantation, and represents a factor in the natural defense against bacterial, viral, fungal, and protozoal diseases, and cancer.

A knowledge of the structure of antibody is necessary in order to appreciate function and diversity. Five classes of immunoglobulins are produced in B cells: IgG, IgM, IgA, IgD, and IgE. These classes are defined by antigenic differences in the C regions of H chains. Antigen binding takes place in the V region.

Human leukocyte antigen (HLA) is the designation for the region in the major histocompatibility complex (MHC) in man, located on chromosome 6, responsible for cellular (T-cell) and humoral (B-cell) immunity. Components of complement and other markers have also been placed in the MHC. HLA loci have been defined by a large and growing number of alleles, making this the most polymorphic system in man. A large number of associations between HLA specificities and disease entities have been discovered. Indeed, disease states having an immune component are becoming increasingly important in medicine—from autoimmune disease to immune deficiency disorders.

REFERENCES

1. Bell, J.I., Todd, J.A., and McDevitt, H.O.: The molecular basis of HLA-disease association. Adv. Hum Genet. 18:1, 1989.
2. Burnet, F.M.: Immunological recognition of self. Science 133:137, 1961.
3. Gill, T.J.: Invited editorial: Influence of MHC and MHC-linked genes on reproduction. Am. J. Hum. Genet. 50:1, 1992.
4. Henderson, R.A., et al.: HLA-A2.1—Associated peptides from a mutant cell line: A second pathway of antigen presentation. Science 255:1264, 1992.
5. Hoffman, M.: Antigen processing: a new pathway discovered. Science 255:1214, 1992.
6. Leder, P.: The genetics of antibody diversity. Sci. Amer. 246:102, 1982.
7. Litwin, S.D. (ed): Human Immunogenetics: Basic Principles and Clinical Relevance. New York, Marcel Dekker, 1989.
8. Milstein, C.: From antibody structure to immunological diversification of immune response. Science 231:1261, 1986.
9. Nossal, G.J.V.: Current concepts: Immunology: The basic components of the immune system. N. Engl. J. Med. 316:1320, 1987.
10. Roitt, I.M.: Essential Immunology, 7th ed. Oxford, Blackwell, 1989.
11. Sinha, A.A., Lopez, M.T., and McDevitt, H.O.: Autoimmune diseases: The failure of self-tolerance. Science 248:1380, 1990.
12. Takemoto, S., et al.: Survival of nationally shared, HLA kidney transplants from cadaveric donors. N. Engl. J. Med. 327:834, 1992.
13. Teillaud, J-L., et al.: Monoclonal antibodies reveal the structural basis of antibody diversity. Science 222:721, 1983.
14. Tonegawa, S.: Somatic generation of antibody diversity. Nature 302:575, 1983.

Chapter 19

Blood Groups and Serum Proteins

ART IN THE BLOOD IS LIABLE TO TAKE THE STRANGEST FORMS.

DR. A. CONAN DOYLE

The fact that people could be classified into groups by the antigens on their red blood cells was first demonstrated by Karl Landsteiner, a German physician, who found that the red blood cells from some people would clump when put in the serum of some, but not all, other people. This led to the discovery of the ABO blood group system, which was the first genetic polymorphism. It also made blood transfusion practical, and the immense benefits to humanity won Landsteiner the Nobel prize 30 years later.

Landsteiner's discovery depended on the fact that there were naturally occurring antibodies to the A and B antigens in the serum. It was another 27 years before the next blood group system (MN) was discovered, when Landsteiner (by then in New York) and his assistant, P. Levine, produced an antibody by immunizing rabbits, and found that it clumped the cells of some people and not of others. By this technique, many other blood group systems have now been identified.[4]

Besides their practical applications in the fields of blood transfusion and forensic medi-

cine (e.g., disputed paternity suits), the blood groups have played an important role in the development of basic genetics. They were used to demonstrate the validity of the Hardy-Weinberg law, and their gene frequencies have been useful in anthropologic genetics—for example, in elucidating the histories of various racial groups. The blood groups have also been useful genetic markers in linkage and disease-association studies.[3]

The invention of starch gel electrophoresis, in 1955, made it possible to separate proteins with a single amino acid difference, provided the substituted amino acid had a different charge. By this technique, many proteins were found to have variants, polymorphisms, that segregated as mendelian traits and provided the same sort of genetic information as the blood groups.[2]

The advantages for genetic investigation offered by blood groups and serum proteins stem from the fact that they are relatively direct expressions of gene action and therefore fall into sharply defined groups with simple inheritance. Codominance is the rule (making heterozygotes as readily detectable as homozygotes), although there are notable exceptions, including the ABO and I systems.

The following sections, because they discuss the various blood groups in succession, may give the impression of being a catalogue, providing more information about blood groups than the average reader cares to know. But some readers will want to have the information, and we hope the average reader can read selectively, skipping lightly over the detail, and noting where the examples illustrate important principles.

ABO BLOOD GROUPS[5]

Landsteiner found that when the red blood cells of certain individuals were mixed with the serum from certain others, the cells became attracted to one another and formed clumps—*agglutination*. This was shown to occur when the serum contained antibody specific to an antigen on the surface of the red cell. By this method, people could be separated into four phenotypes, as illustrated in Table 19–1.

It was soon demonstrated that these antigenic differences showed mendelian inheritance, antigens A and B and lack of either antigen (O) being the expression of three alleles, A, B, and O. Note that a person's serum contains antibodies to whatever antigens are not present on his or her red cells. This is an exception to the rule; antibodies for other blood group systems do not occur unless the person is sensitized by an injection of "foreign" red cells.

Table 19–1. ABO Blood Groups and Frequency in a Representative English Population

Genotype	Pheno-type	Fre-quency %	Red Cell Antigen	Serum Anti-body
AA AO	A	0.42	A	anti-B
BB BO	B	0.09	B	anti-A
AB	AB	0.03	AB	none
OO	O	0.46	none	anti-A, anti-B

The reciprocal relationship between antigen and antibody provides a basis for blood transfusion. If the serum of the recipient contains antibodies against antigens present on the donor cells, the donor cells will be agglutinated and break down, causing a transfusion reaction. Thus group O individuals are called "universal donors"*—their red cells will not be agglutinated by either anti-A or anti-B antibody. Conversely, group AB individuals are "universal recipients"; because their serum has no anti-A and anti-B antibody they can receive cells of any ABO type. Group A people can receive either group A or O blood; group B people either B or O blood, and group O people only O blood.

Why don't the antibodies in the donor serum agglutinate the host's red cells? It seems that they get diluted in the host serum too rapidly to have much effect.

Subtypes

The ABO system can be further divided into subtypes, on the basis of quantitative differences in antigenicity. The most important are A_1 and A_2, increasing the possible phenotypes to 6 (A_1, A_2, B, A_1B, A_2B, and O) B subtypes and other A subtypes also exist. The ABO locus is 9q34.

H Substance

Some group A_1 individuals were found to have an antibody in their serum that agglutinates group O cells, suggesting that the O cells contain an antigen, which was labeled H. Discovery of the Bombay phenotype helped to clarify the situation. In this rare phenotype, discovered in Bombay in 1952, the individual's red cells are not agglutinated by anti-A, anti-B, or anti-H, so they are not group O cells. A family was then discovered in which a woman of this phenotype was shown by family studies to carry the gene for group B because she had a group AB child by an AO father, though she had no antigen B on her

*but only for ABO group differences

red cells. It appears that the Bombay phenotype results from homozygosity for a mutant allele, h, and that the normal allele, H, is responsible for making H substance, which is a precursor of the A and B antigens. With no H, the woman could not make B. This was the first case in humans of a "suppressor" mutant, already well recognized in bacteria, Drosophila, and other organisms.

Biochemical Basis of ABO System

The elegant work of Watkins,[6] and others, has demonstrated the biochemical basis of the ABO system. As illustrated in Figure 19–1, there is a glycoprotein precursor, without any demonstrated antigenic activity. The H gene leads to the presence of an enzyme, H transferase, that adds an L-fucose to the precursor, converting it into H substance. In the Bombay phenotype, the enzyme is missing, so there is no antigen H and thus no substrate from which to make A and B antigens.

Once the H substance is produced, it can be modified by the genes at the ABO locus. The A gene provides an enzyme that adds a sugar, N-acetyl-D-galactosamine, which gives the molecule the configuration that is recognized as antigen A. The B gene provides an enzyme that adds a different sugar, D-galactose, which produces antigen B specificity.

The Secretor Locus

In about 78% of the population, the ABO blood group substances are water-soluble and occur in body fluids (sweat, tears, saliva, semen) as well as in the red blood cells. In the other 22%, the ABO antigens are limited to the red cells. This difference is determined by the secretor gene Se and its recessive allele se which, when homozygous, produces the nonsecretor phenotype. The Se allele appears to be a regulatory gene that allows the H gene to operate in secretory cells; in sese individuals no H substance is produced in those cells, so there are no ABO-type antigens in the secretions.

The secretor locus is linked to the locus of the Lutheran blood group (q.v.) with a 15% recombination frequency. This was the first example of autosomal linkage in man.

Frequency of ABO Groups

The frequency of the ABO blood groups varies widely in different populations reflecting, in part, their origins. For instance, the frequency of the B allele is high in Mongolia and declines towards the West, being lower in Siberia and still lower in Europe, possibly reflecting the invasion of Europe by the Tartars. A is higher in southern England than in Scotland, perhaps as a result of the retreat northward of the aboriginal population (that had a high frequency of O) as continental high-A populations moved in from Europe.

Another interesting feature of the blood groups is their association with certain diseases. These do not represent linkages but are probably pleiotropic effects of the genes concerned. For instance, patients with duodenal ulcers are twice as likely to be group O, nonsecretor, as controls from the same population—for instance, their sibs.[3] There is an excess of group A among patients with cancer of the stomach. Although these differences are highly significant, they are not large enough

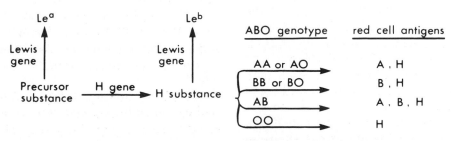

Fig. 19–1.   Possible pathway for biosynthesis of blood groups.

Table 19–2. The Two Notations for the Rh System, and Frequencies of the Various Gene Complexes in an English Population

Fisher/Race	Wiener	Frequency
CDe	R¹	0.41
cde	r	0.39
cDE	R²	0.14
cDe	R⁰	0.03
Cde	r′	0.01
cdE	r″	0.01
CdE	rʸ	low
CDE	Rᶻ	low

to be of predictive value and, so far, their biological basis is not understood.

RH BLOOD GROUPS

In 1940, Landsteiner and Wiener injected blood from Macaca rhesus monkeys into rabbits and prepared an antiserum, antirhesus, which would agglutinate the red cells of other rhesus monkeys. They were delighted to find that this serum would also agglutinate the cells of about 85% of white New Yorkers, and classified them Rh positive. The other 15%, whose cells did not react, were called Rh negative. The Rh-negative quality was soon shown to be recessive to the positive quality. With great perspicacity, Levine associated this difference with erythroblastosis fetalis, more properly termed hemolytic disease of the newborn—a disease caused when an Rh-negative woman is sensitized by an Rh-positive fetus, and makes anti-Rh antibodies. If there is a subsequent Rh-positive baby, these will pass through the placenta and agglutinate the baby's red cells leading to anemia, jaundice, and often death (see the following section for more details).

Other antibodies from sensitized mothers that behave genetically as if they were at the same locus were then found, and the situation began to get complicated. Two interpretations of the results were put forward. Fisher and Race postulated three adjacent loci, each with at least two alleles. These were C and c, D and d, and E and e. D corresponds to the original Rh-positive antigen, now called R⁰. Antibodies have been found against all these antigenic differences except d.

The other interpretation, passionately defended by Wiener, is that the Rh locus is a complex locus with several antigenic sites, characterized by various combinations of the three kinds of antigenic specificity that Race and Sanger call C, D, E, and their alleles. Table 19–2 sets out the two nomenclatures and the frequencies of the eight Rh haplotypes. The frequencies of the various combinations can be calculated by multiplying the frequencies of the individual Rh genes.

As with the ABO groups, the Rh system has several subgroups, such as D^U, an allele with weak D antigenicity, that may be mistyped as d unless a strong anti-D serum is used. There is also a rare phenotype Rh null, comparable to Bombay, with no Rh antigens. Another rare allele is -D-, in which C and E specificities are missing. According to the Fisher-Race model, this would suggest a deletion of the C and E regions and imply that C and E are adjacent. For this reason, the CDE locus is sometimes written DCE.

In the case of hemolytic disease of the newborn, it is important to know whether the father is DD or Dd (the recurrence risk will be 100% in one case and 50% in the other), but there is no anti-d antibody, so this cannot be demonstrated directly. Sometimes family studies detect heterozygosity—for instance, if the father has a dd parent or children. Otherwise, the probability that he is heterozygous can be calculated from his genotype for the other antigens. For example, suppose he types C^-, c^+, D^+, E^-, e^+. Then his genotype must be cDe/cde or cDe/cDe. The frequency of the first genotype (heterozygous D) is 0.03 × 0.39 = 0.0117, and of the second (homozygous D) is 0.03 × 0.03 = 0.0009. The probability of his being heterozygous is 0.0117/0.0126* = 0.9, and of being homozygous is .0009/.0126 = .07; he is 13 (.9/.07) times as likely to be heterozygous as homozygous D. The laboratory would report this as "most probable genotype-cDe/cde."

The Rh genes vary widely in frequency from population to population. The Basques, for instance, have a high frequency of dd individ-

*.0117 + .0009

uals—about 30%—whereas Orientals and North American Indians have almost none.

Hemolytic Disease of the Newborn

It is interesting to consider the serendipitous discovery of the cause of hemolytic disease of the newborn (HDN). This was a mysterious, often lethal disease that caused massive red cell breakdown, jaundice, brain damage, and deafness. It affected about 1 in 200 babies, often occurred in subsequent sibs, but almost always spared the firstborn. Levine was intrigued by a woman who had a stillborn child with HDN, and subsequently had a violent transfusion-reaction to her husband's ABO compatible blood. He demonstrated an antibody in her serum, and when he tested it against his blood-typing panel, he noted that it had the same specificity as the newly identified rabbit anti-rhesus serum. Eureka! Further testing rapidly proved the role of Rh incompatibility in HDN, and paved the way for its prevention.

In the typical case, an Rh-negative, or dd, mother has an Rh-positive child. Red blood cells from the fetus pass across the placenta into the mother's blood stream, particularly during compression of the placenta at birth. The mother may (though not always) become sensitized and begin to make anti-D antibody. This usually does not reach a high enough concentration to cause trouble in the first pregnancy. If the mother then has a second D child, there is a sharp rise in her antibody titer. The anti-D antibodies may then cross the placenta from mother to baby and coat the baby's red cells, causing their destruction—thus the anemia, jaundice, and other features of the disease.

Formerly, the disease was treated by exchange transfusion, in which the baby was transfused with Rh-negative blood, with concurrent removal of its own blood, to try to wash the harmful antibodies out of its system. This was not wholly satisfactory. Now the disease can be prevented by giving the mother RhoGAM, an anti-D antibody preparation. If this is given to the mother when the first D-positive baby is born, the anti-D antibody will coat and destroy any D-positive cells in her blood and thus prevent them from sensitizing her.

Why some incompatible mothers are not sensitized by their babies, whereas others are, is not fully understood. In part, it results from an interaction with the ABO system. If the D baby's cells are also group A, but the mother is dd O, the baby's cells that get into the mother's circulation will be destroyed by her anti-A antibody and so will not be available to sensitize her against the D antigen.

Hemolytic disease of the newborn can also occur as a result of ABO incompatibility, usually in an O mother and A child. The naturally occurring antibody, an IgM globulin, does not cross the placenta, but antibodies resulting from a previous child or an incompatible transfusion are predominantly IgG and cross and attack the baby's cells. However, the resulting disease is usually mild and requires no treatment. Occasionally, a mother develops antibodies against some other blood type antigen, such as K or Fy^a, that may cause HDN in a subsequent child.

MNSs Blood Groups

Landsteiner and Levine discovered the MN blood groups in 1927 after injecting rabbits with human red cells and using the resulting immune serum to distinguish other human red cell samples. They proposed a two-allele mode of codominant inheritance. The two alleles, M and N, produce three genotypes (MM, MN, and NN) and three phenotypes (M, MN, and N) with frequencies in European populations of 28%, 50%, and 22%, respectively.

About 20 years later, another antibody was found, which was associated with M and N, and given the designation S. It was not considered to be an allele of M and N but was thought to be related to them as C and E are related to D. Thus, there are MS, Ms, NS, and Ns combinations. The genes must be close together, although evidence is mounting that recombination can occur occasionally between the MN and Ss sites.

The MNS antigens do not stimulate antibodies in man, so they are not a problem with respect to blood transfusion or maternal-fetal incompatibility. However, because of its relative frequencies and codominance, the MNSs system is the most useful blood group system in medicolegal work and other problems of individual identification.

P Blood Groups

Landsteiner and Levine also discovered the P blood group system in 1927, using the same type of immunization experiments that identified the MN system. This system contains two phenotypes, P_1 and P_2, with frequencies of 79% and 21%, respectively, in Caucasians. P_1 is dominant to P_2. A very rare allele, p, and a p^K allele, perhaps comparable to Bombay, are also known.

Lutheran Blood Groups

The Lutheran blood group system was discovered in 1954 and was named after the person, not the religious sect, in whom the antibody was first found. By this time, the inconsistencies in terminology were great, since many changes had been made as knowledge grew. A new terminology was therefore agreed upon. The phenotypes are designated by the antibodies to which they react. Thus, in this case, there are two antibodies, anti-Lu^a and anti-Lu^b, and three phenotypes $Lu(a+b+)$, $Lu(a+b-)$, and $Lu(a-b+)$. These result from the segregation of two alleles, Lu^a and Lu^b. Thus the phenotype $Lu(a+b-)$ is the expression of the genotype Lu^aLu^a, since the red cells are agglutinated by anti-Lu^a serum but not by anti-Lu^b serum (Table 19–3). This blood group provided the first example in man of autoso-

Table 19–3. Nomenclature of the Lutheran Blood Group System and Frequencies in a Caucasian Population

Genotype	Phenotype	Frequency
Lu^a/Lu^a	$Lu(a+b-)$	0.001
Lu^a/Lu^b	$Lu(a+b+)$	0.08
Lu^b/Lu^b	$Lu(a-b+)$	0.92

mal linkage (with secretor) and suggested that crossing over is more common in the female.

Kell Blood Group

The Kell system consists of three pairs of alleles, Kk, Kp^aKp^b, and Js^aJs^b. The k allele is sometimes referred to as Cellano, after the woman in whom the k antibody was first discovered. The Js alleles (Sutter) were originally thought to be at an independent locus. Js^a is common in Negroes but rare in Caucasians. Hemolytic disease of the newborn is occasionally produced by maternal-fetal interaction in the Kk system.

Lewis Blood Groups

The Lewis blood group was first described in 1946. The common phenotypes in Caucasians are $Le(a+b-)$ (26%) and $Le(a-b+)$ (69%). $Le(a-b-)$ is common in West Africans and Hispanics.

The development of the Lewis antigens usually begins in infancy. Newborn red cells are not agglutinated by either anti-Le^a or anti-Le^b sera, but Lewis antigens are present at birth in the saliva and serum of individuals with the appropriate genotypes. This blood group interacts in a complicated way with the ABO, H, and secretor systems. Individuals with the red cell phenotype $Le(a+b-)$ are nonsecretors of ABH but contain Le^a antigen in their secretions. Individuals with the phenotype $Le(a-b+)$ are secretors.

One proposal is that the precursor substance is converted in the presence of the Lewis (Le) gene into Le^a substance in body secretions. When the H gene and the Se gene are also present, some of the soluble H substance is converted by the Le gene to the Le^b antigen (Fig. 19–1). In nonsecretors, the conversion of Le^a into H in the secretory tissues does not occur—hence the absence of A or B substances in secretions. The inactive allele le when homozygous leads to an H substance without Le activity when the Se gene is present.

It has been observed that red cells that lacked either Le^a or Le^b antigen would ac-quire that antigen if suspended in plasma containing it. This was proved in vivo when Le(a+b−) donor cells were administered to an Le(a−b+) patient. Following transfusion, the donor cells obtained by differential Rh agglutination tested as Le(a+b+). This information has led to a proposal that the Le antigens may be acquired from plasma antigens. There are many theories about the Lewis blood groups that cannot be dealt with within the limited scope of this presentation.

Duffy Blood Groups

The antibody leading to the discovery of the Duffy group was found in the serum of a patient of that name who had hemophilia and who had received multiple transfusions. The gene was designated Fy^a and its allele Fy^b. Later, a silent allele, Fy, was discovered. The homozygous phenotype Fy(a−b−) was present in 85% of New York African-Americans but was rare in Caucasians.

The reason for this racial difference has recently been found. The Duffy antigen appears to be the receptor that permits the malaria vivax parasite to attach itself to the red blood cell. Lack of the antigen greatly decreases susceptibility; hence the negative allele has a selective advantage in areas where malaria is endemic.

The Duffy locus also has the distinction of being the first locus to be assigned to a particular autosome, chromosome 1, now more precisely located at 1q21-q22.

Kidd Blood Groups

Jk^a and Jk^b are the alleles in the Kidd blood group system. The phenotype Jk(a−b−) may be the result of an inhibitory gene or another allele at the Kidd locus. This system is mainly of anthropologic interest. Jk(a+) is present in about 95% of West Africans, about 93% of African-Americans, about 77% of Europeans, and about 50% of Chinese. Both anti-Jk^a and anti-Jk^b have been known to cause HDN, and anti-JK^a has produced transfusion reactions.

Diego Blood Group System

The Diego blood group system was discovered in Venezuela when it produced hemolytic disease of the newborn in a family possessing some physical characteristics of the native Indians. The antigens are called Di^a and Di^b, and their respective antibodies are anti-Di^a and anti-Di^b. The antigens are reported in Chinese, Japanese, South American Indians, Chippewa Indians, and other phenotypically similar populations, with the notable exception of the Eskimo.

I Blood Groups

The I antigen has been studied in patients with acquired hemolytic anemia of the "cold antibody" type—that is, antibodies that are active only at a low temperature (4° C). The I antigen differs in certain respects from other blood group antigens. Almost everyone has some trace of the antigen, and the amount of I antigen on the red cells increases from birth until adult levels are reached at about 18 months of age. The corresponding levels of i decrease as I increases. The i antigen appears to be inherited in a recessive manner, but there is a disturbing excess of i siblings. There are two types of anti-I: auto-anti-I, which occurs in people who have acquired hemolytic anemia with cold antibodies, and natural anti-I, which appears in i phenotype adults. Natural anti-I does not cross the placenta. Examples of the anti-i have been found in persons with some types of reticulosis. Transient anti-i is often present in patients with infectious mononucleosis.

Xg Blood Group System

The Xg blood group is the first recognized X-linked blood group and is presently assigned to Xpter-p22.32. The antibody was discovered in a patient who had had many transfusions. It occurs in 89% of females and 62% of males. (Do you see why the difference? Does it fit the Hardy-Weinberg equilibrium?)

Xg was first discovered at the time when the truth of the Lyon X-inactivation hypoth-

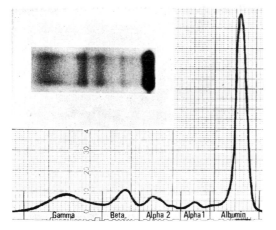

Fig. 19–2. Serum proteins separated by electrophoresis on agar gel with densitometric display.

esis was being hotly debated, and it was hoped that this cell-specific X-linked marker would resolve the question. In fact, it only confused the issue, because it is now clear that the Xg locus does *not* lyonize, nor does the adjacent steroid sulfatase locus, associated with X-linked ichthyosis. This fits in nicely with Ferguson-Smith's suggestion, based on the fact that XO Turner patients have developmental anomalies, that the short arm of the inactive X in females is normally not inactivated. On the other hand, ocular albinism, also on the short arm, does lyonize, so the nonlyonizing segment must be quite short.

Several bits of evidence contribute to the deduction that the Xg locus does not participate in X-inactivation.[4] Firstly, mixtures of red cells from women known to be heterozygous for Xg^a reacted uniformly to anti Xg(a+) antiserum, whereas mixtures of Xg(a+) and Xg(a−) cells from hemizygous males reacted heterogeneously. A second line of evidence comes from studies of women with chronic myeloid leukemia. The leukemia cells are monoclonal, arising from a single progenitor cell. If X-inactivation of the Xg locus occurred, the frequencies of Xg(a+) and Xg(a−) in these cells should correspond to those of males, but in fact the frequency was the same as that in females. Finally, a woman and her daughter carried a translocation of the short arm of the X to an autosome. In both, the normal X was

consistently inactivated, as shown by late-labeling (see Chapter 4). The mother was Xg(a−) and the father Xg(a+), so the daughter's paternal X was inactivated, but she typed Xg(a+), showing that the inactivated X produced the Xg antigen nevertheless.

Other Blood Groups, Public and Private

A number of other "public" antigens have been described. The term *public* antigen is used to describe antigens that are encountered frequently, as opposed to a *private* antigen, which is limited to a single kindred.

Serum Proteins[5]

The invention of physical techniques for separating proteins, chromatography and electrophoresis, led to the identification of many new genetic markers. We have already referred to electrophoretic variants of a number of enzymes, including G6PD, alpha-1-antitrypsin, lactic dehydrogenase, and red cell acid phosphatase. And much of the elegant work on the genetics of hemoglobin and the immunoglobulins was made possible by the existence of these techniques. Indeed, it now seems that electrophoretic polymorphisms are the rule, rather than the exception.

Figure 19–2 is an illustration of a simple electrophoretic separation of serum proteins into albumin and globulin fractions. Further separation is achieved by special methods.

Oliver Smithies, now a prominent geneticist, began his career in genetics when, as an English biochemist working at the University of Toronto, he hit on the idea of using a (potato) starch gel in an electrical field, to separate the serum proteins. He soon noticed a polymorphism in the band representing haptoglobin, a protein that binds hemoglobin. He took the results to a geneticist, Norma Ford Walker, who suggested family studies, and they were off!

In summary, haptoglobin is, like hemoglobin, a tetramere, consisting of α and β chains. The polymorphism resides in the α chain locus. Two major alleles, Hp^1 and Hp^2, result in 3 genotypes, Hp^1Hp^1, Hp^2Hp^2, and Hp^1Hp^2.

The two homozygotes have one band each (types Hp^{1-1} and Hp^{2-2}) the heterozygote has two (Hp^{1-2}). (We are ignoring the initial confusion caused by the fact that the Hp-2 molecule forms polymers, resulting in many bands, which can be gotten rid of by appropriate treatment.) Hp^1 exists in two forms, Hp^{1F} and Hp^{1S} (for Fast and Slow) differing by a single amino acid difference.

Interestingly, the difference between Hp^1 and Hp^2 is of a quite different kind. The Hp-2 molecule is about twice as long as the Hp-1, and amino acid sequencing suggests that it arose as an end to end fusion of Hp^{1F} and Hp^{1S}, in a manner comparable to that of hemoglobin Lepore. Thus it must have arisen in a population already polymorphic for Hp^{1F} and Hp^{1S}. Apes and other "lower" mammals do not have Hp^2, so this polymorphism adds another example of evolution by a combination of point mutation and gene "duplication."[3]

Genetic polymorphisms exist also for other serum proteins including transferrins (an iron-binding protein), ceruloplasmin (a copper-binding protein), the G6 protein (binding vitamin D) and the third component of complement (a series of proteins involved in antigen-antibody reactions).

As we said, genetic polymorphisms of proteins are probably the rule, rather than the exception, and the more one looks, the more one finds. This is not surprising; point mutations altering amino acid sequences are happening all the time and some of the mutants might well have a slight advantage in fitness, or reach the statutory 2% frequency by genetic drift. They have contributed notably to progress in mapping, as well as to understanding of evolutionary mechanisms.

SUMMARY

Blood groups and serum proteins have proved to be highly informative polymorphisms for genetic investigation, family and population studies, linkage analysis and chromosome mapping, and forensic medicine. The ability to identify blood types accurately has made safe blood transfusion possible.

The ABO blood groups were first discovered in 1900. The antigenic specificities A and B are co-dominant, and O (lack of antigen) is recessive. A reciprocal relation exists, in that an individual possessing an antigen (A, for example) has no antibodies against A, but does have antibodies against B—and vice versa. A type AB individual has no antibodies against A or B, and a type O individual has antibodies against both A and B.

The Rh blood groups are next in importance for typing, from the point of view of transfusion. Hemolytic disease of the newborn (HDN) is most often associated with this blood group. A recent advance, the use of RhoGAM, now makes HDN a preventable disease.

A great deal of useful genetic information can be derived from the study of the many other public and private blood groups. Recently, serum proteins such as the haptoglobins and complement polymorphisms have been the subject of useful genetic investigation.

REFERENCES

1. Giblett, E.R.: Genetic polymorphisms in human blood. Ann. Rev. Genet. 11:13, 1977.
2. Harris, H.: The principles of human biochemical genetics, 3rd Ed., New York, Elsevier North Holland Press, 1980.
3. Mourant, A.E., Kopec, A.C., and Domaniewska-Sobsczak, A.: Blood groups and diseases: a study of associations of diseases with blood groups and other polymorphisms. Oxford, Oxford University Press, 1978.
4. Race, R.R., and Sanger, R.: Blood Groups in Man, 6th Ed. Philadelphia, F.A. Davis, 1975.
5. Roychoudhury, A.K., and Nei, M.: Human Polymorphic Genes: World Distribution New York, Oxford University Press, 1988.
6. Watkins, W.M.: Biochemistry and genetics of the ABO, Lewis, and P. blood group systems. Adv. Hum. Genet. 10:1, 1980.

Chapter 20

Somatic Cell Genetics

Somatic cell genetics, which began with the work of Puck in Denver, is based on the ability to grow mammalian cells in cultures outside the body and to manipulate them genetically, much as is done with microorganisms (Fig. 20–1).[30] It is a foundation stone on which the techniques of molecular biology are built. One of the earliest achievements was the attainment of clear and diagnostic preparations of human chromosomes.[32,37–39] A multitude of

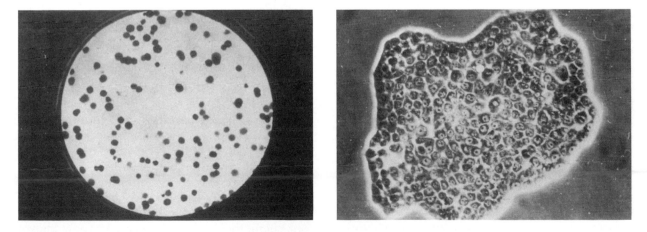

Fig. 20–1. Human cells grown in culture. A shows a Petri dish containing fixed and stained individual colonies of human cells grown in vitro. B shows an enlargement of one such colony in which the individual cells of the colony are visible. Modified with permission from Puck, T.T.: The Mammalian Cell as a Microorganism: Genetic and Biochemical Studies in Vitro. San Francisco, Holden-Day, 1972, p. 219.

operations are now possible with mammalian, including human, cells in culture. Among them are clonal growth of colonies from individual cells, production of single cell survival curves for assessing the sensitivity of various mammalian cell types to physical and chemical agents, isolation of a wide variety of genetic mutants of mammalian cells, biochemical analysis of metabolic pathways in mammalian cells, and biochemical analysis of naturally occurring and induced mutations in mammalian cells. Additionally, various cell types may be fused to create hybrid cells, which permits transfer of isolated genes from one cell type to another and detailed analysis of various types of genetic mutations, either induced or naturally occurring.[21,34] Genetic, cytogenetic, biochemical, and molecular techniques may then be used to investigate inherited diseases, the nature of important biochemical processes, basic genetic mechanisms, and the basis for genetic diseases and chromosomal diseases like Down syndrome, fragile-X syndrome, and cancer. In many cases, somatic cell genetics allows or enhances studies that would otherwise be impossible. It also allows studies to be carried out on cells in culture rather than on animals or on human subjects, thus overcoming ethical as well as technical constraints inherent in research on animals or humans.

CLONAL GROWTH OF MAMMALIAN CELLS

The ability to grow mammalian cells clonally, i.e., to grow cultures of cells from single cells, is the distinguishing feature of somatic cell genetics and its enabling technical operation.[13,28] Clonal growth of mammalian cells depends critically on conditions such as composition of the growth medium, temperature, pH, and CO_2 levels. Scores of different growth media have been designed for a wide variety of purposes ranging from mass culture for preparation of large quantities of cells or their constituents to media designed to maintain or induce a particular state of differentiation in a particular cell type. An interesting example of how critical the exact composition of growth medium on somatic cell cultures can be involves the discovery of the fragile-X syndrome

(see Chap. 4). This is the most common sex-linked genetic cause of major mental retardation known. In cells from patients with this disease, there is an inordinately high tendency for the X chromosome to appear to be broken at a particular site. This fragility of the X chromosome is observed in growth media that are relatively deficient in folate, and, in fact, the reproducibility of induction of the fragile site, an important component of the diagnosis of the disorder, depends on the use of appropriate media.[36] Moreover, the dependence of induction of the fragile site on folate deficiency may give us some clues of the mechanism of formation of the fragile sites. With the use of a combination of molecular and somatic cell genetic techniques, the fragile site on the X chromosome has been identified and isolated.[9] It is hoped that, in the near future, this will bring about the understanding of how the fragile site arises and how it is important in the pathogenesis of fragile-X syndrome.

Being able to grow mammalian cells clonally allows one to assess quantitatively the effects of physical or chemical agents on the growth and survival of these cells. In such an experiment, measured numbers of somatic cells are placed in replicate dishes. Representative samples of the dishes are then exposed to graded doses of the agent in question, and the cells are incubated until visible colonies arise. In this way, a dose response curve for any particular agent can be derived from which one can determine the toxicity of the agent under study.[16,29] These data are often expressed in fraction of surviving cells and plotted as a function of dose of the agent. An illustrative example of this approach is shown in Figure 20–2, in which the survival curve for human cells exposed to increasing doses of x-rays is shown. This particular experiment accurately and quantitatively measured the true sensitivity of mammalian cells to x-rays for the first time. More recently, modifications of this approach have been proposed for assessing the sensitivity of individual tumors to drugs before chemotherapy. Such assays are now known as clonogenicity assays.

A second standard method of somatic cell genetics is the generation of mammalian cell

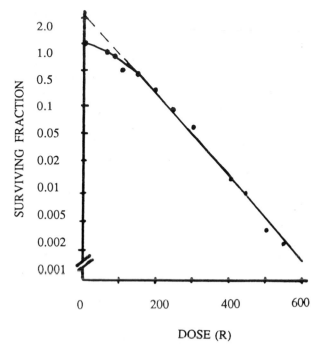

Fig. 20–2. A survival curve demonstrating the lethality of x-rays to mammalian cells as a function of dose. The Y axis shows the surviving fraction of cells on a logarithmic scale plotted against x-ray dose delivered. Modified with permission from Puck, T.T.: The Mammalian Cell as a Microorganism: Genetic and Biochemical Studies in Vitro. San Francisco, Holden-Day, 1972.

mutants in culture. Mutants have been isolated on the basis of resistance to various drugs, on the basis of resistance to killing by macromolecules like diphtheria toxin or antibodies that recognize and bind to important cell surface molecules, or on the basis of induction of additional nutritional requirements not present in the parental cell lines. It has even become possible to isolate mutant mammalian cells by a replica plating protocol patterned after those originally developed for the study of bacteria.[5,14,15,35]

SOMATIC CELL GENETIC ANALYSIS OF BIOCHEMICAL UMP SYNTHESIS

Mutant Isolation by Drug Resistance

An instructive example of many of these approaches of somatic cell genetics and their application is given by the study of the pathway

of uridine monophosphate UMP synthesis, depicted in simplified form in Figure 20–3. Somatic cell mutants have been isolated in all of the genes encoding the enzymes of this crucial biochemical pathway, and often these have been informative regarding medically significant questions and in understanding the basic biochemistry of this pathway in unexpected ways (Fig. 20–4).[22,23,35] For example, many cancer chemotherapy drugs are analogues of pyrimidines or interfere with this pathway. Thus, 5-fluorouracil, a uracil analogue, is commonly used to treat gastrointestinal cancers. Mutant cells resistant to this drug have been isolated that completely lack the last two enzymes of UMP biosynthesis. Ge-

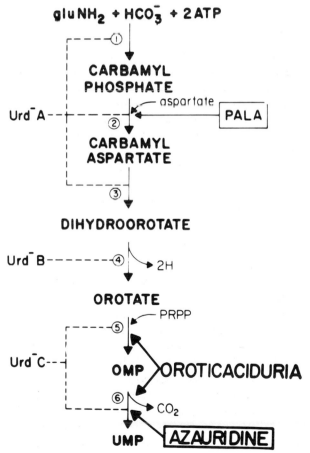

Fig. 20–3. A simplified representation of the biosynthesis of the pyrimidine nucleotide UMP. PALA=phosphonacetyl-L-aspartate, an inhibitor of step 2 of the pathway. Urd⁻A, Urd⁻B, Urd⁻C denote Chinese hamster cell mutants deficient in the enzymatic steps indicated. Azauridine is a pyrimidine analogene that inhibits UMP synthesis as shown.

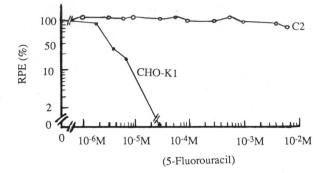

Fig. 20–4. The effect of the anticancer drug 5-fluorouracil on wild-type (CHO-K1) and mutant (CZ) CHO cells lacking the last 2 steps of UMP synthesis (see Fig. 20–3). Modified with permission from Patterson, D.: Isolation and characterization of 5-fluorouracil-resistant mutants of Chinese hamster ovary cells deficient in the activities of orotate phosphoribosyltransferase and orotidine 5′-monophosphate decarboxylase. Somat. Cell Genet. 6:101, 1980.

netic and biochemical analysis of these mutants shows that a single gene encodes a single multifunctional protein carrying out both of these enzymatic steps. Moreover, this enzyme appears to be necessary for the action of 5-fluorouracil, at least in some cell types. The finding that single protein molecules carry out more than one enzymatic step was unsuspected, and is now becoming increasingly observed in the analysis of metabolic pathways. Interestingly, analysis of somatic cells derived from patients with the inherited metabolic disorder orotic aciduria are also lacking the activity of these two enzymes.[19] Both cells resistant to 5-fluorouracil and cells derived from orotic aciduria patients show the expected requirement for uridine as a source of UMP for adequate growth in culture.

Suicide Selection for Mutant Isolation

Uridine requiring mutants of Chinese hamster ovary (CHO) cells have been selected directly using a suicide selection procedure (Fig. 20–5).[22,25] Thus, CHO cells that do not normally require uridine for growth are subjected to mutagenesis with a chemical agent and then grown in medium lacking a source of uridine but containing the light-sensitive thymidine analogue bromodeoxyuridine (BrdU). Under these conditions, growing cells incor-

porate the BrdU into their DNA. However, the mutants defective in synthesis of uridine stop growing and thus do not incorporate the BrdU. Then the culture is exposed to light so that cells that have incorporated the analogue suffer lethal damage to their DNA and are killed. Next, uridine is added back to the growth medium and the uridine-requiring mutants grow and form colonies, which can be isolated and grown up for study.

When such cells were analyzed, they were found to be missing the first three enzymatic steps of UMP synthesis. Detailed molecular analysis of one such mutant has shown that again a single protein carries out these three enzymatic steps and that a single base change in the DNA is responsible for production of a defective protein which cannot supply these activities.[27]

An additional type of mutant involving this same gene has led to similar conclusions regarding the multifunctional nature of the protein carrying out these steps and also has been informative regarding possible mechanisms by which some cancers may become resistant to chemotherapy agents. In this set of experiments, a chemical inhibitor of the second step of the UMP pathway was designed based on a detailed understanding of the mechanism of action of this enzyme, specifically with the hope that it would be useful in treatment of cancer.[6] Mutants resistant to this drug, PALA,

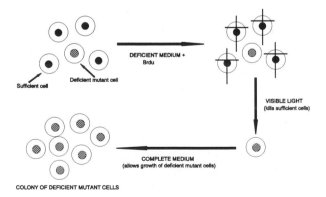

Fig. 20–5. A schematic representation of a "suicide selection" for nutritional mutants of mammalian cells in culture. Modified with permission from Kao, F.-T., and Puck, T.T.: Genetics of mammalian cells. VII. Induction and isolation of nutritional mutants in Chinese hamster cells. Proc. Natl. Acad. Sci. USA 60:1275, 1968.

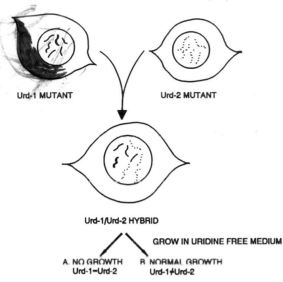

COMPLEMENTATION ANALYSIS OF URIDINE REQUIRING(Urd-) MUTANTS

Urd-1 MUTANT

Urd-2 MUTANT

Urd-1/Urd-2 HYBRID

GROW IN URIDINE FREE MEDIUM

A. NO GROWTH   B. NORMAL GROWTH
Urd-1=Urd-2   Urd-1≠Urd-2

Fig. 20–6. Complementation analysis of uridine requiring mutants of mammalian cells.

were then isolated as a part of the characterization of the drug. Interestingly, these mutants, essentially invariably, were found to have significantly elevated levels of the protein carrying out the three reactions. This was found to be caused by the presence of many copies of the gene encoding the enzyme in the resistant cells.[40] This phenomenon, called gene amplification, has now been documented as a mechanism of resistance of tumors to anticancer drugs.

Replica Plating for Isolating Mutants

The fourth step of UMP biosynthesis, dihydroorotate dehydrogenase, has also been of interest as a possible site of cancer chemotherapy; and drugs thought to inhibit the production or action of this enzyme are under consideration as anticancer agents.[1,4] Mutants defective in this enzyme have been isolated using a replica plating procedure. Thus, cultures of cells are grown up, exposed to mutagen, and then plated out and allowed to produce several hundred colonies on a tissue culture dish. A nylon filter paper is placed over this pattern of colonies, and some cells of each colony are transferred to the nylon, making

an exact replica of the pattern of colonies on the original dish. The original colonies are then stained for the presence of dihydroorotate dehydrogenase using a procedure which produces a colored product in the presence of the enzyme but which kills the cells. Mutant colonies remain colorless. It is then possible to find the cognate colony on the nylon replica, isolate it and grow it up for study.[35]

COMPLEMENTATION ANALYSIS

Using these procedures, mutants in all these steps have been isolated. Such mutants can be used to illustrate another standard somatic cell genetic procedure, complementation analysis by the production of hybrid cells (Fig. 20–6).[17] In this case, cells defective in, for example, the first three steps can be fused with mutants defective in the last two steps of UMP synthesis. In theory, the hybrid cells should have the entire complement of enzymes required for UMP synthesis. In practice, when this experiment is carried out, this is indeed what is observed. The real power of complementation analysis comes when one is confronted with a new mutant with an unknown defect. Then the mutant can be fused with mutants with known defects and classified as to whether it complements or does not complement the known mutants. This procedure has been exceedingly useful in the biochemical genetic analysis of many metabolic pathway mutants of mammalian cells and even in helping to understand inherited metabolic disorders of man, as described in Chapter 6.

HUMAN GENE MAPPING

An extension of complementation analysis has become one of the most powerful methods to map human genes yet developed, and one of the most widely used somatic cell genetic procedures (see Chap. 9). Mapping of human genes is of critical importance for the future of medical genetics as well as for understanding of human genetic diseases and for locating human genes responsible for developmental processes. The location of a gene may be important in determining mechanisms of

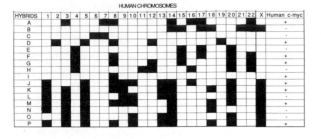

Fig. 20–7. Concordance analysis of somatic cell hybrids demonstrating the mapping of the human *c-myc* proto-oncogene to human chromosome 8. Modified with permission from Dalla-Favera, et al.: Assignment of the human c-myc oncogene to the region of chromosome 8 which is translocated in Burkitt lymphoma cells. Proc. Natl. Acad. Sci. USA 79:7824, 1982.

gene regulation or in determining whether a particular gene might be important in a particular disease like cancer.[31,33]

Thus, it is possible to make a hybrid between a rodent cell with a particular selectable characteristic, like a requirement for uridine for growth, and wild-type human cells and then to select for hybrids.[3,24] In this case, it must be the human gene that complements the selectable marker in the mutant rodent cells. Such a hybrid cell usually contains the human chromosome upon which the gene supplying the selectable marker is located, and may or may not carry other nonselected human chromosomes. If the hybrid contains only a single human chromosome, this maps the gene to that chromosome. In practice, generally some kind of independent verification of mapping, such demonstration that the human gene product is produced in the hybrid, is often sought. Also, another classical genetic procedure, segregation analysis, is applied. In this type of experiment, the selective pressure is removed from the hybrid. Under these conditions, human/rodent hybrids tend to lose the human chromosome. If loss of the human chromosome is invariably accompanied by loss of the marker, this is termed cosegregation of the marker and the chromosome and is taken as further evidence that the gene encoding the marker is located on the chromosome.

Human/hamster hybrids can be used to map any marker for which a discrimination exists between the human and hamster forms of the marker. Human/rodent hybrids with single human chromosomes have been termed monochromosomal hybrids. In the case of monochromosomal hybrids, the presence and absence of the human marker in a battery of hybrids, each containing one of the 24 human chromosomes, will unambiguously assign the marker to a particular chromosome. By now, at least two panels of such monochromosomal hybrids have been assembled.

Panels of hybrids, each containing a few human chromosomes, can also be used for mapping human genes. Such a hybrid mapping panel is constructed in such a way that it is possible to assess the concordant presence of the marker with a particular chromosome and its absence with the presence of all other chromosomes (discordance), thus making it possible to assign any particular marker to a particular chromosome. Again, many such somatic cell hybrid mapping panels have been produced and used for assigning human genes to particular chromosomes. Markers assigned to the same human chromosome are said to be syntenic with each other. Figure 20–7 presents the use of a hybrid mapping panel to assign the c-myc proto-oncogene to human chromosome 8.[7]

Somatic cell hybrids containing translocation or deletion chromosome rearrangements have been used extensively to regionally map human genes on particular human chromosomes. These rearrangements can be derived by making the hybrids from human cells carrying the rearranged chromosomes; or, alternatively, the rearrangements can arise, either spontaneously or through experimental manipulation, after the hybrids are isolated.

A particularly powerful example of this approach has been developed. A somatic cell hybrid containing a single human chromosome is subjected to a highly lethal dose of irradiation so that the chromosome is fragmented. This process kills the hybrid cells. However, the killed cells are then refused with living rodent cells and a collection of new hybrids is produced, each of which retains a fragment of the chromosome under study. Each of the new radiation reduction hybrids (Fig. 20–8) is then checked for the presence or ab-

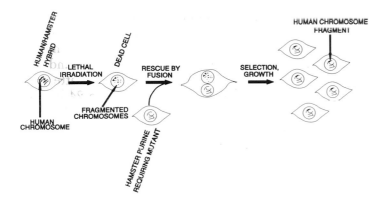

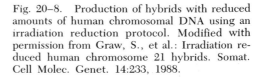

Fig. 20–8. Production of hybrids with reduced amounts of human chromosomal DNA using an irradiation reduction protocol. Modified with permission from Graw, S., et al.: Irradiation reduced human chromosome 21 hybrids. Somat. Cell Molec. Genet. 14:233, 1988.

sence of all the known human genes or markers present on that chromosome. Because, in general, the chance that x-ray will break a DNA molecule, or chromosome, is proportional to the length of the target, markers that are close to each other tend to be present more frequently in the radiation reduction hybrid set than markers that are far apart. By a simple statistical analysis, it is then possible to determine the most likely order of human genes or markers on the chromosome in question, and even to generate some estimate of how far apart they might be.[2,11,12]

SOMATIC CELL GENETIC ANALYSIS OF CHROMOSOME 21

A particularly elegant and instructive example of the application of all of these approaches is the analysis of human chromosome 21. This is the smallest human chromosome, and contains about 1.5% of the human genome, or about 50 million base pairs of DNA. It is estimated to carry about 1000 genes. Chromosome 21, when present in three copies instead of the normal two, is responsible for Down syndrome, the most common chromosomal cause of mental retardation and congenital heart disease in humans. Individuals with Down syndrome also have a markedly increased risk of developing leukemia, virtually always develop the brain neuropathology associated inevitably with Alzheimer disease, and have many other characteristic abnormalities. It is hoped that, by identifying and isolating the genes on chromosome 21, it will be possible to shed light on how Down

syndrome and the disease features associated with it arise.[26]

It is possible to selectively retain chromosome 21 in a CHO cell defective in one of the genes required for purine synthesis, because the human gene for this enzyme is located on human chromosome 21. In fact, many such hybrids have been isolated. Additionally, hybrids containing translocation chromosomes with various fragments of chromosome 21 have been generated, as has a collection of radiation reduction hybrids. These and other reagents have allowed an extremely detailed map of chromosome 21 spanning over 40 million base pairs of DNA to be produced. Many genes thought to be important in the pathology of Down syndrome have been precisely physically mapped in this way.[10] In fact, it seems likely that chromosome 21 will be one of the first human chromosomes mapped in its entirety. Analogous approaches are being used for virtually every other human chromosome, and the number of genetic markers mapped using somatic cell genetic is in the thousands.

Several additional techniques are useful for mapping the human genes, and the most powerful approach is to use a combination of methods. For example, it is now possible to use fluorescently labelled DNA specific for any isolated gene to mark the location of that gene on the human chromosomes. This approach, called fluorescence *in situ* hybridization (Fig. 20–9), is extremely rapid and depends only on having the cloned gene available.[20] It is limited primarily by the cytogenetic resolution of chromosome bands. It can be profitably used in conjunction with somatic cell hy-

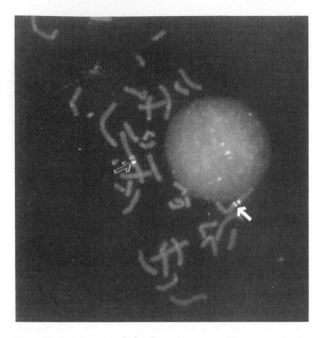

Fig. 20–9. In situ hybridization using fluorescently labeled DNA probes to metaphase chromosomes demonstrating the mapping of a gene encoding the interleukin-1 receptor antagonist (ILIRN) gene to human chromosome 2. The intense single white area (solid arrow) indicates binding of a DNA probe specific for the centromere of chromosome 2. The two dots (dark arrow) indicate binding of a DNA probe for the ILIRN gene.

brid panels for regional mapping. Both approaches can be used in conjunction with family studies, or genetic linkage analysis, to map important human genes physically, genetically, and cytogenetically.

Several laboratories have also reported assessing gene dosage using molecular techniques to help define chromosomal duplications and deletions as well. Again, this approach complements the ability to isolate specific chromosomes carrying the duplications or deletions in somatic cell hybrids for detailed molecular analysis.[8,18]

The success of somatic cell genetics for mapping human genes and the ready availability of somatic cell hybrids for virtually any chromosome combine to form one of the important reasons for the initial proposal to map all the human genes, now known as the Human Genome Project. At present, and for the foreseeable future, somatic cell hybrids and the techniques of somatic cell genetics prom-

ise to play a significant role in this most ambitious human genetics project.

SUMMARY

Somatic cell genetics allows the somatic cells of an animal or a human to be grown in culture outside the body and manipulated much as microorganisms. Thus, it is possible to study the growth characteristics of mammalian cells under extremely well controlled conditions, in some cases using culture media in which all components are chemically defined. It is possible to assess quantitatively the toxicity of many physical and chemical agents, including environmental agents, suspected carcinogens, or chemotherapeutic drugs, on cells in culture. It is possible to isolate mutant somatic cells with a number of important genetic characteristics, either by establishing cultures from organisms with mutations or by experimental manipulation in vitro. It is possible to examine the chromosome content of cells and to perform prenatal diagnosis of various human genetic diseases using somatic cell genetics. One particularly important technique of somatic cell genetics is the ability to create hybrid cells from two different cell types, for example between human and rodent cells. This technique has been a major tool in mapping human genes and in studying their regulation and function. Techniques for introducing foreign genes individually into somatic cells, and more recently into germline cells, have been instrumental in the study of human and mammalian development and malignancy. Recently, somatic cell genetic techniques have played a major role in the human genome project.

REFERENCES

1. Braakhuis, B.J.M., et al.: Antitumor activity of brequinar sodium (Dup-785) against human head and neck squamous cell carcinoma xenografts. Cancer Letters 49:133, 1990.
2. Burmeister, M., et al.: A map of the distal region of the long arm of human chromosome 21 constructed by radiation hybrid mapping and pulsed-field gel electrophoresis. Genomics 9:19, 1991.
3. Chen, K.-C., et al.: Mapping of the gene encoding the multifunctional protein carrying out the first three steps

of pyrimidine biosynthesis to human chromosome 2. Hum. Genet. 82:40, 1989.

4. Chen, S.-F., et al.: Mechanism of action of the novel anticancer agent 6-fluoro-2-(2'-fluoro-1,1'-biphenyl-4-yl)-3-methyl-4-quinolinecarboxylic acid sodium salt (NSC 368390): Inhibition of *de novo* pyrimidine nucleotide biosynthesis. Cancer Res. 46:5014, 1986.

5. Chu, E.H.Y., and Malling, H.V.: Mammalian cell genetics. II. Mutational chemical induction of specific locus mutations in Chinese hamster cells in vitro. Proc. Natl. Acad. Sci. USA 61:1306, 1968.

6. Collins, K.D., and Stark, G.R.: Aspartate transcarbamylase. J. Biol. Chem. 246:6599, 1971.

7. Dalla-Favera, R., et al.: Assignment of the human c-myc onc-gene to the region of chromosome 8 which is translocated in Burkitt lymphoma cells. Proc. Natl. Acad. Sci. USA 79:7824, 1982.

8. Delabar, J.-M., et al.: Gene-dosage mapping of 30 DNA markers on chromosome 21. Genomics 13:887, 1992.

9. Fu, Y.-H., et al.: Variation of the CGG repeat at the fragile-X site results in genetic instability: Resolution of the Sherman paradox. Cell 67:1047, 1991.

10. Gardiner, K., et al.: Analysis of human chromosome 21: Correlation of physical and cytogenetic maps; gene and CpG island distributions. EMBO J. 9:25, 1990.

11. Goss, S.J., and Harris, H.: New method for mapping genes in human chromosomes. Nature 255:680, 1975.

12. Graw, S., et al. Irradiation reduced human chromosome 21 hybrids. Somat. Cell Molec. Genet. 14:233, 1988.

13. Ham, R.G., and Puck, T.T.: Quantitative colonial growth of isolated mammalian cells. Methods Enzymol. 5:90, 1962.

14. Jones, C., et al.: Genetics of somatic cell surface antigens. III. Further analysis of the A_L marker. Somatic Cell Genet. 1:235, 1975.

15. Kao, F.-T., and Puck, T.T.: Genetics of somatic mammalian cells. VII. Induction and isolation of nutritional mutants in Chinese hamster cells. Proc. Natl. Acad. Sci. USA 60:1275, 1968.

16. Kao, F.-T., and Puck, T.T.: Genetics of somatic mammalian cells. IX. Quantitation of mutagenesis by physical and chemical agents. J. Cell Physiol. 74:245, 1969.

17. Kao, F.-T., et al.: Complementation analysis on virus-fused Chinese hamster cells with nutritional markers. Science 164:312, 1969.

18. Korenberg, J.R., et al.: Deletion of chromosome 21 and normal intelligence: Molecular definition of the lesion. Hum. Genet. 87:112, 1991.

19. Krooth, R.S.: Properties of diploid cell strains developed from patients with an inherited abnormality of uridine biosynthesis. CSHSGB 29:189, 1964.

20. Lichter, P., et al.: Analysis of genes and chromosomes by nonisotopic in situ hybridization. GATA 8:24, 1991.

21. Okada, Y.: The fusion of Ehrlich's tumor cells caused by HVJ virus in vitro. Biken J. 1:103, 1958.

22. Patterson, D., and Carnright, D.V.: Biochemical genetic analysis of pyrimidine biosynthesis in mammalian cells: I. Isolation of a mutant defective in the early steps of de novo pyrimidine synthesis. Somat. Cell Genet. 3:483, 1977.

23. Patterson, D.: Isolation and characterization of 5-fluorouracil-resistant mutants of Chinese hamster ovary cells deficient in the activities of orotate phosphoribosyltransferase and orotidine 5'-monophosphate decarboxylase. Somat. Cell Genet. 6:101, 1980.

24. Patterson, D., et al.: Structural gene coding for multifunctional protein carrying orotate phosphoribosyltransferase and OMP decarboxylase activity is located on long arm of human chromosome 3. Somat. Cell Genet. 9:359, 1983.

25. Patterson, D., and Waldren, C.: Suicide selection of mammalian cell mutants. Methods Enzymol. 151:121, 1987.

26. Patterson, D.: The causes of Down Syndrome. Sci. Am. 255:52, 1987.

27. Patterson, D., et al.: A single base change at a splice acceptor site leads to a truncated CAD protein in Urd⁻A mutant Chinese hamster ovary cells. Somat. Cell Mol. Genet. 18:65, 1992.

28. Puck, T.T., et al.: Clonal growth of mammalian cells in vitro. J. Exp. Med. 103:273, 1956.

29. Puck, T.T., and Marcus, P.I.: Action of x-rays on mammalian cells. J. Exp. Med. 103:653, 1956.

30. Puck, T.T.: The Mammalian Cell as a Microorganism: Genetic and Biochemical Studies in Vitro. San Francisco, Holden-Day, 1972, p. 219.

31. Puck, T.T., and Kao, F.-T.: Somatic cell genetics and its application to medicine. Ann. Rev. Genet. 16:225, 1982.

32. Robinson, A.: A proposed standard system of nomenclature of human mitotic chromosomes. JAMA 174:159, 1960.

33. Ruddle, F.H., and Creagan, R.P.: Parasexual approaches to the genetics of man. Ann. Rev. Genet. 9:407, 1975.

34. Sorieul, S., and Ephrussi, B.: Karyological demonstration of hybridization of mammalian cells in vitro. Nature 190:653, 1961.

35. Stamato, T.D., and Patterson, D.: Biochemical genetic analysis of pyrimidine biosynthesis in mammalian cells. II. Isolation and characterization of a mutant of Chinese hamster ovary cells with defective dihydroorotate dehydrogenase (E.C. 1.3.3.1) activity. J. Cell. Physiol. 98:459, 1979.

36. Sutherland, G.R.: Fragile sites on human chromosomes. Demonstration of their dependence on the type of tissue culture medium. Science 197:265, 1977.

37. Tjio, J.H., and Levan, A.: The chromosome number of man. Hereditas 42:1, 1956.

38. Tjio, J.H., and Puck, T.T.: The somatic chromosomes of man. Proc. Natl. Acad. Sci. USA 44:1229, 1958.

39. Tjio, J.H., and Puck, T.T.: Genetics of somatic mammalian cells. II. Chromosomal constitution of cells in tissue culture. J. Exp. Med. 108:259, 1958.

40. Wahl, G.M., et al.: Gene amplification causes overproduction of the first three enzymes of UMP synthesis in N-(phosphonacetyl)-L-aspartate-resistant hamster cells. J. Biol. Chem. 254:8679, 1979.

Chapter *21*
Genetics and Cancer

"NEVERTHELESS, THE SEARCH FOR GENETIC DAMAGE IN CANCER CELLS AND THE EXPLICATION OF HOW THAT DAMAGE AFFECTS BIOCHEMICAL FUNCTION HAVE BECOME OUR BEST HOPE TO UNDERSTAND, AND THUS TO THWART, THE RAVAGES OF CANCER."

J. MICHAEL BISHOP, 1991

It is now clear that cancer is caused by genetic changes in normal cells. Thus, cancer is a genetic disease.[6,20] Virtually every possible genetic lesion has been associated with one or another form of cancer. This is not to say that cancer is always an inherited disease. Often, the genetic lesions associated with cancer are somatic cell mutations.[11] Nevertheless, it has been through the study of inherited cancers that a great deal of knowledge about cancer has been gained.

In general, there are two kinds of cancer inheritance, one in which the damage to the gene or genes involved contributes directly to tumorigenesis, and one in which tumorigenesis is secondary to the genetic lesion.[11] Two examples of the second type are particularly instructive. The first is xeroderma pigmentosa (XP). In this condition, the biochemical defect caused by the mutation is the impaired ability to repair damage to DNA induced by ultraviolet light. Individuals with XP have an extremely high incidence of skin cancer, which can be diminished to some extent by minimizing exposure to sunlight and other sources of ultraviolet radiation. This condition strongly suggests that damage to DNA, or mutation, causes the cancers seen in these individuals.[5]

Another genetic lesion that leads to increased risk of cancer is Down syndrome, or trisomy 21 (Fig. 21–1).[29] Individuals with this disorder have about a 20-fold increased risk of developing childhood leukemia, although the risk of developing other forms of cancer appears to be normal, and the increased risk of adult leukemia is also normal. In this case, the increased risk is associated with the presence of three copies instead of the normal two of the normal complement of genes carried on chromosome 21. Three separate genes have been found on chromosome 21 that may be related to this increased incidence of leukemia,[8,18,21] and one has been identified that is clearly associated with leukemia associated with a chromosomal rearrangement of chromosome 21 that disrupts the gene.[8,17] It is currently unclear whether an extra copy of one or of more than one gene located on chromosome 21 leads to the increased risk of leukemia. In any case, this increased risk would seem to demonstrate clearly that rather subtle genetic changes of a quantitative nature can lead to

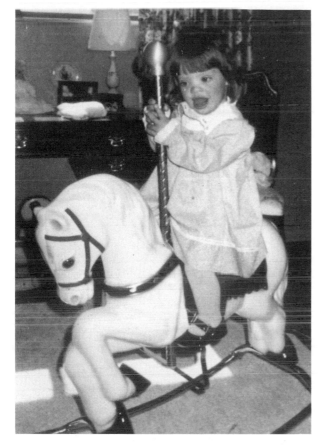

Fig. 21–1.   A child with Down syndrome (trisomy 21). Individuals with this chromosomal disorder have an increased risk of 10 to 20-fold of developing childhood leukemia.

cancer, and that these changes need not damage an individual gene.

Because cancer is a disease in which cells of the tumor undergo unregulated or abnormally regulated growth, genetic lesions that interfere with the normal mechanisms of cellular growth control would seem likely causes of cancer. This hypothesis has now been amply verified. There are, in general, two mechanisms by which this occurs. First, mutations can occur that enhance cell growth directly. These can be thought of as dominant mutations. Second, mutations that eliminate activities that suppress cell growth have been found.

ALTERATIONS IN PROTO-ONCOGENES

Mutations that lead to cancer occur in genes that appear to have some role in controlling cell growth and/or cellular phenotype. The normal counterparts of these genes are called proto-oncogenes. By now there are over 60 proto-oncogenes or suspected proto-oncogenes.[3] So far, they fall into three classes as determined by mode of action, all of which appear to be important for regulation of cell growth. The first type, protein kinases, are genes that control the activities of other proteins by phosphorylation. The second mechanism by which oncogenes have been shown to act is as signal transducers of various types. Finally, there are the transcription factors, which control expression of other genes. This is certainly not meant to imply that other mechanisms for the action of oncogenes will not be found.

Several different types of mutations have been found to cause transformation by this mechanism. The mutations are called dominant because, at the cellular level at least, the mutant functions in the presence of the normal gene product. Occasionally, this appears to be caused by a gain of function. Many different mechanisms can lead to this "gain-of-function" type of mutation. It should be kept in mind that loss of a negative function also appears as a gain of function. Such mutations have also been observed.

One of the common features of most tumors is that they are chromosomally abnormal. In fact, study of chromosomal abnormalities in tumors has provided major insights into tumorigenesis. Often, particular specific chromosomal rearrangements are associated with specific malignancies, and occasionally there are particular chromosomal rearrangements that are essentially always present in particular tumors, either in the presence of other chromosome rearrangements or alone. One example is Burkitt's lymphoma. This tumor is virtually always associated with a translocation between chromosome 8 and chromosome 14 (Fig. 21–2). Detailed molecular analysis of this tumor has revealed that a proto-oncogene, the c-myc gene, normally located on chromosome 8, is juxtaposed with one of the immunoglobulin genes on chromosome 14 in this tumor.[6,7,25] This translocation provokes in-

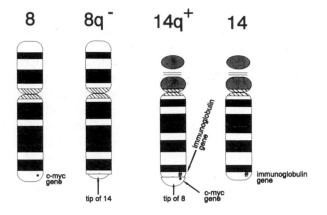

Fig. 21–2. The 8;14 chromosomal translocation associated with Burkitt's lymphoma. This translocation, which is by far the most common (>90% of cases) translocation associated with Burkitt's lymphoma, juxtaposes the c-myc proto-oncogene normally on chromosome 8 with an immunoglobulin gene on chromosome 14, presumably leading to aberrant regulation of the c-myc gene and malignancy.

creased transcription of the c-myc gene and hence increased production of its gene product. Although the evidence is not yet conclusive, it now appears that the product of the myc gene is a transcription factor, so it regulates the activity of other genes.[3] Thus the presence of increased amounts of the normal myc gene product may have a pleiotropic effect and lead to aberrant growth control.

Interestingly, a completely separate mechanism of increasing the amount of the myc-gene product present in cells has also been found to play a role in malignancy, namely amplification of the myc gene. In this case, the number of copies of the myc gene increases from the normal two to up to several hundred. This has been observed, for example, in carcinoma of the lung, breast, and cervix. Mechanisms of gene amplification are unclear, but it does seem that the phenomenon is much more common in malignant cells and that it takes place more easily in cells in which it has already taken place.

Gene amplification was first observed as a mechanism by which mammalian cells can become resistant to the killing action of certain drugs. The first documented case was resistance to the anticancer drug methotrexate.[1] It now seems clear that gene amplification can play a role in the resistance tumors often de-

velop to such drugs used in treatment as well as in the development of malignancy itself.[2,4,26]

Point mutation in individual proto-oncogenes has also been documented. This was done originally using an elegant set of somatic cell genetic and molecular biologic experiments as follows. It is known that most normal mammalian cells show the phenomenon of contact inhibition. Thus, when they are grown in tissue culture on the surface of a tissue culture dish, they grow only to a monolayer of cells and do not pile up on top of one another. Malignant cells, on the other hand, pile up. In a population of normal cells with a few malignant cells, the malignant cells are relatively easily recognized because they form a focus of piled-up cells easily visible on the background monolayer.

Given this observation, the experiment was to add DNA isolated from a malignant human cell, in this case a bladder carcinoma, to normal mouse cells growing in culture using a procedure known to allow the foreign DNA to become incorporated in a functional way into the recipient cells. In any particular recipient cell, however, there is only a small fraction of the input human genome. One then waits for the appearance of transformed foci, grows these up, and isolates the human DNA from these cells on the basis of its containing human DNA-specific repeated DNA sequences. This human DNA should be highly enriched for the transforming gene. Eventually, by two or more rounds of transformation, one should be able to isolate the specific human gene capable of transforming the mouse cells.

When this experiment was carried out, the human proto-oncogene H-ras was isolated (Fig. 21–3). On determining the DNA sequence of the gene, however, it was found to have a single base change leading to a specific amino acid substitution in the H-ras protein.[19,24,24a,27] Many different isolates of transforming ras genes have now been obtained, but the number of sites at which the protein is mutated in these is very limited. Mutant genes have been isolated directly from tumor tissue without in vitro cell culture. This and many other experiments clearly demonstrate that these

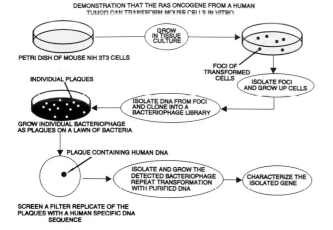

DEMONSTRATION THAT THE RAS ONCOGENE FROM A HUMAN
TUMOR CAN TRANSFORM MOUSE CELLS IN VITRO

Fig. 21–3.   Isolation of the human oncogene H-ras, taking advantage of its ability to transform mouse 3T3 cells in tissue culture.

point mutations are important for development of the malignant phenotype of some human tumors. Unfortunately, thus far the mechanism by which the limited number of specific mutations observed in the ras gene family in a large number of different types of human tumors has not yet led to a coherent idea of the role of the mutated ras protein in tumorigenesis.

ALTERATIONS IN TUMOR-SUPPRESSOR GENES

Tumor-suppressor genes can be defined as genes that encode proteins which normally suppress tumor formation. Thus, when these genes are damaged or removed, a tumor may result. Tumor-suppressor genes are theoretically predicted to be recessive; that is, one functional copy of the gene should be sufficient to suppress tumor growth. This means that damage to both copies of a particular tumor suppressor is essential for tumorigenesis.

Three different lines of evidence first suggested the existence of tumor suppressor genes. In one set of experiments, it was demonstrated that somatic cell hybrids between transformed or malignant cells and normal cells occasionally lost the transformed or malignant phenotype. This implied that some normal gene could suppress the cancer phenotype.

Moreover, loss of normal chromosomes was found to correlate with restoration of malignancy. In fact, by this method, specific chromosomes were identified as carrying putative tumor suppressor genes.[22,27]

A second line of evidence for tumor suppressor genes comes from the existence of rare autosomal-dominant, inherited cancer syndromes such as familial retinoblastoma. In these situations, families have been found in which an otherwise sporadic tumor appears to be inherited as an autosomal dominant genetic condition.

Retinoblastoma provides the most straightforward example. In this case, up to 30% of children have bilateral or multicentric tumors.[9] Moreover, children with bilateral tumors have an earlier age of onset than children with unilateral tumors, and a familial history of the disease. These observations led to the Knudson two-hit hypothesis to explain such situations.[13] Briefly, the hypothesis is that it requires two genetic lesions for a retinoblastoma to develop. In cases of bilateral disease, one of these was hypothesized to be a germline mutation. Then, a second mutation inactivating the other copy of the same gene could occur in a particular somatic cell in a differentiating organ like the retina and give rise to a tumor.

This hypothesis has been amply demonstrated for retinoblastoma. As is often the case, a chromosomal anomaly was important in identifying the gene important for retinoblastoma. It was observed that, in some cases of bilateral disease, there was a constitutive deletion of chromosome region 13q14. Moreover, occasionally, sporadic tumors could be observed with 13q14 deletions. This suggested the presence of a gene in this chromosome region that, when present in one copy in the normal state, could suppress formation of retinoblastoma. This hypothesis received two additional types of support. It was found that in sporadic retinoblastoma, the chromosome region around 13q14 was identical on both chromosomes 13 in the tumor, even though in the other somatic cells of the patient this

*Also see references within reference 9.

region of the chromosome was different on the two different chromosomes. This observation was consistent with mutation of one allele of the retinoblastoma gene and subsequent loss of the normal allele. Indeed, it was later found, in two families in which the disease was inherited, that it was the chromosome region from the nonaffected parent that was lost in the tumor.

This homogenization of regions of chromosomes associated with tumors is called loss of heterozygosity. It represents the third original bit of evidence supporting the concept of tumor-suppressor genes. By now, the retinoblastoma gene has been isolated in its normal and mutant forms, and this analysis has completely verified the concept of tumor-suppressor genes.[12]

Analysis of other familial tumors has been more complex and has given additional insight into the genetics of cancer. Wilms tumor of the kidney is a pediatric tumor that shares some of the characteristics of retinoblastoma. The disease can occur in unilateral and bilateral forms. Occasionally, bilateral Wilms tumor occurs in conjunction with mental retardation, aniridia, and urogenital abnormalities (WAGR syndrome). A deletion of chromosome region 11p13 is associated with some cases of WAGR syndrome. Loss of heterozygosity of this region can be observed in some sporadic tumors. A gene, WT1, which appears to be a Wilms tumor-suppressor gene, has been isolated from 11q13. The product of this gene shares structural features characteristic of a transcription factor.[9]

However, this situation is complicated by the observations that some Wilms tumor patients seem to show chromosomal loss of heterozygosity in 11p15, but have no detected abnormalities in 11p13. Moreover, rarely familial Wilms tumors appear not to be linked to a gene in either of these chromosome locations but to a third gene located elsewhere.[9] These observations are evidence that cancer may often involve a cascade of several defects in different genes. This will be discussed in more detail later.

Retinoblastoma and Wilms tumor are extremely instructive regarding the genetics of cancer. They are, however, relatively rare pediatric tumors. Similar mechanisms do seem to apply to much more common cancers such as lung and colon cancer, and most recently breast cancer.

Some investigators estimate that 5 to 10% of breast cancer is caused by inherited factors. Roughly 150,000 cases are diagnosed each year, and over 40,000 will die from the disease.[10,28] It now appears that, in a select group of families in which breast cancer segregates in an autosomal dominant fashion and in which the disease is bilateral and has an early age of onset, a gene in the chromosomal region 17q21 is likely to be responsible.[10] Although this is extremely provocative from mechanistic and research points of view, it represents a small fraction of all breast cancer cases. Interestingly, though, loss of heterozygosity of loci in this region of chromosome 17 appears to occur in over 60% of sporadic cases of breast cancer analyzed.[14] This brings up the possibility that the gene responsible for the hereditary cases may also be involved in the etiology of the sporadic cases of breast cancer as well. If so, identification of this gene may improve treatment and diagnosis of breast cancer in the majority of cases.

A relatively simple molecular test has been devised that can detect mutation in the ras oncogene in stool samples of patients with colorectal tumors[23] (Fig. 21–4). The test is apparently sensitive enough to detect the presence of nonmalignant, curable tumors. Unfortunately, these ras mutations occur in only 30 to 40% of tumors. Nonetheless, this work demonstrates the potential for understanding of the genetic lesions associated with a particular tumor to lead to simple, noninvasive tests for tumors while they are still curable (i.e., by surgery).

In some families, several types of cancer appear to be hereditary. The first of these for which the genetic lesion has been identified is the Li-Fraumeni syndrome[15] (Fig. 21–5). In these families, the probability of developing invasive cancer reaches roughly 50% by age 30. Both childhood and adult cancers are involved. It has now been shown that a single base substitution in the gene encoding the p53

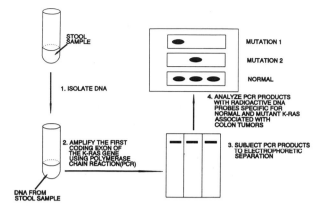

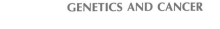

Fig. 21-4. A noninvasive molecular test for RAS mutation. In this assay, DNA is isolated from stool samples of
individuals suspected of having colon cancer (Step 1). The
polymerase chain reaction (PCR) is then used to amplify
the DNA region corresponding to the K-rase oncogene (Step
2). The amplification yields DNA fragments of different sizes,
depending on whether the K-ras gene is normal or carries
mutations associated with malignancy (Step 3). In Step 4,
the different-sized DNA fragments are detected after separation using a radioactive K-ras DNA probe (see reference
23 for details).

protein is the cause of this syndrome. The
mutation appears to inactivate one copy of the
gene in affected individuals.

Many lessons regarding the genetics of cancer can be learned from this finding. Breast
cancer is the most common tumor found in
individuals with Li-Fraumeni syndrome.
Moreover, p53 mutations are often present in
many forms of sporadic cancer, including breast
cancer. The mutations in p53 apparently inactivate the protein. Apparently, certain mutations of p53 cause inactivation of a single
allele, a phenomenon called dominant
suppression, or dominant negative mutation.
Tumors occur in many tissues and over many
years in Li-Fraumeni patients. This suggests
that other mutations may be necessary for the
occurrence of these various tumors.

Instability of Cancer Cells

Taken as a whole, the studies done thus far
suggest that the phenomenon of tumor progression may be attributable to the appearance of several different genetic lesions over
the lifetime of a tumor. Indeed, much evi
dence suggests that a hallmark of cancer cells

may be that they are relatively unstable genetically. Thus, the initial genetic lesions might
be responsible for changing a normal cell into
one that escapes normal growth control but is
nonmalignant, with subsequent changes leading inexorably to a more malignant state, and
perhaps to drug resistance as well. A proposed model of progression for astrocytoma has
been presented Mikkelsen, Cairncross, and
Cavenee and is presented in Figure 21-6.
Variations of this model could apply to many
different tumors.[16]

It is clear that the study of cancer genetics
has allowed fundamental insights into how
cancer arises and evolves. Many different genes
have been identified and demonstrated to be
involved in the malignant process. As yet, in
no case is the entire process fully understood.
Although the process seems complex, the
progress made has already allowed improved
detection of cancer cells based on knowledge
of molecular rearrangements associated with
particular cancers. As our knowledge of the
process and the genes involved increases, the

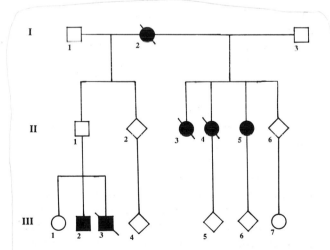

Fig. 21-5. Pedigree of a family afflicted with Li-Fraumeni
syndrome. In this family, individual II-5 shows a germ line
mutation in the p53 gene. A tumor sample from this individual shows loss of the remaining normal p53 gene. Individual I-2 developed carcinoma of the ampulla of Vater
at age 47 and bladder carcinoma at age 53; II-3, ovarian
germ cell carcinoma at age 16; II-4, soft tissue sarcoma at
age 21; II-5, unilateral breast carcinoma at age 34; III-2,
osteosarcoma at age 20; III-3, brain tumor at age 16. Reproduced with permission from Malkin, D., et al.: Germ
line p53 mutations in a familial syndrome of breast cancer,
sarcomas, and other neoplasms. Science 250:1233, 1990.

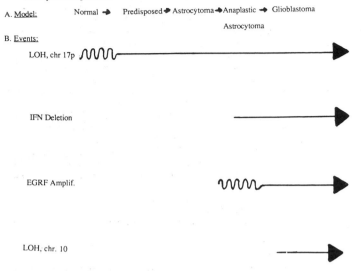

Astrocytoma Progression

A. Model: Normal → Predisposed → Astrocytoma → Anaplastic → Glioblastoma
                                                    Astrocytoma

B. Events:

LOH, chr 17p

IFN Deletion

EGRF Amplif.

LOH, chr. 10

Fig. 21–6.   Proposed genetic alterations leading to malignant progression of astrocytoma. Progression of normal neuroglial cells to malignant astrocytoma (from left to right in this figure) is hypothesized to involve the accumulation of several genetic alterations in the tumor cell lineage. The first event is hypothesized to be loss of heterozygosity of a region of chromosome 17p, followed by deletion of the interferon betagene, amplification of the EGRF gene, and then loss of heterozygosity of a region of chromosome 10. After each lesion, the cells become more malignant. Reproduced with permission from Mikkelsen, T., et al.: Genetics of the malignant progression of astrocytoma. J. Cell. Biochem. 46:3, 1991.

challenge clearly will be to apply this knowledge to improved detection, treatment, and eventually prevention of human cancer.

SUMMARY

Cancer is a disease in which cells of the body lose their normal growth control properties. It is now clear that the vast majority of, and perhaps all, cancer is caused by genetic alterations in the affected cells. Over the last several decades, it has been possible to define specific chromosomal lesions associated with specific malignancies and in some cases to identify the genes altered in these cases. Indeed, specific mutations in cellular genes, proto-oncogenes, have been found that lead to malignancy. Specific types of functions have been assigned to the products of these genes, and both dominant and recessive mutations have been found that lead to malignancy. Study of hereditary cancers such as retinoblastoma and Wilms tumor has led to elucidation of mechanisms by which germline and somatic mutations may interact to lead to cancer. Medical research is now using the powerful tools of molecular biology to understand common cancers like those of the breast, lung, and colon, and genes important for the progression of malignancies are being identified.[30] This knowledge is being applied rapidly to im-

proved accuracy and simplicity of diagnosis of cancer. There is reason to believe that, in the near future, understanding of the genetics of cancer will lead to major advances in diagnosis, treatment, and prevention of this disease.

REFERENCES

1. Alt, F.W., et al.: Selective multiplication of dihydrofolate reductase genes in methotrexate-resistant variants of cultured murine cells. J. Biol. Chem. 253:1357, 1978.
2. Bertino, J.R., et al.: Gene amplification and altered enzymes as mechanisms for the development of drug resistance. Cancer Treat. Rep. 67:901, 1983.
3. Bishop, J.M.: Molecular themes in oncogenesis. Cell 64:235, 1991.
4. Brodeur, G.M., et al.: Amplification of N-*myc* in untreated human neuroblastomas correlates with advanced disease stage. Science 224:1121, 1984.
5. Cleaver, J.E.: Defective repair replication of DNA in xeroderma pigmentosum. Nature (Lond.) 218:652, 1968.
6. Croce, C.M.: Genetic approaches to the study of the molecular basis of human cancer. Cancer Res. (Suppl.) 51:5015s, 1991.
7. Dalla-Favera, R., et al.: Human c-*myc onc* gene is located on the region of chromosome 8 that is translocated in Burkitt lymphoma cells. Proc. Natl. Acad. Sci. USA 79:7824, 1982.
8. Gao, J., et al.: Isolation of a yeast artificial chromosome spanning the 8;21 translocation breakpoint t(8;21)(q22;q22.3) in acute myelogenous leukemia. Proc. Natl. Acad. Sci. USA 88:4882, 1991.
9. Haber, D.A., and Housman, D.E.: Rate-limiting steps: The genetics of pediatric cancers. Cell 64:5, 1991.
10. Hall, J.M., et al.: Linkage of early-onset familial breast cancer to chromosome 17q21. Science 250:1684, 1990.

11. Harris, C.C.: Chemical and physical carcinogenesis: Advances and perspectives for the 1990s. Cancer Res. (Suppl.) 51:5023a, 1991.

12. Horowitz, J.M., et al.: Point mutational inactivation of the retinoblastoma antioncogene. Science 243:937, 1989.

13. Knudson, A.G.: Mutation and cancer: Statistical study of retinoblastoma. Proc. Natl. Acad. Sci. USA 68:820, 1971.

14. Leone, A., et al.: Somatic allelic deletion of nm23 in human cancer. Cancer Res. 51:2490, 1991.

15. Malkin, D., et al.: Germ line p53 mutations in a familial syndrome of breast cancer, sarcomas, and other neoplasms. Science 250:1233, 1990.

16. Mikkelsen, T., et al.: Genetics of the malignant progression of astrocytoma. J. Cell. Biochem. 46:3, 1991.

17. Miyoshi, H.: t(8;21) breakpoints on chromosome 21 in acute myeloid leukemia are clustered within a limited region of a single gene, AML1. Proc. Natl. Acad. Sci. USA 88:10431, 1991.

18. Rao, V.N., et al.: The human erg gene maps to chromosome 21, band q22: Relationship to the 8;21 translocation of acute myelogenous leukemia. Oncogene 3:497, 1988.

19. Reddy, E.P., et al.: A point mutation is responsible for the acquisition of transforming properties by the T24 human bladder carcinoma oncogene. Nature 300:149, 1982.

20. Rowley, J.D.: Identification of the constant chromosome regions involved in human hematologic malignant disease. Science 216:749, 1982.

21. Sacchi, N., et al.: Hu ets-1 and Hu-ets-2 genes are transposed in acute leukemias with (4;11) and (8;21) translocations. Science 231:379, 1986.

22. Sager, R.: Tumor suppressor genes: The puzzle and the promise. Science 246:1406, 1989.

23. Sidransky, D., et al.: Identification of ras oncogene mutations in the stool of patients with curable colorectal tumors. Science 256:102, 1992.

24. Tabin, C., et al.: Mechanism of activation of a human oncogene. Nature 300:143, 1982.

24a. Taparowsky, E., et al.: Activation of T24 bladder carcinoma transforming gene is linked to a single amino acid change. Nature 300:762, 1982.

25. Taub, R., et al.: Translocation of the c-myc gene into the immunoglobulin heavy chain locus in human Burkitt lymphoma and murine plasmacytoma cells. Proc. Natl. Acad. Sci. USA 79:7837, 1982.

26. Trent, J.M., et al.: Cytologic evidence for gene amplification in methotrexate-resistant cells obtained from a patient with ovarian adenocarcinoma. J. Clin. Oncol. 2:8, 1984.

27. Weinberg, R.A.: Tumor suppressor genes. Science 254:1138, 1991.

28. Wright, K.: Breast cancer: Two steps closer to understanding. Science 250:1659, 1990.

29. Zipursky, A., et al.: Hematologic and oncologic disorders in down syndrome. In: Down Syndrome. Advances in Medical Care. Edited by I.T. Lott and E.E. McCoy. New York, Wiley-Liss, 1992.

30. Note added in proof: New developments in colon and breast cancer are discussed on page 9.

Chapter 22
Genetics of Behavior

Man's behavior is probably his most important phenotypic feature, but little is known of its genetic basis. Much of human behavioral genetics deals with normal behavioral traits, such as intelligence, to which the approach has been mainly quantitative, with the emphasis largely on estimates of heritability rather than on the identification of specific segregating factors. An area of increasing interest concerns behavioral traits that deviate sharply from the mean, such as mental retardation resulting from mutant genes and chromosomal aberrations, in which there is a better opportunity to identify specific genes and their biochemical effects. The common behavioral disorders, such as the psychoses and "nonspecific" mental retardation, may be in transit from one to the other. Early studies emphasized their multifactorial nature and contributed heritability estimates; emphasis is now shifting to the identification of specific genetic factors contributing to the final result.

One would expect that genes affecting "normal" behavior would be subtle in their effects and that the primary biochemical effect of the gene at the polypeptide level might be far removed from the behavioral effect. Thus the gene controlling the ability to detect the bitter taste of phenylthiocarbamide presumably affects some enzyme, but it would be hard to deduce the existence of the PTC polymorphism from a genetic study of preference for cabbage or some other food that contains this chemical. Nevertheless, some functional defects resulting in behavioral differences do have a fairly simple genetic basis, such as the specific dyslexias, and some have contributed significantly to the elucidation of normal function, e.g., the defects of color vision. On the other hand, the psychologic effects of phenylketonuria or trisomy 21 will teach us no more about the genetics of normal behavior than tone-deafness will about the genetics of musical ability, or throwing a wrench into a moving engine will teach us about its function.

Pathologic Genes. Several pathologic genes have more or less specific effects on behavior.[1] The phenylketonuric child (untreated) is hyperactive and irritable and has an uncontrollable temper, abnormal postural attitudes, and agitated behavior. About 10% show psychotic behavior. As multiple discriminant analysis of a number of test scores permits discrimination of PKU children from those with other types of mental retardation, the biochemical defect must have certain specific effects on behavior, from which we should be able to learn something. At least the wrench is always thrown into the same part of the engine, so the resulting damage may tell us something of the mechanism. Similarly, characteristic behavioral changes often precede the choreic movements in Huntington disease. Congenital cretinism, which may be recessively inherited, produces its familiar effects on personality. Perhaps the most striking example of a gene-induced behavioral defect is the bizarre tendency to self-mutilation in the Lesch-Nyhan syndrome. We are still far removed from a complete understanding of the relation between the gene-determined biochemical change and the behavioral response, but the rapid advances being made in neurobiochemistry may make this approach rewarding,[16] as will those of molecular genetics—for example, the effect of "knocking out" the thymidine kinase gene on memory (Chap. 11).

Finally, information from animal experiments tells us that mutant genes known by their prominent effects on the physical phenotype, such as albinism, may have much more indirect and subtle effects on behavior, such as docility. Thus a particular behavioral parameter, such as aggression, may be influenced by the indirect effects of a large number of genes with major effects on other traits. In this sense, the genetic basis of the behavioral trait is polygenic.

Chromosomal Aberrations. Chromosomal aberrations also have effects on behavior.[12] Children with Down syndrome tend to be happier and more responsive to their environment than other children of comparable IQ, and they are often musical. Girls with Turner syndrome rate high on verbal IQ tests but lower on performance and seem to have a deficit in perceptual organization.

The psychologic effects of the XYY karyotype has been a subject of heated debate.[8,12] The original suggestion that there are psychologic effects came from a study designed by a Scottish cytogeneticist, Patricia Jacobs, to test the hypothesis that an extra Y chromosome predisposes to aggressiveness. If this were so, males with an extra Y chromosome should have an increased frequency among those of a vi-

olent nature, such as criminals, and a survey of mentally subnormal men with dangerous, violent or criminal propensities in special security institution did, indeed, find a high frequency of the XYY karyotype (7/197). This finding suggested that the XYY karyotype predisposes to criminality. It is not yet clear how. The original study specifically stated that it was not clear whether the increased frequency of XYY males in the institution was related to their aggressive behavior or to their mental deficiency. It was also noted that the XYY males were unusually tall, and subsequent studies of XYY males were made at first mainly in groups selected for tallness and aggression, such as prisoners, and were not representative of XYY men in general. Unfortunately, these findings resulted in some sensational publicity, such as stories about "the criminal chromosome," whereas we still do not know what proportion of XYY males develop anti social behavior, or why. A large study in Denmark which karyotyped a population of tall men ascertained from population records confirmed the association of XYY with height and criminality, but the antisocial behavior did not seem to be a secondary result of the increase in height.[17] The crimes committed tend to be against property rather than people. The XYY men also showed a somewhat decreased score on an Army selection test for intelligence, and low intelligence may be the basis for the predisposition to criminality, rather than aggressiveness or a lowered anxiety threshold, as previously suggested.

When a sex chromosome anomaly is found, either pre- or postnatally, the facts should be discussed frankly with the parents. Results of several prospective studies are now becoming available to provide the necessary information. Although numbers are small, they seem to refute the impression that children with sex chromosome aneuploidies (not including Turner syndrome) have appreciable mental retardation, but they do have an increased risk for developmental problems. It is noteworthy that language and motor deficits and learning problems are less frequent in the group diagnosed prenatally, suggesting that environmental factors may have an important influence on outcome. Prenatally diagnosed babies in one study were more likely to have parents with higher socio-economic status, and therefore likely to be "wanted babies," which may significantly affect their development.[14]

Intelligence. Much of the early work on the genetics of intelligence has considered it as an entity, measured more or less accurately by a variety of performance tests, more or less "culture free." The heritability of "IQ" is discussed elsewhere in Chapter 26. More recently the trend has been toward identification and description of its various components, and this provides an opportunity for defining more specifically the genetic basis for these components.[1]

Several twin studies of specific cognitive abilities suggest that many have a substantial genetic component, but some do not—creativity, for example.[1,12]

Dyslexia. The original concept of dyslexia as simply a reading impairment in children of normal intelligence is now considered simplistic. Dyslexic children are impaired to varying extents in many language skills, and have short-term memory impairments. Twin studies show high heritability for ability to retain sounds in memory, and there are a number of striking autosomal-dominant pedigrees.[4]

Stuttering. Stuttering is another common behavioral trait with a complex etiology.[3] It is more frequent in males (about 4%) than females (1 or 2%). There is a 20 to 25% frequency in fathers, brothers, and sons of male probands, and a 5 to 10% frequency in mothers, sisters, and daughters of male probands, with somewhat higher frequencies in the relatives of female probands. The frequency in sibs is increased if the proband's parent also stuttered—to about 35% for the brothers of male probands, for example. The frequency of stuttering in monozygotic co-twins of stutterers is 75%. Contrary to previous claims, there is no association with left-handedness. The data support a genetic basis for the condition and are compatible with a multifactorial threshold model, with a polygenic genetic contribution, or a single major locus with reduced penetrance.

Psychoneuroses. The psychoneuroses are so common that they might almost be considered normal; their genetic basis is correspondingly complex. The few twin and family studies available agree that the psychoneuroses are familial, with some degree of specificity for subtypes; i.e., if the proband has an anxiety state, most of the affected relatives have an anxiety state, and there is a similar correspondence for hysteria and obsessional neurosis.[7]

THE MAJOR PSYCHOSES

The genetics of the major psychoses is too vast a subject to be dealt with adequately here. The early literature is confused by differences in diagnostic criteria, but recent advances in understanding of the biology and pharmacology of the psychoses are beginning to clarify the picture.

The affective disorders (mania and depression) and schizophrenia are distinguishable by their clinical features, pharmacologic responses, and family distribution. Family, twin, and adoption studies suggest a genetic liability,[10] which appears stronger in the affective disorders. Attempts to map the responsible genes are confounded by genetic heterogeneity and reduced penetrance, and no clear pattern has emerged as yet.[7]

The Affective Disorders. These disorders are strongly familial, with segregation patterns suggesting dominant inheritance with reduced penetrance. There is clearly an X-linked dominant type in up to one third of families. Claims for linkage to autosomal loci (on 11, in particular) are equivocal.[7] The average recurrence risks derived from several studies suggest that bipolar (mania and depression or mania alone) and unipolar (depression alone) affective disorder are genetically related. First-degree relatives of a proband with the bipolar type have about a 7% risk for bipolar and a 7% risk for unipolar disorders, for a total risk of about 14%. For first-degree relatives of a unipolar proband, the risks are about 1% for bipolar and 6% for unipolar disorder. These figures would be substantially higher (about 2×) if both a sib and a parent are affected.[6]

Schizophrenias. The familial nature of schizophrenia is generally recognized, but there has been considerable argument about whether the increased risk for relatives of schizophrenics results from genetic or cultural factors. Recent evidence from adoption studies in Denmark strongly favor the genetic side.[6] A large sample of adults was identified who had been adopted at an early age. Of these, 34 were schizophrenic. The frequency of schizophrenia was then measured in the parents, sibs, and half-sibs of the biologic and the adoptive families. All diagnoses were made without knowledge of which group the individual belonged to. The frequency of definite schizophrenia was much higher in the biologic relatives (6%) than in the adoptive "relatives" (1%). If one includes "uncertain" cases, these numbers rise to 14% and 3%. These rates could hardly be caused by cultural factors in common, as the proband did not share the environment of the biologic relatives.

Possible maternal uterine effects were ruled out by study of paternal half-sibs, who share the same father but have different uterine environments. The frequency of schizophrenic disorders was 22% in the biological paternal half-sibs and 3% in the adoptive paternal half-sibs. Thus there seems to be no doubt that there is a genetic basis for susceptibility to schizophrenia.

Empiric risk figures for near relatives of schizophrenics run about 10 to 15% for sibs, 15% for children of one schizophrenic parent, and 35 to 70% for children of two affected parents.[7] For second-degree relatives, the risk is about 2%. The mode of inheritance is obviously complex. A biochemical marker of the gene(s) for susceptibility would clarify the picture, but, in spite of many claims, none has been found. There appears to be a major locus on chromosome 11q in some families.[5]

Childhood autism seems to have a low recurrence risk and does not behave genetically as a form of schizophrenia.

HOMOSEXUALITY

The situation for homosexuality is unclear. Early studies showing a high concordance of homosexuality in monozygotic twins probably suffered from biases of ascertainment, but more recent twin and family studies still suggest that there is a genetic component.[13]

The finding that a hypothalamic nucleus shows sexual dimorphism (being smaller in females), and that this nucleus is as small in homosexual males as it is in females may, if substantiated, help to clarify the situation.[11]

ALCOHOLISM

For alcoholism, several family studies show a familial tendency; twin studies show that monozygotic pairs have a higher concordance (55%) than dizygotic pairs, but dizygotic pairs also have a fairly high rate (28%).[2] Adoption studies show a striking increase in alcoholism (17%) in the children of alcoholics, who were adopted in infancy by nonalcoholic couples. A large Swedish adoption study suggests two major subtypes, type I being "milieu-limited" and type II "male-limited." Type II has an earlier age of onset, more spontaneous alcohol seeking, more alcohol-related conflicts with the law, less psychologic dependence, less guilt and fear, and a personality that is characterized by high novelty seeking and low harm avoidance and reward dependence. It is highly heritable from father to son; in type I the genetic influence is weaker. Recent progress is summarized by Devor and Cloninger.[2]

PSYCHOPATHY AND CRIMINALITY

Family studies of psychopathy and criminality show that most children with antisocial behavior come from broken homes; thus it is impossible to tell from such studies how much of the antisocial behavior in these children is biologically transmitted and how much culturally acquired. Twin studies seem to have been devoted more to criminality than to the broader category of psychopathy. Monozygotic pairs show a higher concordance rate than dizygotic pairs, but it is clear that criminality must be a highly heterogeneous category. Adoption studies have provided further support for a genetic predisposition. There are undoubtedly predisposing factors, such as EEG abnormalities, low IQ, chromosomal anomalies, and the so-called constitutional psychopathic state—criminals tend to be predominantly mesomorphic. Each of these factors is under some degree of genetic control. This accounts for at least part of the estimated heritability. However, the major group contributing to criminality are those classified as having a psychopathic or sociopathic personality, and the genetics of this condition is still almost completely obscure. In any case, the role of the environment is clearly of major importance in criminality.

ALZHEIMER DISEASE

Most cases of late-onset Alzheimer dementia are sporadic, although there may be a genetic predisposition interacting with environmental factors. Among early-onset cases there is a subset that shows autosomal inheritance with some reduction in penetrance.[15] Within this group there is clearly genetic heterogeneity. In numerous families, there is a mutation in exon 17 of the β-amyloid precursor protein (APP) gene, located on chromosome 21. β-amyloid is the protein that accumulates in the neurofibrillary tangles present in the brains of patients with Alzheimer disease.[9]

PERSONALITY

Finally, there is the question of personality and whether it has any genetic basis. The question is of some eugenic interest in this time of population crisis. For instance, if personality traits such as aggression and altruism were genetically determined, one would expect the former to be selected for and the latter selected against because the altruistic would be more likely to limit their family size than the aggressive.

Personality may be classified along two relatively independent dimensions: various grades of neuroticism or instability on the one hand, and extroversion-introversion on the other.

Unstable extroverts are more likely to become delinquent; unstable introverts are more likely to become neurotic. Several twin studies have shown higher heritability estimates for these dimensions, both by questionnaire and laboratory measurements. Family studies also show significant correlations between near relatives, and there seems little doubt that heredity is important in determining individual differences in personality.[12] Just how important, and by what mechanisms, remains to be seen.

REFERENCES

1. DeFries, J.C., Vandenberg, S.G., and McLearn, G.E.: Genetics of specific cognitive abilities. Ann. Rev. Genet. 10:179, 1976.
2. Devor, E.J. and Cloninger, R.C.: Genetics of alcoholism. Ann. Rev. Genet. 23:19, 1989.
3. Editorial. Speech dysfluency. Lancet I: 530, 1989.
4. Editorial. Dyslexia. Lancet II: 719, 1989.
5. Fletcher, J.M., et al.: Schizophrenia-associated chromosome 11q21 translocation: Identification of flanking markers and development of chromosome 11q fragment hybrids as clonsing and mapping resources. Am. J. Hum. Genet. 52:478, 1993.
6. Gottesman, I.I.: Schizophrenia genesis: The origins of madness. New York, W.H. Freeman & Co., 1991.
7. Gurling, H.M.D.: Recent advances in the genetics of psychiatric disorder. In Human Genetic Information: Science, Law and Ethics. Ciba Foundation Symposium 149. Chichester, John Wiley and Sons, 1990, p. 48.
8. Hamerton, J.L.: Human population cytogenetics: Dilemmas and problems. Am. J. Hum. Genet. 28:107, 1976.
9. Hardy, J., Chartier-Harlin, M.-C., and Mullan, M.: Alzheimer disease. The new agenda. Am. J. Hum. Genet. 50:648, 1992.
10. Kidd, K.K.: Searching for major genes for psychiatric disorders. Ciba Foundation Symposium on Molecular Approaches to Human Polygenic Disease. Chichester, U.K., John Wiley and Sons, 1987, p. 84.
11. LeVay, S.: A difference in hypothalamic structure between heterosexual and homosexual men. Science 253:1034, 1991.
12. Plomin, R., DeFries, J.C., and McLearn, G.E.: Behaviour Genetics. A Primer. 2nd ed. New York, W.H. Freeman and Co., 1990.
13. Puterbaugh, G. (Ed.): Twins and homosexuality. A casebook. New York, Gorland Publishing, Inc., 1990.
14. Robinson, A., Bender, B.G., and Linden, M.G.: Diagnosis of prenatally diagnosed children with sex chromosome aneuploidy. Am. J. Med. Genet. 44:365, 1992.
15. St. George-Hyslop, P.H., et al.: The genetic defect causing familial Alzheimer's disease maps on Chromosome 21. Science 235:885, 1987.
16. Vogel, F.: Research strategies in human behaviour genetics. J. Med. Genet. 24:129, 1987.

23
Cardiovascular Disease

BLESSED ARE THE PURE IN HEART . . .

MATTHEW 5:8

The familial aspects of cardiovascular disease are well recognized.[14] From the beginning of their clinical clerkships, medical students, learn to ask the routine questions in obtaining the history: is there heart disease, high blood pressure, stroke, diabetes in the family? Frequently the questions are asked in such a routine manner that a positive answer is not awaited. This is especially true of history-taking in families with congenital heart diseases. Often the respondent does not know, for instance, that a cousin died in infancy with transposition of the great vessels. The respondent only knows that the cousin (sibling, aunt) died in infancy. All too often, however, the respondent does know that a relative has a heart lesion—if given the time to answer. To demonstrate this point to students and house officers, we frequently ask the parent of a child with a congenital heart lesion who has a relative whom we have also treated for a heart defect: "Is there anyone else in the family with congenital heart disease?" More often than not, if the question is asked hurriedly, the answer is a hurried no. Then we will ask: "Well, what about his cousin, Joe, didn't he have a heart operation here about 6 years ago when he was a baby?"

Patients try to cooperate and to please their busy physicians. Sometimes this takes the form of giving a quick answer (which may be wrong) to "save the physician's valuable time." An occasional patient will get into the spirit of providing a pleasingly positive family history by creating established diagnoses in relatives when none, in truth, exists. Both types of "memory bias" must be avoided in history-taking. The point is that family histories of cardiovascular diseases as recorded in patients' charts are of little or no value. Even if a statement of a positive family history for a congenital heart disease appears in a chart, it is of minimal value unless the degree of relationship to the proband (sib versus third cousin) is stated and the precise anatomic diagnosis established. Family histories for research purposes must be taken by experienced investigators.

Figure 23–1 is an attempt to visualize the interaction between heredity and environment in the etiology of the four major categories of cardiovascular disease. There are few individuals in any category whose disease would be almost exclusively attributable to either heredity or environment alone.

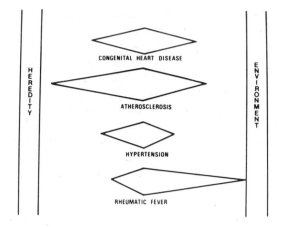

Fig. 23–1. Genetic-environmental interaction and the etiology of the four major categories of cardiovascular disease.

CONGENITAL HEART DISEASES

As has been emphasized in previous chapters, there are essentially three possible genetic bases for a given disease: single mutant gene, chromosomal, and multifactorial. The history of etiologic investigation into congenital heart diseases has followed the devious course pursued by studies of other diseases of complex genetic causation.

Positive family histories in the early decades of this century were interpreted in mendelian terms. Before 1959, if a disease was thought to have a genetic basis, it was a mendelian basis that was considered. Hippocrates and the Doctrine of Diathesis had somehow become obscured. In 1959, the first chromosomal aberration syndromes were recognized, and an effort was made to explain congenital heart diseases on the basis of chromosomal anomalies. Most recently, the cycle has returned to Hippocrates, and data have been accumulated that suggest that most congenital heart lesions are not caused by single mutant genes or by chromosomal aberrations, but appear to be the product of a hereditary predisposition (diathesis) often made manifest by an environmental trigger. About 15% have a chromosomal or mendelian basis and the remaining 85% are presumed to be the result of a genetic-environmental interaction as conceptualized by multifactorial inheritance (encompassing environmental interactions).

Multifactorial Inheritance

Multifactorial inheritance is believed to be the major genetic category in the etiology of congenital heart diseases.[9] It brings together the previously recognized genetic (familial) and the environmentally influenced (e.g., rubella, thalidomide) cases. In the not-too-distant past, the genetic and environmental causes of congenital cardiovascular disease were looked upon as conflicting etiologic interpretations. It is now becoming increasingly obvious that a genetic predisposition to congenital cardiovascular maldevelopment exists in certain families of man and in other animal species, such as mouse and dog.

This predisposition may be visualized in Figure 23–2, in which are inscribed distribution curves. Each one represents a hypothetic genotype with predisposition to a congenital heart lesion—let us say, ventricular septal defect (VSD). The type A family, which is not depicted, has no hereditary predisposition (i.e., it is genetically resistant); the type B family, a moderate predisposition; and the type C family, a marked predisposition. To the far right of the figures is a vertical line representing the threshold of cardiac malforma-

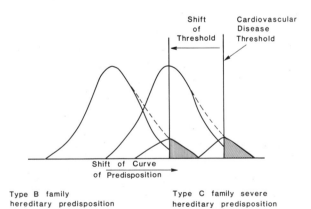

Fig. 23–2. Predisposition to congenital heart disease may be visualized as moderate predisposition (type B family), marked predisposition (type C family). Environmental triggers may be visualized as moving the threshold of predisposition to the left, producing congenital heart disease in a small percentage of individuals in type B families and a larger percentage of individuals in type C families. Blackened areas in type B and type C curves represent the possibility that some cases may follow a mendelian rather than a multifactorial pattern of inheritance.

Table 23–1. Suggested Offspring Recurrence Risk for Congenital Heart Defects Given 1 Affected Parent (percent) (Modified from Nora and Nora[11])

Defect	Father Affected	Mother Affected
Aortic stenosis	3	13–18
Atrial septal defect	1.5	4–4.5
Atrioventricular canal	1	14
Coarctation of aorta	2	4
Patent ductus arteriosus	2.5	3.5–4
Pulmonary stenosis	2	4–6.5
Tetralogy of Fallot	1.5	2.5
Ventricular septal defect	2	6–10

tion *if there is no adverse environmental influence*. The threshold may be moved to the left (or the distribution to the right) by an environmental trigger such as dextroamphetamine or hypoxemia. The important thing is the relationship of the threshold to the distribution. Within the larger curves of the type B and C families are smaller curves that are visualized as representing the possibility that some cases (a small portion of families at risk) follow a mendelian rather than a multifactorial pattern of inheritance.

The type A family is not at risk even when there is maternal exposure to an environmental trigger at the vulnerable period of cardiac development, because their distribution is relatively far from the threshold and most environmental triggers do not push the threshold far enough to the left (or distribution to the right) to cause a congenital heart defect.

To the type B family, it is another story. If there is no adverse environmental influence (threshold to the far right), a congenital heart disease does not usually occur. However, add an environmental trigger and the developing heart is at risk—the threshold moves to the left and produces cardiac maldevelopment in a small proportion of offspring. This may be exemplified by an isogenic animal homology such as the C57/BL6 mouse, which spontaneously has a frequency of VSD of about 1%. This frequency is increased to 11% by dextroamphetamine administration.[11] Type B families represent the vast majority of cases of congenital heart disease.

The type C family illustrates another more marked hereditary predisposition. In this hypothetic example, not only does there appear to be greater risk (with a high frequency of affected offspring) from exposure to environmental triggers, but spontaneous cardiac maldevelopment may occur without a major adverse influence from the environment. What should be recognized is that, in a significant number of high-risk families, a majority of first-degree relatives have congenital heart lesions. The recognition of the prognostic implications of the marked predisposition represented by the type C family is essential if the cardiologist is to offer accurate genetic counseling. What has become apparent is that the risk to offspring of affected mothers is considerably higher than the risk to offspring of affected fathers. The possibility exists that cytoplasmic (or specifically, mitochondrial) inheritance accounts for some high-risk families in which there is maternal transmission to essentially all offspring. The higher risk to offspring of affected mothers may in other instances relate to maternal vulnerability to teratogens, which may or may not be identifiable. Finally, there are clearly mendelian forms of congenital heart disease (as will be discussed), so all of these considerations must enter into the genetic counseling of the so-called type C, high-risk family. Table 23–1, derived from our own investigations combined with data from seven other studies in the literature, shows the substantial difference in risk (2 to 5 times) that we offer to affected parents for recurrence in offspring as related to the sex of the affected parent.[13]

The use of family and twin studies and animal homologies to investigate genetic hypotheses has been presented in Chapters 1 and 24, and the data that favor multifactorial inheritance in the majority of cases of congenital heart disease have been detailed in the literature.[13,14] Therefore, this section will be devoted to empirical and theoretical recurrence risk figures for use in genetic counseling.

As a rule, the more common the cardiovascular lesion, the more likely it is to recur in first-degree relatives. This is consistent with and is predicted by various models of multifactorial inheritance. The risk of ventricular septal defect recurring in a family should be and is much greater than the risk of tricuspid atresia. The next general concept is that if 2 first-degree relatives are affected, the recurrence risk for the next child becomes two to three times as great. If there are three affected first-degree relatives, the recurrence risk is greatly increased. Published empiric risk figures are nonexistent for situations in which three or more members of a single family have congenital heart diseases. These are the type C families (Figure 23–2), and our counseling is that the recurrence risk is likely to be what has already been experienced in the family.

Such counseling may be called into question if one follows theoretic recurrence risks such as those of Smith given in Chapter 13. Please refer to Table 13–1 and note that in high heritability, if the two affected first-degree relatives are parent and sib, the risk is higher than for two affected sibs. To counsel a high recurrence risk if there are no affected parents is not consistent with the usual expectation in multifactorial inheritance *if* one can assume that one or both parents do *not* have a *forme fruste* of the malformation. This assumption is difficult to make for lesions, such as ventricular septal defect, for which there is evidence that 30 to 75% close spontaneously. It is quite likely that there has been spontaneous closure in presumably normal parents of affected children in type C families, and we have some historical evidence of "disappearing murmurs" in such parents. Our position regarding high-risk type C families is to utilize empiric risk data when they exist and theoretic risk data when empiric data are not available. We consider the experience within an individual family to represent the basis for counseling. This concept is essential when one must take into consideration such possibilities as mendelian inheritance, exposure to teratogens, chromosomal microdeletions,[3] and nontraditional inheritance (see Chap. 14).

Nontraditional inheritance is of particular interest as a category of causes of congenital heart diseases as the concepts emerge.[10] Mitochondrial inheritance has the strongest support in epidemiologic data,[10,13] but imprinting may also play a role.[10]

A difficult question that arises in the analysis of families is: What is the underlying mechanism of maldevelopment in a given family? If ventricular septal defect appears to be the anomaly running in the family, is the recurrence risk of 3% the risk for ventricular septal defect alone? Must the population risks for other congenital heart diseases, such as atrial septal defect and patent ductus arteriosus, be added to the empiric risk figure? If the assumption of multifactorial inheritance is correct for a given family, one must also assume an interaction between a genetic predisposition (usually the products of many genes, but perhaps as few as one gene) and an environmental trigger (e.g., drug, virus, maternal nutrition or metabolism, fetal hemodynamics). If the interaction between the same primary gene product "deficiencies" and the same environmental trigger occurs at one gestational age, a ventricular septal defect may result. If the insult is a few days earlier, tetralogy of Fallot could occur or, if a few days later, atrial septal defect could result—*all possibly on the basis of the same genetic predisposition and environmental interaction.*

To stay with the example of ventricular septal defect, human studies and animal experiments do reveal that a specific abnormality tends to run in families. In 30 to 60% of affected sibs of patients with ventricular septal defect, the lesion is also ventricular septal defect, but this means that 40 to 70% of the sibs have another heart lesion. This is similar to what we found in the C57BL/6J mouse with a teratogenic exposure to amphetamine on day 8 of gestation (61% ventricular septal defect; 39% other heart lesions). The closure of the ventricular septum is a critically timed event requiring the simultaneous arrival of contributions from the endocardial cushions, the conus, and the interventricular septum. About 50% of all patients who have congenital cardiovascular lesions have ventricular septal defect alone (25%) or in combination with other anomalies of the heart (25%). But as common as VSD is, it is more of a wonder that 99.5% of older infants do not have persistence of this anomaly because of the critical timing required for the completion of this embryological event. Some mechanism appears to compensate for the failure of the ventricular septum to close at 44 days of conceptional age, which is reflected by the large number of cases of late spontaneous closure.

We assume that the heart lesions in the first-degree relatives are more likely to be related to the same developmental abnormalities rather than to different ones. Clusters of similar anomalies in families appear to support this assumption. A familial recurrence of a heart lesion that apparently bears no developmental relationship to a previously encountered defect may indeed be unrelated (or may be a manifestation of a mechanism of maldevelopment that is obscure to the observer.)

Tables 23–1 and 23–2 list the empiric recurrence risks for congenital cardiovascular malformations derived from a meta-analysis of personal data plus data from the literature. The percentages of suggested risk in the right-hand columns of these two tables are derived from many published sources added together and rounded to the nearest 0.5. In the past, we have relied on our own data exclusively, but we now use combined data in counseling as

Table 23–2. Recurrence Risks in Sibs for any Congenital Heart Defect: Combined Data Published During Two Decades form European and North American Populations. (Modified from Nora and Nora[12]).

Defect	Suggested Risk %	
	if 1 Sib	if 2 Sibs
Venricular septal defect	3	10
Patent ductus	3	10
Atrial septal defect	2.5	8
Tetralogy of Fallot	2.5	8
Pulmonary stenosis	2	6
Coarctation of aorta	2	6
Aortic stenosis	2	6
Transposition	1.5	5
Endocardial cushion	3	10
Fibroelastosis	4	12
Hypoplastic left heart	2	6
Tricuspid atresia	1	3
Ebstein anomaly	1	3
Truncus	1	3
Pulmonary atresia	1	3

providing a broader base of empirical risk. It is useful in genetic counseling to use empirical recurrence risks *when the data base is large enough* and to reserve theoretic risks for those cases in which empiric data are lacking. Thus, the empiric recurrence risk for pulmonary stenosis in a sibling is known and is taken from combined data as 2%. The empiric recurrence risk for anomalous left coronary artery (ALCA) is not known, but for such uncommon lesions a recurrence risk for some form of congenital heart disease of 1% (slightly above the current population risk) is appropriate.

Chromosomal Aberrations

Early investigations sought to link chromosomal anomalies with isolated cardiac malformations (e.g., atrial septal defect), but it has become apparent that, when a congenital heart lesion exists in association with a chromosomal abnormality, it *usually* exists as part of a syndrome of multiple anomalies, such as Down syndrome or the 45, X Turner syndrome. However, a recent study[3] suggests that a chromosomal deletion associated with syndromes (e.g., DiGeorge) that have conotruncal anomalies as part of the clinical picture may occur in patients who have only the conotruncal anomaly, without other noncardiovascular defects. The microdeletion, 22q11.2, has been detected by FISH (see Chap. 2). Table 23–3 summarizes the frequency of occurrence and the characteristic types of cardiac defects for a number of chromosomal aberration syndromes. These syndromes are discussed in more detail in Chapters 3 and 4. Chromosomal syndromes such as XXY Klinefelter syndrome do not appear in the table because there is no substantial increase in congenital heart diseases.

Single Mutant Gene Syndromes

Diseases transmitted by single mutant genes account for about 3% of the total of cardiovascular anomalies. The cardiac defects are usually present as part of a syndrome, such as the Ellis-van Creveld syndrome. It must re-

Table 23–3. Congenital Heart Diseases (CHD) in Selected Chromosomal Aberrations

Population Studied	Incidence of CHD %	Most Common Lesions		
		1	2	3
General population	1	VSD	PDA	ASD
trisomy 21	50	ECD	VSD	ASD
trisomy 18	99+	VSD	PVD	PDA
trisomy 13	90	VSD	PDA	Dex
partial tetrasomy 22 (cat-eye)	40	complex TAPVR	VSD	ASD
4p−	≈40	ASD	VSD	PDA
5p− (Cri-du-chat)	≈20	VSD	PDA	ASD
trisomy 8 (mosaic)	≈50	VSD	ASD	PDA
trisomy 9 (mosaic)	>50	VSD	coarc	DORV
13q−	≈25	VSD		
18q−	<50	VSD		
45,X Turner	35	coarc	AS	ASD
XXXXY	15	PDA	ASD	ARCA

ARCA = anomalous right coronary artery.
ASD = atrial septal defect.
coarc = coarctation of aorta.
Dex = dextroversion.
DORV = double outlet right ventricle.
ECD = endocardial cushion defect.
PDA = patent ductus arteriosus.
PVD = polyvalvular disease
Tet = tetralogy.
TAPVR = total anomalous pulmonary venous return.
VSD = ventricular septal defect.

quire the products of a large number of genes to bring about truncoconal septation, and it is reasonable to doubt that a single gene can be responsible for failure of a ventricular septum to close unless it is a single gene with a specific small effect or more likely a gene of large effect, in which case a single anomaly or a number of associated anomalies could be found. This returns us to the concept of the pleiotropic effect of a mutant gene of large effect.

One example of a single mutant gene in a familial heart lesion is that of idiopathic hypertrophic subaortic stenosis (IHSS). Another is atrial septal defect in a small percentage of families. The gene locus for some familial cases has been provisionally assigned to 6p21.3.

With a few exceptions, such as IHSS and some patients with ASD, congenital heart lesions caused by single mutant genes are usually part of a syndrome. Table 23–4 provides a partial list of syndromes produced by single mutant genes, potent teratogens, and those of unknown etiology that have cardiovascular disease as a feature. The majority of these syndromes are discussed further elsewhere in this text.

CORONARY HEART DISEASE (CHD)

Coronary heart disease (CHD) is the most common cause of death in the U.S.A. (about 550,000 deaths per year). The concept that CHD is the product of genetic and environmental factors is generally accepted. It is the relative contribution of heredity and environment that has remained more obscure. During the past two decades, investigative interest has profitably pursued environmental risk factors, and when genetic factors have been considered, there has been a tendency to limit genetic interest to lipid and lipoprotein abnormalities, particularly to the rare single mutant gene anomalies. However, genetic interest in CHD is over a century old. In the English literature the first mention of the familial aspect of coronary heart disease with xanthomatosis was made by Fagge in 1873. That coronary heart disease, as such, without the emphasis on the sentinel abnormality of familial xanthomatosis, could recur in families was appreciated not by a physician, but by the poet and essayist, Matthew Arnold. While visiting the United States in 1887, he experienced his first attack of angina pectoris and wrote to a friend: "I began to think that my time was really coming to an end. I had so much pain in my chest, the sign of a malady which had suddenly struck down in middle life, long before they came to my present age, both my father and my grandfather." Matthew Arnold lived with chest pain for less than a year before he died on April 15, 1888. One of his biographers disclosed amazingly little scholarship when he described the cause of Arnold's death as "heart failure . . . sudden and quite unexpected." Unexpected—except by Matthew Arnold. Sir William Osler called attention, in 1897, to the Arnold family in discussing the possible genetic features of coronary heart disease. Through successive editions of Levine's widely used textbook, *Clinical Heart Disease*, heredity has been stressed as

Table 23–4.   Mendelian Conditions and Selected Syndromes With Cardiovascular Involvement

Abnormality	Types of Cardiovascular Disease
AUTOSOMAL DOMINANT CARDIOVASCULAR ABNORMALITIES	
Apert syndrome	Ventricular septal defect (VSD), tetralogy, coarctation of the aorta (CA)
Conduction defects, familial	Various levels and types of blocks and dysrhythmias
Crouzon disease	CA, patent ductus arteriosus (PDA)
Ehlers-Danlos syndrome	AV valve regurgitation, rupture of large blood vessels, e.g., carotids, dissecting aneurysms of the aorta
Forney	Mitral insufficiency (MI)
Holt-Oram syndrome	Atrial septal defect (ASD), VSD
Idiopathic hypertrophic subaortic stenosis (IHSS)	Obstructive myocardial disease
Leopard syndrome	Pulmonary stenosis (PS), prolonged P-R interval
Marfan syndrome	Mitral and aortic disease
Mitral click-murmur	MI, dysrhythmias—some families with "dominant" inheritance
Myocardial disease (nonobstructive)	Cardiomegaly, congestive heart failure
Myotonic dystrophy (Steinert)	Conduction defects, myocardial disease
Neurofibromatosis	PS, pheochromocytoma with hypertension, CA
Noonan syndrome	PA, ASD, left ventricular disease
Osteogenesis imperfecta	AI
Periodic paralysis (hypokalemic and hyperkalemic types)	ECG changes, rhythm disturbances
Primary pulmonary hypertension	Primary pulmonary hypertension
Romano-Ward syndrome	Prolonged Q-T, syncope, sudden death
Supravalvar aortic stenosis (with or without elfin facies)	Supravalvar aortic and pulmonary stenosis, peripheral pulmonary stenosis
Treacher Collins syndrome	VSD, PDA, ASD
Tuberous sclerosis	Myocardial rhabdomyoma and angioma
Waardenburg syndrome	VSD
AUTOSOMAL RECESSIVE CARDIOVASCULAR ABNORMALITIES	
Adrenogenital syndrome (21 & 3)	Hyperkalemia, broad QRS, arrhythmias
Alkaptonuria	Aortic and mitral disease, ? premature arteriosclerosis
Carpenter syndrome	Patent ductus arteriosus (PDA), ventricular septal defect (VSD), pulmonary stenosis (PS), transposition of the great arteries (TGA)
Chondrodysplasia punctata	VSD, PDA
Conduction defects (familial)	Various levels of blocks
Cutis laxa	Pulmonary hypertension, peripheral pulmonary artery stenosis (PPAS)
Cystic fibrosis	Cor pulmonale
Ellis-van Creveld syndrome	Atrial septal defect (ASD), most commonly single atrium, other congenital heart lesions
Fanconi pancytopenia	ASD, PDA
Friedreich ataxia	Myocardiopathy and conduction defects
Glycogenosis IIa (Pompe)	Myocardiopathy
Glycogenosis III (Cori) and IV (Andersen)	Myocardiopathy
Ivemark syndrome	Asplenia with cardiovascular anomalies
Jervell and Lange-Nielsen syndrome	Prolonged QT, sudden death
Laurence-Moon (Bardet-Biedl) syndrome	VSD and other structural defects
Meckel-Gruber syndrome	Both complex and simple structural defects
Mucolipidosis II and III	Valvar disease
Mucopolysaccharidosis (MPS) IH, IS, IV, VI	Coronary artery and valvar disease
Muscular dystrophy I, II	Myocardiopathy
Pseudoxanthoma elasticum	Generalized vascular disease, coronary insufficiency, mitral insufficiency (MI), hypertension
Refsum syndrome	Atrioventricular (AV) conduction defects
Seckel syndrome	VSD, PDA
Sickle cell disease	Myocardiopathy, mitral insufficiency
Smith-Lemli-Opitz syndrome	VSD, PDA, and other congenital heart diseases
Thalassemia major	Myocardiopathy
Thrombocytopenia absent radius (TAR)	ASD, tetralogy, dextrocardia
Thyroid defects	Myocardial function
Weill-Marchesani syndrome	PS, VSD, ?PDA
Zellweger syndrome	PDA, VSD, ASD
X-LINKED RECESSIVE AND DOMINANT (R AND D) SYNDROMES WITH ASSOCIATED CARDIOVASCULAR ABNORMALITIES	
MPS II (Hunter) X–R	Coronary artery disease, valvar disease
Muscular dystrophy (Duchenne and Dreifuss types) X–R	Myocardiopathy
Focal dermal hypoplasia X–D	Occasional congenital heart defects, telangiectasia
Incontinentia pigmenti X–D	PDA, primary pulmonary hypertension

Table 23–4.   Mendelian Conditions and Selected Syndromes With Cardiovascular Involvement (continued)

Abnormality	Types of Cardiovascular Disease
CARDIOVASCULAR DISORDERS OR UNDETERMINED ETIOLOGY	
Arthrogryposis multiplex congenita	Patent ductus arteriosus (PDA), ventricular septal defect (VSD), coarctation of the aorta (CA), aortic stenosis (AS)
Asymmetric crying face	Tetralogy of Fallot (TOF), VSD
Atrial myxoma, familial	Myxoma, rheumatic fever
Biliary-hepatic and cardiovascular disease	Peripheral pulmonary artery stenosis (PPAS), PDA, VSD
C syndrome	PDA, ? other defects
Cardio-auditory syndrome of Sanchez-Cascos	? Myocardial disease
Chromosomal phenocopies	Atrioventricular (AV) canal, dextroversion, VSD, PDA
DeLange syndrome	VSD, TOF, PDA, double outlet right ventricle
DiGeorge syndrome	VSD, interrupted aortic arch, truncus
Goldenhar syndrome	TOF, VSD, atrial septal defect (ASD)
Kartagener syndrome	Dextrocardia
Klippel-Feil syndrome	VSD with pulmonary hypertension, total anomalous pulmonary venous return (TAPVR), transposition of the great arteries (TGA), TOF, ASD, PDA
Klippel-Trenaunay-Weber syndrome	Hemangiomata
Limb-skin-heart syndrome of Falek	Complex anomalies
Linear sebaceous nevus	CA, VSD
Maffucci syndrome	Hemangiomata
Mitral click-murmur	Mitral prolapse or redundancy
Ophthalmoplegia with AV block	First, second, or third degree AV block, fascicular blocks
Poland anomaly	CA, VSD
Polydactyly-chondrodystrophy 1 (Majewski) and II (Saldino-Noonan)	TGA and other truncoconal anomalies
Robin anomaly	Pulmonary hypertension secondary to hypoxia
Rubinstein-Taybi syndrome	PDA, ASD, VSD
Silver syndrome	TOF, VSD
Sturge-Weber anomaly	Hamangiomata, CA
Williams syndrome	Supravalvar aortic and pulmonic stenosis, PPAS

"the most important etiologic factor." A study of our own reveals that heritability of ischemic heart disease is 63% if one includes single gene disorders, and 56% if familial cases that appear to conform to mendelian patterns are excluded.[12]

Table 23–5.   Etiologic Factors in Ischemic Heart Disease

Heredity	interaction ⟷	Environment
Metabolism		Diet
Cholesterol, etc.		Stress
Diabetes		Striving
Personality		Inadequate exercise
Hypertension		Overweight
Coronary artery		Cigarettes
anatomy		
Cellular mechanisms		Socioeconomic level
Immunologic factors		Education
Coagulation		Culture

Examples of familial aggregates abound in the literature as well as in the practice of almost any physician who treats patients with coronary artery disease. Twin studies, such as the National Danish Study, show a significantly higher concordance between monozygotic than dizygotic twins. A variety of animal homologies, including rabbit, pigeon, dog, and monkey, have been found to be susceptible to atherosclerosis. There are few diseases, if any, in which the etiologic factors have been more vigorously investigated (and contested) than coronary artery disease. This high priority is entirely justified. Atherosclerotic diseases are unequaled as a cause of morbidity and mortality in Western society.

In preparing this chapter, an effort was made to list some of the hereditary and environmental factors in the etiology of coronary artery disease (Table 23–5). It became obvious that these factors could not be categorized so

Table 23–6. Nomenclatures of Phenotypes of Hyperlipoproteinemias

Type I	hyperchylomicronemia
Type IIa	hyperbetalipoproteinemia
Type IIb	hyperlipoproteinemia with multiple lipoprotein types (familial combined hyperlipidemia)
Type III	broad beta disease
Type IV	hyperglyceridemia (familial hypertriglyceridemia)
Type V	mixed hyperlipidemia

simply. Although certain causes of coronary artery occlusion are secondary to factors that are predominantly hereditary (e.g., mendelian forms of hyperlipoproteinemia, Hunter syndrome) or predominantly environmental (smoking), most causes do not comfortably fit under heredity or environment, but depend more on the interaction between factors. For example, considering personality, diabetes mellitus, hypertension, and coronary artery anatomy under heredity is merely a judgment that, perhaps, the hereditary basis of these factors exceeds the environmental—although both are known to be important.

A brief discussion of only some of the hereditary factors will be undertaken together with a consideration of how environment may interact with heredity. Because cardiovascular diseases are so widespread, need for their cure and prevention is most urgent. Although genetic manipulation may provide some eventual solution, the immediate attack on the problem has most judiciously been on the environmental factors as they interact with the hereditary predisposition.

Metabolism

The association of elevated serum cholesterol with atherosclerosis has been repeatedly documented for decades, although there has not been broad agreement regarding its etiological role until recently with the publication of the Lipid Research Clinics Primary Prevention Trial.[6] Other lipid abnormalities, such as elevated triglycerides, beta-lipoproteins, pre-beta-lipoproteins, chylomicrons, and total plasma lipids, have been studied in an effort to define phenotypes of individuals and families at risk. High levels of one form of lipoprotein, high density lipoprotein (HDL) appear to be associated with "protection" against coronary disease. A lipoprotein is a conjugated protein consisting of moieties of a simple protein and a lipid. As will be discussed later, interest is now focusing on components of the lipoproteins and gene markers to define more precisely individuals and families at increased risk of atherosclerotic disease.

Lipoprotein Phenotypes

In the 1960s, the Fredrickson group proposed a valuable phenotypic classification of hyperlipoproteinemias as a means of reaching a genetic definition of lipid disorders, some of which underlie coronary heart disease. In Table 23–6 we present the current WHO version of the Fredrickson phenotypes, together with the Goldstein terminology in parentheses. A relatively simple screening procedure, obtaining serum (or plasma) cholesterol and triglyceride levels and looking at the serum or plasma of the patient after the red blood cells have settled, is the initial step. By this screening procedure, patients who are normal or abnormal according to present criteria may be distinguished with sufficient confidence to assign them to groups of those requiring no further investigation and those needing more definitive study. In fact, it is usually possible to predict the phenotype by screening alone. Because of notable exceptions, more extensive examination, preferably using ultracentrifugation, provides the more definitive phenotype of those who are suspected of having a lipoprotein abnormality by screening.

However, it has become apparent that these phenotypes are several steps removed from primary gene products and are subject to considerable variability. For example, three or four phenotypes of hyperlipoproteinemia may be present within the same family. Even the same individual may be phenotyped differently under varying circumstances (e.g., diet and alcohol consumption the previous day). Because the phenotypes in most cases do not relate directly to primary gene products, the terminology of Goldstein has merit for the 3 most common conditions (i.e., hypercholesterolemia, combined hyperlipidemia, and hypertriglyceridemia). However, the goal of more specific phenotyping remains viable. Biochemical definition should extend to the primary gene product in the case of single gene disorders. Polygenic disorders should also be distinguished and specified as such. A much more detailed presentation of the Fredrickson phenotypes and the Goldstein terminology will be found in *The Metabolic Basis of Inherited Disease* (see Appendix B). What will be presented in the following section is a brief description of hyperlipoproteinemias.

Type I Hyperlipoproteinemia—Hyperchylomicronemia. This disease is characterized by striking chylomicronemia (producing a "creamy" plasma after the blood cells have settled), extremely high plasma triglyceride levels (2000 to 3000 mg/mL is common), and normal or high plasma cholesterol. One form of this rare autosomal recessive disorder, a defect in removal of chylomicrons, is secondary to a deficiency in activity of lipoprotein lipase. Another recessive form is a deficiency of apo C-II (a cofactor for lipoprotein lipase). The more definitive biochemical evaluation reveals that the elevated triglycerides and cholesterol are not accomplished by abnormally high beta, low density lipoproteins (LDL) or high pre-beta, very low density lipoproteins (VLDL). The excess lipids are carried in the chylomicrons. Clinically, the disorder is recognized in childhood because of the presentation of episodic abnormal pain (with sometimes fatal pancreatitis), xanthomatosis, and hepatosplenomegaly. The gene locus for the lipoprotein lipase deficiency is 8q22.

Subgroups include cases associated with dysglobulinemia, diabetes, disseminated lupus erythematosus, hypothyroidism, and administration of oral contraceptives. The relative contribution of polygenic predisposition and environmental triggers in these conditions has not been assessed. It is essential to look for the presence of associated diseases before assuming that a patient has a monogenic form of the disease, such as the lipoprotein lipase deficiency or apo C-II deficiency.

Type IIa—Hyperbetalipoproteinemia, Hypercholesterolemia, Familial Hypercholester- olemia **(FH).** This is the group that is of greatest interest and concern. In 1970, a WHO committee split Type II into IIa, those with high beta (LD) lipoproteins alone; and IIb, those with high pre-beta (VLD) lipoproteins in addition to the high betalipoproteins. There are both monogenic (uncommon) and polygenic (common) forms of Type II phenotypes. The Type IIa monogenic disease (familial hypercholesterolemia) represents a model of receptor disorders and led to the award of the 1985 Nobel Prize to Brown and Goldstein.[2] Figure 23–3 illustrates the defects in cell membrane receptors and in the regulation of 3-hydroxy-3-methylglutaryl coenzyme A (HMG CoA) reductase. The autosomal dominant forms of the disease (population frequency 0.2%) are of serious clinical consequence and produce coronary heart disease as early as the third and fourth decades of life, but it is the homozygous manifestation of the disease that is disastrous. Children in the second and even first decades of life die of coronary heart disease, and it is the exceptional homozygote who survives long into adult life. Tuberous xanthomas are present in the homozygotes in infancy and childhood and in the heterozygotes in the third and fourth decades. Angina pectoris, congestive heart failure, progressive aortic stenosis, and frank myocardial infarction ensue.

In cultured fibroblasts, it has been possible to show that the activity of HMG CoA reductase is regulated by a feedback mechanism involving low-density lipoprotein receptors and that the activity is low in normal fibroblasts and high in homozygotes. Brown and Goldstein have demonstrated a basic abnormality in cell surface LDL receptor sites, which control the binding, degradation, and suppression of reductase activity.

Heterozygotes with familial hypercholesterolemia have half the number of LDL receptors and FH homozygotes have few or no functioning LDL receptors. As may be visualized in Figure 23–3, the absence or diminished number of receptors located in coated pits on the cell surface decreases the binding of LDL molecules, which should be transported to the lysosomes where the cholesterol is split from the protein and free cholesterol

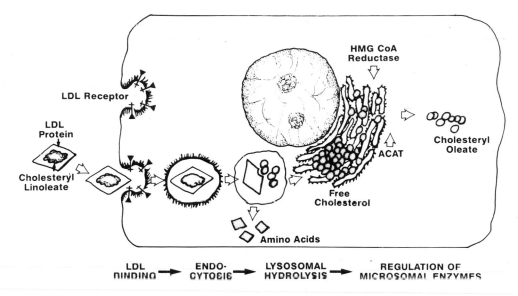

Fig. 23-3. Receptor model of cholesterol metabolism. (Courtesy of Dr. Michael S. Brown and modified from Brown, M.S. and Goldstein, J.L.: Science 191:150, 1976.)

accumulates to suppress HMG CoA reductase (to prevent cholesterol synthesis). However, in the absence of free cholesterol, the synthesis continues unchecked. FH heterozygotes are only able to catabolize LDL at about two-thirds the normal rate and homozygotes can remove LDL from their plasma at only about one-third the rate in normals.

Many different mutant receptors (resulting from multiple alleles) have been identified in patients with heterozygous or homozygous familial hypercholesterolemia. The FH gene, which is responsible for the formation of LDL receptors, is located on the short arm of chromosome 19 (19p13.2-13.1). The allelic mutations are divided into four classes. In class I mutations, the receptor protein is simply not synthesized. In class 2, receptor proteins are synthesized in the rough endoplasmic reticulum, but are transported slowly to the golgi apparatus to pick up additional carbohydrate necessary for them to become incorporated into the cell membrane. In class 3 mutations, receptors are processed and reach the cell surface, but have a reduced ability to bind LDL. In class 4, receptors reach the cell surface and bind LDL, but fail to cluster in the coated pits where the receptor-bound LDL is internalized.

Prenatal diagnosis of the homozygote using cells cultured from amniotic fluid has been accomplished. The LDL receptor gene has also been cloned and shown to be polymorphic.

A breakthrough in the exploration and management of this problem was provided by Starzl and co-workers when they demonstrated a dramatic decrease in plasma cholesterol (from 1000 mg/100 mL to 300 mg/100 mL), striking regression of xanthomas (Fig. 23–4) and the gradient of aortic stenosis, and improvement in the coronary arteriograms in a 12-year-old homozygous type IIa patient following portacaval shunt. The investigation of the role of hepatotrophic factors, specifically insulin, in cholesterol and LDL metabolism in these patients has been stimulated by this case. This is an early example of documented regression of a genetic disease following "metabolic surgery."

The majority of patients with hypercholesterolemia do not have the monogenic familial form. Depending on where one sets the threshold to define hypercholesterolemia, from 10 to 75% of American adults have elevated cholesterol levels (a commonly accepted figure is 15%). The relationship of diet, exercise, and stress to the level of plasma cholesterol requires precise evaluation. Medical condi-

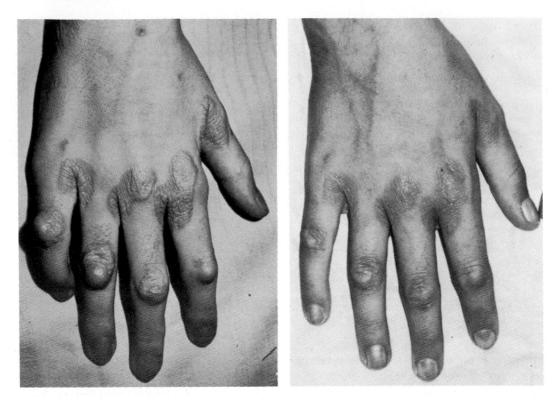

Fig. 23–4. Typical xanthomatous skin lesions in child with severe homozygous type IIa hyperlipoproteinemia before portacaval shunt (on left) and after shunt has dramatically lowered plasma cholesterol (on right). See text. (From Nora, J.J.,
and Nora, A.H.: Genetics and Counseling in Cardiovascular Diseases. Charles C Thomas, Springfield, Ill., 1978. Used by
permission.)

tions known to be associated with hypercholesterolemia include hepatic disease, porphyria, diabetes, nephrosis, hypothyroidism, and
dysglobulinemia.

Type IIb—Combined Hyperlipidemia. This
disorder has been proposed as a discrete entity caused by a single gene, which can produce within different individuals: elevated
levels of cholesterol and triglycerides, elevation in cholesterol alone, or elevations in triglycerides alone. There is debate as to whether
a monogenic form of this disease exists. Our
experience is compatible with such a proposal. For the purposes of this presentation,
the type IIb phenotype will be elevation of
both cholesterol and triglycerides in the same
individual, whether or not a single gene or
multifactorial etiology is proposed, and irrespective of the other phenotypes which may
occur in the family. In our family studies, first-
degree relatives ascertained through proband

having type IIb disease were almost evenly
divided between type IIb, type IV and type
IIa phenotypes. Type III and type V phenotypes are also occasionally found in combined
hyperlipidemia families. If a proband with type
IIa or type IV hyperlipoproteinemia is found
to have a first-degree relative with combined
hyperlipidemia, we have arbitrarily classified
the entire family as combined hyperlipidemia.

Type III—Broad-Beta Disease. This disorder is characterized biochemically by the
presence of an abnormal lipoprotein which has
a high content of both triglycerides and cholesterol and which appears as a broad-beta band
on electrophoresis and intermediate density
on ultracentrifugation. Clinically, the orange-
yellow lipid deposits in the creases of the hands
are highly characteristic. As in patients with
type I and type IIa, there are also large tub-
eroeruptive and planar xanthomas. Premature
coronary and especially peripheral vascular

disease are features of this disorder, as are abnormal glucose tolerance and hyperuricemia.

Rather than being a monogenic disorder, it is thought that this condition results from the presence of the genes for type III disease occurring with any of the genes for other monogenic or polygenic forms of hyperlipoproteinemia. The absence of apoE3 is a consistent finding in type III disease. As in other hyperlipoproteinemias, medical conditions that may play an etiologic role (or are at least associated) include diabetes, dysglobulinemia, and hypothyroidism.

Type IV—Hyperglyceridemia, Hypertriglyceridemia. This common disorder is characterized biochemically by abnormally high levels of triglycerides, VLDL, and pre-beta lipoproteins. Early-onset coronary heart disease and peripheral vascular disease are found in familial and nonfamilial cases of hypertriglyceridemia, but not with the high frequency that coronary disease is found in Type IIa. In the majority of patients, triglyceride levels are raised by dietary carbohydrate and lowered by carbohydrate restriction. Abnormal glucose tolerance is common. Xanthomas are not a feature, but hyperuricemia and diabetes are frequently associated with it.

There are autosomal dominant pedigrees in which this mode of inheritance clearly appears, and in one form a gene assignment has been confirmed at 11q13. This is the apoA-1 locus (which will be discussed later). Most familial cases, however, do not fit a dominant mode. The interaction of obesity and carbohydrate indiscretion with a familial predisposition is well recognized.

Type V—Mixed Hyperlipidimia. Exogenous chylomicrons, increased beta (LD), and pre-beta (VLD) lipoproteins appear in patients with this type of disease. Eruptive xanthomas, abdominal pain, pancreatitis, hyperuricemia, abnormal glucose tolerance, and possibly some prematurity of vascular disease occur. The phenotype appears to be highly heterogeneous.

Patients with the type V phenotype not infrequently appear in families in which the predominating phenotype is type IV and the frequent mode of inheritance is autosomal dominant. Autosomal recessive inheritance has been proposed on the basis of a pedigree in which inbreeding was identified and on the somewhat tenuous findings of affected siblings without apparent phenotypic expression in the parents. Patients with apolipoprotein C-II deficiency may show a type V pattern.

This phenotype even more than some of the other hyperlipoproteinemias is associated with other diseases, such as lupus erythematosus, diabetes, nephrosis, and alcoholism. Some type IV individuals may readily convert to type V (or type III) after a sizable consumption of alcohol the day before their blood is drawn— even following the traditional 12- to 14-hour fast.

Current Recommendations

Because of the possibility of yet to be discovered risk factors, the hope for refinement of established risk factors, and the development of new therapeutic modalities, recommendations for preventive strategies require frequent revision.

The European Atherosclerosis Society published a policy statement which captures the thinking of many investigators.[4] The report stresses the complementary relationship of the population strategy of mass intervention and the high-risk strategy of selective intervention. The population strategy reiterates the need to eradicate smoking, control hypertension, and promote suitable exercise and nutrition. In the area of selective intervention, the Consensus Conference goal of 200 mg/dL of serum cholesterol[8] is emphasized along with attention to control of diabetes and monitoring of HDL cholesterol and triglycerides. Low HDL cholesterol attracts even more attention at many centers as a dominant risk factor independent of high total cholesterol and high LDL cholesterol.

The recommendation that one sees repeatedly is that of early intervention, preferably starting in early childhood, as part of both mass and high-risk strategies.[4,12] It is in this context that the genetic identification of those at risk, which is possible at any age, becomes obviously relevant.

Advances in the diagnosis, treatment, and prevention of atherosclerotic disease. Traditional risk factors suitable for use by practicing physicians and in community health programs were described earlier. What is needed is the development of new tools for case finding that are economical and well accepted. Advances in sensitivity and specificity may be increased through the study of new genetic risk factors. Apolipoproteins A, B, E, Lp(a) lipoprotein antigen, and DNA markers are among the candidates for informative analysis.

Apolipoproteins.[18] An apolipoprotein is the lipid-free protein moiety of a plasma lipoprotein. The better characterized apolipoproteins are apoA-I, A-II, A-III (D), A-IV, B, C-I, C-II, C-III, and E. ApoA-I and A-II are the major protein constituents of human high density lipoproteins (HDL). HDL is the lipoprotein that exerts a protective influence against the deposition of cholesterol in arterial walls that lead to atherosclerosis, heart attacks, and strokes. Thus, high levels of HDL cholesterol correlate well with resistance to coronary artery disease. ApoB is the major protein in low density lipoproteins (LDL) and is increased in patients with hypercholesterolemia. An increased level of LDL cholesterol is felt to be more informative of risk of coronary heart disease than is simply an increase in total cholesterol. ApoB is also a major constituent in chylomicrons and very low density lipoproteins (VLDL). ApoC-I, C-II, and C-III are major components of chylomicrons and VLDL and apoE is prominent in VLDL.

Apolipoprotein A. A DNA polymorphism flanking the apoA-I gene has been found to be associated with a ten-fold increase in premature coronary artery disease and low levels of HDL.[15] In another study, an apoA-I related DNA polymorphism was found to be present in less than 10% of healthy controls, but in 47% of people with atherosclerosis. An increasing number of RFLPs for the gene cluster on chromosome 11 that encompasses apoA-I, apoC-III, and apoA-IV are being investigated and should be productive in studying coronary risk factors. Hypertriglyceridemia and hypercholesterolemia (without receptor defect) have been reported in the apoA-1 to

apoC-III gene cluster in DNA polymorphisms. Homozygotes for a restriction site polymorphism at apoA-II have such high HDL that they may actually be resistant to coronary disease.

Apolipoprotein B. An association between myocardial infarction and alleles at three RFLs involving the apoB gene has been reported.[5] Oddly enough, in this study, rather than higher levels of LDL being found in the myocardial infarction group, it was lower levels of HDL, apoA-I, and apoA-II that emerged. Other studies have shown an association between DNA variants at the apoB locus and *increased* levels of cholesterol, triglycerides, and apoB.

Apolipoprotein B. An association between myocardial infarction and alleles at three RFLs involving the apoB gene has been reported.[5] The apoE4 allele raises LDL cholesterol and the apoE2 allele lowers it. Nearly every type III hyperlipoproteinemia patient is homozygous for apoE2 (E2/E2); however, 95 to 99% of persons with this phenotype do not have type III disease. ApoE3 is absent in patients with type III hyperlipoproteinemia.

Lp(a) lipoprotein. Lp(a) lipoprotein is proving to be an important independent risk factor in early onset coronary disease as has been demonstrated by Berg and associates.[1] Men in the upper quartile of Lp(a) concentration have a population attributable risk of 28% for myocardial infarction before age 60.

RHEUMATIC FEVER[19]

The familial aspects of rheumatic fever have been recognized for several decades, even to the extent that one prominent worker in the field attempted to interpret the family clusters of this disease in mendelian terms, concluding that this was an autosomal recessive disorder. Data from the National Danish Twin Study support a hereditary predisposition to rheumatic fever on the basis of higher concordance in monozygotic twins as compared to dizygotic twins, which is significant at a probability level of 0.01%. However, no data from twin or family studies provide evidence of mendelian inheritance of this disease and no active investigators in this area are willing to discount that the streptococcus is the essential environmental trigger in rheumatic fever.

Rheumatic fever appears to be an excellent example of a disease produced by a genetic-environmental interaction. Certain families have a hereditary predisposition, but rheumatic fever does not result unless there is an infection (almost always respiratory) with a group A betahemolytic streptococcus. (See Chapter 18 for immunologic considerations in rheumatic fever.)

ESSENTIAL HYPERTENSION

Evidence has been accumulated by a number of investigators to support the concept of a multifactorial mode of inheritance.[16] Other investigators propose a monogenic etiology.[17] Our review of the subject strongly favors multifactorial inheritance in the majority of cases, but does not exclude that a minority of patients may have hypertension attributed to single mutant genes.

An individual's systemic blood pressure, like his height and intelligence, appears to be determined by many genes. A "normal" distribution curve for systolic blood pressure in adults runs from 90 to 140 mm Hg (and a diastolic curve from 50 to 90 mm Hg). The tail at the lower end can extend further, but not as far as the tail at the upper end of the curve, because a minimum blood pressure is required to sustain life. Thus it can be visualized that some individuals can have systolic blood pressures of 160, 180, or even 200 and be at the far end of a now skewed distribution curve.

This concept alone probably does not account for the relatively large number of people with hypertension. A polygenic predisposition to hypertension interacting with environmental triggers (most importantly, sodium, stress, and obesity), a genetic-environmental interaction, is as conceptually sound an etiologic proposal for hypertension as for congenital heart diseases, rheumatic fever, and coronary artery diseases.

Of course, there are pathologic conditions that, when superimposed on a genetic predisposition to normal or even low blood pressure, will result in severe systemic hypertension. Renal diseases are in this category. However, this is no longer within the definition of essential hypertension.

Salt sensitivity, influenced by genetic variance, plays a major role in many but not all patients with essential hypertension. Haptoglobin phenotypes may prove useful in identifying salt-sensitive subjects.[7]

SUMMARY

A genetic-environmental interaction appears to operate in the production of the majority of cases in the four major categories of cardiovascular diseases: ischemic heart disease, hypertension, congenital heart disease, and rheumatic fever. Within the categories, however, there are entities in which the contribution of heredity greatly outweighs the role of environment (e.g., type IIa familial hypercholesterolemia, Marfan syndrome) or the contribution of environment is the essential factor (e.g., rheumatic fever).

REFERENCES

1. Berg, K. In: Lp(a) Lipoprotein. 25 Years of Progress. Edited by A. Scanu. San Diego, Academic Press, 1990.
2. Brown, M.S. and Goldstein, J.L.: A receptor-mediated pathway for cholesterol homeostasis. Science 232:34, 1986.
3. Emanuel, B.S., et al.: Detection of microdeletions of 22q11.2 with FISH: Diagnosis of DiGeorge, velo-cardiofacial syndromes, CHARGE association and conotruncal cardiac malformations (Abst.). Am. J. Hum. Genet. 51:A3 (suppl.), 1992.
4. European Atherosclerosis Society: Strategies for the prevention of coronary heart disease. Europ. Heart J. 8:77, 1987.
5. Hegele, R.A.: Apolipoprotein B-gene DNA polymorphisms associated with myocardial infarction. N. Engl. J. Med. 315:1509, 1986.
6. Lipid Research Clinics Program: Lipid Research Clinics Primary Prevention Trial. JAMA 251:351, 1984.
7. Luft, F.C. et al.: Heritable aspects of salt sensitivity. Am. J. Cardiol. 61:1H, 1988.
8. NIH Consensus Development Conference: Lowering blood cholesterol to prevent disease. JAMA 253:2080, 1985.
9. Nora, J.J.: Multifactorial inheritance hypothesis for the etiology of congenital heart diseases: the genetic-environmental interaction. Circulation 38:604, 1968.
10. Nora, J.J.: Causes of congenital heart diseases: Old and new modes, mechanisms, and models. Am. Heart J. 125:1409, 1993.

11. Nora, J.J., Sommerville, R.J., and Fraser, F.C.: Homologies for congenital heart diseases: Murine models influenced by dextroamphetamine. Teratology 1:413, 1968.
12. Nora, J.J., et al.: Genetic-epidemiology of early-onset ischemic heart disease. Circulation 61:503, 1980.
13. Nora, J.J. and Nora, A.H.: Maternal transmission of congenital heart diseases: New recurrence risk figures and the questions of cytoplasmic inheritance and vulnerability to teratogens. Am. J. Cardiol. 59:459, 1987.
14. Nora, J.J., Berg, K., and Nora, A.H.: Cardiovascular Diseases: Genetics, Epidemiology and Prevention. New York, Oxford University Press, 1991.
15. Ordovas, J.M. et al.: Apolipoprotein A-I gene polymorphism associated with premature coronary artery disease and familial hypoalphaproteinemia. N. Engl. J. Med. 314:671, 1986.
16. Pickering, G.W.: High Blood Pressure, 2nd ed. London, Churchill, 1968.
17. Platt, R.: Heredity in hypertension. Lancet 1:899, 1963.
18. Stampfer, M.J., et al.: A prospective study of cholesterol, apolipoproteins, and the risk of myocardial infarction. N. Engl. J. Med. 325:373, 1991.
19. Stevenson, A.C., and Cheeseman, E.A.: Heredity and rheumatic fever. Ann. Hum. Genet, 21:139, 1956.

Chapter *24*
Pharmacogenetics

Physicians know from experience that patients vary in their responses to drugs. This is not surprising; the fate of a drug in the body depends on its rate of absorption, how much it is bound to the serum proteins, its distribution to organs and transfer across cell membranes, its interaction with cell receptors and organelles, and its metabolism and excretion. Not only are many of these processes modified by the environment (diet, other drugs, and so on), but it is reasonable to suppose that they will be modified by genes, as they involve many enzymes and other proteins.

Twin studies show that the heritability of drug clearance is very high for most of the drugs tested, suggesting that the determination of dosage for chronically administered drugs should be based not on body weight but on systemic monitoring of blood level and adjustment of dose to the patient's individual response.

Occasionally, the response of an individual to a drug is dramatically different from the norm and perhaps life-threatening, and it was the discovery that some of these marked deviations in response showed simple mendelian inheritance that led the German geneticist, Vogel, in 1952, to coin the term *pharmacogenetics*.

The pharmacogenetic disorders are a special type of inborn error of metabolism, involving proteins that function in drug metabolism or drug action; they are considered a special subcategory because of their pharmacologic implications and because they represent an interesting kind of gene-environment interaction.[6,9] We will discuss several conditions involving aberrant reactions to drugs and showing simple mendelian inheritance (Table 24–1). We have also included examples of gene-determined diseases that may be precipitated or exacerbated by certain drugs (periodic paralysis, porphyria).

These disorders represent rather extreme genetic variations in response to drugs and are usually rare. They may serve to remind the physician that there are also genetically determined five-to-tenfold variations in the disposition of many commonly used drugs such as phenylbutazone (for arthritis), phenytoin (for epilepsy), ethanol (an anesthetic), salicylate, and amobarbital. These may be important in studies of toxicity and emphasize the importance of treating each patient as a unique individual.

One genetic difference that modifies our responses, not only to drugs but to many other

Table 24–1.   Examples of Inherited Conditions with Altered Response to Drugs[6,9]

Trait or Deficient Enzyme	System Affected	Drug or Factor	Frequency of Trait	Clinical Effect
Acatalasia	Tissues	H_2O_2	High in Japanese	No response to peroxide
Alcohol dehydrogenase atypical	Liver	Alcohol	?	Increased tolerance
Alpha-I-antitrypsin deficiency	Plasma	Smoking	Moderately rare	Emphysema (cirrhosis)
Debrisoquine hydroxylase	Nervous	Debrisoquine	5–10%	Parkinson's
Diabetes mellitus	Vasomotor	Chlorpropamide	Common	Flushing after alcohol ingestion
Dicumarol resistance	Clotting	Dicumarol	Rare	Decreased response
Glucose-6-phosphate dehydrogenase	RBC	Fava beans, primaquine, others	High in Mediterraneans, Negroes	Hemolysis
Gout	Uric acid metabolism	Chlorothiazide (diuretic)	Frequent	Exacerbation of gout
Hemoglobins, unstable	RBC	Sulfonamides, oxidants	Very rare	Hemolysis
INH transacetylase	Liver	Isoniazid	Common	Polyneuritis
Malignant hyperthermia	Sarcoplasmic reticulum	Anesthetics	Very rare	Rigor, hyperthermia
Methemoglobin reductase	RBC	Nitrites, oxidants	Variable	Methemoglobinemia
Periodic paralysis	? Cell membrane	Insulin, adrenalin, others	Rare	Paralysis
Porphyria (some kinds)	Liver	Barbiturates, sulfas, others	Variable	Acute "attacks"
Pseudocholinesterase deficiency	Plasma	Succinylcholine	Moderately rare	Apnea

toxic substances including teratogens, mutagens, and carcinogens, relates to the cytochrome P-450-mediated monooxygenases.[4] These are a group of liver enzymes involved in the detoxification of foreign chemicals, many of which are so hydrophobic that they would remain in the body indefinitely if not metabolized. The first step in the detoxification process is to introduce one or more polar groups, such as hydroxyls, into the molecule, which make it accessible to attack by various conjugating enzymes. One such hydroxylating system, the cytochrome-P-450-mediated monooxygenases has been referred to in relation to genetic susceptibility to lung cancer (Chapter 21). Most of the genetic analysis has been done in the mouse, but there are important implications for man.

In the mouse, the Ah locus controls the induction of cytochrome P-450 and more than 20 associated monooxygenase activities. The locus controls a cytosol protein receptor that combines with environmental toxins (inducers), such as polycyclic aromatic hydrocarbons, biphenyl halogenated hydrocarbons, insecticides, aflatoxins, drugs, and steroids, many of which are carcinogenic and/or mutagenic. The receptor-inducer complex activates the structural genes for the cytochrome P-450 and other enzymes. In the noninducible mutant, no receptor is present, and the enzyme activities are not increased. It appears that the active carcinogen, mutagen, or toxin is often an intermediate in the detoxification process, not the original molecule. Thus an exposed individual, with the inducible phenotype, breaks down the parent compound into toxic metabolites quickly and is therefore exposed to high concentrations; that is, he is susceptible. The noninducible individual is not exposed to high concentrations of the toxic products and is relatively resistant. This genetic difference appears to affect susceptibility of cigarette smokers to bronchogenic carcinoma. In mice, it also affects susceptibility to other carcinogens, and to teratogens. It provides, for example, one possible explanation for the fact that some babies exposed to a teratogen are malformed and others, similarly exposed, are not. Unfortunately, the assays on lymphocytes are difficult to standardize, but further study should be productive.

For simplicity's sake, we have arranged the following pharmacogenetic disorders alphabetically rather than attempting a classification by organ system or class of drug or according to whether the gene alters the way the body acts on the drug (e.g., acatalasia, pseudocholinesterase deficiency, isoniazid inactivation) or the way the drug acts on the body (e.g., G6PD deficiency, dicumarol resistance, ocular response to steroids, malignant hyperthermia).

ACATALASIA

This odd example of a gene-drug interaction was discovered in 1959 by a Japanese otolaryngologist, Takahara, who removed some diseased tissue from the mouth of a patient and applied hydrogen peroxide to disinfect the wound. The usual bubbling of oxygen did not occur, and the tissue turned black, presumably because of oxidation of hemoglobin by the drug. Takahara, who must have been unusually knowledgeable in biochemistry, deduced that the tissue must lack the enzyme catalase and demonstrated that this enzyme deficiency showed autosomal inheritance, the heterozygote having intermediate enzyme levels. There is genetic heterogeneity, with five different types described so far, severity ranging from mild (ulcers of the tooth sockets) to severe (gangrene of the gums and recession of the tooth socket). The condition is not uncommon in Japan, but it has not yet been reported in North Americans. A rare type of acatalasia has been discovered in Switzerland. In the Swiss type, the small amount of residual enzyme differs in its physicochemical properties from the normal, whereas the residual enzyme is normal in the Japanese type, suggesting that the Swiss type represents a structural gene mutation and the Japanese type a mutation of a controller gene.

ALCOHOL DEHYDROGENASE

Ethyl alcohol is metabolized in the liver by alcohol dehydrogenase. A variant has been found with increased activity in Swiss (20%) and English (4%) populations, which results in more rapid clearance of alcohol from the system. The genetic basis for this polymorphism and its possible relationship to alcoholism are unclear. Research is impeded by a certain reluctance of healthy individuals to provide liver biopsies.

Racial differences in alcohol metabolism have been demonstrated, but the relationship to alcohol dehydrogenase type or to alcoholism is not clear. White volunteers showed a more rapid fall in blood level after a standard dose of alcohol than did Eskimos or Canadian Indians.

Finally, it has been reported that Japanese, Taiwanese, and Koreans show facial flushing and other unpleasant effects after drinking amounts of alcohol that produce no detectable effect in Caucasians. These reactions are related to deficiencies in alcohol dehydrogenase or aldehyde dehydrogenase that cause rapid increases in blood acetaldehyde after drinking alcohol. These mutant alleles are less frequent in Oriental alcoholics than in nonalcoholic controls, and thus appear to have a protective effect against alcoholism.[8]

There is no clear-cut evidence that alcoholism is related to a pharmacogenetic difference. However, there are enough suggestions that alcohol metabolism and the reactions to alcohol are genetically influenced to warrant its inclusion in this chapter.

ALPHA-1-ANTITRYPSIN DEFICIENCY[2]

This condition can be considered a pharmacogenetic disorder if cigarette smoking can be considered a form of drug-taking, although it is not known what constituent of cigarettes is the interacting factor in this case. In any case, it is an interesting example of a gene-environment interaction, where a genetically determined disease can be ameliorated by modifying the environment. The genetics and physiology of alpha-1 antitrypsin has been extensively reviewed elsewhere.[2]

When cells are damaged by inflammation or trauma, the body's defense mechanisms include proteases, enzymes that break down the proteins that must be removed as part of the clearing up process, leucocyte elastase in this case. But the proteases must be prevented from attacking normal cells, so there are protease inhibitors, including alpha-1 antitrypsin. When the inhibitors are deficient, the proteases run amok and destroy normal tissues. This explains why individuals deficient in the inhibitor are prone to emphysema, a disease in which the elasticity of the lung alveoli is destroyed so that the alveoli remain dilated and air exchange is diminished, with all its consequences. Smoking and probably other kinds of air pollution provide the irritation leading to protease release and tissue destruction in deficient individuals.

Extensive genetic studies have shown that the locus for α-1 AT is on 14q. It is named Pi (protease inhibitor), the major allele being Pi^M. There are some 30 codominant alleles producing electrophoretic variants, with varying frequencies in different populations, making it a useful tool for population genetics studies. The most important variant, medically, is Pi^Z. Homozygotes (PiZZ) have a severe, and heterozygotes (PiMZ) an intermediate, deficiency. Homozygotes have a high risk for emphysema in mid-life if they smoke. They also have about a 10% risk for prolonged obstructive jaundice or cirrhosis of the liver, possibly because the molecular defect prevents completion of the carbohydrate side chains and leads to retention of the molecule in liver globules. The homozygote frequency is about 0.03% in US whites, and accounts for about 1% of all emphysema patients.

Whether the MZ heterozygote is at risk is still a matter of debate. There is some evidence that it causes some impairment of respiratory function in smokers.

DEBRISOQUINE HYDROXYLATION

An important example of a cytochrome P450 pharmacogenetic polymorphism is the hydroxylation of the antihypertensive drug debrisoquine, as well as that of numerous other drugs including sparteine, nortriptyline, phenacetin, phenformin, dextromorphan and propranolol.[6] About 5 to 10% of Caucasians are deficient metabolizers, homozygous for the mutant gene, and are prone to toxic side effects as well as having the highest antihypertensive responses. The gene (CYP2D6) has been mapped to chromosome 22, sequenced, and the mutant identified as an aberrant splice recognition site. This will facilitate screening for the mutant phenotype.

It has been shown that the mutant phenotype is increased more than twofold in patients with Parkinson's disease, suggesting that the inability to metabolize medications, or other environmental agents, exposes the substantia nigra to neurotoxins.[7]

GLUCOSE-6-PHOSPHATE DEHYDROGENASE (G6PD) DEFICIENCY (FAVISM, PRIMAQUINE SENSITIVITY)[3]

The structural gene for G6PD is on the X chromosome, about 5 centimorgans from the locus for colorblindness. Its deficiency is the most common abnormal genetic trait in man, and its study has contributed notably to our knowledge of human genetics. Deficiency of the enzyme in the red blood cell renders the cell sensitive to certain drugs, for reasons not yet well understood. This is the cause of *favism*, long recognized as a hemolytic condition peculiar to Mediterranean peoples and related to the eating of uncooked fava beans, a Mediterranean delicacy. The enzymatic basis was not recognized until the antimalarial drug primaquine was issued to American troops in malarial regions during World War II, following which a number of hemolytic reactions were noted, particularly in blacks; the affected men were found to be deficient in G6PD.

G6PD is involved in a minor pathway for red cell glycolysis, the hexose monophosphate shunt, and plays a role in maintaining the concentration of reduced glutathione, which, in turn, is necessary for stability of the red cell in the presence of certain drugs, although the mechanism for this is not clear.

There are over 150 G6PD allelic variants. They can be classified according to their electrophoretic characteristics, their enzymatic activity, or the clinical severity of the enzyme deficiency. A deficiency can result from decreased production of enzyme molecules, decreased catalytic activity, or reduced stability of the molecule. The most common electrophoretic type is B, and a faster-migrating type A is present in about 20% of American black males. A single amino acid substitution determines the difference. Clinically there are three major groups.

Mild G6PD deficiency. Mild G6PD deficiency, common in persons of African origin, involves only type A (a curious association, not understood) and results in enzymatic activity of 8 to 20% of normal. The deficiency appears to result from decreased stability. It is asymptomatic except under stress, such as exposure to certain drugs, infection, or diabetic acidosis. Because enzyme levels decrease with increasing age of the red cell, the deficient cells do not become susceptible until they are about 50 days old. Thus an exposed mutant individual may have mild hemolysis, with dark urine and perhaps jaundice, but if the drug is continued, the episode passes and the patient gets better, because most of his red cells are now young and resistant.

Severe G6PD deficiency. Severe G6PD deficiency, the Mediterranean or B⁻ type, also occurs in Orientals. The enzyme has only 0 to 4% activity, and there is a more severe hemolysis following exposure. Over 340 drugs are listed that will cause hemolytic crises, including aspirin, acetanilid, sulfanilamide and other sulfa drugs, several antimicrobials, quinidine, primaquine and several other antimalarials, and naphthalene. One infant had a hemolytic crisis when he "inherited" his brother's diapers, which had been stored in moth balls. Occasionally hemolysis occurs spontaneously.

G6PD deficiency with congenital hemolytic anemia. G6PD deficiency with congenital hemolytic anemia (nonspherocytic) occurs with some rare, usually unstable or kinetically grossly abnormal, variants. Varying degrees of anemia and reticulocytosis occur without drug administration. Neonatal jaundice may occur, and hemolysis is increased by drugs and infection.

Various other mutant types have been described, particularly in East and Southeast Asia.

One variant has increased enzyme activity. In general, severity of hemolysis correlates with the degree of enzymatic deficiency. The population frequency correlates with malaria frequency, suggesting that the gene confers an advantage against malaria, as in the case of hemoglobin S. In some populations (e.g., Sardinians), the gene is so frequent that patients are screened routinely before being treated with sulfa drugs or other drugs known to cause hemolysis in mutant subjects.

Because the gene is X-linked, heterozygous females are mosaics for two populations—in fact, the demonstration of this mosaicism by cloning of fibroblasts was one of the first convincing demonstrations of the Lyon hypothesis in man. The ratio of the two populations of cells is about 50:50 on the average, but there is wide variation, from as high as 99% to as low as 1% in occasional heterozygotes. Thus heterozygote detection may be difficult. This would be expected if a fairly small number of cells made up the anlage of the blood-forming tissues. As lyonization is random, if n cells were involved, there would be a 2^n chance that all would have either the X carrying the mutant gene or the X carrying the normal gene inactivated. If the latter, the female would be just as susceptible to hemolysis as a mutant male. About one third of heterozygous females have enough mutant cells to predispose them to clinically significant hemolysis on exposure.

By reversing the argument, one can calculate from the variation in proportions of mutant to normal red cells in various mutant females how many cells must have been present in the anlagen of the blood-forming tissues—probably about 5. The role of G6PD in supporting the somatic mutation hypothesis for cancer is mentioned in Chapter 21. Thus this pharmacogenetic trait has advanced our knowledge in several areas of human genetics.

HEMOGLOBIN MUTANTS, UNSTABLE[6,9]

Several rare mutant hemoglobins are known in which the carrier is predisposed to hemolytic crisis when exposed to certain drugs, mainly of the same types that affect G6PD-deficient males. These include hemoglobin Zurich and Torino.

ISONIAZID INACTIVATION[6]

The observation that some patients excreted the antituberculosis drug isoniazid rapidly and others relatively slowly led to the discovery of a pharmacogenetic polymorphism (see Fig. 12–1), rapid inactivation of isoniazid being transmitted as an autosomal dominant trait. There are marked differences in frequency between populations, the proportion of rapid inactivators being about 45% among North American Caucasians and African-Americans, 67% among Latin Americans, and 95% among Eskimos.

The responsible enzyme is an acetylase (N-acetyltransferase) in the liver that acetylates isoniazid and a few related drugs including several sulfas, and nitrazapam, a sleeping pill. The polymorphism is of some importance, as the drug interacts with pyridoxine (a B vitamin) and may cause a pyridoxine deficiency with peripheral neuritis, but only in slow inactivators. Treatment with pyridoxine is effective. Furthermore, when the drug must be given intermittently, as in some Eskimo and Native American communities, rapid inactivators have a poorer therapeutic response. For these, a slow-release form of the drug has been developed.

In patients with both tuberculosis and epilepsy, a curious pharmacogenetic drug interaction may occur. When the epilepsy is treated with phenytoin (diphenylhydantoin, DPH), high levels of isoniazid may inhibit the metabolism of DPH by the liver oxidases, and the DPH may reach toxic levels, but this happens only in slow inactivators of isoniazid.

MALIGNANT HYPERTHERMIA[1]

This pharmacogenetic trait is a dominantly inherited tendency to react to certain anesthetics, including ether, nitrous oxide, and halothane, with a rapid rise in body temperature, progressive, muscular rigidity, and often death from cardiac arrest. The population frequency is about 1 in 15,000 in Canada. Some

cases also show an ill-defined muscular disease.

The condition also occurs in swine, in which the gene has been cloned and the defect shown to be in the ryanodine receptor, involved in the Ca^{2+} release channel (CRC) of skeletal muscle sarcoplasmic reticulum. In many (but not all) human families, the RYRI gene has been shown to cosegregate with the MH gene and mapped to chromosome 19q13.1.[1] Because of the genetic heterogeneity, DNA testing does not detect all cases, but is useful in families in which the RYRI linkage exists (about 50% of European families tested). In the other families, one must rely on the invasive, expensive, and sometimes inconclusive test of muscle fiber contraction following in vitro exposure to caffeine and halothane.

Susceptible individuals requiring operation can be safely anesthetized by some combination of barbiturates, nitrous oxide, narcotics, neuroleptanalgesics, or local anesthetics.

PERIODIC PARALYSIS

There are three types of periodic paralysis, all autosomal-dominant, in which the plasma potassium rises, falls, or remains unchanged, respectively. *Low-potassium paralysis* may be precipitated, in gene carriers, by prolonged rest after vigorous exercise, a heavy carbohydrate meal, anxiety, cold, and a variety of drugs, including insulin, adrenalin, ethanol, some mineral corticoids—and licorice. *High-potassium paralysis* may be brought on by vigorous exercise followed by rest, potassium chloride, and some kinds of anesthesia. The third type has no pharmacogenetic significance.

PSEUDOCHOLINESTERASE DEFICIENCY[5]

One of the most dramatic pharmacogenetic disorders involves a deficiency of serum cholinesterase, or "pseudocholinesterase" (now known as butyrylcholinesterase), a defect that seems to have no harmful effect whatsoever unless the patient is given the drug succinylcholine or suxamethonium as a preoperative muscle relaxant or before electroconvulsive therapy. This drug causes paralysis of striated muscle, which, at the doses used, lasts only a minute or two, because it is rapidly broken down by the serum cholinesterase. In the absence of the enzyme, the paralysis may be greatly prolonged, and the patient may stop voluntary breathing for half an hour or more, causing somewhat of a flap in the operating room.

Genetic analysis shows a system of multiple alleles. The locus is called E_1 (E for esterase, and 1 because it was the first esterase to show genetic variation). The E_1 locus is linked to the transferrin locus. The normal allele is E_1^U (for "usual") and the mutant allele is E_1^A (for "atypical"). The mutant homozygote has a structurally abnormal enzyme, which is resistant to inhibition by dibucaine (Cinchocaine). A standard concentration of dibucaine causes 80% inhibition of the normal enzyme (the dibucaine number), 60% inhibition in the $E_1^U E_1^A$ heterozygote, and 22% inhibition in the E_1^A homozygote, who is sensitive to succinylcholine.

Another allele, E_1^S, is the "silent" allele, the homozygote having no activity and being extremely sensitive to succinylcholine. As one would expect, the $E_1^S E_1^A$ heterozygote is also sensitive to succinylcholine. The use of other inhibitors has led to the detection of other alleles, for example, E_1^f, in which the resulting enzyme is inhibited by fluoride, but not by dibucaine.

The "atypical" allele has a frequency of about 3% in the general U.S. population and 10% in Oriental Jews, with homozygote frequencies of 1 in 2500 and 1 in 400, respectively. The "silent" allele may be quite frequent in some Eskimo populations. Thus, although only about half the reported cases of succinylcholine sensitivity are caused by detectable abnormalities in serum cholinesterase, the genetic trait is frequent enough to justify routine screening of patients to be exposed to this drug. A simple screening test exists.

The gene has been mapped to chromosome 3q26, and the specific mutational sites of many of the alleles have been identified.[5]

The high frequency suggests that the gene has, or had, some selective advantage, but this is difficult to study because we do not even know why the normal enzyme is there; presumably, it was not evolved simply to degrade succinylcholine. One theory for the high frequency of this mutant gene is that tomatoes, potatoes, and related plants may sometimes produce toxic amounts of an alkaloid, solanine, which is a potent cholinesterase inhibitor. Because the mutant enzyme is less sensitive to this inhibition, mutant gene carriers would be more resistant to solanine poisoning.

SUMMARY

Pharmacogenetics concerns itself with a special type of inborn error of metabolism, the response of individuals to drugs. Aberrant responses may be manifested only in a need for a dose different from that usually given to achieve a desired therapeutic effect or may be responsible for marked deviations from normal that may have mild, moderate, or serious untoward effects, including death. A number of mendelian disorders have been identified and are discussed. One of the most informative loci in human genetics is the X-linked gene determining the red blood cell enzyme glucose-6-phosphate dehydrogenase. Over 90 mutant alleles are known, many of which determine enzyme deficiencies, resulting in a hemolytic response to more than 20 drugs, as well as infection. This locus has also been useful in the investigation of the Lyon hypothesis and in linkage studies.

It is likely that further genetic differences influencing responses to drugs will be found, thus permitting increasing accuracy in determining doses, choosing appropriate drugs, and avoiding undesirable side reactions. For example, of women taking oral contraceptives, those of blood group O are least likely to develop thromboembolism, perhaps because they have reduced levels of antihemophilic globulin. (On the other hand, they are more prone to bleeding peptic ulcers.) Another example involves antidepressant drugs: Patients seem to fall into two classes, those who respond well to tricyclics and those who do best on monoamine oxidase inhibitors. This difference seems to be family-specific—probands and their near relatives respond best to the same group of drugs—suggesting that there are at least two genetically different kinds of depressive disorders. Thus pharmacogenetic principles may be an aid to disease classification.

The examples given in this chapter, besides demonstrating the truth of the adage that one man's medicine is another man's poison, remind us that our genes make us unique pharmacologically, as in so many other ways, that pharmacogenetic differences may make it desirable to screen high-risk families and high-risk populations before exposing them to certain agents, and that patients being treated with drugs should be regarded as individuals, not just as so many kilograms of body mass.

REFERENCES

1. Ball, S.P., and Johnson, K.J.: The genetics of malignant hyperthermia. J. Med. Genet. 30:89, 1993.
2. Lieberman, J.: Alpha 1-antitrypsin deficiency and related disorders. *In* Principles and Practice of Medical Genetics. 2nd ed. Edited by A.E.H. Emery and D.L. Rimoin. New York, Churchill Livingstone, 1990, vol. 2, p. 1179.
3. Luzzato, L., and Mehta, A.: Glucose-6-phosphate deficiency. *In* The metabolic basis of inherited disease. Edited by Scriver, C.R., Beaudet, A., Sly W.S., and Valle D. New York, McGraw-Hill, 1989.
4. Nebert, D.W., and Weber, W.W.: Pharmacogenetics. *In* Principles of drug action. 3rd. ed. Edited by Pratt, W.B. and Taylor, P.W. New York, Churchill-Livingstone, 1990, p. 252.
5. Nogueira, C.P., Bartels, C.F., McGuire, M.C., et al.: Identification of two different point mutations associated with the fluoride-resistant phenotype for human butyrylcholinesterase. Am. J. Hum. Genet. 51:521, 1992.
6. Price Evans, D.A.: Pharmacogenetics. *In* Principles and Practice of Medical Genetics. 2nd ed. Edited by A.E.H. Emery and D.L. Rimoin. New York, Churchill Livingstone, 1990, vol. 2, p. 1869.
7. Smith, C.A.D., Gough, A.C., Leigh, P.N., et al.: Debrisoquine hydroxylase gene polymorphism and susceptibility to Parkinson's disease. Lancet 339:1375, 1992.
8. Thomasson, H.R., Edenberg, H.J., Crabb, D.W., et al.: Alcohol and aldehyde dehydrogenase genotypes and alcoholism in Chinese men. Am. J. Hum. Genet. 48:677, 1991.
9. Vesell, E.S. Pharmacogenetics. Pediatric Pharmacology. Therapeutic principles in practice. Edited by Yaffe, S.J. and Aranda, J.V. Philadelphia, W.B. Saunders Co., 1992, p. 29.

Chapter 25
Normal Traits

I AM THE FAMILY FACE;
FLESH PERISHES, I LIVE ON,
PROJECTING TRAIT AND TRACE

THOMAS HARDY

NORMAL PHYSICAL FEATURES

Nearly everyone is interested in the inheritance of physical features, and it is rather disappointing that so few of them show clear-cut mendelian pedigree patterns. One difficulty is that normal physical differences often do not fall into sharply different classes, so that it is difficult to know how to classify individuals in the overlap range. Nevertheless, there is a great deal of data about the inheritance of normal traits, as well as a good many misconceptions. The reader is referred to Amram Scheinfeld's book, *Your Heredity and Environment,* for an interesting and detailed coverage of inherited normal variations.[5] We will touch only lightly on the subject, and admit that much of the data is uncritical and should not be taken too seriously.

Eye Color

Probably the example of "simple mendelian inheritance" in man most frequently cited in elementary texts and popular articles is eye color. This has the advantage of being a trait with which almost everyone is familiar, but it also has a disadvantage. It is *not* an example of *simple* mendelian inheritance, as a modicum of observation and a little thought will tell you. Eye color is clearly a graded character, with many possible shades of color as well as innumerable patterns. That it is genetically determined is clear from the striking resemblances in color and pattern between monozygous (genetically identical) twins. The color is determined by the amount and distribution of melanin in the iris. Complete albinos have little or none, so the iris appears red because it transmits light reflected from the fundus. "True blue" eyes have virtually no pigment in the anterior part of the iris, but some in the posterior layers, and darker colors have progressively more melanin (yellow or brown) present. The structure of the iris also modifies the shade.

In general, the genes for the darker colors tend to be dominant to those for the lighter, but the situation is complex: A child with eyes darker than those of both parents is not necessarily cause for divorce. Remember, also, that the iris may darken considerably for some months, or even years, after birth.

Hair Color

The innumerable shades of hair color also attest to complex inheritance, as well as a considerable amount of environmental modification, at least in some populations. Again, the various shades of blonde through black are determined by the concentration and type of melanin, and the genes causing the darker colors tend to dominate those for the lighter ones.

Red hair results from another pigment, which appears to be under the control of a separate gene locus. The gene for presence of the red pigment is recessive to its "not-red" allele, but of course the difference between red and not-red is visible only if the hair is fair. The dark-hair genes are epistatic to the red hair locus.

Hair Form

The form or texture of the hair depends on its cross-sectional shape, which is round in straight hair and elliptical in curly hair. A case has been made for a single locus, with curly hair resulting from homozygosity for one allele, straight hair from homozygosity for the other allele, and the heterozygote having wavy hair, but the situation is hardly as simple as that because there are many degrees of waviness. Kinky hair in Caucasians shows dominant inheritance, and the straight hair of Orientals is also said to be dominant, but there is a lack of critical data.

Baldness

Hair loss in older age is presumably determined multifactorially. Pattern baldness, with onset before about 30 years of age, is one of the few common traits that seem to fit mendelian expectations. It is caused by an autosomal gene that expresses itself in the heterozygote in males but not in females. Presumably, androgen makes the difference, and its lack may also prevent expression of the gene in homozygous females; otherwise, there should be more pattern-bald women than there appear to be.

Skin Color

It should be evident that skin color is multifactorially determined, since there is a continuous range of shades from "black" to "white." Davenport's original proposal that the black-Caucasian skin color difference is due to two independent loci, each showing intermediate dominance, is an oversimplification. Gates' scheme, involving three loci contributing different amounts of melanin (dark, beige, and dark brown), allows 18 possible shades and fits observed family patterns reasonably well. Either scheme implies that a "dark" person and a "white" mate cannot have a baby much darker than the dark parent, contrary to the myth that African ancestry on only one side of the family can result in a "black" baby, even though both parents are light-skinned.

Little information is available on the genetic control of skin color in the "red-skinned" and "yellow-skinned" peoples.

Attached Ear Lobes

Most ear lobes extend below the lower point of attachment of the ear, but some merge with the facial skin along the anterior border, making it difficult to wear earrings. The attached lobe is said to be recessively inherited, but in some people it is difficult to decide whether the lobe is attached or not.

Ear Pits

Pinhead-sized depressions in the skin just in front of the pinna's upper attachment or on the pinna itself near its attachment are present in about 1% of people. They sometimes show dominant inheritance, and may occur as part of numerous syndromes, for example, the BOR syndrome (see Fig. 8–6).

Tongue Rolling

The ability to roll the tongue into a trough, or even tube, is said to be dominant to the inability, but there are exceptions—e.g., occasional discordant monozygotic twins.

Handedness[3]

Left-handedness is certainly familial, but how much of the tendency to resemble parents is cultural is not at all clear. In one study, the frequency of left-handedness was about 6% when both parents were right-handed, 17% when one parent was left-handed, and 50% when both parents were left-handed. This can be made to fit a single-locus scheme if the right- or left-handedness of heterozygotes is postulated as depending on subtle environmental variations. Associations with twinning and with malformations have been noted.[1]

Hand Clasping

When you fold your hands, which thumb is on top? This is a sharply determined characteristic, with about 50% of Caucasians preferring one hand to be uppermost, and 50% the other. It does not seem to be related to handedness and has only a slight tendency to be familial, though there are racial variations in frequency. It is curious that this discrete difference does not seem to have a simple genetic basis.

"Hitch-Hikers' Thumb"

The ability to extend the terminal phalanx of the thumb more than 30 degrees from the axis of the second phalanx is said to be recessive, but some people fall close to this value and are therefore hard to classify.

Dental Anomalies

Inherited variations in tooth morphology are numerous and cannot be reviewed adequately here. One of the most striking is the dominant gene that causes peg-shaped or missing lateral incisors.

Webbed Toes

Partial webbing of the second and third toes is an anomaly so frequent that it may be included among the normal variations. Autosomal dominant inheritance is the usual pattern, although in some families it appears only in females.

NORMAL PHYSIOLOGIC VARIATIONS

In addition to "normal" morphologic variants, a number of interesting physiologic variants have been identified. We will exclude the biochemical polymorphisms here.

PTC Taste Threshold

The ability to taste phenylthiocarbamide, or related goitrogenic chemicals with the N-C-S group, shows marked variation among individuals. The majority of people can taste weak concentrations of the compound (tasters), but (in Caucasians) about one out of three people can taste only much higher concentrations (nontasters). This striking physiologic difference is determined by a single locus, the nontaster allele being recessive. It is not related to taste acuity in general. If taste thresholds are carefully measured, a few individuals fall into the intermediate range, but if allowance is made for general taste sensitivity, good discrimination can be achieved, and the heterozygotes can be shown to have somewhat higher taste thresholds for PTC than the homozygous tasters.[4] As with other polymorphisms, there are wide variations in gene frequency in different populations, and there is some evidence to suggest that the nontaster genotype predisposes to the development of toxic goiter.

Ear Wax

Almost all Caucasians and Africans have brown, wet, sticky ear wax, but in the Japanese the common type is gray, dry, and flaky. The dry type is also frequent in American Indians and Eskimos and appears to be recessively inherited.

Color Blindness

About 8% of Caucasian males have X-linked red-green color vision anomalies. These result from deficiencies in the retinal cone pigments sensitive to light in the green-yellow or red region of the spectrum. The genes for these pigments have now been cloned and mapped to Xq28. Defective red color perception is called protanopia if severe (1% of males) and protanomaly if moderate or mild (1%). For green perception defects, the terms are deuteranopia (5%) and deuteranomaly (1.5%). The genes for the two pigments are highly homologous and are located in tandem; unequal crossing over between them may result in mutants with varying degrees of color vision defect.[2] A much rarer form, X-linked blue cone monochromacy, results from such mutants, which lead to inactivation of both genes.

Beetroot Urine

An autosomal recessive gene results in the appearance of red pigment in the urine after eating beets.

SUMMARY

The inheritance of physical features and normal variation is a subject of general interest attended by a considerable number of misconceptions. Selected physical features are briefly discussed.

REFERENCES

1. Boklage, C.E.: Twinning, non right-handedness and fusion malformations. Am. J. Med. Genet. 28:67, 1987.
2. Deeb, S.S., Lindsey, D.T., Hibiya, Y., et al.: Genotype-phenotype relationships in human red/green color-vision defects: Molecular and psychophysical studies. Am. J. Hum. Genet. 51:687, 1992.
3. Hicks, R.E., and Kinsbourne, R.M.: Human handedness: A partial cross-fostering study. Science 192:908, 1976.
4. Kalmus, H.: Improvements in the classification of taster genotypes. Ann. Hum. Genet. 22:200, 1958.
5. Scheinfeld, A.: Your Heredity and Environment. Philadelphia, J.B. Lippincott Co., 1964.

Chapter *26*

Twins and Their Use in Genetics

Twins have always been a subject of interest, particularly to their surprised parents, but also as mythical, historical, and literary figures. Yet it was only in 1875 that Galton pointed out their value in estimating the relative importance of heredity and environment—or, as he put it, of "nature and nurture." "Identical" or monozygotic (MZ) twins result from the splitting of a fertilized egg, giving rise to two genetically identical individuals. "Fraternal" or dizygotic (DZ) twins result from fertilization of two different eggs and are therefore no more similar genetically than sibs. Galton saw that this experiment of nature allowed comparison of genetically identical and genetically different individuals in similar environments.

A third type of twin has been postulated to arise from fertilization of an egg and its polar body by two sperm.[3]

In Caucasian populations, about 1 in every 87 deliveries is a twin birth, and the proportion of monozygotic to dizygotic pairs is about 30:70.[4] This proportion was first estimated by Weinberg, who reasoned that for dizygotic twins there should be equal numbers of like-sex and unlike-sex pairs (1 boy/boy:2 boy/girl:1 girl/girl). Because MZ twins are always like-sexed, the excess of like-sexed twins in a representative series of twin pairs measures the proportion of MZ twins.

The frequency of MZ twins is remarkably constant, ranging from 3.5 to 4 per 1000 deliveries in various populations. Virtually nothing is known about the causes of MZ twinning.

The frequency of DZ twins is much more variable. It varies with maternal age from near 0 at puberty to 15/1000 at age 37 in Caucasians, and then falls sharply to near 0 again just before the menopause. The frequency is low in Mongoloid races (about 4/1000), higher in Caucasians, (8/1000), and higher still in Negroes (16/1000 or more).

Whereas MZ twinning does not show any familial tendency, DZ twinning does. As one would expect, the predisposition to have DZ twins is a maternal characteristic. The probability of recurrence of DZ twins in subsequent deliveries of mothers who have had a pair is about 3%—about a fourfold increase. After "trizygotic" triplets, the recurrence rate for DZ twins is increased about ninefold.

DETERMINATION OF ZYGOSITY

In any study in which twins are used to estimate heritability, it is necessary to determine whether each pair is monozygotic or dizygotic. This can be done in several ways, of varying degrees of reliability: examination of fetal membranes, physical similarity, dermatoglyphic patterns, genetic markers, and skin grafts.

Fetal Membranes

The fetal membranes can sometimes be useful in the diagnosis of zygosity. To show how, a brief digression into embryology is necessary.[2]

At about the fourth day after fertilization, the ovum has developed into a 16-celled solid ball, the morula. By the sixth day, this has progressed to a hollow sphere, the blastula, which contains an outer layer of cells, the trophoblast, and an inner cell mass. The trophoblast develops into the *chorion*, a heavy outer membrane which eventually lines the uterus and in one area forms the fetal component of the placenta. About 7 days after fertilization, the trophoblast begins to implant itself in the uterine wall. The inner cell mass forms the embryo proper and also, in the second week, develops the amnion, a thin membrane which forms a fluid-filled sac around the embryo, thus providing a protective barrier for the developing baby.

The splitting of the egg to form monozygotic twins may occur at several stages. If (as occasionally happens) it occurs at the two-celled stage, or at any point before the end of the morula stage, each resulting embryo will form a complete set of membranes. Thus there will be two amnions, two chorions, and two placentas, *just as there are in dizygotic twins* (Fig. 26–1A). If the inner cell mass splits after the trophoblast has formed but before the amnion appears, the twins will have a common chorion (and placenta), but separate amnions (Fig. 26–1C). Finally, if the embryonic disc splits after the amnion has developed (a rare event), the twins will share both placenta, chorion, and amnion. Table 26–1 shows the relative frequencies of the various types.

Dizygotic twins always have separate chorions and amnions, although if they implant close together, the placentas may fuse and ap-

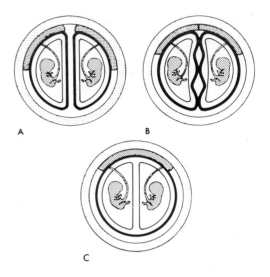

Fig. 26–1. Arrangements of placentas and fetal membranes in twins. The placenta, umbilical cord, and fetus are heavily stippled; the thick line is the chorion, and the thin line enclosing the fetus is the amnion. *A*, 2 placentas, 2 chorions, 2 amnions. *B*, 2 placentas fused, 2 chorions fused, 2 amnions. *C*, 1 placenta, 1 chorion, 2 amnions. (After Thompson, J.S., and Thompson, M.W.[12])

pear to be single (Fig. 26–1B). Occasionally, the membranes separating DZ twins may break down (because of mechanical pressure?), leaving the twins in a common sac.

Thus, examination of the fetal membranes is sometimes, but not always, useful in establishing zygosity. If there is only one chorion, the twins are almost certainly monozygotic. If there are separate chorions and amnions, the twins may be either monozygotic or dizygotic. The distinction between a fused dichorial placenta (Fig. 26–1B) and a monochorial diamniotic placenta (Fig. 26–1C) requires careful examination, preferably histologic.

Table 26–1. Placentas and Fetal Membranes in Twins

Placenta	Chorion	Amnion	Percent of All Twins	
			MZ	DZ
1	1	1	rare	—
1	1	2	~22.5	—
1 (or fused)	2	2	~ 7.5	~35.0
2	2	2	rare	~35.0
			30.0	70.0

Physical Similarity

In most cases, the zygosity of pairs of twins can be estimated fairly reliably from their physical similarity alone. If the twins look so much alike that they are difficult to tell apart, they have about a 95% probability of being monozygotic (Fig. 26-2). However, if they are discordant for a congenital malformation such as cleft lip or for a chromosomal anomaly, this criterion becomes unreliable. If twins differ in some trait known to be genetically determined, such as eye color, or webbed toes also occurring in other family members, they are almost certainly dizygotic.

Dermatoglyphics

The dermatoglyphic patterns (Chapter 17) are determined largely by the genetic constitution and can be used for zygosity determination. The corresponding hands of MZ twins should be just as similar, dermatoglyphically, as the right and left hands of each twin, whereas this is not so for DZ pairs. The degree of dissimilarity and the corresponding probability of dizygosity have been put on a statistical basis and presented in tabular form for convenient reference.[9] For instance, if the mean ridge count differs by 33 or more, the twins have a relative probability of 34:1 of being DZ.

Genetic Markers

A more reliable method than physical or dermatoglyphic similarity is the use of genetic

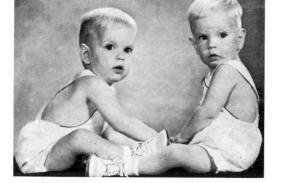

Fig. 26-2. Monozygotic twins with atrial septal defect.

markers such as blood groups, serum proteins (Chapter 19) and, of course, sex. If the twins differ by even one such marker, they must be dizygotic—ignoring the minute possibility of mutation. If they are similar for a particular marker, they may be MZ or may have just happened to inherit the same marker. Obviously, the more markers are the same, the higher the probability that the twins are monozygotic.

The exact probability can be calculated if the genotypes of twins and parents are known.[9] Consider a pair of twin boys who are both blood group MM and whose parents are group MM and MN, respectively. To begin with, a pair of twins has an a priori chance of $7/10$ of being DZ because this is the proportion of DZ to MZ twins in the population. If the twins are DZ, they have one chance in four of being boys, two in four of being a boy and a girl, and one in four of being girls, so the chance of being like-sexed is $1/2$. The possible genotypes of DZ twins would be one in four of being MM-MM, two in four of being MM-MN and one in four of being MN-MN, so the chance of being alike in their MN groups is also $1/2$. Thus the probability of the twins being DZ and alike for sex and MN blood group is $7/10 \times 1/2 \times 1/2 = 7/40$.

If the twins are MZ, they must be like-sexed and have the same blood groups, so the probability of these twins being MZ is $3/10 \times 1 \times 1 - 3/10$ or $12/40$. So the relative probability of being MZ is $12/(7 + 12) = 12/19 = 63\%$.

Each additional marker for which the twins are identical (provided there is an opportunity for segregation) increases the probability of monozygosity. For instance, if both parents are group AB and the twins are alike for this group, one can calculate that DZ twins have 3 chances in 8 of being alike for this locus (work it out). The probability of being DZ then becomes $7/40 \times 3/8 = 21/320$, the probability of being MZ is $12/40 \times 1 = 96/320$, and the relative probability of being MZ is $96/(21 + 96) = 96/117 = 82\%$. Of course, if there is no opportunity for the twins to be different—e.g., if both twins and parents are group O—this marker will not contribute any information.

If the parental genotypes are not known, they can sometimes be deduced from those of their other children or their parents. If not, they can be estimated from the known population frequencies of the genes concerned, but the arithmetic is complex. Tables of probabilities for such situations are available.[9] DNA "fingerprints" are very useful markers.

Skin Grafts

If a piece of grafted skin contains an antigen different from the host's, the host will make antibodies against it, and the graft will be rejected (Chapter 18). Dizygotic twins are almost certain to be antigenically different, since there are several histocompatibility loci, with many alleles, that will result in skin graft rejection if graft differs from host. Monozygotic twins, on the other hand, are antigenically alike and will therefore accept grafts from their co-twins. Thus, skin grafting provides the ultimate test of zygosity and may be used when zygosity determination is important, as in the case of a contemplated kidney transplant.

A somewhat less sensitive, but easier and faster method is the mixed lymphocyte assay, which also depends on antigenic dissimilarity. The lymphocytes from one of a pair of MZ twins will not stimulate division of lymphocytes from the other, whereas there is often a response if the twins are DZ (Chapter 18).

USE OF TWINS IN ESTIMATING HERITABILITY

Quantitative Characters

Twin studies have contributed a great deal to our knowledge of the genetic component in many quantitative characters, particularly intelligence. The statistical methodology is complicated, and its detailed discussion is not within the authors' competence or the scope of this book. We will present some of the concepts involved and refer the reader to textbooks of quantitative genetics for the technical aspects.[5,6] Let us begin with some definitions.

In twin studies designed to estimate heritability, the aim is basically to measure how much more closely members of MZ pairs resemble one another than do members of DZ

pairs. This can be done by determining mean pair difference, variance, or correlation.

Mean Pair Difference. The tendency of pairs (of twins, sibs, parent—child, and so on) to resemble each other can be measured by obtaining the difference between the members of each pair by subtraction and calculating the mean of these values. If y is the value of the measurement for one twin and y^* for the other, the mean pair difference of n pairs is $\Sigma(y - y^*)/n$. The smaller the mean pair difference, the greater the similarity.

Variance. Variance (V) is a measure of the variation, calculated by squaring the difference (d) of each value from the mean, summing the squared differences, and dividing by the number of observations: $V = \Sigma d^2/n$. The greater the tendency of pairs to resemble each other, the smaller will be the mean pair difference and the variance of the mean pair differences.

Correlation. Correlation (r) is another measure of the tendency of pairs to resemble each other. Several methods of calculation exist. For twin pairs, it may be calculated from the variance of the mean pair difference, $V(y - y^*)$, as compared to the variance of the population, $V(y)$, by the formula

$$r = 1 - \frac{\frac{1}{2}V(y-y^*)}{V(y)}$$

The formula shows that the smaller the variance of the mean pair difference, the greater the correlation. A perfect correlation (complete resemblance) has a value of 1. For a quantitative character that is completely determined by additive genes, MZ twin pairs would have a correlation of 1, and parent-child, sib-sib, and DZ twin pairs would have a correlation of 0.5.

Partitioning of the Variance. Suppose we want to determine the degree to which a given quantitative character is genetically determined. We will assume that the character is normally distributed. The questions can be framed in terms of the total variation shown by the character in the population and how much of this variation is caused by genetic factors. The following discussion will deal with the conceptual basis of this approach to the estimation of heritability, without getting into the complexity of the mathematics. The subject is well reviewed elsewhere.[7]

The observed value of the character (y) for a particular individual will deviate from the population mean ($\bar{y}$) by an amount determined by genetic factors (g) and an amount determined by environmental factors (e). That is,

$$y = \bar{y} + g + e.$$

For the population as a whole, the variance of y will be similarly determined by the variance of g and the variance of e. This can be symbolized as

$$V = V_G + V_E.$$

The degree of genetic determination can be estimated by the heritability (H), which was defined in Chapter 8 as the amount of variation resulting from genetic differences as a proportion of the total variation. Thus,

$$H = V_G/(V_G + V_E).$$

For a character determined completely by genes, the heritability would be 1 because V_E would be 0. Similarly, if genes played no part in determining the value of the character, H would be 0.

Assortative mating (the tendency for people to choose mates similar to themselves) increases the genetic variance by increasing the proportion of offspring falling in the tails (extremes) of the distribution. There is considerable assortative mating for several characteristics. For instance, the correlation between mates is about 0.3 for height and 0.4 or more for intelligence.[6]

The genetic variance can in turn be partitioned into V_A, that due to additive genes (where the heterozygote is intermediate between the two homozygotes), and V_D, that due to genes showing dominance. If there is dominance, the children will not be intermediate between the parents. The dominance variance tends to reduce parent-child correlation relative to sib-sib correlation and can be estimated from this comparison. Other deviations from additive gene action can also be considered as contributing to the variance in a complex way. Epistasis, or the interaction of different loci in a nonadditive way, also contributes to lack of resemblance between parents and offspring.

Furthermore, there may be a correlation between genetic and environmental factors. For instance, children with a better than average genotype for intelligence have a better than average chance of having relatively intelligent parents, who will provide a relatively better environment for fostering the intellectual endowment. This is referred to as the *covariance* of heredity and environment. Distinct from this is the *interaction* of heredity and environment, which refers to the fact that different genotypes may respond differently to changes in the environment. For instance, two genetically different individuals may have the same caloric intake and activity levels, but one may become fat and the other stay thin, because their different genotypes cause them to metabolize their food differently. In an "annotation," which anyone interested in the subject should study, Lewontin points out that the complexities of the interaction between the genotype and environment may render conclusions about heritability based on the partitioning of variance virtually meaningless.[8]

Thus the estimation of how much of the variation in the population is caused by genes is a complicated procedure and, in man, entails the use of many untested assumptions. (The procedure and the limitations are well described elsewhere.[6,7]) Nevertheless, the partitioning of variance can be a rough guide to the relative importance of genetic factors, which is necessary if we are to interpret what has happened to, or predict what may happen to, the genes influencing quantitative characters.

It should also be emphasized that any such estimate of heritability *refers to a particular population and its particular range of environments*. In the case of intelligence, for instance, a poor environment will prevent the expression of some favorable genetic potential, and a good environment will allow the full expression. Thus, for the same population, the heritability (proportion of variation due to genes) will be greater in the better environment.

Twin Studies

A major contribution of twin studies to genetics has been the estimation of H for various quantitative characters. Because monozygotic twins are genetically identical, any differences between them must result from environmental variation. Thus the measurement of differences between MZ twins provides a direct estimate of V_E. Differences between DZ pairs represent $V_G + V_E$ (although this will be a biased estimate, since V_G for DZ twins will be less than that for the general population). For any sex-influenced character, of course, one should compare only like-sexed pairs.

Another bias is introduced by the fact that the environment is more similar for twins than for unrelated pairs, and perhaps for MZ than for DZ pairs; for postnatal measurements, this can be partly compensated for by using twins reared apart, but these are relatively uncommon. It must be emphasized that the statistical models are necessarily oversimplifications. Table 26–2 gives some examples of similarities between pairs of MZ and DZ twins for quantitative characters, along with estimates of heritability.

For characters that are classified as present or absent, rather than measured, heritability can be estimated from the frequency with which pairs are *concordant* (both affected) or *discordant* (only one affected). If the trait is determined in part by genes, the concordance rate will be higher in MZ than in DZ twins.

Table 26–2. Heritability Estimates for Some Quantitative Traits Based on MZ-DZ Twin Comparisons

| Trait | Sex | | |
	Male	Female	Both
Height (child)			0.92
Height (adult)	0.79	0.92	
Weight (child)			0.83
Weight (adult)	0.05	0.42	
Arm length	0.80	0.87	
Age at menarche		0.93	
Alcohol clearance			0.88
Stanford-Binet IQ			0.83
Arithmetic			0.25
School achievement			0.09

However, as with ordinary sib studies, the concordance rate should be corrected for the method of ascertainment. If the concordance rate is defined as the proportion of affected individuals among the co-twins of previously defined index cases (called the proband concordance rate), the corrected concordance rate, c', will be

$$c' = \frac{c + 2c^*}{c + 2c^* + d}$$

where c is the number of concordant pairs ascertained through only one of the affected twins, c^* is the number of concordant pairs in which both members were ascertained independently, and d is the number of discordant pairs.[1] In other words, concordant pairs ascertained twice (once for each twin) are counted twice.

Gottesman provides a useful guide to the management and interpretation of data on concordance rates for discontinuous characters in twin pairs.[7] Discontinuous familial traits not due to single mutant genes are likely to be multifactorial threshold characters, and it therefore seems appropriate to use the threshold model to estimate heritability from twin-concordance rates. It turns out that even when MZ concordance rates are relatively low, heritability can be high. In an individual whose genes place him near the threshold, relatively small environmental differences will place him on one side of the threshold or the other and determine whether he is affected or unaffected. Table 26–3 gives examples of concordance and heritability estimates for a number of discontinuous traits (diseases and malformations).

Remember that these estimates are subject to sampling error and are only approximations. For instance, it is most unlikely that the heritability of manic depressive psychosis is really 1. We should conclude only that it is high. Similarly, the heritability of death from acute infection is obviously not a negative value, but it must certainly be low.

An interesting new approach to the use of twins in genetic analysis compares the offspring of monozygous twin pairs for the character being studied. The children of monozy-

Table 26–3. Twin Concordance and Heritability Estimates for Various Diseases (Assuming No Dominance)*

Disease	% Concordance		
	MZ	DZ	H
Manic depressive psychosis	67	5	1
Congenital hip dislocation	40	3	0.90
Club foot	33	3	0.88
Cleft lip ± cleft palate	38	8	0.87
Rheumatoid arthritis	34	7	0.74
Bronchial asthma	47	24	0.71
Tuberculosis	37	15	0.65
High blood pressure	25	7	0.62
Rheumatic fever	20	6	0.55
Cancer, same site	7	3	0.33
Death from acute infection	8	9	−0.06

*Estimate from Cavalli-Sforza, L.L., and Bodmer, W.F.: The Genetics of Human Populations. San Francisco, W.H. Freeman, 1971 and Smith, C.: Concordance in Twins: methods and interpretation. Am. J. Hum. Genet. 26:454, 1974.

gous twins are full sibs, of course, and also half-sibs of the children of the co-twin.[11] This makes it possible to sort out, more effectively than in orthodox twin studies, the contributions to variance of maternal effects (which would make the offspring of female pairs more similar than the offspring of male pairs) and the effects of dominance and epistasis (avoiding parent-child comparisons that may be confounded by intergenerational effects), common environment (often ignored in ordinary twin studies) and assortative mating. Space does not permit further discussion here, and the reader is referred to Walter Nance's review for more details.[11] Studies so far suggest that environmental and maternal effects and gene-environment interactions have been underestimated in previous studies.

Twin studies have their limitations. They cannot determine the mode of inheritance of a character. For prenatal traits, and particularly malformations, assumptions about similar environments are complicated by the mechanical effects of having two babies growing in the same confined space, the relations of the fetal membranes, and the fact that monozygotic twins may have vascular connections between the placentas that may favor one twin at the expense of the other. Other difficulties have been referred to previously. Neverthe-

less, careful studies of twins, their sibs, and their parents are the most valuable method available for demonstrating whether the familial tendencies observed in many quantitative traits and common diseases have a genetic basis and, if so, its relative magnitude.

Finally, MZ twins can be useful in therapeutic trials and other experimental situations in which absence of genetic variation is an advantage—for example, to test the effect of vitamin C on the common cold.[10]

SUMMARY

Twins have proved useful in weighing the relative importance of heredity and environment in normal variation and in disease. Traits or disorders having an important genetic component are found in higher frequency in the co-twins of affected monozygotic (MZ, identical) twins than in the co-twins of affected dizygotic (DZ, fraternal) twins. The frequency of identical twins in various populations is about 3.5 per 1000 deliveries; the frequency of dizygotic twins varies greatly depending on race and maternal age.

The zygosity of twins may be determined by many methods, including examination of fetal membranes, physical similarity, dermatoglyphics, genetic markers, immunologic reactions, and skin grafts.

Twin studies have been useful in the study of the genetic component of quantitative characters, such as intelligence and threshold characters, such as common diseases. Statistical methods have been employed; the results must be evaluated within the context of their limitations.

REFERENCES

1. Allen, G., Harvald, B., and Shields, J.: Measures of twin concordance. Acta Genet. 17:475, 1967.
2. Benirschke, K.: Origin and clinical significance of twinning. Clin. Obstet. Gynecol. 15:220, 1972.
3. Boklage, C.E.: Twinning non-righthandedness, and fusion malformations: evidence for heritable causal elements held in common. Am. J. Med. Genet. 28:67, 1987.
4. Bulmer, M.G.: The Biology of Twinning in Man. Oxford, Clarendon Press, 1970.
5. Bodmer, W.F., and Cavalli-Sforza, L.L.: Genetics, Evolution, and Man. San Francisco, W.H. Freeman, 1975.

6. Cavalli-Sforza, L.L., and Bodmer, W.F.: The Genetics of Human Populations. San Francisco, W.H. Freeman, 1971.

7. Gottesman, I.I., and Carey, G.: Extracting meaning and direction from twin data. Psychiatr. Dev. 1:35, 1983.

8. Lewontin, R.C.: The analysis of variance and the analysis of causes. Am. J. Hum. Genet. 26:400, 1974.

9. Maynard-Smith, S., and Penrose, L.S.: Monozygotic and dizygotic twin diagnosis. Ann. Hum. Gen. 18:273, 1955.

10. Miller, J.Z., et al.: Therapeutic effect of vitamin C. A co-twin control study. J.A.M.A. 237:248, 1977.

11. Nance, W.E., et al.: Monozygotic twin sibships: A new design for genetic and epidemiologic research. *In* Genetic Epidemiology, edited by N.E. Morton and C.S. Chung. New York, Academic Press, 1978.

12. Thompson, J.S., and Thompson, M.W.: Genetics in Medicine, 4th ed. Philadelphia, W.B. Saunders Co., 1986.

Chapter 27
Syndromology

WHAT IS THIS FACE, LESS CLEAR AND CLEARER
THE PULSE IN THE ARM, LESS STRONG AND STRONGER . . .?

T. S. ELIOT, MARINA

One of the most frustrating problems a genetic counselor meets is to decide whether a patient with multiple anomalies represents simply a coincidental association of several independent defects or a syndrome and, if so, which syndrome. The difference may be important, for both the genetic and the clinical prognosis. If a baby's hypospadias, webbed toes, and cleft palate represent the Smith-Lemli-Opitz syndrome, the outlook is different than if these defects occurred together by chance. In one case, the risk of mental retardation is high and so is the risk of recurrence in sibs (one in four). In the other case, these risks are comparatively low.

There is no problem if the cause is defined, as in the case of a chromosomal trisomy or an enzyme defect. However, often this is not the case: no single diagnostic test is conclusive. The situation is further confused by differences of opinion as to what constitutes a "syndrome." Some take the "syndrome-by-definition" approach; i.e., a syndrome is that association of defects described by whoever first described the syndrome, particularly if the syndrome is named after that person. This simplifies the matter for those who are interested mainly in categorizing, but represents difficulties to those interested in assigning causes or making prognoses, either clinical or genetic. In cases in which the cause is known, such as the autosomal recessive gene causing the Laurence-Moon-Biedl syndrome or the trisomy 21 of Down syndrome, it is perfectly clear that the same etiology does not always produce the same effect. In the geneticist's jargon, the various features of the syndrome somewhat independently show reduced penetrance and variable expressivity. The sibs affected by the same gene that caused the Laurence-Moon-Biedl syndrome in the proband do not always have the same array of features.

This brings us to the "syndrome-by-cause" approach, which holds that a syndrome should include all combinations of anomalies known to result from whatever causes the syndrome. Thus, not all cases of Marfan syndrome have arachnodactyly, not all cases of Down syndrome have a simian crease, and not all cases of rubella syndrome have a patent ductus arteriosus. In other words, syndromes are *polythetic* classes, in which the members share a number of features, but not necessarily any one feature, or any specific combination of them.[9] This definition is all very well when the etiology is known, but in many syndromes the etiology is not known. In such cases, we are left in the unsatisfactory position of having to make an arbitrary judgment as to how many and which features a patient must have before he or she can reasonably be considered an example of the syndrome.

The syndrome-by-definition approach results in another difficulty—ascertainment bias. If we decide arbitrarily that all cases of a given syndrome must have all the features possessed by the original group of cases, and if in fact the same cause can produce an array of defects that does not include one or more of the original array, we are ruling out as examples of the syndrome some cases with the same cause as those we accept as having the syndrome. This, to say the least, reduces the value of the syndrome concept.

When a new syndrome is described, the course of events often proceeds somewhat as follows: Dr. Eponi, in describing the first group of cases, shows that they all have features A, B, C, and D and that the individual features are rare enough that the association is not likely to be coincidental. Thus the association of features becomes the "Eponi syndrome." Other workers start to report cases of the syndrome, and they show that in addition to A, B, C, and D, features E, F, and G may also be associated with the syndrome. Then someone observes a case with features, A, C, D, E, F, and G. Is this a case of the Eponi syndrome? No, according to the syndrome-by-definitionists, because it does not have B, and Eponi syndrome always has B. Why does Eponi syndrome always have B? Because if it does not have B it is not a case of Eponi syndrome. We hope the circular reasoning is apparent. Thus there are those who will not accept a patient as a case of the Rubinstein-Taybi (or "broad-thumb-and-great-toe syndrome") unless he has broad thumbs, even though he may have all the other characteristic features. If this view prevailed, the frequency of broad thumbs in the Rubinstein-Taybi syndrome would always be 100%. We prefer the view that probably no one feature is a sine qua non of a syndrome. This is true in many syndromes of known cause. Presumably it is also true in syndromes of unknown cause.

Consider the history of Turner syndrome, which was originally recognized by the association of shortness, edema, webbed neck, and increased carrying angle in female children. Sexual infantilism was recognized later, and other features later still. Sex chromatin analysis and, later, karyotyping revealed the cause of the syndrome. Only then was it recognized that about half the cases of Turner syndrome do not have webbed neck, some are not strikingly short, and, in fact, an appreciable number of cytologically diagnosed cases would not fit the original criteria for Turner syndrome.

What can be done about this difficult situation? The best solution would be to discover the specific cause of each syndrome. For instance, some may be the result of presently unrecognizable chromosome rearrangements, and others the result of a specific prenatal insult at a particular stage of gestation. Secondly, we can try to understand the basis for the variability of syndromes. One source may be the timing of an embryologic insult, as demonstrated for the rubella and the thalidomide syndromes. Another may be variation in the genetic background. Are the relatively not short cases of Turner syndrome not short because they come from tall families? Do persons who have Marfan syndrome without arachnodactyly fail to show arachnodactyly because they have an otherwise short stocky build? Finally, we must be aware of the ascertainment bias mentioned previously and recognize, for instance, that cases of Turner syndrome diagnosed in a cardiology clinic will have the highest frequency of heart defects, whereas those diagnosed at birth will have the highest frequency of webbed neck and puffy feet, and those diagnosed in endocrinology clinics are most likely to be short. Being aware of these biases and keeping an open mind on the question of atypical syndromes will at least leave the way open toward a better understanding of syndromology.

Patients may be identified as having a particular syndrome either by having a characteristic combination of major anomalies, as in the Laurence-Moon and Apert syndromes, or by having a particular combination of minor anomalies or other physical characteristics that give the patient a "characteristic" appearance, as in the de Lange or Rubinstein-Taybi syndromes.

In attempting to make a diagnosis of a patient with a suspected but unidentified dysmorphic syndrome, one may search through the various catalogues, compendia, and atlases[1-4,7,10-12] for the syndromes that have the most features displayed by the patient, or the facies most similar to that of the patient. But because syndromes are polythetic, it is not unusual for a patient to lack some of the features listed in the description of a syndrome and to have some not listed and deciding whether a patient should be diagnosed as having a certain syndrome becomes a matter of judgment.

Progress towards a more objective approach to classifying patients into groups according to their similarities is being made by applying the principles of numerical taxonomy. A large number of dysmorphic patients are coded with respect to a large number of characters. Each character may be considered to lie on an axis in a multi-dimensional space, or hyperspace. With the aid of a computer, each patient is placed in the hyperspace according to the similarity (number of characters in common) of each patient to all the other patients. Patients with a syndrome should be closer to one another than to other patients, and clustering methods are available that divide the nonrandom distribution of points into groups, according to how similar they are.[6] This approach makes no assumption about what features constitute the syndrome and therefore gets around the bias of ascertainment referred to above. Further progress will depend on the accumulation of systematically recorded data on large numbers of syndromic patients and should result in a more objective definition of syndromes, and of communities of syndromes.[5]

Reference should also be made to the several computer-assisted systems for the diagnosis of dysmorphic syndromes now available.[2,8] The problem of access to the overwhelming volume of information is being facilitated by several computerized data bases, including one in Australia (Possum; A. Bankier, Murdoch Institute, Victoria, FAX (03) 345-5789); London (R. Winter et al., J. Med. Gen. 25:118, 1988); Marseille (Gendiag, S., Aymé, Hopital d'Enfants, 13385 Marseille Cedex S); and Boston (M.L. Buyse, Center for Birth Defects Information Services, Dover, MA 02030). These systems can act as a guide to diagnostic thinking by providing a list (sometimes quite long) of syndromes having the features that occur in the patient in question, but they require some syndromic expertise in choice of features to be entered, terminology, and interpretation of results.[8]

REFERENCES

1. Buyse, M.L. (Ed.): Birth Defects Encyclopedia. Dover, MA, Centre for Birth Defects Information Services, 1990.
2. Gorlin, R.J., Cohen, M.M., and Levin, L.S.: Syndromes of the Head and Neck. Oxford, Oxford University Press, 1990.
3. Jones, K.L.: Smith's recognizable patterns of human malformation. Philadelphia, W.B. Saunders Co., 1988.
4. McKusick, V.. Mendelian Inheritance in Man, 9th ed. Baltimore, The Johns Hopkins Press, 1990.
5. Pinsky, L.: Informative morphogenetic variants. Minor congenital anomalies revisited. Issues and Reviews in Teratology 3:135, 1985.
6. Preus, M.: Numerical classification of syndromes. Hospital Practice 20(6):111, 1985.
7. Schinzel, A.: Catalogue of Unbalanced Chromosome Aberrations in Man. New York, Walter de Gruyter, 1984.
8. Schorderet, D.F.: Using OMIM (On-line Mendelian Inheritance in Man) as an expert system in medical genetics. Am. J. Med. Genet. 39:278, 1991.
9. Sokal, R.: Classification: Purposes, principles, progress, prospects. Science 185:1115, 1974.
10. Taybi, H., and Lackman, R.S.: Radiology of syndromes, metabolic disorders and skeletal dysplasias. 3rd edition. Chicago, Year Book Medical Publishers, Inc., 1990.
11. Warkany, J.: Congenital Malformations. Notes and Comments. Chicago, Year Book Publishers, Inc., 1971
12. Winter, R.M., and Baraitser, M.: Multiple congenital anomalies. London, Chapman and Hall, 1991.

Chapter 28
Genetic Counseling

GOOD COUNSELLORS LACK NO CLIENTS.

SHAKESPEARE

Thirty years ago, most genetic counseling recognized as such was done by nonmedical geneticists, as a sideline to their main interest, research and teaching. Counseling consisted mainly of applying the mendelian laws to a particular family situation. Much information about the inheritance of human diseases was misleading because of the tendency to choose strikingly familial cases for publication, failure to correct for ascertainment bias, and overenthusiastic attempts to fit segregation data to mendelian patterns. There were few textbooks on human genetics, and none that made reference to genetic counseling. Since then, the dramatic growth in knowledge of human genetics has made the genetic counselor's task tremendously more complex.

THE GROWTH OF GENETIC COUNSELING

Patients with a great variety of diseases and syndromes are now referred for evaluation and counseling, and the relevant literature has expanded exponentially. Keeping track of the enormous volume of relevant information in molecular, biochemical, population, and clinical cytogenetics is a formidable task. Furthermore, genetic counseling depends on accurate diagnosis, and this depends on the

expertise of various medical and surgical specialists, as well as laboratories expert in cytogenetic and appropriate biochemical techniques. In short, a single person can no longer be familiar with the relevant fund of knowledge and competent in the techniques necessary to provide good genetic information. The genetic evaluation and counseling of a patient (family) has become a team affair, requiring the resources of a genetics center. Most major medical centers now include a department of medical genetics in their system of health care services. Figure 28–1 depicts the stages of the genetic counseling process.

WHO IS IT FOR?

Genetic counseling usually begins with someone wanting to know whether a disease suspected of being genetic will recur in the near relatives of someone with the disease. The traditional role of the counselor is to estimate P, the probability of recurrence, and to assist the person concerned in deciding what the appropriate action would be. However, the final decision must be left to the family.

Most counseling involves the occurrence of a particular disorder in a child and the question of whether future children may be sim-

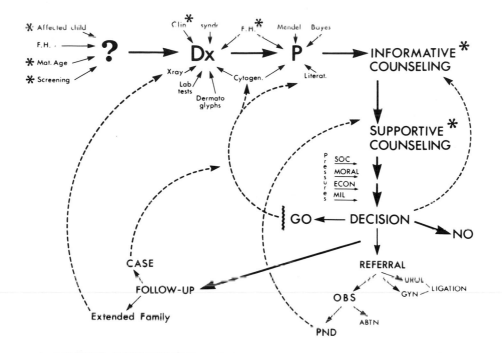

A GENETIC COUNSELING MAP

Fig. 28–1.   Map of the genetic counseling process. It begins with a question, raised by the advent of a child with a ? genetic disorder, other aspect of the family history, etc. There must be a diagnosis (Dx), which may depend on information from clinicians, syndromologists, X-ray studies, laboratory tests, dermatoglyphics, cytogenetics, and the family history (FH). To answer the question usually requires estimating a probability (P), using information from the family history, cytogenetics, the literature, the mendelian principles and Bayesian calculations. Following informative and supportive counseling (often influenced by social, moral, economic, and family pressures) the counselee may reach a decision either to refrain from reproduction or to go ahead. Both of these may require appropriate referral. If the "GO" decision results in a recurrence, further counseling may be required. Follow-up of the counselee and the extended family may result in reentry into the process.

ilarly affected. The parents may be referred because they have expressed their concern to a physician or because the physician thinks the disease has an appreciable recurrence risk, or they may approach the counselor directly. Parents may also want to know about the risk for affected children's children, or for the children of the unaffected brothers and sisters. Prenatal diagnosis has added a new complexity (Chapter 15). A person contemplating marriage may be concerned about a specific disease or history of racial admixture in the fiancé's family. Cousins contemplating marriage may be worried about the possible hazards of consanguinity. Occasionally, the question may involve a child being considered for adoption and the presence of a disease or racial admixture in the family. And sometimes the counselor may be concerned with the near relatives of people he has counseled, who are at risk for, or for having children with, a particular disease.

In certain populations in which a severe genetic disorder is unusually high, screening programs have been organized to detect and counsel heterozygotes. This procedure involves "prospective" counseling rather than retrospective (when the affected child already has been born); it requires a quite different approach and raises quite different problems. See page 414 for further discussion.

THE GENETIC COUNSELOR

A good counselor needs a sound grasp of genetic principles, a wide knowledge of the scientific literature on diseases of possible genetic origin, and much sympathy, tact, and good sense. No longer is counseling simply a sideline in which a geneticist applies the mendelian laws to specific family situations. Increasingly, the counselor is being recognized as a specialist, who has undergone formal training.[7]

In some cases, the family physician is the most appropriate person to do the counseling because he knows the family, its attitudes, and its socioeconomic background. However, he may have neither the genetic knowledge nor the time for several interviews, and sometimes the family does not have a family physician. Finally, some cases may be so complex or may require sufficiently specialized tests that the services of a medical genetics center are desirable.

Genetic associates are a newly recognized group of "genetic care-providers." They are trained at the master's degree level to participate in the genetic counseling process in a variety of ways which include taking family histories, gathering information from hospital records, searching the literature, interpreting information to the family, following up of families, and acting as a liaison between various other members of the team.[18,19]

In many countries, medical genetics is now a recognized medical specialty, in recognition of the need to ensure that those providing health care services are competent to do so. To this end, the Canadian College of Medical Geneticists has been incorporated as an accrediting body for geneticists—both M.D. and Ph.D—providing health-care services in Canada, and the American Society of Human Genetics has, more recently, set up the American Board of Medical Genetics for the same purpose.

Genetic counselors are still doing a considerable amount of soul-searching about the role of the counselor. The book, *Genetic Counseling: Facts, Values and Norms*, presents an instructive spectrum of views.[1] The counselor may play the role of information giver (Hsia), facilitator of the counselee's decision process (Antley), psychotherapist (Kessler) or moral advisor (Twiss). These are by no means mutually exclusive. The traditional attitude is that presenting the genetic facts and options is the essence of genetic counseling, which should be nondirective, nonpsychoanalytic, and nonjudgmental. The decision-facilitator model claims, on the other hand, that the counselor must choose the most relevant parts of the genetic information available to present to the counselee, that his own biases will inevitably influence these choices, and that the facts presented will inevitably influence the counselee's value system. The counseling process is therefore psychodynamically fluid, involving a series of decisions on the part of both counselor and counselee, and the counselor, to be effective, must be aware of this. Most counselors probably employ a mix of these two approaches, in varying proportions.

The psychologic aspects of genetic counseling in various situations are usefully discussed in several review volumes.[1,4,5,9,14,15]

GENETIC EVALUATION OF THE PATIENT

The physician's approach to genetic evaluation can be formulated as a series of questions:

1. Does the patient have a disease of clearly nongenetic origin, such as infection or birth trauma? Microcephaly, cataracts, retinopathy, heart defects, and other abnormalities should raise the question of prenatal infection with rubella, toxoplasma, cytomegalic inclusion disease virus, herpes, or other teratogenic organisms. Did the mother take any drugs suspected of being teratogenic? It is useful to inquire about nonmedical drugs such as LSD and marijuana at this point. With the exception of alcohol and cocaine, there is little evidence that these are teratogenic, but parents who have taken them may fear that this was the cause of the baby's disorder and may need reassurance.

2. Does the baby have a disease of clearly genetic etiology, such as hemophilia, an inborn error of metabolism, or a chondrodystrophy? The clinical and laboratory features will obviously provide the most important diagnostic information, and the family history may also be use-

ful. Genetic heterogencity should be kept in mind, that is, the conditions with similar clinical features may be genetically distinct.

3. If the patient's disorder does not fall into either of the above categories, does the patient have features that suggest a syndrome? If so, the subsequent investigation and management will depend on the nature of the syndrome. Some syndromes are well known to physicians; others are so rare as to be "once-in-a-lifetime" events for the medical geneticist, and one must resort to appropriate compendia, atlases, and catalogues or to consultation with other clinical geneticists experienced in syndromology. It should be recognized, however, that many children with combinations of dysmorphic features so unusual, and a facies so striking, that one feels sure they have a syndrome, nevertheless defy classification by even the most experienced syndromologists. Furthermore, many dysmorphic features are age-dependent, and an infant who, as he grows older, will develop the facies associated in the physician's mind with a particular syndrome may have a quite different appearance at birth. Conversely, in some children, collections of minor anomalies that may lead one to suspect a syndrome may simply represent the "family facies," be normal variants, and may even disappear in childhood.

4. When a syndrome cannot be identified, one must consider what further investigations are necessary. Is examination of the chromosomes indicated? The indications for karyotyping have continued to expand as improved methods of staining have allowed detection of progressively more subtle deletions, duplications, and rearrangements of chromosomal material. Except when a specific, nonchromosomal syndrome has been identified, karyotyping should be considered for the patient who has multiple malformations, ambiguous genitalia, or hypospadias of moderate or severe degree, or

who exhibits unexplained small size, failure to thrive, or mental retardation, especially when these are accompanied by dysmorphic features.

5. In any case, the *family history* should be screened for clues to the possible genetic basis for the baby's problem. For hospital patients, taking a detailed family history is usually neither feasible nor justified at the time of admission. On the other hand, following the time-honored practice of asking whether there are any relatives with "diseases of hereditary tendency," such as allergy, cancer, epilepsy, heart disease, insanity, or tuberculosis, is not likely to be rewarding. If the cause of the patient's disease is not obviously environmental, a minimal family history should be taken early, with elaboration later if indicated.

The most useful question to ask when taking the family history is whether problems similar to the present one have occurred in other members of the family. The answer will usually be negative, even when the disease is clearly genetic (because inherited diseases are rare, and the majority of patients with genetic diseases have a negative family history). Nevertheless, when it is positive the family history can be helpful. For example, a little girl was admitted in coma, following a measles infection. The fact that she had been acidotic was noted on the discharge summary, but its significance was not realized until review of the family history uncovered the fact that a sib had died of acidotic coma. The parents had been told (in another country) that this was caused by renal tubular acidosis, which was stated (incorrectly) to be nongenetic. Investigation of this clue led to correct diagnosis, methylmalonic aciduria.

In older patients, a question about near relatives with such familial diseases as early coronary disease, or several relatives with cancer, may alert the physician to the need for increased vigilance. When surgery is contemplated, it is also wise to inquire about relatives with bleeding tendencies or unusual reactions to anesthetics.

The patient's sibs should be listed by age and sex, and their state of health noted. The main reason for this is that parents may not recognize what constitutes a "similar problem," as the example demonstrates. The causes of any deaths in sibs should be established. For example, the mother of a child admitted for "cerebral palsy" said that a previous child had died of "pneumonia," but did not mention that the underlying cause was Tay-Sachs disease, which the second child also had.

Finally, one should ask about the possibility of parental consanguinity as this can be a clue that the patient's problem is caused by a recessively inherited disease.

THE COUNSELING INTERVIEW

It is difficult for anyone who has not had the experience of having a baby who is defective to imagine the feelings of parents in this situation. They may be shocked, bewildered, scared, and often angered. Counseling at this point is directed largely to explaining the nature of the baby's disorder and the short-term prognosis and to providing as much emotional support as possible. This can, and probably should, be done by the family physician, who knows the parents, although it is sometimes left to the genetic counselor, particularly in cases of chromosomal problems and inborn errors of metabolism where the geneticist is involved in making the diagnosis. During this initial stage, the cause of the disorder is not one of the most important worries of the parents, except that they will often feel that the child's defect is a sign that they themselves are defective in some way and may benefit by having these feelings aired. This is usually not the time to go deeply into the question of recurrence risks for future children, for in most cases the parents will not be listening. They should, however, be made aware that such information will be available later.

When the initial crisis is over and the parents become aware of the long-term significance of their baby's disorder, they may begin to wonder more about the cause of the child's disease and, in particular, whether it may happen again. This is the time for the specifically *genetic* counseling. If it is delayed too long, the parents may have already started another pregnancy, unaware of a high risk or burden, or have been sterilized, unaware that the risk and burden are low. To inform the parents that there is a risk of recurrence is particularly important if prenatal diagnosis is possible. Even if prenatal diagnosis is not relevant, parents must still be made aware of what the risks are so that they will be neither shocked by an unforeseen recurrence nor deterred from having children when the risk is negligible, but be able to make an informed decision. Obviously, the parents should seek counseling before the baby at risk is conceived but, people being only human, sometimes they do not.

The first interview in the medical genetics center usually takes the better part of an hour or more; in addition to the collection of information, it allows the counselor a chance to begin to get to know the parents and vice versa. For this reason, the counselor, rather than an assistant, may wish to take the family history, time-consuming though it may be. It is also preferable to interview both parents; together they may present a more accurate family history than separately, and the counselor has a chance to get some impression of how they interact, which may be helpful later in the counseling process. This also guards against the interviewed parent misinterpreting what the counselor said, when relaying the information to the other parent. The facts given by the counselor should be placed on record in the patient's hospital chart and in a letter to the family physician or the parents, or both.

The first requirement, of course, is that the disease causing the concern be accurately diagnosed. The diagnosis may already have been made, in which case the counselor need only be able to evaluate the reliability of the diagnosis and know when to ask for confirmatory tests or opinions. In other cases, the counselor may aid in making the diagnosis, either by performing special tests, such as examination of the chromosomes, or through her or his familiarity with diseases so rare that the practicing physician may not know of them. For instance, he or she must take into account the problem of genetic heterogeneity—

the fact that diseases that present very similar features may have different causes and therefore different risks of recurrence. Further special tests and interpretation of the family history may permit a distinction to be made. Thus, taking the family history may help to establish a diagnosis, and it is usually essential to the estimation of P, the probability of recurrence.

Taking the Family History

Taking the family history involves making a pedigree and listing the patient's near relatives by sex, age, and state of health, particularly with reference to the occurrence of relevant diseases in the family. A special form is used to ensure systematic recording of the data. It is often necessary to correspond with doctors and hospitals or to examine medical records directly to confirm diagnoses of possible relevant disease occurring in family members. In most cases, carrying the family study beyond first cousins and grandparents is not useful (unless there are affected relatives in this group), both because the information gets progressively less reliable with increasing distance of relationship and because diseases only in relatives more distantly removed than this are not likely to be relevant to the patient. Depending on the nature of the disease involved, the counselor may want to amplify the family history by doing special examinations or tests on particular family members (e.g., to detect whether certain individuals are carrying a mutant gene or a chromosomal rearrangement).

The counselor may be able to estimate P reliably by the end of the first interview, and if the estimate is reassuringly low and the parents are happy about it, there may be no need for further interviews. However, if test results are not back, the risk is not reassuring, or the parents have any doubts about it or show any signs of uneasiness, a second interview is indicated. The interval provides an opportunity for the parents to absorb the information given, clarify their thoughts, and define the questions they want to ask.

Establishing the Recurrence Risk

The process by which the counselor establishes the recurrence risk in question has been reviewed in Chapter 5 and elsewhere.[3,16,24] It involves placing the disease in one of four etiologic categories: major mutant genes, chromosomal aberrations, major environmental agents, and multifactorial. The recurrence risk can then be calculated either from mendelian laws with appropriate Bayesian modification, or by selection of the appropriate empirical estimate, as outlined in previous chapters.

Interpreting the Recurrence Risk

The next step in the counseling process is to make certain that the parents know what the probability figure means in their situation. Some have trouble understanding the very concept of probability, and some, even though they have an affected child, may not grasp the full implications of having another one.

For one thing, statement of the fact that the risk is a probability introduces an element of uncertainty.[5,12] Whatever the odds given, parents may tend to see them in a binary form— "either it will happen or it won't" or, as one parent put it, "No matter how big the number in the bottom of the fraction, 1 in 100, or 1000, or 10,000, that *one* is still there, and it could be my child." Uncertainty is greater if the risk given is not based on a simple segregation ratio but, as so often happens, is an average of two or more such ratios—for example, either you are a carrier and the risk is 1 to 3 or you are not, with a risk near zero, so your average is somewhere between these extremes, the "somewhere" being estimated with varying degrees of precision depending on the current state of knowledge. Or, your brothers may have had the X-linked form of the disease, in which case your son has a 1 to 7 chance of getting it, or the recessive form, in which your children are at negligible risk, and we cannot tell which. Further uncertainty is added if the prognosis is variable—your child would have a 1 to 1 chance of inheriting the mutant gene, and if (s)he does (s)he may have anything from a few trivial features to severe mental retardation or death.

Once parents clearly understand the meaning of the probability they have been given, they must convert the probability into a decision—whether to try for another baby, seek sterilization or artificial insemination, marry, adopt, or whatever their particular problem indicates (Fig. 28–1). The counselor may be able to help the family reach a wise decision, but he should avoid making it for them. For instance, he can point out the various factors to be considered: the severity of the disease in relation to the risk of recurrence, the impact of the disease on the rest of the family, the social and moral pressures they may feel, the present number of children, the possibility of adoption or artificial insemination as an alternative to having their own children, the pros and cons of sterilization, and the possibility of prenatal diagnosis. Increasingly important factors are the availability and effectiveness of treatment. One reason why families do not choose prenatal diagnosis for disorders such as Huntington disease and cystic fibrosis as often as expected is the hope that gene therapy may soon provide a cure.

The parents may handle the uncertainties by focusing more on the consequences than on the statistical risk. They may approach the process of decision-making by imagining the various possible outcomes of each decision, what each would be like, and how and whether they would be able to cope with it. The characteristic "scenario" involves trying out the worst: making use of the available factual information and trying to determine how they would manage, not just the affected child, but all the other issues perceived as problematic were chance to go against them. They search for an alternative with a maximum loss that would be acceptable—a "least-lose" option—and if they find one they may be able to reach a decision to take a chance. During this process, the statistical risk that the event will occur (Will the child be abnormal?) becomes so intertwined with the other uncertainties (How serious will it be? How long will he suffer? Will I be able to handle it?) that the distinction between risk and consequences is lost, and the risk is perhaps being considered as part of the consequences. It is important to

realize that this process may lead to a decision that does not seem "rational," in the sense of being reached by a conscious weighing of the benefits, risks, and burdens[11] but still may be the best for that particular family.

The counselor should not try to impose his view of the appropriate decision on the parents. However, it is not enough simply to present the required probability and leave it at that. In the ensuing discussion, the parents may eventually ask the counselor what he would do in the same situation. When they ask his opinion, they may not be so much asking the counselor to tell them what to do, but asking for guidelines. They may never have heard of the situation they are in, much less known anyone who has been in it, and they have no norms, no idea of what is "done."[12] In this circumstance, we feel that the counselor should say that no one really knows what he would do without actually being in the same situation and then he may be justified in saying what he thinks others *might* do. More than one of our counselees has expressed a wish in retrospect that we *had* been more directive, at least in emphasizing what an affected child meant in terms of daily living. "I understood the statistics in my head, but I didn't *feel* it."

Taking Action

The decision reached may demand definitive action. A decision not to have further babies will require further decisions by the parents about contraceptives, sterilization, artificial insemination, adoption, and so on. If contraception fails, the question of abortion may arise. Several recent developments have changed the situation radically with respect to this kind of decision.

The Pill. The advent of contraceptive pills has made it easier for those who wish to avoid having further children to do so. Diaphragms, condoms, and (even more so) the rhythm method were sufficiently unreliable to make the prospect of another—potentially diseased—baby a constant menace. The pill has provided increased security, but on the other hand, for a young woman, the prospect of years "on the pill" and the fear of a single instance of forgetfulness resulting in a high-risk pregnancy can be formidable.

Changing Attitudes toward Abortion. There has been a radical change in social and legal attitudes toward abortion in recent years, from a generally proscriptive to a generally permissive one. In some groups, the mere fact that a pregnancy is unwanted is sufficient grounds for termination; in others, there must be danger to the life of the mother to justify killing an unborn human being. The counselor must respect the religious and moral attitudes of the parents, but in many cases the suggested action may be in conflict with the law or the church. That is, the parents in good conscience may wish to have the pregnancy terminated, but may find it difficult to do so because of legal or religious restrictions. This situation has improved greatly in many areas, but there are still many regions where the law, or the prevailing mores, does not allow parents who wish to prevent the birth of a child with a high risk of severe disease from taking the necessary steps.

Prenatal Diagnosis. Finally, the advent of prenatal diagnosis has introduced an important new option which has radically changed the counseling for certain diseases (Chapter 15).

The Follow-up

One or more follow-up interviews are usually desirable for several reasons. First, they may reinforce the parents' understanding of the information given and correct any misapprehensions resulting from reinterpretation of the information. Not infrequently, follow-up interviews reveal that the figures given have been modified upward or downward, either through reinterpretation with the "aid" of friends and relatives or perhaps in response to the parents' own wishes, subconscious or otherwise. For instance, when 1-to-3 is translated into 3-to-1, one wonders whether this reflects the parents' desire not to have more children for any reason.

Secondly, a significant portion of couples (43% in one study[8]) have difficulty in making reproductive decisions after counseling, or have doubts about the decision they made, or fail

to reach a decision at all. Follow-up interviews are helpful in such cases.

Finally, there are situations in which the mutant gene or chromosomal rearrangement segregating in the family places certain relatives at high risk. In the case of dominant, X-linked, and, occasionally autosomal recessive disorders, and chromosomal rearrangement, certain family members other than the parents may be at risk for developing the disease or having affected children. Arranging that these individuals receive counseling may be troublesome, involving questions of breach of confidence or invasion of privacy, but in failing to do so, the counselor may be criticized for not providing information that could prevent a tragedy. There are no clear guidelines and no legal precedents to resolve such conflicts of interest. With tact, and the help of the proband's parents and the appropriate family physicians, the persons at risk can usually be notified without indiscretion.

Our family follow-ups have also discredited the opinion that "people are going to go ahead and have children no matter what you tell them." Most attempts to evaluate the effectiveness of genetic counseling have used subsequent reproductive behavior as the main criterion (perhaps because it is the easiest to measure) rather than how well the counseling has met the parents' needs.[11] It is true that some parents seem to ignore the genetic hazards to the point of irresponsibility. On the other hand, the decision to take what may seem to us a rather inordinate risk may emerge from well-informed and responsible consideration and should be respected. Whatever decision is reached, our experience is that the majority do heed the risks, and several surveys indicate that, when the risk is low (less than 10%), most parents are prepared to take a chance even with a severe disease, but when the risk is high, the majority take steps (however inadequate) to stop having children. Also, a crippling disease with long-term survival is regarded as more formidable than one that results in early death. It is important, however, to distinguish between parents who have been counseled routinely (e.g., as part of a clinic procedure) and those who have actively sought counseling. Parents who have not sought counseling may not pay much attention to it. Those who have are usually grateful for the knowledge and the counselor's sympathetic ear, making the counselor's task rewarding indeed.

GENETIC SCREENING

Genetic counseling programs usually have an input from genetic screening programs, so genetic screening programs should certainly include genetic counseling resources; therefore a brief discussion of genetic screening is included here. Further discussion will be found in several recent reviews.[1,9,14,17,21,22]

Genetic screening refers to the application of tests to groups of individuals for the purpose of detecting the carriers of deleterious genes or chromosome rearrangements. Its goals are (1) to identify individuals with genetic disease, so that they may receive treatment to obviate the effects of the mutant phenotype (e.g., PKU), or (2) to identify individuals or couples at increased risk for having offspring with genetic disorders. Additional benefits may be the collection of epidemiologic data and expansion of our knowledge of these diseases.

The choice of what groups to screen depends on the nature of the disease. In some cases it is the family, although in this context, the procedure is more properly referred to as genetic testing. If a counselee has a genetic disease or has a near relative with such a disease, the family becomes a group of individuals potentially at increased risk for having affected offspring (e.g., hemophilia, Duchenne muscular dystrophy, Tay-Sachs disease, neurofibromatosis, tuberous sclerosis) or for being affected themselves (e.g., early coronary artery disease, peptic ulcer, G6PD deficiency). In other cases the group may be a subpopulation with characteristics that put its members at increased risk, such as blacks (sickle cell disease), Mediterranean races (beta thalassemia, G6PD deficiency), Ashkenazi Jews and French-Canadians (Tay-Sachs disease), and older mothers (trisomies). Or screening may involve the whole population, as in the case of PKU and other inborn errors of metabolism.

With respect to mass screening, various other factors are important in determining who should be screened for what diseases. These revolve around the question of resource allocation: since funds are not unlimited, what investments will bring about the best returns in prevention of disease and reduction of suffering? Among these factors are disease frequency and severity, availability and efficacy of treatment, cost and accuracy of tests, and benefits.

Disease Frequency. If the condition is too rare, the effort of mass screening may not be justified. If common, it may be better to treat everyone than to screen (e.g., fluoride and caries).

Disease Burden. The greater the burden, the greater the pay-off per case found. Burden includes severity, duration, and the cost of support services.

Availability and Efficacy of Treatment or Preventive Measures. Availability of prenatal diagnosis, for example, is a strong argument for programs aimed at detecting high-risk couples, and absence of treatment is an argument against screening to identify affected individuals (e.g., Duchenne muscular dystrophy).

Cost of Test. Time-consuming or expensive tests are difficult to justify for mass screening programs.

Accuracy of Diagnostic Tests. Specificity should be high—that is, ideally there should be no false positives—and sensitivity should be high—there should be no false negatives. Many screening tests are not ideal in these respects; in general it is better to have some false positives that can be identified by more precise follow-up tests than to have false negatives, which would not be followed up.

Evidence That the Program Will Be Beneficial. For example, there would be no point in a heterozygote detection program if the heterozygous individuals detected paid no attention to the findings.

Screening programs have been instituted for various genetic diseases, with varying degrees of success. The earliest was that for phenylketonuria (PKU). The discovery that dietary control could ameliorate the effects of the enzymatic block created a demand for mass screening programs. In spite of some controversy, mandatory screening programs were set up for various populations—44 of the United States passed such laws between 1962 and 1971, and over 14 million children have been screened in these programs. These may have been premature; genetic heterogeneity was not yet appreciated and some hyperphenylalaninemics were inappropriately treated, with tragic results. Nevertheless, there is no question that these programs have led to the prevention of mental retardation in hundreds of children. Over 20 nations now have screening programs for PKU and various other inborn errors of metabolism. Many of them are not mandatory, and it seems that compliance rates in voluntary programs are comparable to those of legislated ones.

Screening for sickle cell disease has a much more complex history. In this case, the aim was to identify matings at risk for having children with sickle cell disease, but there was neither successful treatment nor prenatal diagnosis, and the only preventive measure was for heterozygotes not to marry other heterozygotes or for high-risk couples to refrain from having children. Nevertheless, numerous mandatory screening programs were set up, either for preschool children or couples before marriage. Unfortunately, many of these were ill-conceived and ill-conducted. The first state law requiring screening for the sickle cell trait in the United States was passed in 1971; 17 states rapidly followed suit, but by 1973, 8 of these laws had been repealed.[10] Part of the trouble was inadequate public education. There was confusion as to the difference between the trait (heterozygote) and the disease (homozygote), for example, "there are two forms of the disease." Because screening was aimed primarily at blacks and implied having fewer babies, there were accusations of racial discrimination and even genocide. Certainly, a legislative classification based on race is constitutionally suspect. The trait was misrepresented as a health hazard, leading to unnecessary anxiety and sometimes discrimination with respect to insurance premiums and eligibility for certain jobs. The early laws did not require adequate genetic counseling (and what counseling there was, was sometimes highly directive) or the privacy of records. In short, it has been suggested that the early programs were a lesson in how *not* to legislate genetic screening.[17]

Tay-Sachs screening programs have generally been better planned and better executed. None of them is compulsory, although some states require that couples be informed that screening for Tay-Sachs trait is available.

Genetic screening involves many complex practical, legal, and ethical issues, which we have been able to do no more than mention here. For more detailed discussions the reader is referred to various reviews.[9,14,15,17,21,22]

In summary, it is generally agreed that optimal genetic screening programs would meet the following requirements. There would be an adequate public education program before screening began, with evidence of community support of and involvement in the program; those screened (or their guardians) would be informed of the purpose of the test and consent to it; the results would be conveyed with appropriate nondirective counseling; and the results would be kept confidential. The screening tests would be accurate, simple, and inexpensive, and evidence would be provided that the expected benefits would justify the cost (a complex and difficult task). There would be assurance of the necessary manpower and laboratory facilities. Finally, the program would provide a means of assessing its effectiveness.

LEGAL, MORAL, AND ETHICAL ISSUES

Throughout this book, we have referred to various ethical, moral, and legal issues that the genetic counseling process may raise. They are so complex that to summarize them would take several volumes, and no clear-cut answers would emerge. In many cases they arise because our social, ethical, and legal development lags behind our technological progress.[4] A number of review volumes present useful discussions of the complex physiological, moral, legal and practical issues that the genetic counselor will meet.[1,4,5,9,14,15,21] Our hope is that these issues will continue to be reviewed and debated, that our norms will continue to evolve, and that our values will never harden into dogma.

Probably the most controversial issues concern prenatal diagnosis. Firstly, prenatal diagnosis implies abortion which, in the eyes of some, is taking an innocent life, and therefore unacceptable. Others view it as the lesser of two evils when the fetus has a serious disorder. Secondly, abortion of a fetus because it has a disabling disorder implies devaluation of individuals with that disorder which is viewed by some as practicing eugenics. This is taken to the extreme in the case of prenatal diagnosis of sex for non-medical reasons. Another concern is the question of whether women are coerced into having prenatal diagnosis, or having an abortion when a disorder is diagnosed.[2,10] Other ethical issues, such as the conflict between the right to privacy of those with genetic problems and their relatives' right to know, how much genetic information to reveal, and when (if ever) directive genetic counselling is justified concern counsellors more than the public.[23] It must be recognized that there are, indeed, dangers that genetics can be abused in the form of eugenics programs downgrading those with disabilities, or exploitation of women. These are social problems that must be recognized and guarded against.

HOW TO LOCATE A GENETIC COUNSELOR

As awareness of genetic counseling and what it can do becomes more widespread, the demand for it increases. Most medical schools and some large hospitals now have departments or divisions of medical genetics or have affiliations with a university genetics department through which referral to an experienced counselor can be arranged. Furthermore, an increasing amount of counseling may be done by specialized clinics—diabetes clinics may provide counseling for diabetes, cystic fibrosis clinics for pancreatic cystic fibrosis, and so on.

SUMMARY

Genetic counseling depends on accurate diagnosis and definition of etiology when pos-

sible. On the basis of the family history, appropriate tests, and a knowledge of the literature, an estimate of the recurrence risk is made. The counselor may then assist in the process of reaching a decision and taking appropriate action, as desired by the family. Decisions include whether to marry, have another baby, use contraceptive measures, seek sterilization, adopt, have antenatal diagnosis, or have a therapeutic abortion. The counseling process may extend to other members of the family, who are (or think they are) at risk for developing the disorder in question, or having affected children. The genetic counseling center is preferably connected with a university medical center with its extensive diagnostic and consultative resources. The counselor should be prepared to provide the complete counseling service or to support the primary physician who wishes to handle the case himself. Follow-up studies suggest that most families react responsibly to the information given.

Genetic screening programs, to identify individuals with treatable genetic diseases and couples at increased risk for having children with severe genetic diseases, are an important element of genetic counseling programs. The development of genetic counseling as a health care service raises complex legal, moral, and ethical issues.

REFERENCES

1. Capron, A.M., et al. (Editors): Genetic counseling: Facts, values and norms. Birth Defects 15(2):1979.
2. Clarke, A.: Is non-directive counselling possible? Lancet 338:1001, 1991.
3. Emery, A.E.H.: Methodology in Medical Genetics. An Introduction to Statistical Methods. New York, Churchill Livingstone, 2nd ed., 1986.
4. Emery, A.E.H., and Pullen, J., Editors: Psychological aspects of genetic counseling. London, Academic Press, 1984.
5. Evers-Kieboons, G., Cassiman, J.-J., van den Berghe, H., and d'Ydewalle, G. (Eds.): Genetic risk, risk perception, and decision making. Birth Defects Original Article Series 23, 1987.
6. Fraser, F.C.: On being a medical geneticist. Am. J. Hum. Genet. 15:1, 1963.
7. Fraser, F.C.: The Development of Genetic Counseling. In Genetic Counseling: Facts, Values and Norms. Birth Defects 15(2):5, 1979.
8. Frets, P.G., Duivenvoorden, H.J., Verlage, F., et al.: Analysis of problems in making the reproductive de-

cision after genetic counselling. J. Med. Gen. 28:194, 1991.

9. Hsia, Y.E., et al. (Editors): Counseling in Genetics. New York, Alan R. Liss, 1979.

10. Lippman, A. Prenatal genetic testing and screening: constructing needs and reinforcing inequities. Am. J. Law and Med. 17:15, 1991.

11. Lippman-Hand, A., and Fraser, F.C.: Genetic counseling: Provision and reception of information. Am. J. Med. Gen. 3:113, 1979.

12. Lippman-Hand, A., and Fraser, F.C.: Genetic counseling: The postcounseling period. I. Parents perceptions of uncertainty. Am. J. Med. Genet. 4:51, 1979.

13. Lippman-Hand, A., and Fraser, F.C.: Genetic counseling: The postcounseling period. II. Making reproductive choices. Am. J. Med. Genet. 4:73, 1979.

14. Lubs, H.A., and de la Cruz, F. (Editors): Genetic Counseling. New York, Raven Press, 1977.

15. Milunsky, A., and Annas, G.J. (Editors): Genetics and the Law. New York, Plenum Press, vol I, 1976; vol II, 1979; vol III, 1985.

16. Murphy, E.A. and Chase, G.A.: Principles of Genetic Counseling. Chicago, Year Book Publishers, Inc., 1975.

17. National Research Council, Committee for the Study of Inborn Errors of Metabolism: Genetic Screening: Programs, Principles and Research. Washington, D.C., National Academy of Science, 1975.

18. Opitz, J.M.: Genetic caring. The professionalization of genetic services in the U.S.A. Am. J. Med. Gen. 3:1, 1979.

19. Powledge, T.M.: Genetic Counselors without Doctorates. In Genetic Counseling: Facts, Values, and Norms. Birth Defects 15(2):103, 1979.

20. Reilly, P.: Professional identification: Issues in licencing and certification. In Genetic Counseling: Facts, Values, and Norms. Birth Defects 15(2):291, 1979.

21. Royal College of Physicians (London). Prenatal diagnosis and genetic screening, 1989.

22. Weiss, J.O., et al.: Genetic disorders and birth defects in families and society. Birth Defects 20(4):1, 1984.

23. Wertz, D.C., Fletcher, J.C., and Mulvihill, J.J. Medical Geneticists confront ethical dilemnas: cross-cultural comparisons among 18 nations. Am. J. Hum. Genet. 465:1200, 1990.

24. Young, I.D.: Introduction to risk calculations in genetic counseling. Oxford, Oxford University Press, 1991.

Glossary

Abiotrophy. A disease resulting from a genetic defect that causes progressive failure of some previously normal state or process, and therefore has a postnatal onset—e.g., muscular dystrophy, Huntington's disease.

Acrocentric. Refers to a chromosome with the centromere near one end, so that one arm is very short.

Active site. A region of a protein (particularly enzyme) directly involved in interaction with another molecule.

Adaptor molecules. See *Transfer RNA*.

Adenylcyclase. Enzyme that catalyzes production of cyclic AMP from ATP.

Affinity, cellular. Tendency of cells to adhere specifically to cells of same type, but not of different types. This property is lost in cancer cells.

Alleles. Alternative forms of a gene. If more than two alleles exist for a given locus, they are called multiple alleles—for example, all the mutant genes at the hemoglobin beta chain locus.

Allograft. A tissue graft from a donor of one genotype to a host of the same species but another genotype. Contrast *Isograft*.

Allosteric. Refers to a protein in which the activity of the active site is changed by the binding of a specific small molecule (allosteric effector) at another site.

Alpha-fetoprotein. A protein made in the fetal liver and present in fetal serum, which appears in excessive amounts in the amniotic fluid in the presence of a neural tube defect or certain other fetal abnormalities.

Amino acids. The building blocks of proteins. Each has an amino group on one end, a carboxyl group on the other, and a side group (R) that gives it its specificity.

Amino acids, acidic. Amino acids having a net negative charge at neutral pH (aspartic acid, glutamic acid).

Amino acids, aromatic. Amino acids whose side chains include a derivative of a phenyl group. The aromatic amino acids found in protein are phenylalanine, tyrosine, and tryptophan.

Amino acids, basic. Amino acids having a net positive charge at neutral pH (arginine, lysine, hydroxylysine, histidine).

Amniocentesis. The procedure of withdrawing fluid from the amniotic sac for prenatal diagnosis.

Amplification. The production of multiple copies of a sequence of DNA.

Anaphase. The phase of mitosis or meiosis in which the chromosomes are drawn by their centromeres from the equatorial plate and pass to the poles of the cell

Androgen(s). A group of male-determining hormones produced mainly by the testis and adrenal cortex.

Aneuploid. A chromosome number that is not an exact multiple of the haploid number.

Antibody. A gamma globulin formed by immune-competent cells in response to an antigenic stimulus, and reacting specifically with that antigen.

Anticipation. The term used to describe the apparent tendency of certain diseases to appear at earlier onset ages and with increasing severity in successive generations. It usually appears to be a statistical artifact.

Antigen. A substance having the power to elicit antibody formation by immune-competent cells and to react specifically with the antibody so produced.

Antigenic determinant. Chemical structure (small compared to macromolecule) recognized by the active site of an antibody. Determines specificity of antibody-antigen interaction.

Antisense strand of DNA. The noncoding DNA strand that serves as a template for RNA synthesis and is complementary to nRNA.

Ascertainment. The selection through an individual (the proband) of families for inclusion in a genetic study.

Association. The occurrence together, in a population, of two characteristics with a frequency greater than would be predicted on the basis of chance, that is, with a frequency greater than the product of the frequency of each. Not to be confused with linkage, where the association occurs only within families when the relevant genes are in coupling.

Assortative mating. Nonrandom mating; a tendency of parents with a particular characteristic to select mates with that characteristic (positive assortative mating) or shun such mates (negative assortative mating).

Autoimmunity. The formation of antibodies to an individual's own proteins, leading to autoimmune disease.

Autoradiography. A technique whereby the precise location of a radioactively labeled molecule in a cell or tissue can be demonstrated by applying a photographic emulsion to the histological section or cytological slide; the film will be sensitized wherever the label is present. Applied in cytogenetics particularly to delineating DNA synthesis by the chromosome by adding tritium-labeled thymidine to the culture—the label will be incorporated wherever DNA synthesis is proceeding.

Autosome. Any chromosome other than the sex chromosomes.

Backcross. Term from experimental genetics to indicate mating between F_1 hybrid and one of the two parental strains.

Bacteriophage. A virus that infects bacteria and is used as a vector for cloning.

Barr body. See *Sex chromatin*.

Base pair. The guanine-cytosine and adenine-thymine pairs of purine (guanine, adenine) and pyrimidine (cytosine, thymine) bases that make up DNA. In RNA, uracil substitutes for thymine. One of the pair is on one chain of the DNA double helix, the other on the complementary chain.

β-galactosidase. An enzyme catalyzing the hydrolysis of lactose into glucose and galactose; in *E. coli*, the classic example of an inducible enzyme.

Bivalent. A pair of homologous chromosomes associated in meiotic pachytene.

Breakage and reunion. The classic model of crossing over between chromatids by physical breakage and crossways reunion of complete chromatids during meiosis. This model has recently been shown to be applicable in at least one case on the molecular level—crossing over between phage-DNA molecules proceeds by breakage and reunion.

Cancer. Strictly refers to carcinomas, but loosely used for diseases characterized by uncontrolled invasive cellular growth. See *Neoplasm*.

Candidate gene. A gene whose product has properties that may cause a disease under investigation and is located in a region of interest.

Cap. The nucleotide added to the 5′ end of a growing mRNA chain for processing and translation.

Cap site. The site of transcription initiation.

Carcinogen. An agent that induces cancer.

Carrier. An individual who carries a gene but may not manifest it—i.e., either an autosomal or X-linked recessive gene or a dominant mutant gene that has not yet resulted in overt disease.

Catalyst. A substance that can increase the rate of a chemical reaction without being consumed in the reaction (e.g., enzymes catalyze biological reactions).

CCAAT box. A DNA sequence upstream from the transcription initiation site of many genes that is important in transcription.

cDNA. Complementary DNA. Synthetic DNA transcribed through the action of the enzyme reverse transcriptase from a specific RNA.

Centimorgan. See *Map unit*.

Cell cycle. The cycle undergone by the nuclear DNA from one cell division to the next. It consists of: G1, a period of growth; S, a period of chromosomal DNA replication; G2, a period of further growth; and mitosis. (G stands for "gap" in DNA replication activity, and S stands for "synthesis.")

Centriole. One of the pair of small organelles that form the points of focus of the spindle during cell division in animal cells. The centrioles lie together outside the nuclear membrane at prophase and migrate during cell division to opposite poles of the cell.

Centromere (kinetochore, primary constriction). The constricted portion of the chromosome, separating it into its two arms. It is situated in a heterochromatic region, is the last part of the chromosome to divide, and is attached to the spindle fibers at mitosis and meiosis.

Chiasma. Refers to the X-like crossing of chromatid strands of homologous chromosomes, seen at diplotene of the first meiotic prophase. Chiasmata are evidence of interchanges of chromosomal material (cross-overs) between members of a chromosome pair.

Chimera. An individual composed of cells derived from different zygotes; in human genetics, especially with reference to blood group chimerism, in which dizygotic twins exchange hematopoietic stem cells in utero and continue to form blood cells of both types. Distinguish from mosaicism, in which the two genetically different cell lines arise after fertilization.

Chorionic villus sampling. The procedure of obtaining fetal tissue from the villus area of the chorion for prenatal diagnosis at an earlier time than regular amniocentesis.

Chromatid. After the chromosome has made a replica of itself at the beginning of mitosis or meiosis, it consists of two strands, called chromatids, held together at the centromere. Each will become a separate chromosome when the centromere divides.

Chromatin. The material of the chromosomes that stains with nuclear (basic) stains—more or less synonymous with DNA.

Chromatography. A technique of separating compounds from a mixture, by their rate of migration through a medium, followed by appropriate staining.

Chromomeres. Areas of increased optical density and/or increased diameters along the length of a chromosome, especially clearly discernible in prophase of meiosis.

Chromosomes. The carriers of the genes, consisting of long strands of DNA in a protein framework. The exact structure of mammalian chromosomes is still not known. In nondividing cells they are not individually distinguishable in the nucleus, but at mitosis or meiosis they become condensed into visible strands that stain deeply with basic stains.

Chromosome jumping. Molecular cloning of DNA sequences up to 100 kb away from a starting clone.

Chromosome walking. A method of trying to locate a specific gene within a defined region by sequential isolation of overlapping clones of DNA sequences.

Cis configuration. See *Linkage*.

Cleavage division. Mitotic divisions of the fertilized egg that divide it into smaller and smaller units, until the stage when the original regions of the egg begin to shift relative to one another.

Clinodactyly. Crooked finger, resulting from angulation at interphalangeal joint(s).

Clone. A group of cells all derived from a single cell by repeated mitosis and all having the same genetic constitution (in somatic cell genetics). Now refers also to a cloned gene, when the gene sequence has been excised and grown in a bacterial or viral vector.

Coding strand. The "sense" (as opposed to "antisense") strand of DNA that has the same 5'-to-3' sense as does mRNA (except that T substitutes for U). It is not transcribed by RNA polymerase.

Codominance. See *Dominant*.

Codon. A triplet of three nucleotide bases in a DNA or messenger RNA molecule that codes for a specific amino acid, or the initiation or termination of transcription.

Coefficient of inbreeding. The probability that an individual has received both alleles of a pair from an identical ancestral source; or the proportion of loci at which he is homozygous for such alleles.

Coefficient of relationship. The probability that two persons have inherited a certain gene from a common ancestor; or the proportion of all their genes that have been inherited from common ancestors.

Colinearity. The relationship between two macromolecules (DNA and protein) in which the sequence of components (bases) of the former specifies the sequence of components (amino acids) of the latter.

Complementary DNA (cDNA). DNA produced from an RNA template by the action of reverse transcriptase (RNA-dependent DNA polymerase).

Complementation test. The bringing together of two mutant genes, either by crossing, co-culturing of cell lines, or cell hybridization, to see if together they can produce a normal phenotype. From this, tentative conclusions can be drawn as to whether they are alleles.

Compound heterozygote. The presence of two different mutant alleles at the same locus.

Concordant. If both members of a twin pair exhibit a certain trait, they are said to be concordant for that trait. Contrast *Discordant*.

Conditional lethal. A class of mutants whose viability is dependent on growth conditions (e.g., temperature-sensitive lethal mutants).

Congenital. Present at birth. Does not imply either genetic or nongenetic causation.

Consanguinity. Relationship by descent from a common ancestor.

Constitutive enzymes. Enzymes that are synthesized independently of an inducer.

Consultand. The person, in a genetic counseling situation, whose genotype is being evaluated—often the parents of an affected child.

Contact inhibition. The cessation of cell membrane movement that may occur when freely growing cells come into physical contact with each other.

Contiguous gene syndrome. The clinical result of microdeletions of two or more contiguous loci of chromosomal DNA (also called segmental aneusomy).

Cosmid. Plasmid vector designed for cloning large fragments of DNA.

Coupling. See *Linkage*.

CRM—Cross-reacting material. A term used to refer to a molecule that has antigenic specificity for a particular antigen.

Crossing over. The process of exchange of genetic material between homologous chromosomes. The chiasmata seen at the diplotene of meiosis are the physical basis of a previous crossover. See *Breakage and reunion*.

Cyclic AMP. Adenosine monophosphate group bonded internally (phosphodiester bond between 3' and 5' carbon atoms) to form cyclic molecule. Plays an important role in the mechanism by which hormones (and other compounds) regulate the activity of specific genes. See *Hormone*.

Cytogenetics. The branch of genetics concerned mainly with the appearance and segregation of the chromosomes and their relation to phenotype.

Degenerate code (genetic). One in which two or more codons code for the same amino acid.

Deletion. A chromosomal aberration in which a portion of a chromosome is missing.

Deme. A group defined by the population from which members select their mates—an effective breeding population.

Deoxynucleoside. The condensation product of a purine or pyrimidine with the five-carbon sugar, 2-deoxyribose.

Deoxyribonucleotide. A compound that consists of a purine or pyrimidine base bonded to the sugar, 2-deoxyribose, which in turn is bound to a phosphate group.

Dermatoglyphics. The patterns formed by the ridges of the skin of the palms, fingers, soles, and toes.

Determination. The commitment of an embryonic tissue to a particular development fate.

Diakinesis. The final stage of prophase of the first meiotic division. During diakinesis the chromosomes become tightly coiled and darkly staining.

Dicentric. A structurally abnormal chromosome with two centromeres.

Dictyotene. The stage in which the oocyte persists, in arrested prophase from late fetal life until ovulation.

Differentiation. The process whereby the developmental and functional abilities of a cell become restricted to a specific structure and major function.

Dimer. Molecular structure resulting from association of two subunits.

Diploid. Having two complete sets of chromosomes, double the number in the gametes. In man, the diploid number is 46. Contrast, *Haploid, Triploid*.

Diplotene. The stage of first meiotic prophase during which the paired centromeres begin to repel one another and the chromosomes begin to separate, exhibiting chiasmata.

Discordant. The converse of *Concordant*.

Disulfide bond. Covalent bond between two sulfur atoms in different amino acids of a protein. Important in determining secondary and tertiary structure.

Dizygotic (dizygous, fraternal). Twins produced by two separate ova and sperm.

DNA (deoxyribonucleic acid). A polymer of deoxyribonucleotides that is the genetic material of all eukaryote cells.

DNA methylation. The process of adding a methyl residue to a cytosine base and thus influencing gene regulation.

DNA polymerase. An enzyme that catalyzes the formation of new deoxyribonucleotide (DNA) strands from deoxyribonucleoside triphosphates, using DNA as a template.

DNA-RNA hybrid. A double helix that consists of one chain of DNA hydrogen bonded to a chain of RNA by means of complementary base pairs.

Domain. A discrete part of a polypeptide sequence that can be equated with a particular function.

Dominant. A gene is said to be dominant if the phenotype of the heterozygote is the same as that of the homozygote for that gene. In human genetics the term is used, more loosely, for a mutant gene that is expressed in the heterozygote. If the mutant homozygote is more severely affected than the heterozygote (which is often unknown), there is "intermediate" dominance, and if both alleles are expressed independently, there is "codominance." Traditionally, the term refers to traits, but is now commonly applied to genes as well. See also *Incomplete dominance*.

Dosage compensation. A term, usually used in relation to sex determination, when the effects of structural genes on the X chromosome are the same, whether the X chromosome is represented once, or twice. In many species, including man, the Lyon hypothesis provides a mechanism.

Drift, genetic. Chance variation in gene frequency from one generation to another. The smaller the population, the greater are the random variations.

Drumstick. A small protrusion from the nucleus of a polymorphonuclear leukocyte, found in 3 to 5% of these cells in females but not in males.

Duplication. The recurrence of a segment of chromosome.

Dysmorphism. Developmental morphologic abnormality as seen in clinical syndromes.

Ecogenetic. Interaction of an environmental factor with a genetic predisposition.

Electrophoresis. A method of separating large molecules by their rate of migration through a medium (e.g., filter paper, starch gel) in an electrical field.

Empiric risk. Probability based on past experience rather than on knowledge of cause that an outcome will occur.

Endonuclease. An enzyme that makes internal cuts in DNA backbone chains.

Endoreduplication. A process in which the chromosomes replicate without cell division.

Enzymes. Protein molecules capable of catalyzing specific chemical reactions.

Epigenesis. The influence on development through the regulation of gene function and differentiation without altering the genotype.

Epistasis. The masking of the effects of one gene or set of genes by the action of a gene at another locus—e.g., the albino gene is epistatic to the genes determining the normal color of the iris.

Erythroblast. Nucleated cell in bone marrow that differentiates into red blood cell.

Estrogen. Female sex hormone produced mainly by the ovary.

Euchromatin. Most of the chromosomal material, which stains uniformly. Contrast *Heterochromatin*.

Eukaryote. An organism in which the cells have a nuclear envelope, as contrasted to prokaryotes (e.g., bacteria, blue-green algae). Eukaryotes also have larger cells than prokaryotes and have cytoplasmic organelles.

Euploid. A chromosome number that is an exact multiple of the number in a haploid gamete.

Exon. The region of a gene that is transcribed to mature mRNA.

Exonuclease. An enzyme that digests DNA from the ends of strands.

Expressivity. The variability in the degree to which a mutant gene expresses itself in different mutant individuals.

F. Coefficient of inbreeding.

Familial trait. A trait that occurs with a higher frequency in the near relatives of individuals with the trait than in unrelated individuals from the same population.

Feedback (end-product) inhibition. Inhibition of the enzymatic activity of the first enzyme in a metabolic pathway by the end product of that pathway.

Fertilization. Fusion of gametes of opposite sex to produce a diploid zygote.

FISH (fluorescent in situ hybridization). A technique used for fine localization in genome mapping and now in clinical cytogenetics.

Fingerprint. (1) The pattern of the ridged skin of the distal phalanx of a finger. (2) The pattern of spots on a two-dimensional chromatogram produced by the peptides of a hydrolyzed polypeptide. (3) Pattern of DNA bands on a gel formed by VNTRs.

Fitness (Darwinian). The probability that an individual of a given phenotype will transmit his (her) genes to the next generation, relative to the average for the population.

Flanking sequence. A region of a gene on either side of a transcribed region.

Founder effect. A comparatively high frequency of a mutant gene in a population derived from a small group of ancestors of which one or more carried the mutant gene. A special case of genetic drift.

Frameshift mutation. A deletion or insertion that is not an exact multiple of three base pairs and thereby alters the reading frame of the gene. The stop codon will thus not be the normal one, and the polypeptide formed will be elongated or shortened.

Fraternal twins. See *Dizygotic*.

G1, G2. See *Cell cycle*.

Gamete. A mature sperm or egg cell normally with haploid chromosome number.

Gene. A portion of a DNA molecule that is the code for the amino-acid sequence of a particular polypeptide chain.

Gene family. A set of genes containing related exons that have evolved from an ancestral gene.

Gene flow. Transfer of genes by migration of individuals from one population to the other and mating between individuals of the two populations.

Gene map. An assignment of gene loci to specific chromosomes.

Gene pool. All the genes at a given locus in a population.

Gene redundancy. Presence in cell of many copies of a single gene. Multiple copies may be inherited or result from selective gene duplication during development.

Genetic. Determined by differences between genes.

Genetic code. The relation between the nucleotide triplets in the DNA or RNA and the amino acids in the corresponding polypeptides.

Genetic death. The failure of a mutant gene to be passed on to the next generation because of the phenotypic effects of that gene on an individual.

Genetic drift. The fluctuation, either directed or undirected, in gene frequencies in a population.

Genetic engineering. Technologies used to alter the genome of a living cell.

Genetic heterogeneity. The production of the same phenotype by more than one genotype.

Genetic load. See *load, genetic*.

Genetic marker. A readily recognizable genetic difference that can be used in family and population studies.

Genocopy. A trait genetically different from a phenotypically similar one. See also *Genetic heterogeneity*. Contrast *Phenocopy*.

Genome. The complement of genes found in a set of chromosomes or comparable unit of inheritance.

Genotype. The genetic constitution of an individual, with respect either (a) to his/her complete complement of genes or (b) to a particular locus. Contrast *Phenotype*.

Germ cell. The gametes (sperm and ovum) or the cells giving rise to them.

Germline. The cell line that produces gametes.

Germline mosaicism. The presence of two or more genetically different types of germline cells.

Glycoprotein. Protein in which a carbohydrate is covalently bonded to the peptide portion of the molecule.

Gonosome. Term now rarely used, referring to sex chromosome. Contrast *Autosome*.

Haploid. Having only one complete set of chromosomes. Contrast, e.g., *Diploid*. In man, the haploid number is 23.

Haplotype. That aspect of the phenotype determined by closely linked genes of a single chromosome region—particularly with respect to the HLA region.

Haptoglobin. A serum protein that binds hemoglobin; it exists in several polymorphic variants.

Hardy-Weinberg law. Law relating the frequency of genotypes to the frequency of alleles in a population.

HeLa cells. An established line of human cervical carcinoma (cancer) cells from a patient named Henrietta Lacks; used extensively in the study of biochemistry and growth of cultured human cells.

Hemizygous. Having only one member of a gene pair or group of genes in an otherwise diploid individual. Since males have only one X, they are said to be hemizygous with respect to X-linked genes.

Hemoglobin. The protein carrier of oxygen in red blood cells. A tetramere of two pairs of polypeptide chains, each with an iron-containing heme group.

Hepatoma. A form of liver cancer.

Hereditary, heritable, heredofamilial. Essentially synonymous terms for genetic traits. Formerly *hereditary* was sometimes used in the sense of dominant. *Heredofamilial* is archaic.

Heritability. The proportion of phenotypic variance that is genetically determined.

Hermaphrodite. An individual with both ovarian and testicular tissue (not necessarily functional).

Heterochromatin. Chromosomal material with variable staining properties different from that of the majority of chromosomal material, the euchromatin.

Heterogametic. Producing gametes of two types with respect to sex determination. In man the heterogametic sex is the male, who produces sperm bearing X and Y chromosomes, respectively. The female is the homogametic sex, producing only X-bearing ova.

Heterogeneous nuclear RNA. The RNA molecules of various sizes, found in the nucleus, that include the precursors of the messenger RNAs.

Heterograft. A tissue graft from a donor of one species to a host of a different species—called a xenograft in the modern terminology.

Heterokaryon. A cell with two genetically different nuclei.

Heteropyknosis. A state in which a region of chromosome is heavily condensed and darkly staining.

Heterozygous (heterozygote). Possessing different alleles at a given locus. Double heterozygote refers to heterozygous state at two separate loci. An individual heterozygous for two mutant alleles, such as those for hemoglobin S and C, is a compound heterozygote. Contrast *Homozygous*.

Histocompatibility genes. Genes for antigens that determine the acceptance or rejection of tissue grafts.

HLA. Human leukocyte antigen that determines major histocompatibility.

Histones. Proteins rich in basic amino acids (e.g., lysine) found in chromosomes except in sperm, where the DNA is complexed with another group of basic proteins, the protamines.

Holandric. The pattern of inheritance of genes on the Y chromosome; transmission from father to all his sons but none of his daughters.

Homeobox. A conserved 180 base pair coding region encoding a DNA binding domain important in regulating gene expression.

Homogametic. See *Heterogametic*.

Homograft. A graft of tissue between two genetically dissimilar members of the same species.

Homologous chromosomes. Chromosomes that pair during meiosis, have essentially the same morphology, and contain genes governing the same characteristics.

Homozygous (homozygote). Possessing identical alleles at a given locus. Contrast *Heterozygous*.

Hormone. Chemical substance (often small polypeptide) synthesized in one organ of body that stimulates functional activity in cells of other tissues and organs. Many hormones act by stimulating adenylcyclase in the cell membrane to produce cyclic AMP.

Housekeeping genes. Genes whose products provide basic functions in cells.

^{3}**H (tritium)**. A radioactive isotope of hydrogen, a weak β-emitter, with a half-life of 12.5 years, useful in radioautography.

Hybrid cell. A cell formed by the fusion of two cells of different origin.

Hybridization. In somatic cell genetics, the fusion of two cells of different origin. In molecular genetics, the complementary pairing of an RNA and a DNA strand or two different DNA strands.

Hydrogen bond. A weak attractive force between one electronegative atom and a hydrogen atom that is covalently linked to a second electronegative atom.

Hydrolysis. The breaking of a molecule into two or more smaller molecules by the addition of a water molecule.

Hydrophilic (polar). Pertaining to molecules or groups that readily associate with water.

Hydrophobic (nonpolar). Literally, water hater. Describes molecules or certain functional groups in molecules that are insoluble or only poorly soluble in water.

Hydrophobic bonding. The association of nonpolar groups with each other in aqueous solution, arising because of the tendency of water molecules to exclude nonpolar molecules.

Hypertelorism, ocular. An increase, beyond the normal range, of the distance between the orbits. Hyperteloric individuals are always telecanthic, but not necessarily vice versa.

Idiogram. A diagram of a chromosome complement.

Immune competent. Capable of producing antibody in response to an antigenic stimulus.

Immunoglobulin. Protein molecule, produced by plasma cell, that recognizes and binds a specific antigen. Also called antibody.

Immunological incompatibility. Donor and host are incompatible if, because of genetic difference, the host rejects cells from the donor.

Immunological tolerance. Absence of immune response to antigens.

Immunosuppressive drug. Drug that blocks normal response of antibody-producing cells to antigen.

Imprinting (genomic). The differential expression of genetic material, at either the chromosomal or allelic level, depending on whether the genetic material has come from the male or female parent.

Inborn error of metabolism. A genetically determined biochemical disorder in which a specific enzyme defect produces a metabolic abnormality that may have pathological consequences.

Inbreeding. The mating of closely related individuals.

Incomplete dominance. A term used sometimes as a synonym for intermediate dominance (see *Dominant*), and sometimes as referring to a mutant gene that is expressed in some heterozygotes and all homozygotes.

Index case. See *Proband*.

Inducer. A small molecule that increases the production of the enzymes involved in its metabolism.

Inducible enzyme. An enzyme whose rate of production is increased by the presence of an inducer.

In situ hybridization. Molecular hybridization of a cloned DNA sequence to a chromosome spread on a slide. Used in gene mapping.

Intergenic DNA. The DNA of unknown function that is untranscribed and makes up a large proportion of total DNA.

Intermediary metabolism. The chemical reactions in a cell that transform food molecules into molecules needed for the structure, growth and function of the cell.

Interphase. The stage of the cell cycle between two successive divisions during which the normal metabolic processes of the cell proceed.

Intersex. An individual whose genitalia or gonads, show characteristics of both sexes or are ambiguous.

Intron. The noncoding region of a gene, which is initially transcribed but then removed from the RNA transcript by splicing together the coding regions (exons) on either side of it.

Inversion. End-to-end reversal of a segment within a chromosome; *pericentric* if it includes the centromere and *paracentric* if it does not.

In vitro (Latin: in glass). Refers to experiments done on biological systems outside the intact organism. Contrast *In vivo*.

In vivo (Latin: in life). Refers to experiments done in a system such that the organism remains intact. Contrast *In vitro*.

Isochromosome. An abnormal chromosome with two arms of equal length and bearing the same loci in reverse sequence, formed by crosswise rather than longitudinal division of the centromere.

Isogenic. Refers to grafts with identical histocompatibility antigens.

Isograft. A tissue graft in which donor and host have identical genotypes. Contrast *Allograft*.

Isolate. A population in which mating does not occur outside the group. See also *Deme*.

Karyotype. The chromosome set of an individual. The term also refers to photomicrographs of a set of chromosomes arranged in a standard format.

Kindred. Family in the larger sense, as contrasted to the nuclear family (parents and children).

Kinetochore. See *Centromere*.

Lampbrush chromosome. Giant diplotene chromosome found in some species in the oocyte nucleus with loops projecting in pairs from certain regions. Loops are sites of active messenger RNA synthesis.

Leptotene. The first stage of prophase of the first meiotic division, in which individual chromosomes appear as unpaired threads.

Lethal equivalent. A gene that, if homozygous, would be lethal; or a combination of two genes, each of which, if homozygous, would have a 50% chance of causing death; or any equivalent combination.

Leukemia. Form of neoplasm characterized by extensive proliferation of nonfunctional immature white blood cells (leukocytes).

Ligase, polynucleotide. Enzyme that covalently links DNA backbone chains.

Linkage. Gene loci are linked if they are close enough to each other on the same chromosome that they do not segregate independently, but tend to be transmitted together. Genes are linked in coupling if they are on the same chromosome (the *cis* configuration) and in repulsion if they are on homologous chromosomes (the *trans* configuration). See also *Syntenic*.

Linkage disequilibrium. The tendency for alleles at one locus to occur with alleles at another locus on the same chromosome with a greater frequency than can be attributed to chance alone.

Load, genetic. The sum total of death and disease caused by mutant genes.

Locus. The position of a gene on a chromosome. Different forms of a gene (alleles) may occupy the locus.

Lod score. The logarithm of the odds in favor of linkage. A lod score of 3 is accepted as proof of linkage and of -2 as proof that loci are unlinked.

Lymphoblast. A precursor of a lymphocyte. The lymphocytes transformed by phytohemagglutinin resemble lymphoblasts.

Lymphocyte. A type of white blood cell important in the immunological system.

Lymphoma. Neoplasm of lymphatic tissue.

Lyonization (Lyon hypothesis). The process by which all X chromosomes in excess of one are made genetically inactive and heterochromatic. In the female, the decision as to which X (maternal or paternal) is inactivated is taken independently for each cell, early in embryogeny, and is permanent for all descendants of that cell.

Lysosome. A cytoplasmic organelle, bounded by a single membrane, that contains a variety of acid hydrolytic enzymes.

Map unit (centimorgan); map distance. The measure of distance between two loci on a chromosome as inferred from the frequency (%) of crossing over (recombination) between them. Accurate only for small distances, as double cross-overs will not appear as recombinations. Fifty percent recombination is the maximum, corresponding to independent segregation.

Meiosis. The special type of cell division by which gametes, containing the haploid number of chromosomes, are produced from diploid cells. Two meiotic divisions occur. Reduction in number takes place during meiosis I.

Messenger RNA (mRNA). RNA that serves as a template for protein synthesis.

Metabolic cooperation. The correction of the metabolic defect in mutant cells lacking an enzyme, by coexistence, in culture or in vivo, with cells that produce the enzyme.

Metacentric. Refers to chromosomes with the centromere near the middle.

Metaphase. The stage of mitosis or meiosis when the centromeres of the contracted chromosomes are arranged on the equatorial plate.

MHC. Major histocompatibility complex located on chromosome 6p and containing the HLA genes.

Micron (μ). A unit of length convenient for describing cellular dimensions; it is equal to 10^{-3} mm or 10^5 Å.

Microsatellites. Also known as simple sequence repeats (SSR). A class of genomic sequences with unusually high polymorphic content.

Missense mutation. A mutation that changes a codon specific for one amino acid to specify another amino acid.

Mitochondrial DNA (mtDNA). The genome of the mitochondrion; inheritance is matrilineal.

Mitogen. A substance that stimulates cells to undergo mitosis.

Mitosis. Somatic cell division resulting in the formation of two cells, each with the same chromosome complement as the parent cell.

Monoclonal antibody. An antibody produced by genetic engineering that has only one antigenic specificity.

Monomer. The basic subunit from which, by repetition of a single reaction, polymers are made. For example, amino acids (monomers) condense to yield polypeptides or proteins (polymers).

Monosomy. The absence of one chromosome of a pair from the complement.

Monozygotic (monozygous, identical). Refers to twins derived from one egg and thus genetically identical.

Mosaic. An individual or tissue with two or more cell lines differing in genotype or karyotype, derived from a single zygote.

Multifactorial. Determined by multiple genetic and nongenetic factors, each making a relatively small contribution to the phenotype. See also *Polygenic*.

Multiple allele. See *Alleles*.

Mutagen. An agent that increases the mutation rate.

Mutant. (1) A gene altered by mutation. (2) An individual bearing such a gene.

Mutation. A permanent change in the genetic material. Usually refers to point mutation, i.e., change in a single gene, but includes the occurrence of chromosomal aberrations. **Germinal** mutations, occurring in the germ cells, are relevant to gene frequencies and the genetic load. **Somatic** mutations are important in neoplasia and aging.

Mutation rate. The rate at which mutations occur at a given locus; expressed as mutations per gamete per locus per generation.

Myeloma. Cancer arising from a clone of plasma cells, and producing a pure immunoglobulin.

Neoplasm. Literally "new growth," a general term for cancers and other tumors in which there has been loss of the normal regulation of mitotic activity.

Nondisjunction. The failure of two members of a chromosome pair to disjoin during anaphase of cell division, so that both pass to the same daughter cell.

Nonpolar. See *Hydrophobic bonding*.

Northern blot. Analogous to Southern blotting for detection of RNA molecules by hybridization to a complementary DNA probe.

Nu body. The microscopically visible structure of a nucleosome.

Nucleic acid. A nucleotide polymer. See also *DNA* and *RNA*.

Nucleolus. Round granular structure found in the nucleus of eukaryotic cells, usually associated with a specific chromosomal site, involved in rRNA synthesis and ribosome formation.

Nucleolus organizer. Secondary constrictions of chromosomes, particularly those related to satellites, seem to have this function.

Nucleoside. The combination of a purine or pyrimidine base and a sugar.

Nucleosome. The repeating nucleoprotein unit of chromatin containing a histone core and a length of compacted DNA.

Nucleotide. The combination of a purine or pyrimidine base, a sugar, and a phosphate group. The monomers from which DNA and RNA are polymerized.

Obligate heterozygote. An individual who, on the basis of pedigree analysis, must carry a mutant allele even if there is no clinical evidence.

Oligonucleotide. A short fragment of DNA or RNA, of a dozen or so bases, of defined sequence, used as a probe for a specific mutant or normal gene segment.

Oncogene. A gene involved in unregulated cell growth, responsible for tumor development.

Oocyte. Unfertilized egg cell.

Oogenesis. The process of formation of the female gametes.

Operator. A chromosomal region capable of interacting with a specific repressor, thereby controlling the function of an adjacent series of genes (operon). See also *Regulator, Repressor*.

Operon. According to the Jacob and Monod theory of gene regulation, a group of closely linked genes, with related functions, and an adjacent locus, the *operator*, that regulates them. See also *Regulator gene*.

Organelle. Membrane-bound structure found in eukaryotic cells, containing enzymes for specialized function. Some organelles, including mitochondria and chloroplasts, have DNA and can replicate autonomously.

Pachytene. A stage of first meiotic prophase during which the bivalents (paired chromosomes) shorten and thicken and may be seen to consist of two chromatids per chromosome.

Palindrome. A nucleotide sequence that reads the same (5' to 3') on complementary strands of DNA, and serves as a recognition site for restriction enzymes.

Panmixis. Random mating.

Paracentric. See *Inversion*.

PCR (polymerase chain reaction). A technique to amplify $>10^6$ times a short DNA or RNA sequence, using flanking oligonucleotide primers and DNA polymerase to permit analysis from very small quantities.

Pedigree. A diagram of a family with relationships to a proband and status regarding a hereditary condition.

Penetrance. The percentage frequency with which a heterozygous dominant, or homozygous recessive, mutant gene produces the mutant phenotype. Failure to do so is (loosely) called "nonpenetrance," and penetrance less than 100% is "reduced penetrance."

Peptide bond. A covalent bond between two amino acids in which the a-amino group of one amino acid is bonded to the a-carboxyl group of the other with the elimination of H_2O.

Pericentric. See *Inversion*.

PHA. See *Phytohemagglutinin*.

Pharmacogenetics. The area of biochemical genetics dealing with drug responses and their genetically controlled variations.

Phenocopy. An environmentally induced mimic of a genetic disorder, with no change in the corresponding gene.

Phenotype. (1) The observable characteristics of an individual as determined by his genotype and the environment in which he develops. (2) In a more limited sense the outward expression of some particular gene or genes. Thus a heterozygote and homozygote for a fully dominant gene will have the same phenotype, but different genotypes.

Phytohemagglutinin (PHA). A compound, extracted from beans, that stimulates circulating lymphocytes to enter mitosis. Used in the standard techniques for cytogenetic study of human chromosomes from peripheral blood.

Plasma cell. An antibody-producing cell derived from a lymphocyte (a kind of white blood cell).

Plasmid. Extra-chromosomal double-stranded DNA molecules found in a variety of bacterial species and used in manipulating DNA in genetic engineering.

Pleiotropy. A mutant gene or gene pair that produces multiple effects is said to exhibit pleiotropy (as seen in hereditary syndromes).

Polar. See *Hydrophilic*.

Polyadenylation site. A site at which the polyA tail (a sequence of adenosine residues) is added to the 3' end of an RNA transcript to aid transport out of the nucleus.

Polygenic. Refers to determination by many genes, with small additive effects.

Polymer. A regular, covalently bonded arrangement of basic subunits (monomers) produced by repetitive application of one or a few chemical reactions.

Polymorphism. The occurrence of two or more genetically determined alternative phenotypes in a population, in relatively common frequencies ("common" is defined as 98% or less for the most common phenotype). When maintained by heterozygote advantage, it is referred to as a balanced polymorphism.

Polynucleotide. A linkage sequence of nucleotides in which the 3' position of the sugar of one nucleotide is linked through a phosphate group to the 5' position on the sugar of the adjacent nucleotide.

Polyoma virus. An RNA virus that will transform cells into a neoplastic state in culture.

Polypeptide. A chain of amino acids, held together by peptide bonds between the amino group of one and the carboxyl group of an adjoining one. A protein molecule may be composed of a single polypeptide chain, or of two or more identical or different polypeptides.

Polyploid. Any multiple of the basic haploid chromosome number, other than the diploid number.

Polyribosome. Complex of a messenger-RNA molecule and ribosomes actively engaged in polypeptide synthesis.

Positional cloning. Cloning of a gene based on the knowledge of its map position without knowing the gene product.

Primary constriction. See *Centromere*.

Primary transcript. The first RNA transcript, which contains introns as well as exons.

Proband *(propositus, proposita)*. The affected family member through which the family is ascertained—the index case. Originally a proband was not necessarily affected and a propositus was, but by current usage the terms are synonymous.

Probe. A labeled DNA or RNA sequence used in molecular hybridization to detect a complementary sequence. Also a reagent capable of identifying a clone in a mixture of DNA or RNA sequences.

Promoter. A region on a DNA molecule located at the 5′ end of a gene to which an RNA polymerase binds and initiates transcription.

Prophase. The first stage of cell division, during which the chromosomes become visible as discrete structures and subsequently thicken and shorten. Prophase of the first meiotic division is further characterized by pairing (synapsis) of homologous chromosomes.

Propositus *(female, proposita; plurals, propositi and propositae)*. Synonyms are *proband* or *index case*. (Proband is preferred.)

Protamines. Proteins rich in basic amino acids found in the chromosomes of sperm.

Prota-oncogene. A normal gene that can be activated by a mutational event to become an oncogene.

Pseudogene. A region of the DNA with a base sequence very close to that of a structural gene, but which is not transcribed.

Pseudohermaphrodite. An individual who has gonadal tissue of only one sex, but who has ambiguous genitalia. Pseudohermaphrodites are designated as male or female by the type of gonadal tissue present.

Quasicontinuous variation. A term applied to discrete traits classified as present or absent (i.e., discontinuous) that are determined by an underlying continuous distribution, multifactorially determined, separated into two parts by a developmental or other threshold.

R. See *Roentgen*.

Rad. The unit of absorbed dose of ionizing radiation (100 ergs per gram). Roughly equivalent to 1R (roentgen).

Radioactive isotope. An isotope with an unstable nucleus that stabilizes itself by emitting ionizing radiation.

Random mating. Selection of a mate without regard to the genotype of the mate (except for sex, of course).

Reading frame. The sequence of codons by which translation may occur, depending on the location of the start codon.

Recessive. Refers to a trait that is expressed only in individuals homozygous for the gene concerned. Usage now justifies applying the term to the gene as well. The definition is an operational one—whether a "recessive" gene is expressed in the heterozygote may depend on the means used to detect it.

Reciprocal translocation. An exchange of segments between nonhomologous chromosomes.

Recombinant DNA. A DNA molecule constructed from more than one parental DNA molecule. The basis of gene-splicing and genetic engineering.

Recombination. The formation of new combinations of linked genes by the occurrence of a cross-over at some point between them.

Reduction division. The first meiotic division, so called because at this stage the chromosome number per cell is reduced from diploid to haploid.

Regulator gene. A gene that synthesizes a repressor substance that inhibits the action of a specific operator gene, thus preventing the synthesis of mRNA by that operon. See also *Operator, Operon.*

Regulatory genes. Genes whose primary function is to control the rate of synthesis of the products of other genes.

REM Roentgen equivalent man. The dose of any ionizing radiation that has the same biological effect as 1R of X rays.

Repressible enzymes. Enzymes whose rates of production are decreased when the intracellular concentration of certain metabolites increases.

Repressor. In the operon model, the product of a regulatory gene, now thought to be a protein and to be capable of combining both with an inducer (or corepressor) and with an operator.

Repulsion. See *Linkage.*

Restriction enzyme. An enzyme that cuts the DNA at specific short base sequences, or recognition sites.

Restriction fragment length polymorphism. (RFLP). A fragment of DNA following cleavage by a restriction enzyme, that exists in two alternate lengths depending on whether a specific recognition site is present. RFLPs constitute a new class of genetic markers.

Reticulocyte. Immature red blood cell that has lost its nucleus but is actively synthesizing hemoglobin.

Retrovirus. A virus that has an RNA genome and propagates by conversion of the RNA to DNA by the enzyme reverse transcriptase.

Reverse (back) mutation. A heritable change in a mutant gene that restores the original nucleotide sequence.

Reverse genetics. See *Positional cloning.*

Reverse transcriptase. An enzyme that catalyzes the synthesis of DNA on an RNA template.

RFLP. See *Restriction fragment length polymorphism.*

Ribonucleotide. A compound that consists of a purine or pyrimidine base bonded to ribose, which in turn is esterified with a phosphate group.

Ribosome proteins. A group of proteins that bind rRNA by noncovalent bonds to give the ribosome its three-dimensional structure.

Ribosomes. Small cellular particles (200 Å in diameter) made up of rRNA and protein. Ribosomes are the site of transcription of polypeptide chains from the mRNA.

RNA (ribonucleic acid). A nucleic acid formed upon a DNA template and taking part in the synthesis of polypeptides. Instead of thymine, RNA contains uracil. Three forms are recognized: (1) messenger RNA (mRNA), which is the template upon which polypeptides are synthesized; (2) transfer RNA (tRNA or sRNA, soluble RNA), which in cooperation with the ribosomes brings activated amino acids into position along the mRNA template; (3) ribosomal RNA (rRNA), a component of the ribosomes, which function as nonspecific sites of polypeptide synthesis. See also *Heterogeneous nuclear RNA.*

RNA polymerase. An enzyme that catalyzes the formation of RNA from ribonucleoside triphosphates, using DNA as a template.

Robertsonian translocation. A translocation between two acrocentric chromosomes by fusion at the centromeres and loss of the respective short arms.

Roentgen (R). The unit of ionizing radiation dose. The amount of radiation that will produce 2×10^5 ionizations in 1 cm^3 air.

rRNA. Ribosomal RNA (See *RNA*).

S (svedberg). The unit of ultracentrifuge sedimentation (S). S is proportional to the rate of sedimentation of a molecule in a given centrifugal field and is thus related to the molecular weight and shape of the molecule.

Satellite, chromosomal. A small mass of chromatin attached to the short arm of each chromatid of a human acrocentric chromosome by a relatively uncondensed stalk (secondary constriction). Not to be confused with satellite DNA.

Satellite DNA. DNA containing many tandem repeats of a short basic unit.

Second set response. The rapid rejection of grafted tissue by a host already sensitized to tissue of that genotype.

Secondary constriction. Narrowed, heterochromatic area in a chromosome. A secondary constriction separates the satellite from the rest of the chromosome. Probably associated with nucleolus formation. See *Nucleolus organizer*. The centromere is the primary constriction.

Secretor. (1) A trait characterized by the presence of the appropriate ABO blood group substance in saliva and other body fluids. (2) The gene responsible for this trait.

Segregation. In genetics, the separation of allelic genes by meiosis, into different gametes, and consequently their occurrence in different offspring.

Selection. In population genetics, the effect of the relative fitness of a genotype in a population on the frequency of the genes concerned.

Sendai virus. A parainfluenza virus isolated in Sendai, Japan, which, in killed suspension, increases cell fusion in somatic cell cultures

Serum proteins. Proteins found in serum (cell-free component of blood). Includes immunoglobulins, albumin, haptoglobins, clotting factors, and enzymes.

Sex chromatin. A chromatin mass in the nucleus of interphase cells of females of most mammalian species, including man. It represents a single, condensed X chromosome inactive in the metabolism of the cell. Normal females have sex chromatin, thus are chromatin positive; normal males lack it, thus are chromatin negative. Synonym: Barr body.

Sex chromosomes. Chromosomes responsible for sex determination. In man, the X and Y chromosomes.

Sex-influenced. Refers to a genetically determined trait in which the degree of manifestation of the responsible gene is different in males and females.

Sex-limited. Refers to autosomal traits that occur only in either males or females.

Sex-linked. Determined by a gene located on the X or Y chromosome. Since most sex-linked traits are determined by genes on the X chromosome, the term is often assumed to refer to these; X-linked is the preferable term in such cases.

Sex ratio. The ratio of males to females. The primary sex ratio refers to that at fertilization; the secondary sex ratio to that at birth.

Sibs, siblings. Brothers and sisters. Brevity makes *sib* the preferred term.

Sibship. Group of brothers and/or sisters.

Silent allele. An allele that has no detectable product.

Sister chromatid exchange. The crossing over and exchange of DNA segments between sister chromatids.

Snurps. Small nuclear RNA particles that may be involved in splicing.

Somatic mutation. A mutation occurring in a somatic cell.

Southern blot. The method developed by Southern for transferring DNA fragments previously separated by agarose gel electrophoresis to a nitrocellulose filter to detect specific fragments by their hybridization to radioactive probes.

Spermatogenesis. The process of formation of spermatozoa.

Spermiogenesis. That part of spermatogenesis in which spermatids develop into spermatozoa.

S phase. See *Cell cycle*.

Splicing. The removal of introns and joining of exons in the generation of mature RNA from the primary transcription.

SSCP. Single strand conformation polymorphism. A method for scanning regions of genes for mutations.

SSR. Simple sequence repeat. (see Microstellate.)

Structural gene. One that specifies the amino acid sequence of a polypeptide chain, as opposed to regulator genes, which may not.

Substrate. A compound acted on by an enzyme in a metabolic pathway.

Synapsis. The process by which homologous chromosomes come to pair side-by-side early in meiosis.

Syndactyly. Soft tissue webbing between digits. Loose usage includes bony fusion or zygodactyly.

Syndrome. A characteristic association of several anomalies in the same individual implying that they are causally related.

Syntenic. Two genetic loci on the same chromosome. Linked genes are syntenic, but not all syntenic genes show linkage.

Tandem repeats. Two or more copies of a DNA sequence arranged head to tail.

TATA box. A segment in the promoter region about 25 kb upstream from the start site that determines the site of transcription. The nucleotides most commonly found are TATAAAA.

Telecanthus. An increase, beyond the normal range, in the distance between the inner corners of the eye. Not to be confused with hypertelorism.

Telocentric. Refers to chromosome with its centromere at the end.

Telomere. The end of each chromosome arm.

Telophase. The last stage of cell division, from the time the centromeres of the daughter chromosomes reach the poles of the dividing cell until cell division is complete.

Temperature-sensitive mutant. Mutant that is functional at one temperature but inactivated at another.

Teratogen. An agent that causes congenital malformations.

Termination codon. One of the three codons (UAG, UAA, and UGA) that terminate synthesis of a polypeptide.

Tetramer. Structure resulting from association of four subunits.

Trait. Any specific, classifiable characteristic.

Trans configuration. See *Linkage*.

Transcription. The process whereby the genetic information contained in DNA is transferred, by the ordering of a complementary sequence of bases, to the messenger RNA as it is being synthesized.

Transduction. The transfer of bacterial genes from one bacterium to another by a bacteriophage particle.

Transfection. The process whereby a cell is transformed by DNA from a virus.

Transfer RNA (tRNA, sRNA). Any of at least 20 structurally similar species of RNA, all of which have a MW 25,000. Each species of RNA molecule is able to combine covalently with a specific amino acid and to hydrogen-bond with at least one mRNA nucleotide triplet.

Transferases. Enzymes that catalyze the exchange of functional chemical groups between substrates.

Transformation, cell. A permanent change in cell phenotype occurring in somatic cell cultures, in which the resulting cell strain manifests neoplastic features, including many, but not necessarily all, of the following: loss of contact inhibition, and thus change in cell and colony morphology; progressive changes in karyotype; formation of neoplasms on transplantation to host.

Transformation, DNA. The genetic modification induced by the incorporation into a cell of DNA from a genetically different source.

Transgenic mice. Mice that carry a foreign gene (transgene) produced by injection of oocytes. If the DNA is integrated into the genome, it is expressed; and if incorporated into the germ-line, it may be transmitted to the progeny.

Translation. The process whereby the genetic information present in an mRNA molecule directs the order of the specific amino acids during protein synthesis.

Translational control. Regulation of gene expression by control of the rate at which specific mRNA molecules are translated.

Translocation. (1) The transfer of a piece of one chromosome to another. (2) The transferred piece. If two chromosomes exchange pieces, the translocation is reciprocal. See also *Robertsonian translocation*.

Triplet. See *Codon*.

Triploid. Having three sets of the normal haploid chromosome complement.

Triradius. In dermatoglyphics, a point from which the dermal ridges course in three directions at angles of approximately 120 degrees.

Trisomy. The presence of a complete extra chromosome homologous with one of the existing pairs.

Tritium. See ^3H.

Truncate selection. The selection of families of parents with given genotypes in such a way that one or more kinds of sibship are not ascertained—those in which no member is affected.

Tumor-suppressor gene. A normal gene involved in the regulation of cell growth. Tumor development can result from recessive mutations, such as in the retinoblastoma or p53 genes.

Tumor virus. A virus that induces the formation of a tumor.

Ultracentrifuge. A high-speed centrifuge that can attain speeds up to 60,000 rpm and centrifugal fields up to 500,000 times gravity and thus is capable of rapidly sedimenting macromolecules and separating them by differences in migration along a gradient.

Ultrasonography. Examination of internal body structures by high-frequency sound waves.

Ultraviolet (UV) radiation. Electromagnetic radiation with wavelength shorter than that of visible light (3900–20,000 Å). Causes DNA base-pair mutations and chromosome breaks.

Unequal crossing over. The cause of many genetic variants as a result of misalignment from crossing over of similar DNA sequences.

Uniparental disomy. The presence of two chromosomes of a pair inherited from one parent with no homologous chromosome from the other parent.

Vector. The plasmid or phage used to carry a cloned DNA segment.

Viruses. Infectious disease-causing agents, smaller than bacteria, possessing a DNA or RNA genome and a protein coat; they require intact host cells for replication.

VNTRs. Variable number of tandem repeats. Sequences of 11 to 60 base pairs repeated several times producing patterns of bands of such specificity that they may be used for "DNA fingerprinting." (Also known as microsatellites.)

Western blot. Similar to Southern blotting, used to detect proteins, usually by immunologic methods.

Wild type. The normal allele of a rare mutant gene, sometimes symbolized by +.

Xenograft. A tissue graft from a donor of one species to a host of a different species.

X-inactivation. The repression of genes on one X-chromosome in somatic cells of female mammals at an early embryonic stage.

X-ray crystallography. The use of diffraction patterns produced by x-ray scattering from crystals to determine the 3-D structure of molecules.

YAC. Yeast artificial chromosome, a vector for cloning large fragments of DNA.

Zygodactyly. Bony fusion of digits. See also *Syndactyly*.

Zygote. The fertilized ovum or (more loosely) the organism developing from it.

Zygotene. The stage of prophase of the first meiotic division in which pairing (synapsis) of homologous chromosomes occurs.

Appendix A. High-Resolution Chromosome Banding and the Morbid Anatomy of the Human Genome

We wish to thank Dr. Harold P. Klinger, who provided the high-resolution chromosome banding illustrations, which appear in *An International System for Human Cytogenic Nomenclature* (1985), ISCN Basel, Switzerland, S. Karger, 1985. Reproduced with permission.

We thank Dr. Victor A. McKusick for the illustrations of the morbid anatomy of the human genome, which are updated frequently in his computer and are published every two years in *Mendelian Inheritance in Man*, Baltimore, Johns Hopkins University Press. Reproduced with permission.

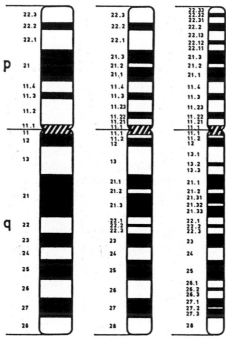

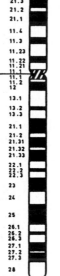

X

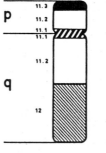

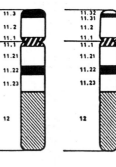

Y

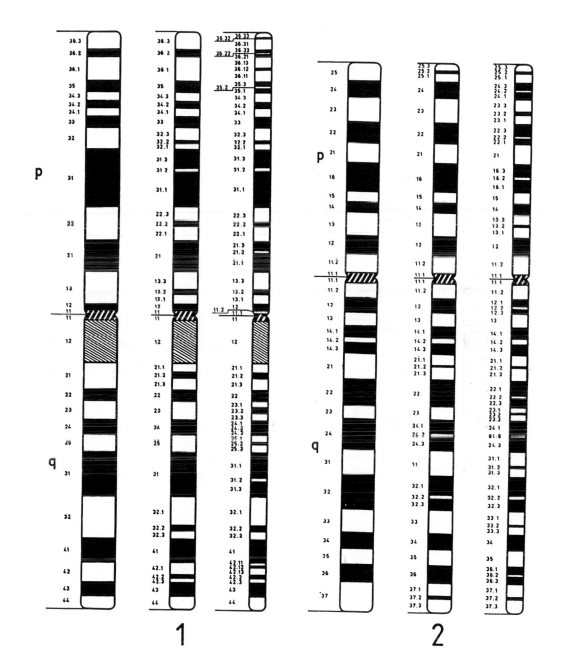

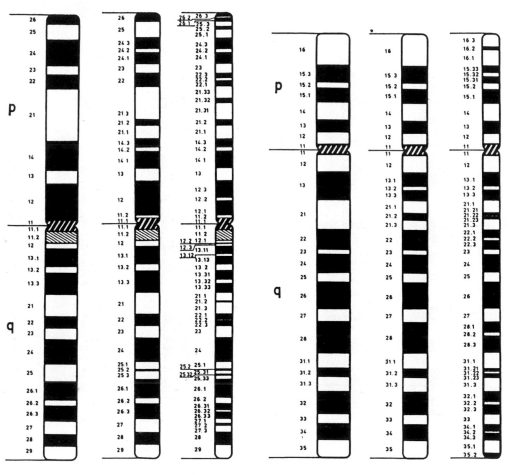

5

6

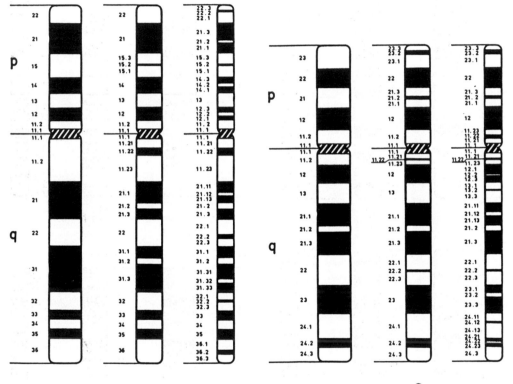

7

8

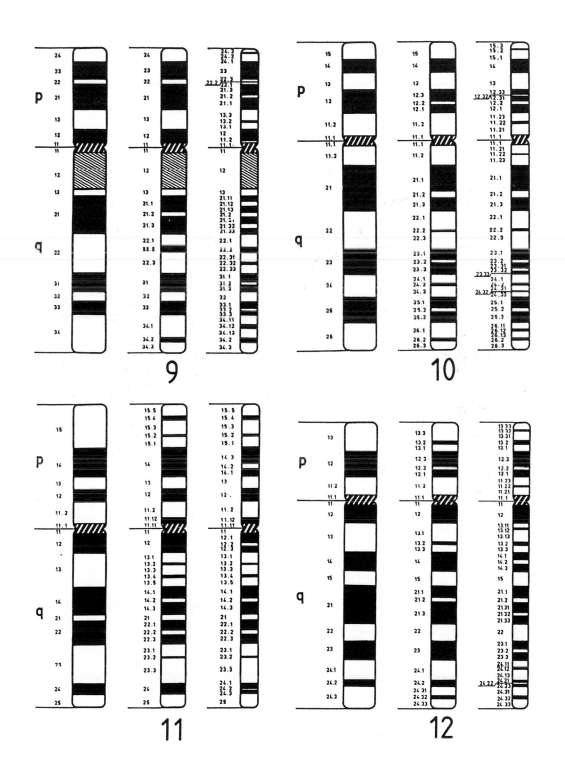

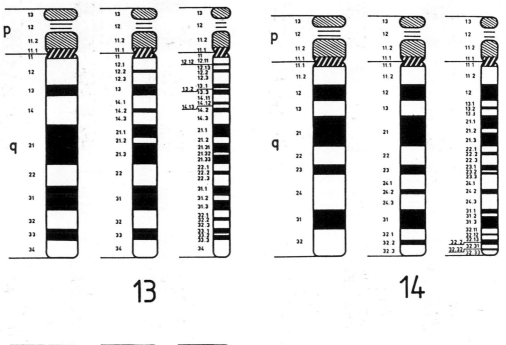

13

14

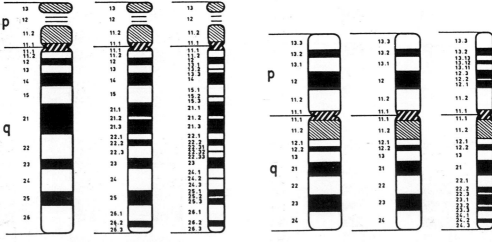

15

16

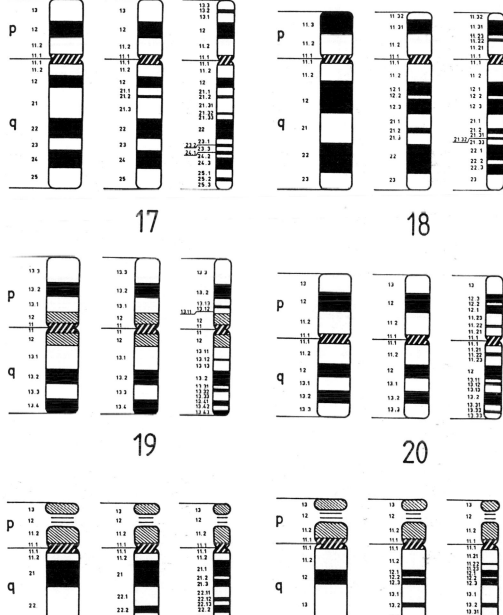

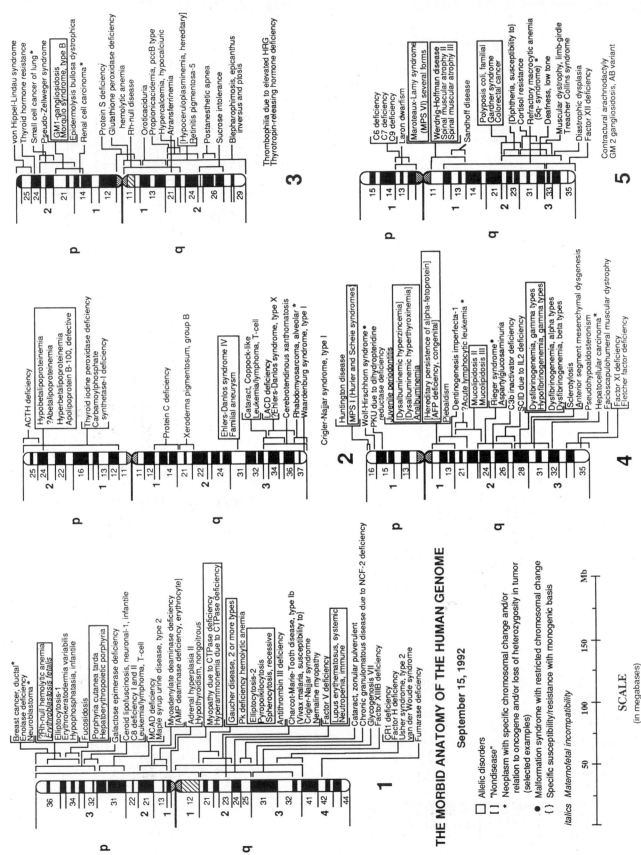

THE MORBID ANATOMY OF THE HUMAN GENOME

September 15, 1992

☐ Allelic disorders
[ ] "Nondisease"
* Neoplasm with specific chromosomal change and/or relation to oncogene and/or loss of heterozygosity in tumor (selected examples)
● Malformation syndrome with restricted chromosomal change
{} Specific susceptibility/resistance with monogenic basis
italics *Maternofetal incompatibility*

SCALE
(in megabases)

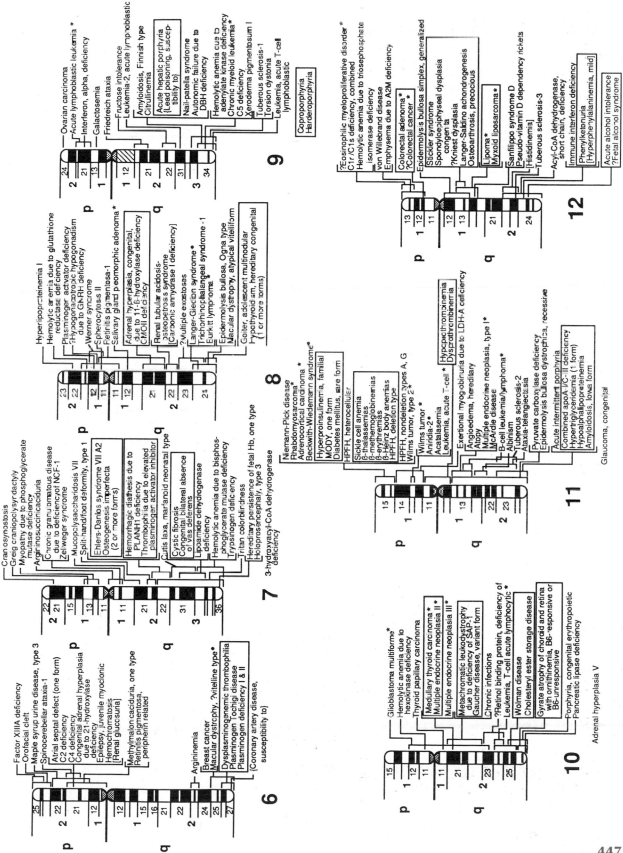

447

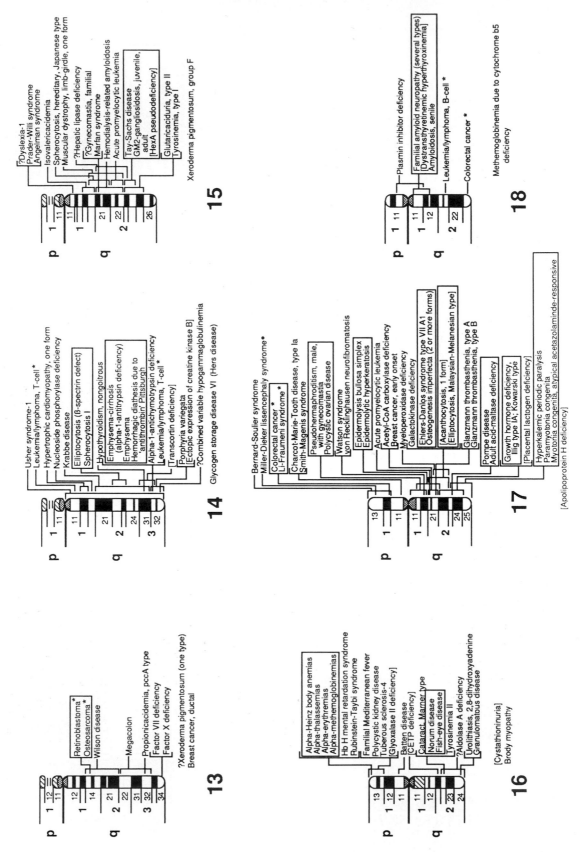

448

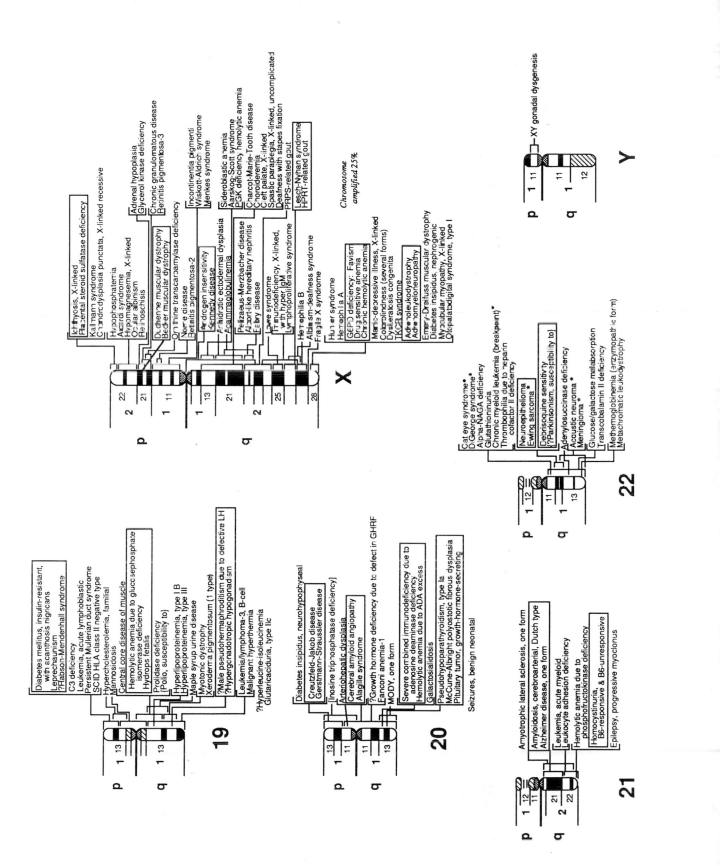

449

Appendix B. Selected Sources of Information on Medical Genetics and General Genetics

REVIEW ARTICLE SERIES

1. Harris, H., and Hirschhorn, K. (eds.): Advances in Human Genetics. New York, Plenum Press.
2. Steinberg, A.G., Bearn, A.G., Motulsky, A.G., and Childs, B. (eds.): Progress in Medical Genetics. New Series. New York, Grune and Stratton.
3. Oxford Monographs on Medical Genetics. Oxford, Oxford University Press.

HUMAN GENETICS TEXTS AND SOURCE BOOKS

4. Emery, A.E.H., and Rimoin, D.L. (eds): Principles and Practice of Medical Genetics. 2 vols. 2nd ed. New York, Churchill Livingstone, 1990. Multi-authored source book.
5. McKusick, V.A.: Mendelian Inheritance in Man. A Catalogue of Autosomal Dominant, Autosomal Recessive and X-linked Phenotypes. 10th ed. Baltimore, Johns Hopkins Press, 1992. (The most complete catalogue of mendelian traits, with references.)
6. Scriver, C.S., et al. (eds).: The Metabolic Basis of Inherited Disease. 6th ed. New York, McGraw-Hill Book Co., 1989. (A detailed description of the major inborn errors of metabolism and their underlying biochemistry.)
7. Thompson, M.W., McInnes, R.R., and Willard, H.F.: Thompson & Thompson Genetics in Medicine, 5th ed. Philadelphia, W.B. Saunders, 1991 (Basic introductory text, completely revised).
8. Vogel, F., and Motulsky, A.G.: Human Genetics, Problems and Approaches. 2nd ed. New York, Springer Verlag, 1986: In depth treatment, particularly of quantitative and population aspects.

SYNDROMES AND BIRTH DEFECTS

9. Baraitser, M., and Winter, R.: A colour Atlas of Clinical Genetics. London, Wolfe Medical Publications, 1983. Good pictures and short descriptions of the not-too-rare genetic diseases and syndromes.
10. Encyclopedia of Birth Defects, Ed.-in-Chief M.L. Buyse. New York, 1990 (comprehensive source book on birth defects).

11. Gorlin, R.J., Pindborg, J.J., and Levan L.S.: Syndromes of the Head and Neck, 3rd ed. New York, Oxford University Press, 1989. (An atlas overlapping Smith's somewhat, but with more emphasis on adults.)

12. National Foundation—March of Dimes. Birth Defects Original Article Series. New York. Alan Liss. Proceedings of a series of conferences on birth-defect-related topics. Much information on syndromes if you can find your way around.

13. Jones, K.L.: Smith's Recognizable Patterns of Human Malformations. 4th ed. Philadelphia, W.B. Saunders Co., 1988. (An excellent review of the problems of "dysmorphogenesis" and catalogue, well-illustrated and annotated, of syndromes, particularly those of the pediatric group.)

14. Warkany, J.: Congenital Malformations. Chicago, Year Book Medical Publishers, 1971. (An exhaustive source book of information and wisdom.)

CHROMOSOMES

15. Grouchy, J de, and Turleau, C.: Clinical Atlas of Human Chromosomes. 2nd ed. New York, John Wiley & Sons, 1984. (A definitive source.)

16. Hamerton, J.L.: Human Cytogenetics, Vols. I and II. New York, Academic Press, 1971.

17. Schinzel, A.: Catalogue of unbalanced chromosome aberrations in man. New York, Walter de Gruyter, 1984. (Catalogue of chromosomal syndromes.)

TERATOLOGY

18. Wilson, J.G., and Fraser, F.C. (eds.): Handbook of Teratology (4 volumes). New York, Plenum Press, 1977. (A comprehensive treatment of the subject.)

19. Shepherd, T.H.: Catalog of Teratogenic Agents, 7th ed. Baltimore, Johns Hopkins University Press, 1992. (Comparable to McKusick's catalogue of mendelian disorders.)

20. Persaud, T.V.N. (ed.): Advances in the Study of Birth Defects. New York, Alan R. Liss. Periodic collections of reviews, with a practical orientation aimed at physicians of birth defects embryology and causation.

21. Schardein, J.L.: Chemically Induced Birth Defects. 2nd ed. New York, Marcel Dekker, 1992.

Index

Note: Page numbers in *italics* indicate figures; page numbers followed by t indicate tables.